Sphingolipids,
Sphingolipidoses
and Allied Disorders

ADVANCES IN EXPERIMENTAL MEDICINE AND BIOLOGY

Sphingolipids, Sphingolipidoses and Allied Disorders

Proceedings of the Symposium on Sphingolipidoses and Allied
Disorders held in Brooklyn, New York, October 25-27, 1971

Edited by
Bruno W. Volk
*Isaac Albert Research Institute of the Kingsbrook Jewish Medical Center
and Department of Pathology, State University of New York
Downstate Medical Center
Brooklyn, New York*

and

Stanley M. Aronson
*Department of Pathology
Miriam Hospital and Brown University
Providence, Rhode Island*

Ⴔ SPRINGER SCIENCE+BUSINESS MEDIA, LLC 1972

Library of Congress Catalog Card Number 71-188925
ISBN 978-1-4757-6572-4   ISBN 978-1-4757-6570-0 (eBook)
DOI 10.1007/978-1-4757-6570-0

© 1972 Springer Science+Business Media New York
Originally published by Plenum Press, New York in 1972
Softcover reprint of the hardcover 1st edition 1972

ACKNOWLEDGMENTS

The Editors wish to acknowledge the invaluable assistance of Mr. Herbert Fischler, Chief Medical Photographer, Mrs. Renee Brenner and Mrs. Sarah Ginsberg in the preparation of this book.

PREFACE

This text contains the scientific contributions to the
Fourth International Symposium on Sphingolipids, Sphingo-
lipidoses and Allied Disorders held at the Kingsbrook Jewish
Medical Center on October 25-27, 1971. These meetings were
conducted under the auspices of the Isaac Albert Research
Institute of the Kingsbrook Jewish Medical Center and the
National Tay-Sachs and Allied Diseases Association, Inc.

Four symposia, held in 1958, 1961, 1965 and 1971 were
designed to gather the most relevant and innovative of the
laboratory and field studies concerned with these hereditary
disorders. The texts generated by these periodic meetings
have mirrored the increasing absorption of the scientific
community in the problems of sphingolipid metabolism.

The first meeting in 1958 consisted of but twelve presentations, the majority emanating from local laboratories.
The current sessions contain 48 scientific presentations by
scientists from nine countries and demonstrate the increas-
ingly diversified techniques and approaches employed in the
study of these diseases. Many of the authors, in exploring
data on the mucopolysaccharidoses and leucodystrophies, as
well as the sphingolipidoses, have given recognition to those
biochemical areas held in common by these otherwise diverse
disease processes.

The problems of prevention and therapy of these diseases
have been considered by some of the contributors. Laboratory
screening procedures designed to detect carriers of the various lipidoses are now available and the experiences of
some laboratories in this area are summarized within this
volume. The prospective identification of heterozygotes may
indeed become a powerful adjunct in genetic counseling.

The editors hope that the prompt publication of these
proceedings will encourage others not only to direct their

scientific attention to the still unsolved problems, but also
to pose those questions as yet unasked regarding the systemic
sphingolipidoses.

                                                    B.W.V.
                                                    S.M.A.

Brooklyn, New York
October 27, 1971

CONTRIBUTORS AND PARTICIPANTS

MASAZUMI ADACHI, Department of Neuropathology, Isaac Albert Research Institute of the Kingsbrook Jewish Medical .Center, Brooklyn, New York; Department of Pathology, New York University School of Medicine, New York, New York

DANIEL AMSTERDAM, Isaac Albert Research Institute of the Kingsbrook Jewish Medical Center, Brooklyn, New York; Department of Microbiology, Mt. Sinai School of Medicine, New York, New York

STANLEY M. ARONSON, Department of Pathology, Miriam Hospital-Brown University, Providence, Rhode Island

JAMES A. AUSTIN, Division of Neurology, University of Colorado Medical Center, Denver, Colorado

YECHEZKEL BARENHOLZ, Department of Biochemistry, The Hebrew University-Hadassah Medical School, Jerusalem, Israel

ROBERT W. BARTON, National Institute of Arthritis and Metabolic Diseases, National Institutes of Health, Bethesda, Maryland

ROLF BLOMSTRAND, Karolinska Institute, Stockholm, Sweden

SAMUEL BOGOCH, Boston University School of Medicine, Foundation for Research on the Nervous System, Boston, Massachusetts; and Dreyfus Medical Foundation, New York, New York

ILANA BORKOVSKI-KUBILER, Department of Biochemistry, The Hebrew University-Hadassah Medical School, Jerusalem, Israel

ROSCOE O. BRADY, Laboratory of Neurochemistry, National
Institute of Neurological Diseases and Stroke,
National Institutes of Health, Bethesda, Maryland

JAN L. BRESLOW, Molecular Disease Branch, National
Heart and Lung Institute, National Institutes of
Health, Bethesda, Maryland

ROBERT M. BURTON, Departments of Pharmacology, Pediatrics
and Pathology, The Beaumont-May Institute of Neurology, Washington University Medical School, St.
Louis, Missouri

MICHAEL CANTZ, National Institute of Arthritis and
Metabolic Diseases, National Institutes of Health,
Bethesda, Maryland

J. A. CIFONELLI, Departments of Pediatrics and Biochem-
istry, Joseph P. Kennedy, Jr. Mental Retardation
Research Center and La Rabida-University of Chicago
Institute, University of Chicago, Chicago, Illinois

JOE T.R. CLARKE, The Donner Laboratory of Experimental
Neurochemistry, Montreal Neurological Institute,
McGill University, Montreal, Canada

ALLEN C. CROCKER, Departments of Medicine and Surgery,
Children's Hospital Medical Center; Department of
Pediatrics, Harvard Medical School, Boston,
Massachusetts

JOEL A. DAIN, Department of Biochemistry, University of
Rhode Island, Kingston, Rhode Island

GLYN DAWSON, Departments of Pediatrics and Biochemistry,
Joseph P. Kennedy, Jr. Mental Retardation Research
Center, University of Chicago, Chicago, Illinois

JEFFERY G. DERGE, National Institute of Arthritis and
Metabolic Diseases, National Institutes of Health,
Bethesda, Maryland

ROBERT J. DESNICK, Department of Pediatrics and Dight
Institute for Human Genetics, University of Minnesota Medical School, Minneapolis, Minnesota

S.J. DESNICK, Department of Pediatrics and Dight Institute for Human Genetics, University of Minnesota
Medical School, Minneapolis, Minnesota

ALBERT DORFMAN, Departments of Pediatrics and Biochemistry, Joseph P. Kennedy, Jr. Mental Retardation Research Center and La Rabida-University of Chicago Institute, University of Chicago, Chicago, Illinois

SAMUEL DUNKELL, Medical Advisory Board, National Tay-Sachs Ass'n.; Department of Psychiatry, Post Graduate Center for Mental Health, New York, New York

JAMES E. EVANS, Eunice Kennedy Shriver Center at the Walter E. Fernald State School, Waltham, Massachusetts

PH. EVRARD, Département de Neurologie Infantile, Université de Louvain, Louvain, Belgique

ROBERT M. FILLER, Department of Surgery, Children's Hospital Medical Center; Harvard Medical School, Boston, Massachusetts

JOSEPH N. FISHER, Department of Pediatrics, Children's Hospital Medical Center; Harvard Medical School, Boston, Massachusetts

THOMAS F. FLETCHER, Department of Veterinary Anatomy, College of Veterinary Medicine, University of Minnesota, St. Paul, Minnesota

JORDI FOLCH-PI, Department of Neurochemistry, Harvard Medical School, Boston, Massachusetts; McLean Hospital, Belmont, Massachusetts

STANLEY S. FRANKLIN, Department of Medicine, University of California, Los Angeles, California

DONALD S. FREDRICKSON, Molecular Disease Branch, National Heart and Lung Institute, National Institutes of Health, Bethesda, Maryland

SHIMON GATT, Department of Biochemistry, The Hebrew University-Hadassah Medical School, Jerusalem, Israel

HANS H. GOEBEL, Department of Pathology, Indiana University Medical Center, Indianapolis, Indiana

ARTHUR GORDON, Department of Medicine, University of California, Los Angeles, California

CARL G. GROTH, Department of Surgery, Karolinska Institute, Stockholm, Sweden

LARS HAGENFELDT, Department of Clinical Chemistry, Karolinska Institute, Stockholm, Sweden

CLARA W. HALL, National Institute of Arthritis and Metabolic Diseases, National Institutes of Health, Bethesda, Maryland

SHIZUO HANDA, Biochemistry Department, Tokyo University, Tokyo, Japan

MADELEINE D. HARBISON, Eunice Kennedy Shriver Center at the Walter E. Farnald State School, Waverley, Massachusetts

DON R. HARRIS, Division of Pediatric Neurology, University of California at Los Angeles and Brentwood V.A. Hospital, Los Angeles, California

HENRI-GERY HERS, Laboratoire de Chimie Physiologique, Université de Louvain, Louvain, Belgique

MAE WAN HO, Department of Neurosciences, University of California at San Diego School of Medicine, La Jolla, California

ROBERT E. HOWARD, Department of Pathology, Texas University, San Antonio, Texas

GEORGE HUG, The Children's Hospital Research Foundation, University of Cincinnati College of Medicine, Cincinnati, Ohio

ALAN R. HULL, Department of Internal Medicine, University of Texas Southwestern Medical School, Dallas, Texas

DAVID HUTTON, Department of Medicine, School of Medicine, University of California, San Diego, La Jolla, California

B.I. IVEMARK, Department of Medical Chemistry, Royal Veterinary College, Stockholm, Sweden

HORST JATZKEWITZ, Max-Planck-Institut für Psychiatrie, Neurochemische Abteilung, München, Germany

GEORGE A. JERVIS, Institute for Basic Research in
    Mental Retardation, Staten Island, New York

W.G. JOHNSON, Laboratory of Neurochemistry, National
    Institute of Neurological Diseases and Stroke,
    National Institutes of Health, Bethesda, Maryland

PARVIN JUSTICE, Department of Pediatrics, Stritch
    School of Medicine, Loyola University of Chicago,
    Chicago, Illinois

MICHAEL M. KABACK, Department of Pediatrics, Johns
    Hopkins University School of Medicine, Baltimore,
    Maryland

SHIGEHIKO KAMOSHITA, Department of Pediatrics, Univer-
    sity of Tokyo School of Medicine, Tokyo, Japan

JULIAN N. KANFER, Eunice K. Shriver Center at the Walter
    E. Fernald State School, Waltham, Massachusetts

DENISE KARCHER, Laboratory of Neurochemistry, Fondation
    Born-Bunge, Berchem-Antwerpen, Belgium

ALFRED G. KASSELBERG, Department of Pediatrics, Johns
    Hopkins University School of Medicine, Baltimore,
    Maryland

PETER KOHLER, Division of Clinical Immunology, Univer-
    sity of Colorado Medical Center, Denver, Colorado

EDWIN H. KOLODNY, Eunice Kennedy Shriver Center for
    Mental Retardation, Inc., at the Walter E. Fernald
    State School, Waltham, Massachusetts; and J.P.
    Kennedy Memorial Laboratories, Massachusetts General
    Hospital, Boston, Massachusetts

HANS KRESSE, National Institute of Arthritis and Meta-
    bolic Diseases, National Institutes of Health,
    Bethesda, Maryland

GENE KRITCHEVSKY, Division of Neurosciences, City of
    Hope National Medical Center, Duarte, California

WILLIAM KRIVIT, Department of Pediatrics, University of
    Minnesota Medical School, Minneapolis, Minnesota

BENJAMIN H. LANDING, Departments of Pathology and Pedia-
    trics, Childrens Hospital of Los Angeles and Univer-

sity of Southern California School of Medicine, Los Angeles, California

MARIE-ANNE LA RAMEE, Research Institute, The Hospital for Sick Children, Toronto, Ontario, Canada

ROBERT W. LEDEEN, Departments of Neurology, Biochemistry and Pathology, Albert Einstein College of Medicine, Bronx, New York

DONALD LEEBER, Department of Internal Medicine, University of Texas Southwestern Medical School, Dallas, Texas

ZELINA LEIBOVITZ-BEN GERSHON, Department of Biochemistry, The Hebrew University-Hadassah Medical School, Jerusalem, Israel

J. ALEXANDER LOWDEN, Research Institute, The Hospital for Sick Children, Toronto, Ontario, Canada

ARMAND LOWENTHAL, Department of Neurochemistry, Fondation Born-Bunge, Berchem-Antwerpen, Belgium

CAROL A. MAPES, Department of Biochemistry, Michigan State University, East Lansing, Michigan

REUBEN MATALON, Departments of Pediatrics and Biochemistry, Joseph P. Kennedy, Jr., Mental Retardation Research Center and La Rabida-University of Chicago Institute, University of Chicago, Chicago, Illinois

ROBERT H. McCLUER, Eunice K. Shriver Center at the Walter E. Fernald State School, Waltham, Massachusetts

JOHN H. MENKES, Division of Pediatric Neurology, University of California at Los Angeles and Brentwood V.A. Hospital, Los Angeles, California

HUGO W. MOSER, Eunice Kennedy Shriver Center at the Walter E. Fernald State School, Waverley, Massachusetts; Department of Neurology, Harvard University; Department of Neurology, Massachusetts General Hospital, Boston, Massachusetts

NTINOS C. MYRIANTHOPOULOS, Section on Epidemiology and Genetics, Perinatal Research Branch, National Institute of Neurological Diseases and Stroke, National Institutes of Health, Bethesda, Maryland

ELIZABETH F. NEUFELD, National Institute of Arthritis
    and Metabolic Diseases, National Institutes of
    Health, Bethesda, Maryland

HARRY B. NEUSTEIN, Department of Pathology, Childrens
    Hospital of Los Angeles and University of Southern
    California School of Medicine, Los Angeles, Cali-
    fornia

EDWARD NEUWELT, Division of Neurology, University of
    Colorado Medical Center, Denver, Colorado

ALEX B. NOVIKOFF, Department of Pathology, Albert Ein-
    stein College of Medicine, Bronx, New York

JOHN S. O'BRIEN, Department of Neurosciences, University
    of California at San Diego School of Medicine, La
    Jolla, California

PER-ARNE ÖCKERMAN, Department of Clinical Chemistry,
    University of Lund, Lund, Sweden

SHINTARO OKADA, Department of Neurosciences, University
    of California at San Diego School of Medicine, La
    Jolla, California

VIMALKUMAR PATEL, Department of Pathology, Indiana
    University Medical Center, Indianapolis, Indiana

ALAN K. PERCY, Departments of Pediatrics and Neurology,
    Johns Hopkins University School of Medicine,
    Baltimore, Maryland

GUTA PERLE, Department of Biochemistry, Isaac Albert
    Research Institute of the Kingsbrook Jewish Medical
    Center, Brooklyn, New York

MICHEL PHILIPPART, Mental Retardation Center, The Neuro-
    psychiatric Institute and Departments of Pediatrics,
    Neurology and Psychiatry, University of California,
    Los Angeles, California

JANE M. QUIRK, Laboratory of Neurochemistry, National
    Institute of Neurological Diseases and Stroke,
    National Institutes of Health, Bethesda, Maryland

NORMAN S. RADIN, Mental Health Research Institute,
    University of Michigan, Ann Arbor, Michigan

RICHARD RELKIN, Department of Medicine, Isaac Albert
    Research Institute of the Kingsbrook Jewish Medical
    Center, Brooklyn, New York

GEORGE ROUSER, Section of Lipid Research, City of Hope
    National Medical Center, Duarte, California

ABRAHAM SAIFER, Department of Biochemistry, Isaac Albert
    Research Institute of the Kingsbrook Jewish Medical
    Center, Brooklyn, New York

KARIN SAMUELSSON, Department of Chemistry, Royal
    Veterinary College, Stockholm, Sweden

KONRAD SANDHOFF, Max-Planck-Institut für Psychiatrie,
    Neurochemische Abteilung, München, Germany

LARRY SCHNECK, Department of Neurology, Kingsbrook
    Jewish Medical Center-Veterans Administration Hos-
    pital; Department of Pediatrics, State University
    of New York, Downstate Medical Center, Brooklyn,
    New York

WILLIAM K. SCHUBERT, Department of Pediatrics, The
    Children's Hospital Research Foundation, University
    of Cincinnati College of Medicine, Cincinnati, Ohio

JAMES F. SCOTT, National Institute of Arthritis and
    Metabolic Diseases, National Institutes of Health,
    Bethesda, Maryland

ROBERT G. SENIOR, The Donner Laboratory of Experimental
    Neurochemistry, Montreal Neurological Institute,
    McGill University, Montreal, Canada

HARVEY L. SHARP, Department of Pediatrics, University of
    Minnesota Medical School, Minneapolis, Minnesota

ARISTOTLE N. SIAKOTOS, Department of Pathology, Indiana
    University Medical Center, Indianapolis, Indiana

HOWARD R. SLOAN, Molecular Disease Branch, National
    Heart and Lung Institute, National Institutes of
    Health, Bethesda, Maryland

PAUL D. SNYDER, Department of Pediatrics, University of
    Minnesota Medical School, Minneapolis, Minnesota

SHIRLEY SOUKUP, The Children's Hospital Research Foundation, University of Cincinnati College of Medicine, Cincinnati, Ohio

CHRISTINE SPIELVOGEL, Eunice K. Shriver Center at the Walter E. Fernald State School, Waltham, Massachusetts

MARCIA STEIN, Eunice K. Shriver Center at the Walter E. Fernald State School, Waltham, Massachusetts

NATALIE STEIN, Division of Pediatric Neurology, University of California at Los Angeles and Brentwood V.A. Hospital, Los Angeles, California

DANIEL STEINBERG, Department of Medicine, School of Medicine, University of California, San Diego, La Jolla, California

JACK STERN, Department of Pathology, Albert Einstein College of Medicine, Bronx, New York

DAVID STUMPF, Division of Neurology, University of Colorado Medical Center, Denver, Colorado

MUTSUMI SUGITA, Eunice Kennedy Shriver Center at the Walter E. Fernald State School, Waverley, Massachusetts; Department of Biochemistry, Massachusetts General Hospital, Boston, Massachusetts

KUNIHIKO SUZUKI, Department of Neurology, University of Pennsylvania School of Medicine, Philadelphia, Pennsylvania

YOSHIYUKI SUZUKI, Department of Neurology, University of Pennsylvania School of Medicine, Philadelphia, Pennsylvania

LARS SVENNERHOLM, Department of Neurochemistry, University of Gothenburg, Gothenburg, Sweden

CHARLES C. SWEELEY, Department of Biochemistry, Michigan State University, East Lansing, Michigan

JOHN F. TALLMAN, Laboratory of Neurochemistry, National Institute of Neurological Diseases and Stroke, National Institutes of Health, Bethesda, Maryland; Department of Biochemistry, Georgetown University, Washington, D.C.

L. TENNANT, Department of Neurosciences, University of California at San Diego School of Medicine, La Jolla, California

ROBERT D. TERRY, Department of Pathology, Albert Einstein College of Medicine, Bronx, New York

JERRY THOMPSON, Departments of Pediatrics and Biochemistry, Joseph P. Kennedy, Jr., Mental Retardation Research Center and La Rabida-University of Chicago Institute, University of Chicago, Chicago, Illinois

JUNZO TORII, Isaac Albert Research Institute of the Kingsbrook Jewish Medical Center, Brooklyn, New York

ROBERT S. TYZBIR, Department of Biochemistry, University of Rhode Island, Kingston, Rhode Island

CARLO VALENTI, Department of Obstetrics and Gynecology, State University of New York, Downstate Medical Center, Brooklyn, New York

FRANCOIS VAN HOOF, Laboratoire de Chimie Physiologique, Université de Louvain, Louvain, Belgium

MARIE THÉRÈSE VANIER, Hôpital Sainte-Eugénie, Lyon, France

M.L. VEATH, Department of Neurosciences, University of California at San Diego School of Medicine, La Jolla, California

TERESA VIETTI, Departments of Pharmacology, Pediatrics, and Pathology and The Beaumont-May Institute of Neurology, Washington University Medical School, St. Louis, Missouri

BRUNO W. VOLK, Isaac Albert Research Institute of the Kingsbrook Jewish Medical Center; Department of Pathology, State University of New York, Downstate Medical Center, Brooklyn, New York

ITARU WATANABE, Department of Pathology, Indiana University Medical Center, Indianapolis, Indiana

MARCIA WILLIAMS, Eunice Kennedy Shriver Center at the Walter E. Fernald State School, Waverley, Massachusetts

HENRYK WISNIEWSKI, Departments of Neurology, Biochemistry
    and Pathology, Albert Einstein College of Medicine,
    Bronx, New York

LEONARD S. WOLFE, The Donner Laboratory of Experimental
    Neurochemistry, Montreal Neurological Institute,
    McGill University, Montreal, Canada

PAUL W.K. WONG, The Infants' Aid Perinatal Research
    Laboratories, Mount Sinai Hospital, The Chicago
    Medical School, Chicago, Illinois

ROBERT K. YU, Departments of Neurology, Biochemistry
    and Pathology, Albert Einstein College of Medicine,
    Bronx, New York

ROBERT S. ZEIGER, Department of Pediatrics, Johns
    Hopkins University, School of Medicine, Baltimore,
    Maryland

WOLFGANG ZEMAN, Department of Pathology, Indiana Univer-
    sity Medical Center, Indianapolis, Indiana

ROLF ZETTERSTRÖM, Department of Pediatrics, S:t Görans
    Sjukhus, Karolinska Institutet, Stockholm, Sweden

K. ZIELKE, Department of Neurosciences, University of
    California at San Diego School of Medicine, La
    Jolla, California

CONTENTS

xxiii

FINE STRUCTURE OF EARLY TAY-SACHS DISEASE

M. Adachi, J. Torii, L. Schneck and B.W. Volk

Isaac Albert Research Institute of the Kingsbrook Jewish

Medical Center, Brooklyn, New York

Tay-Sachs disease is an inborn error of glycolipid. It is characterized by massive accumulation of G_{M2}-ganglioside (4), mainly in the brain and by the absence of the enzyme hexosaminidase A (5). Despite the significant increase of our knowledge of the biochemical aspects of this disorder during the past few years, the ultrastructural alterations of the neuronal organelles related to the accumulation and the evolution of the intracytoplasmic deposited lipid material at the early stage of Tay-Sachs disease are unknown.

The present report will demonstrate the development of the abnormal ganglionic bodies within the cisternae of the endoplasmic reticulum in the brain from a 14 week old Jewish boy afflicted with the clinical and biochemical characteristics of Tay-Sachs disease.

Case History

A two months old Jewish male was admitted to another hospital with a tentative diagnosis of infantile spasms. At four weeks of age, the infant had recurring episodes of flexion spasms described as "jack-knife" in character. These lasted for several seconds and occurred in clusters of 10 to 15 times a day. Except for head lag, the neurological examination, including ophthalmoscopic examination were said to be negative. The EEG was diffusely abnormal and the child was placed on ACTH gel. A week following the institution of steroid therapy, the seizures decreased in frequency and the EEG showed some improvement. However, the child's response to visual stimuli remained poor and

1

ophthalmoscopic examination at age three months revealed suspicious cherry-red maculae. A percutaneous needle biopsy of the
cerebrum was performed for evaluation. Hexosaminidase A levels
were found to be absent and a diagnosis of Tay-Sachs disease was
made. At three months of age, the child showed an abnormal startle response to sound, bilateral cherry-red maculae with persis-
tant head lag and weakness of pelvic and pectoral girdle. The
child was hospitalized at this institution for further diagnostic
studies and care. At the time of admission, the above findings
were confirmed. A sleep EEG record was interpreted as normal for
the age. Brain and liver biopsies were performed. The child's
clinical course in the hospital since admission followed the
stereotype clinical deterioration characteristic of Tay-Sachs disease. The family history was significant in that both mother and
father have intermediate levels of hexosaminidase activity. One
sibling, aged five, is alive and well. The rest of the history
was noncontributory.

METHODS

Ultrastructural studies were carried out on a biopsy from
the right cerebral frontal lobe and from the liver. The tissue
was immediately minced in cold 3% buffered glutaraldehyde solution,
fixed for three hours and post-fixed in cold 1% buffered osmium
tetroxide for 90 minutes. After fixation, the tissues were rinsed
briefly in distilled water, dehydrated quickly in a graded series
of ethanol, and embedded in Epon resin. Ultrathin sections were
obtained with glass or diamond knives, stained with uranyl acetate
and lead hydroxide and viewed with an electron microscope (RCA EMU
3G). Portions of the biopsies were fixed in 10% formalin and embedded in paraffin for histological studies and stained in hematoxylin and eosin, periodic acid Schiff (PAS), Luxol fast blue
(LFB), toluidine blue, alcian blue, phosphotungstic and hematoxylin (PTAH), trichrome, Nissl, Mahon and Romanes preparations.
Frozen sections were stained with Sudan black B, Sudan IV and Oil
red O techniques.

Biochemical Studies

Biochemical studies were carried out on frozen tissue with
the ganglioside isolation technique of Rouser, et al (6). Similar
tissues of Tay-Sachs cases and of non-neurological patients served
as controls. The gangliosides prepared from normal and pathologic
brains were dissolved in chloroform-methanol (2:1) for a concentration of about 8 mg./ml. The individual gangliosides were
separated by means of thin layer chromatography on silica gel G
plates (250μ thick) using chloroform:methanol:2.5N NH_4OH (60:40:9)
as the first ascending developing solvent. After allowing the
solvent to evaporate at room temperature, the plates were placed

in a dessicator overnight. The chromatograms were then redeveloped ascendingly in a saturated atmosphere of n-propanol-water (70:30). The separated gangliosides were visualized and the amount of each fraction determined by the method of Suzuki (7).

RESULTS

Gross Findings

The removed tissue consisted of a small portion of the cerebral cortex and subcortical white matter which were markedly pale, although the demarcation between them was well-defined. The entire tissue was soft, and on sectioning appeared to be of normal consistency. A small portion of the liver was grossly unremarkable.

Light Microscopy

The cortical neurons were moderately reduced in number, but were not distended (Fig. 1A). Under higher magnification, however, the neuronal cytoplasm contained fine round vacuoles which varied in size (Fig. 1B and 1C). These vacuoles gave positive reactions with PAS and LFB stains (Fig. 2). The cortex showed only a minimal degree of reactive astrocytic and microglial proliferation (Fig. 1A). Macrophages containing sudanophilic material were only slightly increased. The white matter showed a moderate reduction of the axonal fibers (Fig. 3A) which were similar to those observed in the fetal cerebrum at 21 weeks of gestation (Fig. 3B). With LFB-PAS and Mahon preparations, no visible myelin sheaths were demonstrated. In the white matter, a moderate increase of reactive astrocytes was noted (Fig. 4). Microglial cells and macrophages containing sudanophilic material were present in small numbers only. The leptomeninges and blood vessels were unchanged.

The cytoarchitecture of the liver was normal, although the Kupffer cells contained similar fine vacuoles as were seen in cerebral neurons. They also exhibited positive reactions in PAS and LFB preparations (Fig. 5).

Electron Microscopy

Most of the neurons showed marked dilatation of the cisternae of the endoplasmic reticulum (Figs. 6 and 7). They were filled with a fine granular or moderately dense homogeneous material (Figs. 7 and 8), which occasionally contained a few layers of concentric lamellae (Fig. 9). These lamellae seemed to originate from the most peripheral layers of the membranes of the cytosomes (Figs. 9 and 10). At this stage the cisternae of the endoplasmic reticulum were frequently identifiable, though closely applied to the membranous inclusion bodies (Fig. 10A and 10C).

In the liver, the Kupffer cells exhibited abnormal intracytoplasmic inclusion bodies which were membrane-bound and contained fine dense granules (Fig. 11). Membranous inclusion bodies
were absent. The hepatocytes were unchanged.

Biochemical Studies

Thin layer silica gel patterns obtained from the cerebrum
and liver showed a sialic acid positive glycolipid which had similar Rf values to G_{M2}-ganglioside (Fig. 12).

DISCUSSION

The role of the subcellular organelles in neurons during
accumulation of the abnormal cytoplasmic inclusion bodies in
various lipidoses is unknown. In the past few years, the morphogenesis of these inclusion bodies in lipidoses has been investigated (1-3). Since the advanced stage of these disorders showed
abundant neuronal lipid bodies, it was difficult to observe clear
details of the relationship between the subcellular organelles
and the intracytoplasmic bodies. Recently, ultrastructural studies
were carried out on ganglion cells in the myenteric plexus and
cerebral astrocytes in lipidoses. The myenteric ganglia showed
dilatation of the cisternae of the endoplasmic reticulum which contained the well-developed membranous cytoplasmic bodies (MCB), although the evolution of these bodies could not be traced. On the
other hand, in astrocytes of various lipidoses ranging in age from
nine months to 12 years, those areas of the cytoplasm which contained only few or no lipid bodies showed marked dilatation of the
cisternae of the endoplasmic reticulum, although in the more involved areas, the abnormal cytosomes were adjacent to or contiguous
with the smooth portion of the endoplasmic reticulum (1). In these
astrocytes the abnormal material, however, was not present within
the cisternae of this organelle.

In recent studies, further details of the subcellular alterations were observed in cerebral neurons of a 21 week old fetus
with Tay-Sachs disease, which showed an abnormal dense granular
material within the dilated cisternae of the endoplasmic reticulum.
The phylogenetically older areas, such as the spinal cord, however,
contained loosely arranged membranous bodies (2). Typical MCB's
were not present in the central nervous system. While these previous observations strongly suggested, but never clearly indicated,
that the endoplasmic reticulum is the site of origin of the lipid
cytosomes in Tay-Sachs disease, in the present study, the complete
evolution of the inclusion bodies in cerebral neurons from finely
granular material to the MCB's within the dilated cisternae could
be observed (Figs. 6-10).

The small amount of biopsied material was insufficient for additional enzyme histochemical studies. However, previous studies have demonstrated absence of acid phosphatase reaction product in cytoplasmic bodies in the fetal brain with Tay-Sachs disease (2), while those of the well developed MCB's in the advanced stage of the disease gave a strongly positive reaction (8,9). These histochemical observations, therefore, indicate that these lysosomal activities are a secondary cellular reaction involving the elimination of the accumulated abnormal inclusion material.

SUMMARY

Despite the significant increase of knowledge of the biochemical aspects of Tay-Sachs disease during the past few years, the ultrastructural alterations of the neuronal organelles related to the accumulation and evolution of the intracytoplasmic deposited lipid material at the early stage of the disorder are unknown.

Electron microscopic and biochemical studies were carried out on brain and liver from a three month old Jewish male who had clinical and biochemical features of Tay-Sachs disease. There was absence of hexosaminidase A in cerebral tissue. Furthermore, thin layer chromatographic studies showed a sialic acid positive glycolipid which had similar Rf values as G_{M2} (Tay-Sachs) ganglioside.

Histologically, the cortical neurons contained fine vacuoles, but were not distended. The vacuoles gave positive reactions with periodic acid Schiff and Luxol fast blue stains. The white matter showed no visible myelin sheaths and moderate reduction of axonal fibers which were similar to those observed in the fetal cerebrum. The liver showed similar vacuoles in the Kupffer cells which also exhibited positive reactions in periodic acid Schiff and Luxol fast blue preparations.

Electron microscopically, most of the neurons showed marked dilatation of the cisternae of the endoplasmic reticulum which were filled with a fine granular or moderately dense homogeneous material and occasionally contained a few layers of concentric lamellae. The majority of the membranous cytoplasmic bodies seemed to form from the peripheral layers of these lamellae within the cisternae of the endoplasmic reticulum. The liver showed abnormal intracytoplasmic inclusion bodies in the Kupffer cells which were membrane-bound and contained fine dense granules, but membranous inclusion bodies were absent. The hepatocytes were unchanged.

This work was supported by a grant from the National Tay-Sachs and Allied Diseases Association, Inc.

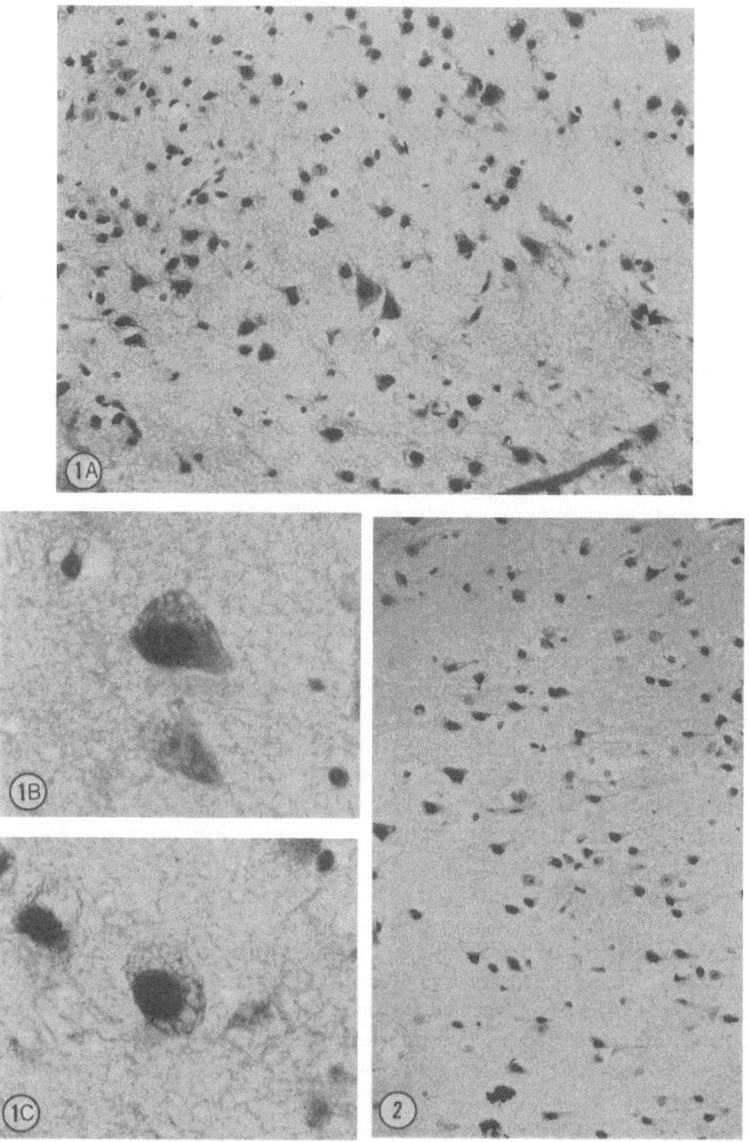

FIGURES 1A, B, C: Several cortical neurons. They are not distended (A) but contain fine vacuoles within the cytoplasm which
vary in size (B and C). Hematoxylin-Eosin Stains. A) X 280;
B) X 1,280; C) X 1,280.

FIGURE 2: The vacuoles within the neuronal cytoplasm give positive reaction in Luxol fast blue preparations. X 280.

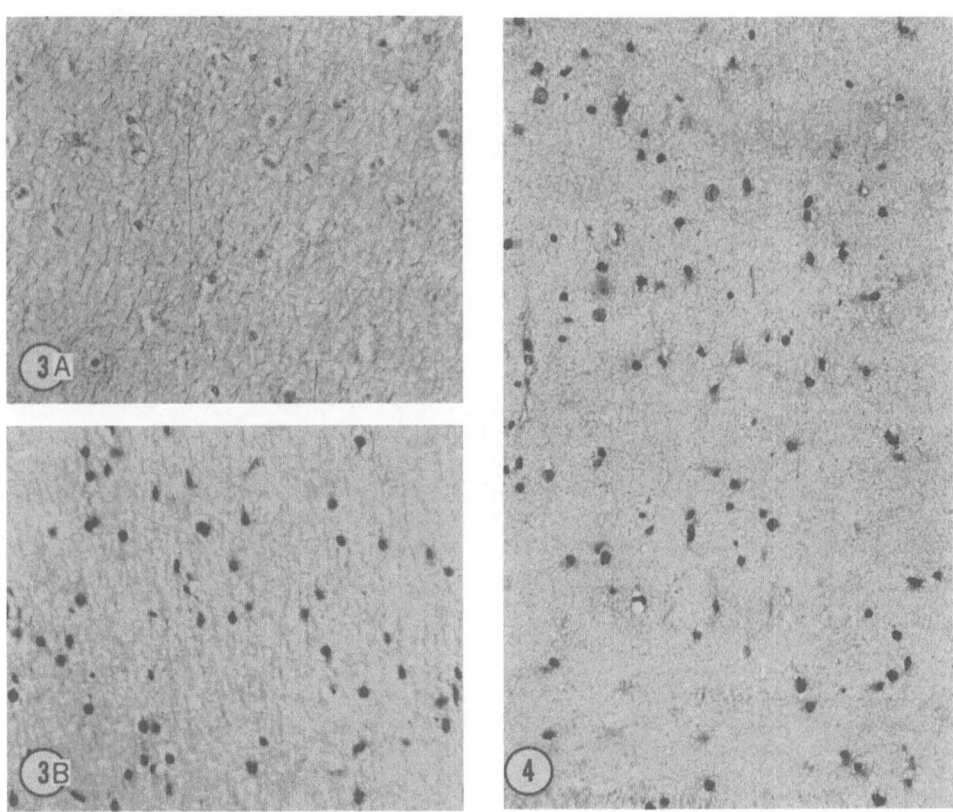

FIGURES 3A, B: Cerebral white matter, showing moderate reduction
of the number of axons (A). The amount of axonal fibers is similar to that observed in the fetal cerebrum at 21 weeks gestation
(B). Romanes Stain. A) X 280; B) X 280.

FIGURE 4: White matter of present case showing proliferation of
reactive astrocytes, while microglial cells and macrophages are
only slightly increased in number. Hematoxylin-Eosin Stains. X 280.

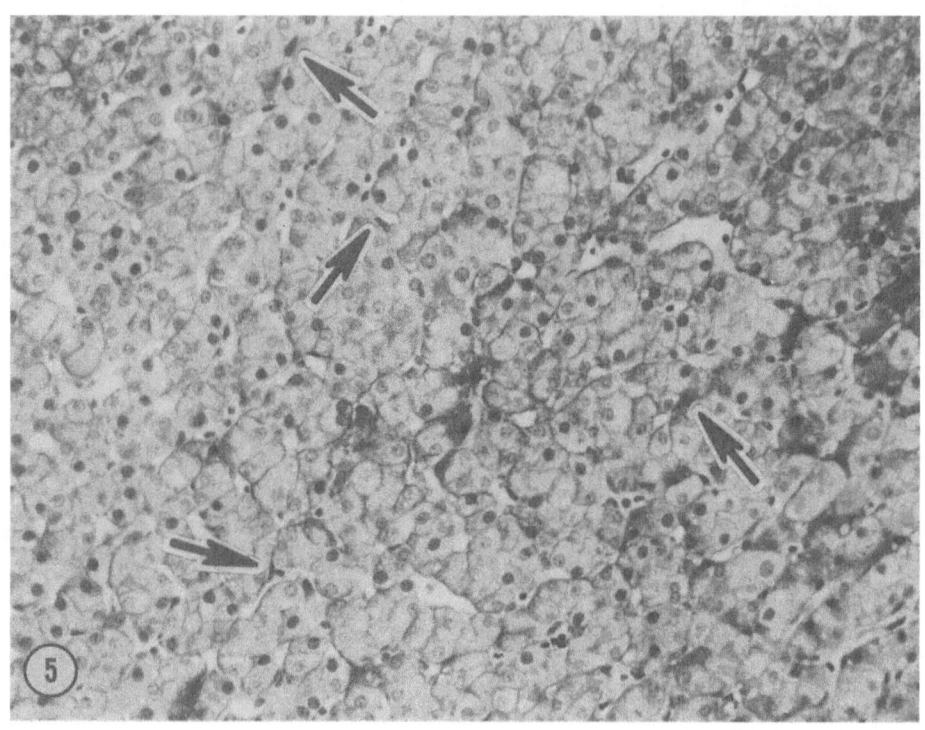

FIGURE 5: Section from liver showing Luxol fast blue positive material in Kupffer cells (arrows). The hepatocytes are unchanged. Luxol Fast Blue Stain. X 280.

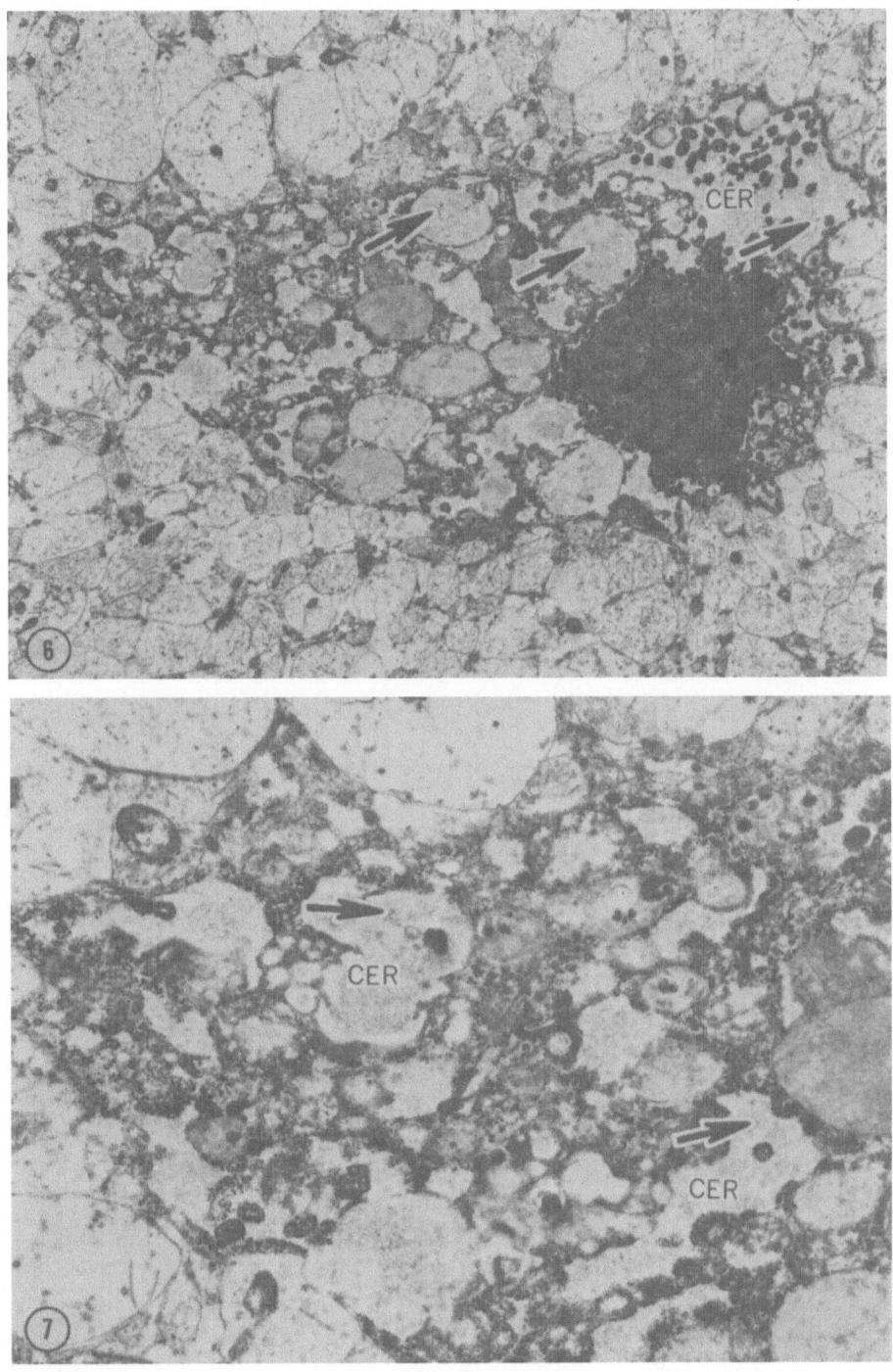

FIGURES 6 and 7: Electron microphotograph of cerebral neuron showing marked dilatation of the cisternae of the endoplasmic reticulum
(CER) which contains a fine dense granular material (arrows).
6) X 7,000; 7) X 17,000.

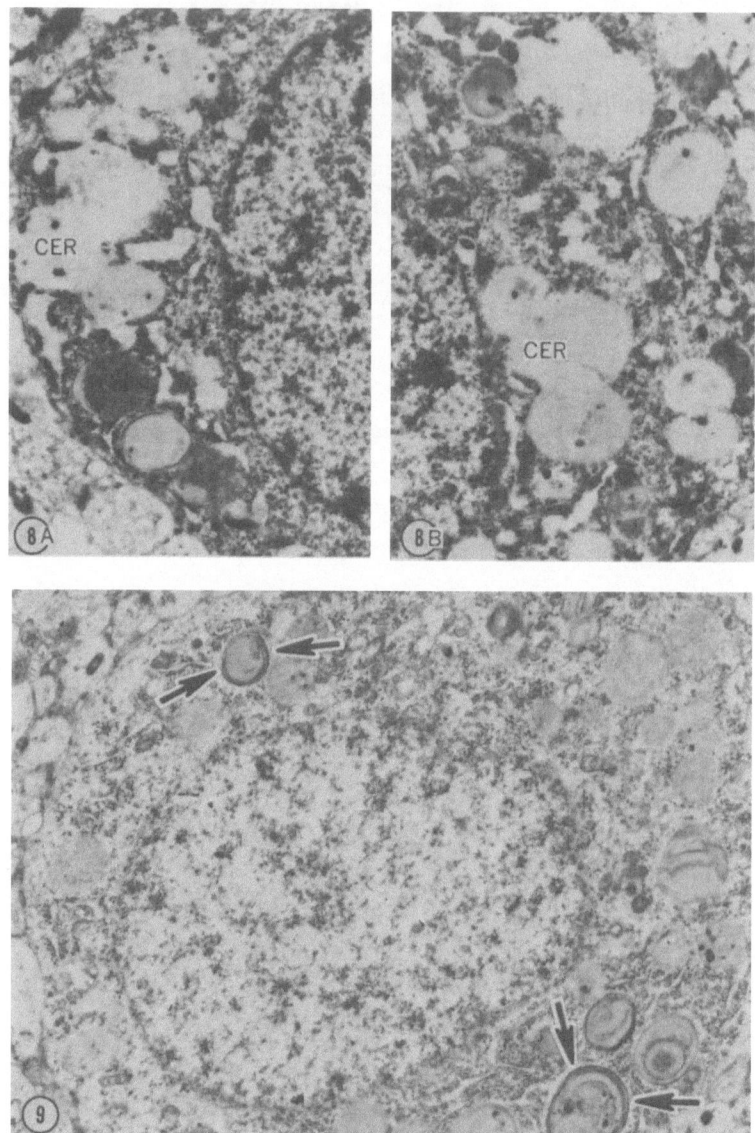

<u>FIGURES 8A, B</u>: In many areas the cisternae of endoplasmic reticu-
lum (CER) are rounded and distended and are filled with a moderately electron-dense, homogeneous material. A) X 8,500; B) X 8,500.

<u>FIGURE 9</u>: There are occasionally a few layers of concentric mem-
branes in the homogeneous material (arrows) within the endoplasmic
reticulum. X 8,400.

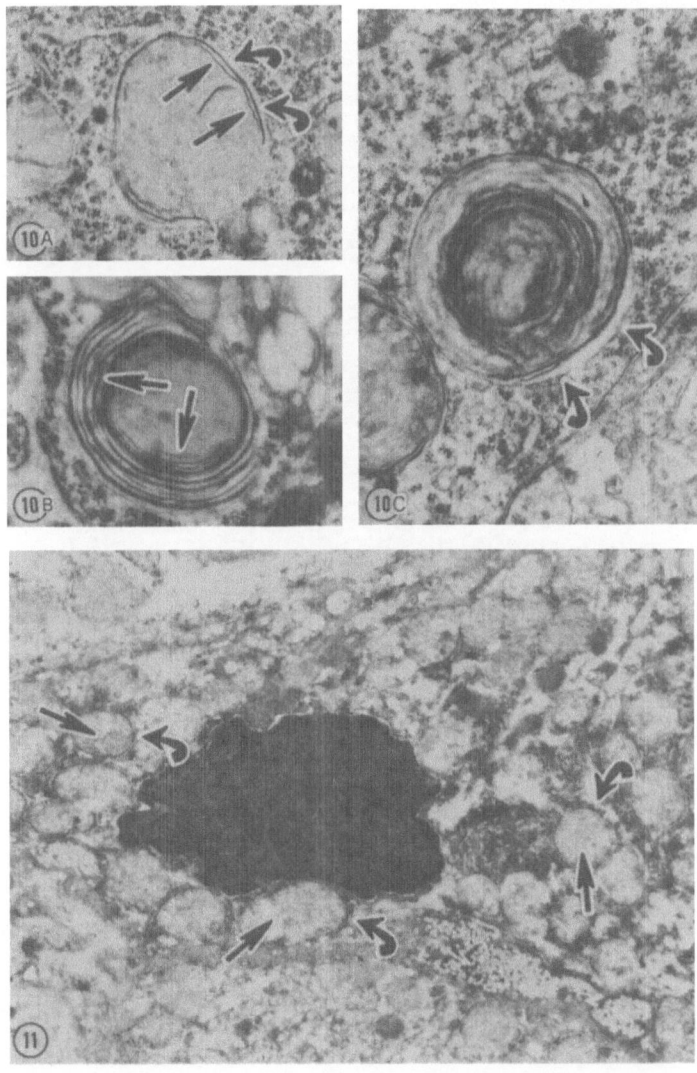

FIGURES 10A, B, C: Concentrically arranged membranous structures
are present which seem to derive from the periphery of the cytosomes (straight arrows) (A and B). The cisternae of the endoplasmic reticulum can still be differentiated from the membranous
inclusions at this stage (curved arrows) (A and C). A) X 19,800;
B) X 9,800; C) X 34,700.

FIGURE 11: Portion of Kupffer cells. The cytoplasm contains inclusion bodies (curved arrows) which are membrane-bound and contain fine dense granules (straight arrows). X 15,200.

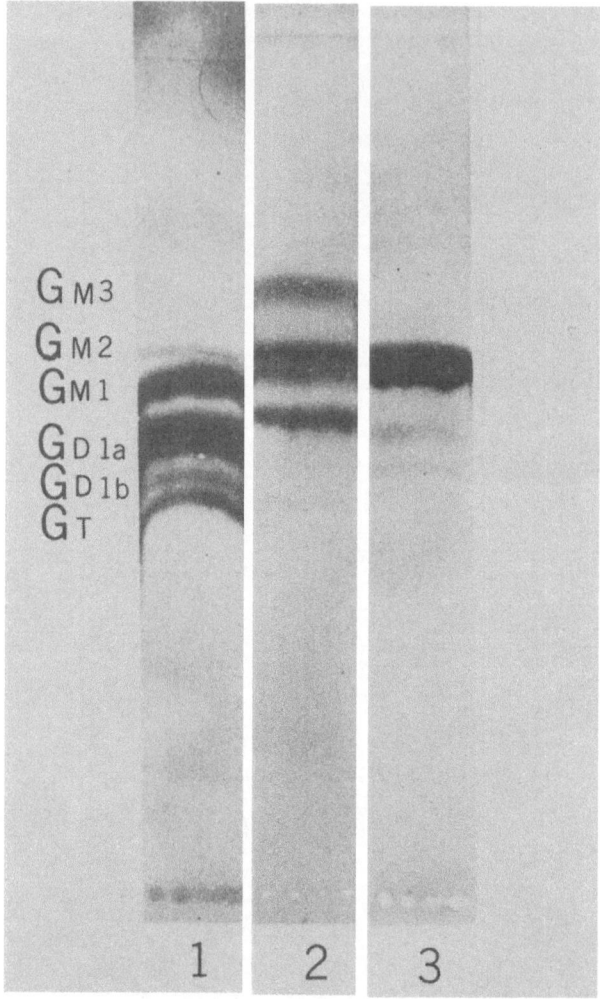

FIGURE 12: Silica gel thin layer chromatograms. 1) Normal cerebrum, 2) cerebrum, present case, 3) liver, present case.

REFERENCES

1. Adachi, M., Torii, J., Karvounis, P.C., and Volk, B.W.: Al-
    terations of Astrocytic Organelles in Various Lipidoses and
    Allied Diseases. Acta Neuropath., 18, 74, 1971.

2. Adachi, M., Torii, J., Schneck, L., and Volk, B.W.: The Fine
    Structure of Fetal Tay-Sachs Disease. Arch. Path., 91, 48,
    1971.

3. Adachi, M., Volk, B.W., Schneck, L., and Torii, J.: Fine
    Structure of the Myenteric Plexus in Various Lipidoses.
    Arch. Path., 87, 228, 1969.

4. Klenk, E., Vater, W., and Bartsch, G.: Storage of Ganglio-
    sides in Nervous Tissue in Tay-Sachs Disease and Changes in
    Material Preserved in Formalin. J. Neurochem., 1, 203, 1957.

5. Okada, S., and O'Brien, J.S.: Tay-Sachs Disease: General
    Absence of a B-D-N-Acetyl Hexosaminidase Component. Science,
    165, 698, 1969.

6. Rouser, G., Kritchesky, G., and Yamamoto, A.: Lipid Chromato-
    graphic Analysis. Marinetti, G.V. (Ed.), New York; M.
    Dekker, Inc., 1967, p. 99.

7. Suzuki, K.: The Pattern of Mammalian Brain Gangliosides: II.
    Evaluation of the Extraction Procedures, Postmortem Changes
    and the Effect of Formalin Preservation. J. Neurochem.,
    12, 629, 1965.

8. Wallace, B.J., Volk, B.W., and Lazarus, S.S.: Fine Structural
    Localization of Acid Phosphatase Activity in Neurons of Tay-
    Sachs Disease. J. Neuropath. Exp. Neurol., 23, 676, 1964.

9. Wallace, B.J., Volk, B.W., Schneck, L., and Kaplan, H.: Fine
    Structural Localization of Two Hydrolytic Enzymes in the
    Cerebellum of Children With Lipidoses. J. Neuropath. Exp.
    Neurol., 25, 76, 1966.

BIOPSY DIAGNOSIS OF LIPIDOSES: Background Considerations, General Concepts and Practical Aspects

Benjamin H. Landing, M.D.,[1,2] Harry B. Neustein, M.D.[1]
and Shigehiko Kamoshita, M.D.[3]

Departments of Pathology[1] and Pediatrics[2], Childrens
Hospital of Los Angeles and University of Southern
California School of Medicine, Los Angeles, California
Department of Pediatrics, University of Tokyo School
of Medicine, Tokyo, Japan[3]

General Concepts of Biopsy Diagnosis of Lipidoses and Other Storage Diseases

Selection of the site for diagnostic biopsy of a patient with lipidosis or other storage disease depends in good part on the clinical picture, whether neurologic, generalized visceral (hepatomegaly, splenomegaly) or other (e.g., cardiomegaly, muscular weakness, renal insufficiency, skeletal disease). The site, and method of biopsy (needle vs. surgical specimen), also depend on the analytic procedures to be employed, the possibilities which may be available including: chemical analysis for the nature of the stored material (e.g., lipid, acid mucopolysaccharide); chemical determination of enzyme defect (e.g., galactosidase, hexosaminidase, "acid maltase"); histologic and histochemical study; electron microscopic study; and, tissue culture followed by one or more of these methods. The nature of the specimen to be procured, and the procedures employed, are also influenced by the precise purpose of the diagnostic procedure, the various types of situations which are encountered including: 1) initial diagnosis of a patient without "strong" clinical diagnosis; 2) confirmation of diagnosis in a patient with "strong" clinical diagnosis, in a patient, whether symptomatic or not, with known disease in the family, or in a patient with presumptive chemical evidence (e.g., aryl sulfatase or hexosaminidase determination) or with non-specific abnormal findings (e.g., lipid histiocytosis of bone marrow, acid mucopolysaccharide in urine), 3) establishment of diagnosis antenatally (see paper of Dr. O'Brien and co-workers). The type of procedure and specimen are also influenced, although perhaps to a lesser extent, by whether the differential diagnostic points to be resolved are clinical (e.g., apparent gray

15

matter or apparent white matter disease of nervous system) or pathologic (e.g., lipofuscin accumulation in histiocytes, or neutral polysaccharide histiocytosis.[13]

Space does not permit detailed analysis of the obviously complicated inter-relations of clinical situation, clinical picture of the patient, precision and type of laboratory methods available, and differential issues, whether clinical or laboratory, which influence the practice of biopsy diagnosis in this field. It is obvious that initial or presumptive diagnosis is often best performed with a specimen of tissue with high probability of abnormality (e.g., bone marrow), from which a large enough specimen can be obtained to permit use of several analytic methods (e.g., brain or liver), or which contains several different cell types (e.g., rectum[15], appendix). Validation or confirmation of a presumptive diagnosis, conversely, can often be done from a specimen of tissue with diagnostically more distinctive lesions (e.g., peripheral nerve in metachromatic leukodystrophy, kidney in Fabry's or von Gierke's diseases, jejunal mucosa in Wolman's disease or a-beta-lipoproteinemia).

Table I attempts to summarize the possible sites for diagnostic biopsy in this sphere of disease, the situations in which the procedure may be performed in children (whether for these or other purposes), and the methods of histologic and histochemical study we have employed in our laboratory.

Table II attempts to set the scene for much of the material to be presented in later papers in this symposium, by listing presently defined entities with known or presumptive lysosomal storage disease, and other diseases involved in their clinical or pathologic differential diagnosis, with indication as to whether the most probably useful diagnostic site is nervous system (usually cerebral or rectal biopsy; for some, peripheral nerve), reticuloendothelial system (usually bone marrow, liver or rectal lamina propria), or other tissue (e.g., kidney, skin, skeletal muscle, small intestine, etc.).

Practical Applications of Diagnostic Biopsy

Table III analyzes the relevant specimens processed in the Surgical Pathology Laboratory of the Department of Pathology, Children's Hospital of Los Angeles, during the ten-year period, 1961-1970. The spectrum of biopsy sites and diagnosable disorders covered in Table I and II is well represented. The single largest group, rectal biopsy, comprises 156 biopsies on patients with clinical neurologic disease, of which 26 (17%) were productive of a "positive" diagnosis. These results compare with those of Brett and Berry[2], who found 20% positive of 165 rectal biopsies. As

TABLE I

Diagnostic biopsy for neural lipidosis, or other conditions involved in clinical or laboratory differential diagnosis.

Possible Biopsy Sites
1) Brain, myenteric plexus (rectum, appendix) peripheral nerve
2) Reticuloendothelial system (spleen, lymph node, bone marrow, tonsil/adenoid, lamina propria of rectum or appendix)
3) Other sites less often useful - liver, kidney, skin, jejunum, periarticular tissue, peripheral blood, etc.

Purposes of Cerebral Biopsy in Children
1) Differential diagnosis of gray matter diseases (e.g., neural lipidoses, kinky-hair disease)
2) Differential diagnosis of white matter diseases (e.g., metachromatic leukodystrophy, spongy degeneration)
3) Diagnosis of neuroaxonal dystrophy

Purposes of Rectal Biopsy in Children
1) Establishment of presence or absence of neurons (e.g., Hirschsprung's disease)
2) Demonstration of stored material in neurons (e.g., neural lipidoses, metachromatic leukodystrophy)
3) Demonstration of stored material in reticuloendothelial cells (e.g., lipid histiocytosis)
4) Study of plasma cells, etc. (e.g., agammaglobulinemia)
5) Study of inflammatory processes (e.g., ulcerative colitis, granulomatous colitis)
6) Other (rare) - demonstration of schistosomiasis, amyloid

Purposes of Peripheral Nerve Biopsy in Children
1) Demonstration of abnormal myelin (e.g., metachromatic leukodystrophy)
2) Demonstration of abnormal axons (e.g., neuroaxonal dystrophy)
3) Demonstration of abnormal sheath (e.g., Refsum's heredopathia atactica, hypertrophic neuritis)

Histochemical Procedures for Brain or Rectal Biopsy for Neurologic Disease
Formalin-fixed tissue, paraffin section
    H&E, PAS, Sudan (4 or black), luxol blue
Unfixed (preferable) or formalin-fixed tissue, frozen section
    PAS, Sudan, toluidine blue, acetic cresyl violet (Hirsch-Pfeiffer)
Either - Autofluorescence

Histochemical Procedures for Peripheral Nerve Biopsy
Formalin-fixed tissue, paraffin section
    H&E, luxol blue (trichrome, PTAH, Bodian, etc., optional)
Unfixed (preferable) or formalin-fixed tissue, frozen section
    Sudan, toluidine blue, acetic cresyl violet, luxol blue
(Procedures for liver, spleen, etc., in patient with presumed neurovisceral storage disease - same as for brain-rectal biopsy)

TABLE II
Lysosomal and Other Storage Diseases

	Biopsy Sites		
Glycolipid Storage Diseases	RE System	Nervous System	Other
Cerebroside Storage Diseases:			
Gaucher -			
Acute infantile	x	-	-
Chronic ("adult")	x	-	-
Juvenile with CNS disease	x	x	-
? chronic form, dominant	x	-	-
Krabbe's disease	-	x	-
Lactosyl ceramidosis (Dawson)	x	x	-
Fabry's trihexosyl ceramidosis	x	±	kidney, heart
Sphingomyelin Storage Diseases			
Niemann-Pick disease -			
Congenital	x	x	-
Acute infantile	x	x	-
Chronic (juvenile) without CNS disease	x	-	-
Chronic with CNS disease	x	x	-
Chronic with CNS disease (Yarmouth epicenter type)	x	x	-
"adult" visceral disease	x	-	-
Visceral disease with hepatoma	x	-	-
Ganglioside Storage Diseases			
GM I - generalized, Type I	x	x	kidney
generalized, Type II	x	x	-
GM II - fetal "Tay-Sachs" disease	x	-	-
infantile amaurotic idiocy (Tay-Sachs)	-	x	-
infantile generalized (Sandhoff)	x	x	-
late infantile generalized	x	x	?
GM III -			
Sulfatide Storage Diseases			
Metachromatic leukodystrophy, late infantile	(colon)	x	kidney, liver peripheral nerve
Metachromatic leukodystrophy, juvenile type	(colon	x	"
Metachromatic leukodystrophy, adult type	?	x	?
Acid Mucopolysaccharidoses			
Hurler (Type I)	x	x	kidney, skin
Hunter (Type II)	x	x	skin
Sanfilippo (Type III)	x	x	

	Biopsy Sites		
	RE System	Nervous System	Other
Morquio (Type IV)	x	-	
Scheie (Type V)	x	-	
Moroteaux - Lamy (Type VI)	x	-	? skin
Lipofuscin Storage Diseases			
Neural - late infantile amaurotic idiocy (Jansky-Bielschowsky)	-	x	-
juvenile amaurotic idiocy (Spielmeyer-Vogt)	-	x	-
adult amaurotic idiocy (Kufs)	-	x	-
leukodystrophy with "pigmented ortho-chromatic lipid"	-	x	-
Visceral - Septic granulomatosis, sex-linked recessive form	x	-	-
septic granulomatosis, "female" form	x	-	-
Ford syndrome	x	-	-
ceroid storage disease (? one entity)	x	-	?
Also - ceroid storage of - malabsorption, cystic fibrosis, other vitamin E deficiency hemochromatosis, hemosiderosis (e.g., thalassemia)			
Triglyceride/Cholesterol Storage Diseases			
Analphalipoproteinemia (Tangier)	x	-	-
Abetalipoproteinemia (Bassen-Kornzweig)	±	x	intestine
Hyperlipoproteinemia, Type I (Bürger-Grütz)	x	-	-
Hyperlipoproteinemia, Type III	x	-	-
Hyperlipoproteinemia, Type V	x	-	-
Wolman's acid lipase deficiency	x	±	intestine, adrenal
Cerebello-peduncular cholesterinosis	-	x	-
Cholesterol ester storage disease (hepatic)	-	-	liver
Others			
Lipogranulomatosis (Farber)	x	±	intestine lung, skin joint
Mucolipidosis, Type I (Spranger-Wiedemann)			

	Biopsy Sites		
	RE System	Nervous System	Other
Mucolipidosis, Type II (Leroy-Opitz) (I-cell disease)			
Mucolipidosis, Type III (pseudopolydystrophy)			
Fucosidosis	x	x	-
Mannosidosis			
Infantile familial myoclonic epilepsy (Unverricht-Lundborg; Lafora)	-	x	liver, muscle, heart

Glycogen Storage Diseases

	RE System	Nervous System	Other
Type 1 - Glucose-6-phosphatase deficiency (von Gierke)	-	-	liver, kidney
2 - Alpha - 1, 4- glucosidase ("acid maltase") def. (Pompe)	x	-	muscle
3 - Debrancher enzyme def. (Forbes)	-	-	liver, muscle
4 - Brancher enzyme def. (Andersen-Cori)	x	-	liver, heart
5 - Myophosphorylase def. (McArdle)	-	-	muscle
6 - Hepatophosphorylase def. (Hers)	-	-	liver
7 - Phosphoglucomatase def.	-	-	muscle
8 - Phosphorylase inactivation, responsive in vivo (Hug)	-	±	liver
9 - Phosphorylase kinase def.	-	-	liver
10 - Juvenile cardiac form	-	-	heart
11 - Phosphofructokinase def. (Nishikawa)	-	-	muscle
12 - Muscular acid maltase def. (Zellweger)	-	-	muscle
13 - ? systemic form with phosphorylase def.	?	±	muscle
14 - ? "phosphorylase kinase kinase" def.	-	-	liver

Miscellaneous

	RE System	Nervous System	Other
Acid phosphatase def. (Nadler)	x	x	x
Myopathy with lysosome accumulation	-	-	muscle

Disorders in differential diagnosis of neural lipidosis and metachromatic leukodystrophy:

	RE System	Nervous System	Other
Spongy degeneration (Canavan; van Bogaert-Bertrand) (cf., also maple syrup urine dis.)	-	x	-

	Biopsy Sites		
	RE System	Nervous System	Other
Megalobarencephaly (Alexander)	-	x	?
Sudanophilic leukodystrophy (Schilder)	-	x	-
Sex-linked "Schilder's" with adrenal atrophy	-	x	adrenal
Pelizaeus-Merzbacher	-	x	-
Kinky-hair disease (Menkes)	-	x	-
Sudanophilic leukodystrophy with meningeal angiomatosis (Divry-van Bogaert)	-	x	-
Leukodystrophy with Smith-Opitz-Inhorn (Zellweger) syndrome	-	x	liver, kidney
Infantile neuroaxonal dystrophy	-	x	-
Cockayne syndrome	-	x	kidney
Phytanic acid storage disease (Refsum)	-	x	peripheral nerve

TABLE III

Diagnostic Biopsies - Patients with neurologic disease and/or lysosomal storage disease (Surgical Pathology series, Childrens Hospital of Los Angeles, 1961-1970)

Reticuloendothelial System - 40
(see also: liver, appendix,
 rectal biopsy)

```
Bone Marrow - 21
    Niemann-Pick                    - 6
    Gaucher                         - 5
    Positive for lipid histiocytes, ? type - 5 (?Sanfilippo, 1)
    Negative                        - 4
    GM I gangliosidosis, Type 2     - 1
Tonsil - 3
    Fucosidosis                     - 1
    Pigmented lipid histiocytosis (septic granulomatosis) - 1
    Negative                        - 1
Lymph Node - 9
    Pigmented lipid histiocytosis   - 5
    Gaucher                         - 1
    Niemann-Pick                    - 1
    Positive for lipid histiocytes,
                        ? type      - 1
    Negative                        - 1
Spleen - 7
    Niemann-Pick                    - 3
    Gaucher                         - 1
```

```
         Positive for lipid histiocytes, ? type - 2 (? Sanfilippo - 1)
         Pigmented lipid histiocytosis      - 1
    Liver - 20
         Negative                           - 8
         Niemann-Pick                       - 4
         GM I gangliosidosis, Type 1        - 3
         Pigmented lipid histiocytosis      - 2
         Gaucher                            - 1
         Metachromatic leukodystrophy       - 1
         Positive, ? Sanfilippo             - 1
    Kidney - 4
         Fabry's disease                    - 1
         Metachromatic leukodystrophy       - 1
         GM I generalized gangliosidosis,
                         Type 1             - 1
         Positive, ? type                   - 1
Nervous System
    Brain - 16
         Negative                           - 5
         Metachromatic leukodystrophy       - 3
         Menkes' kinky-hair disease         - 3
         Neural lipidosis, ? type           - 3
         Canavan's spongy degeneration      - 2
    Sural Nerve - 10
         Negative                           - 8
         Abnormal, ? type                   - 1
         Metachromatic leukodystrophy       - 1
    Appendix - 2
         Tay-Sachs disease                  - 1
         Pigmented lipid histiocytosis      - 1
    Rectal Biopsy - 161
         No specific neurologic diagnosis   - 125
         Positive for "storage disease,"
                         ? type             - 10
         Inadequate for study               - 5
         Pigmented lipid histiocytosis      - 5
         Metachromatic leukodystrophy       - 4
         Jansky-Bielschowsky                - 4
         Tay-Sachs disease                  - 3
         Fucosidosis                        - 2
         Spielmeyer-Vogt disease            - 1
         Niemann-Pick disease               - 1
         GM I generalized gangliosidosis,
                         Type 1             - 1
         (biopsy called negative, later autopsy positive - 1)
Miscellaneous
    Skin - 4
         Negative                           - 3
         Farber's disease                   - 1
```

```
Testis - 1
   Testicular lipidosis              -  1
Heart - 1
   Tuberose sclerosis                -  1
Larynx - 1
   Farber's disease                  -  1
Joint - 1
   Farber's disease                  -  2
Placenta - 1
   Negative for pigmented lipid
       histiocytosis                 -  1
```

with the data of Brett and Berry, this series shows that rectal biopsy is most likely to be productive when there is probability of neurovisceral lipidosis, or of metachromatic leukodystrophy, and that diagnostic features do not exist, or have not yet been recognized, for many other neurologic diseases of children. For instance, antecedent or subsequent neurologic diagnoses on patients whose rectal biopsies were not considered diagnostic have included tuberose sclerosis, Cockayne syndrome, autism, Menkes' kinky-hair disease, leprechaunism, Duane syndrome, DeLange syndrome, Rubinstein-Taybi syndrome, subacute necrotizing encephalopathy, cri-du-chat syndrome, Schilder's disease, subacute sclerosing panencephelitis (Dawson), and hypsarrhythmia. Ultimate diagnosis has not been established on many of the patients in this rectal biopsy series; to date, only one patient whose rectal biopsy was called negative has subsequently been shown to have a neural lipidosis (Jansky-Bielschowsky disease).

Examples of the findings in selected biopsies are shown in Figs. 1-17. Additional comment is warranted on aspects of the material from certain of the specimens on which Table III is based.

FUCOSIDOSIS: Fig. 6 illustrates the findings in rectal biopsy of a 4 7/12 year old male, one of two affected male sibs, with fucosidosis proven chemically by Dr. J. S. O'Brien. These patients are to be reported in detail by Dr. Martin Rosenfeld. PAS - positive histiocytes have been demonstrated in one or both these patients in tonsil (Fig. 7), rectal lamina propria, nasal mucosa and esophageal mucosa, and myenteric plexus neurons show cytoplasmic granules typical of lysosomal storage disease. Skeletal muscle fibers contain PAS - positive granules, and smooth muscle cells may also. Figs. 8 and 9 show examples of fibroblasts in tissue culture from his skin; ultrastructural features of these cells are shown in Figs. 10 and 11.

LIPOFUSCIN STORAGE DISEASE (Jansky-Bielschowsky type): This is the neural lipidosis most commonly fatal in childhood in the non-jewish caucasian population of the United States. The neuronal

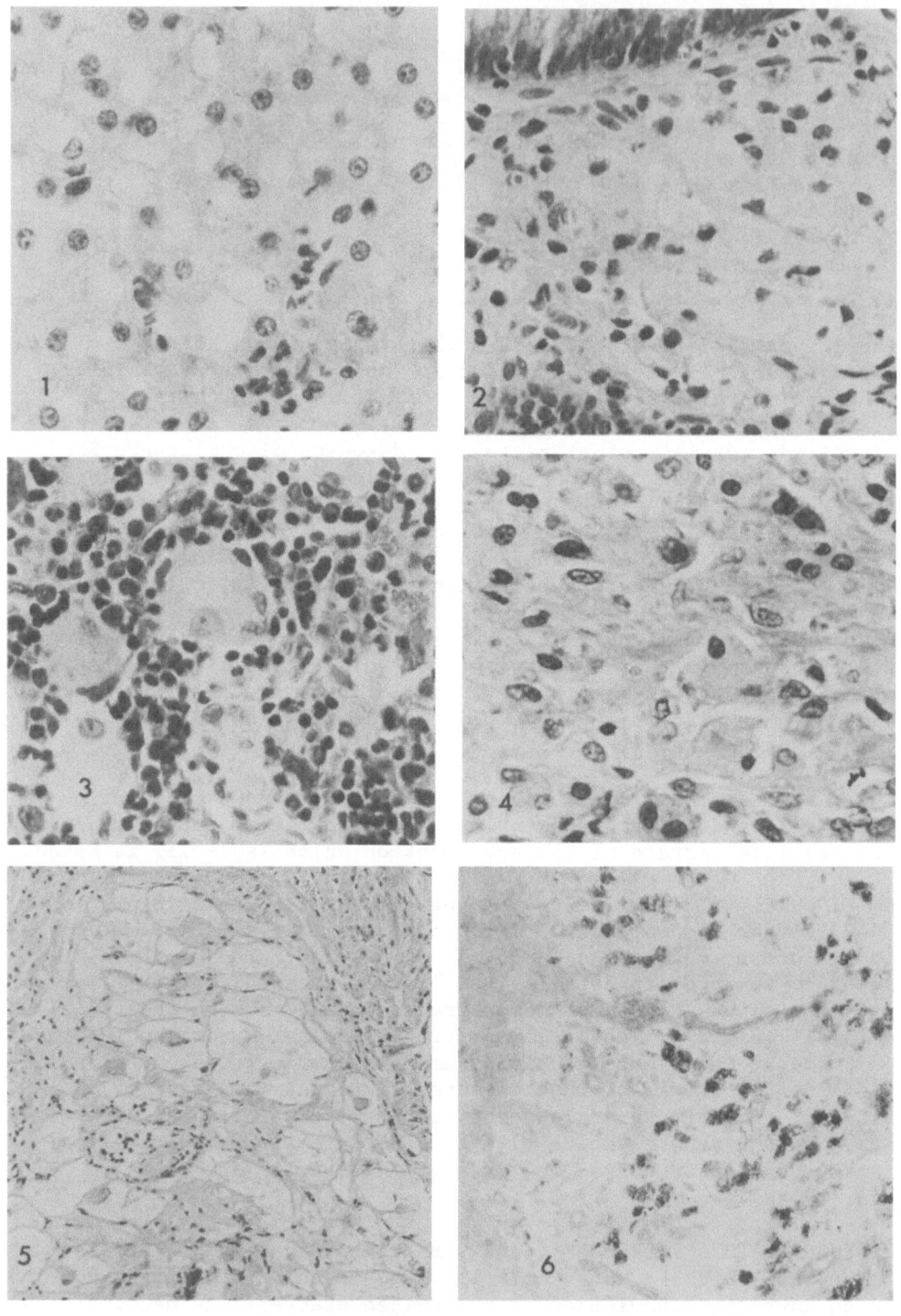

<u>Fig. 1</u> Liver biopsy of 6-month-old male with GM I generalized ganliosidosis, Type 1 (9,16,18), showing vacuolation of both hepatocytes and Kupffer cells. (H&E, X 515)

<u>Fig. 2</u> Rectal biopsy of same patient as in Fig. (1), at age 7 months, to show the massive vacuolar histiocytosis of the lamina propria, (cf. Figs. 16 and 17) (H&E, X 515)

<u>Fig. 3</u> Bone marrow biopsy of 16 7/12 year old girl with "adult" Gaucher disease, showing the typical histiocytes with opaque striated cytoplasm. (H&E, X 515)

<u>Fig. 4</u> Periarticular tissue of male infant with Farber's disease (lipogranulomatosis) showing massive infiltration by histiocytes with granular cytoplasmic deposit. (H&E, X 515)

<u>Fig. 5</u> Rhabdomyoma in surgical specimen of pulmonary outflow tract of 1 3/12 year old girl with tuberose sclerosis. (H&E, X 130)

<u>Fig. 6</u> Rectal biopsy of 4 7/12 year old male with fucosidosis, showing infiltration of both lamina propria and submucosa by PAS-positive (weakly Sudan positive, metachromasia negative) histiocytes. (PAS, X 130)

<u>Fig. 7</u> Tonsil of same patient as Fig. (6), at age 3 years, showing histiocytes with weakly acidophilic cytoplasmic granules (H&E, X 515)

<u>Fig. 8</u> Cell from skin fibroblast tissue culture of same patient as in Figs. (6) and (7) (PAS, X 515)

<u>Fig. 9</u> Cell from skin fibroblast tissue culture (same biopsy as in Fig. 8), showing cytoplasmic granules (colloidal iron stain, X 515)

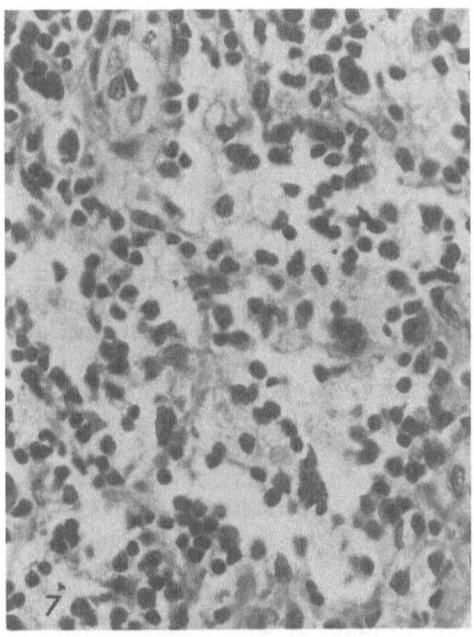

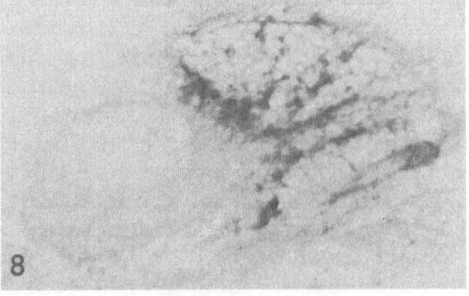

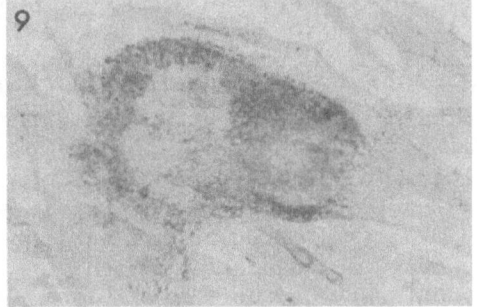

lipofuscin in this disease shows a typical "curvilinear" pattern
(Fig. 12-14), different from that seen in the lipofuscin in
Bürger-Grütz disease[5] or septic granulomatosis [1,7], for example.
That lipofuscin is a class term, and that different lipofuscins
need not show the same ultrastructural features, is discussed below.
Our studies confirm those of Seitelberger, et al.[19], that a small
but abnormal amount of lipofuscin can be demonstrated in reticuloendothelial and other cells in this disorder. The diagnostic ultrastructural specificity of this extraneuronal lipofuscin requires
further study.

JUVENILE METACHROMATIC LEUKODYSTROPHY: In the second volume of
this symposium series, Landing and Rubinstein reported massive
non-metachromatic rectal histiocytosis in a 14-year-old boy with
progressive neurologic disease of, at that time, unknown nature.
This patient has subsequently died, and been shown (by Dr. E. V.
Perrin) to have metachromatic leukodystrophy. Fig. 17 shows the
rectal biopsy of a 16-year-old boy with proven familial metachromatic leukodystrophy; the massive histiocytosis in this patient is
also not metachromatic with toluidine blue or cresyl violet. In
contrast, the histologically similar rectal histiocytes in infantile
metachromatic leukodystrophy (Fig. 16) are metachromatic. The chemical and ultrastructural differences between these two cell populations require further study, which may shed light on differences
in sulfatase specificity which explain the differences between the
two disorders.

ADDITIONAL DIAGNOSTIC METHODS:
1) Tissue Culture - The diagnosis of lipidoses and other metabolic
disorders by tissue culture methods is discussed in greater detail
in this symposium by Dr. Hug and co-workers, by Dr. O'Brien and
co-workers and by Dr. Philippart. To emphasize the potential value
of such methods, Figs. 8 to 11 illustrate the findings in skin
fibroblast tissue culture of a 10-year-old boy with fucosidosis
whose biopsy specimens are shown in Figs. 6 and 7 (see above).
2) Direct Tissue Chromatography - This procedure, as described
by Rogers and Berton [17], is a simple and rapid screening method
for acid mucopolysaccharide storage. Its potential for demonstration of other stored lipids and glycosides appears not to have been
explored. Fig. 18 shows a direct tissue chromatogram prepared
from a 13-year-old male with Hurler's disease. In this technique
small "biopsy-sized" pieces of tissue are pressed into the chromatography paper, an ascending chromatogram is performed with normal
saline as the solvent, and the paper is stained with .04% toluidine
blue at pH 2-2.2. Our experience with Hunter syndrome (mycopoly-
saccharidosis Type 2) and Scheie syndrome (mucopolysaccharidosis
Type 5) is limited to one patient each; the results were that Hunter
syndrome tissues showed much less acid mucopolysaccharide stainable
at this pH than do tissues from Hurler syndrome, and Scheie syndrome

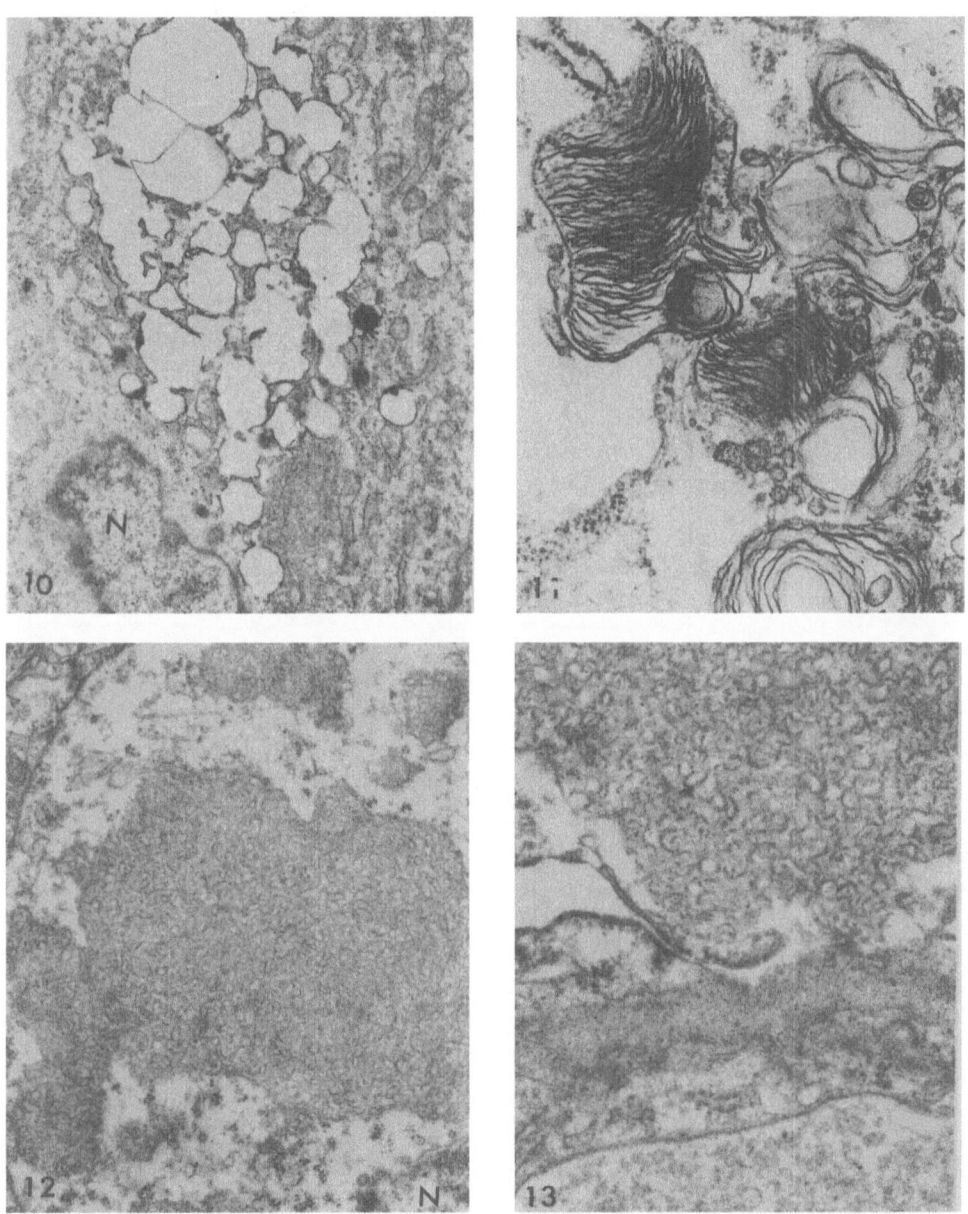

Figs. 10,11 - Fucosidosis, tissue culture fibroblast. In Fig. 10
the cytoplasm shows the numerous vacuoles found in these cells.
Fig. 11 shows some of the numerous cytoplasmic membranous structures.
                    Fig. 10 - X 2000, Fig. 11 - X 36,000
Fig. 12,13 Jansky-Bielschowsky disease - Brain; Fig. 12 shows the
cytoplasmic curvilinear bodies in a glial cell and Fig. 13 shows
similar membrane-bound material in the perithelial cell. Same
patient as Fig. 14.   Fig. 12 - X 18,000 Fig. 13 - X 30,000

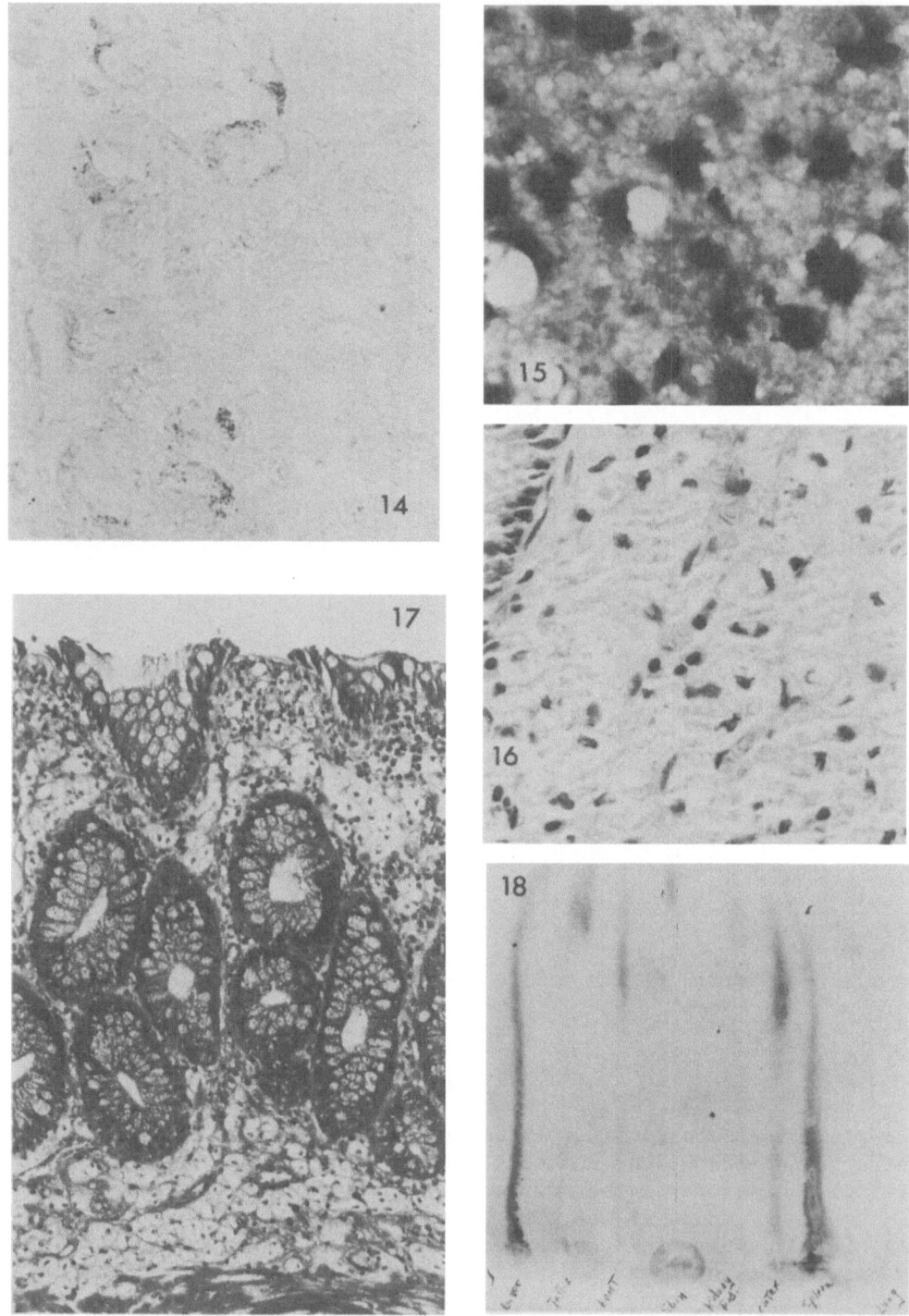

Fig. 14 - Rectal biopsy of 4 3/12 year old boy with Jansky-
Bielschowsky disease, showing lipofuscin granules in cytoplasm of
myenteric plexus neurons (Sudan black stain of paraffin section,
X 515)
Fig. 15 - Cerebral biopsy of 4-year-old male with infantile-onset
metachromatic leukodystrophy, showing abundant metachromatic de-
posit in cerebral white matter (acetic cresyl violet, X 515)
Fig. 16 - Rectal biopsy at age 2 7/12 years from same patient as
Fig. 15, showing heavy histiocytosis of lamina propria. The intracellular material is less clearly vacuolar than is the material in
GM I generalized gangliosidosis (cf. Fig. 2) (H&E, X 515)
Fig. 17 - Rectal biopsy of 16-year-old male with juvenile metachromatic leukodystrophy, showing massive histiocytosis of lamina
propria. This histiocytosis is a repetitive finding in this disease,
in our experience; the material is much less metachromatic than is
that in infantile metachromatic leukodystrophy (H&E, X 130)
Fig. 18 - Direct tissue chromatogram of 13-year-old male with Hurler's
disease. The ascending chromatogram with normal saline as the
solvent is stained with toluidine blue at pH 2.2.

---

none. Since these two diseases are more slowly progressive than
Hurler syndrome, quantitative difference in the degree of acid
mucopolysaccharide storage compared to Hurler syndrome can probably
be expected, but the results to date may indicate more fundamental
difference in the visceral lesions of the various acid mucopolysaccharidoses[12,21].
3) Sites for Diagnostic Biopsy - The various biopsy sites found
useful, by ourselves or by others, for diagnosis of the various
lipidoses and other lysosomal storage diseases to date have been
summarized above. Not hitherto considered as a possible diagnostic site is the testis. Since testicular biopsy is a simple procedure, its consideration in the context of the lipidoses appears
appropriate. Figs. 19-22 show the testicular findings in an
11-month-old male with Niemann-Pick disease and in an 8 9/12 year
old male with Hurler's disease. Foam-cell infiltration of the
testis has also been observed in Tangier disease (analphalipopro-
teinemia) and Wolman's disease[6]. The value of testicular biopsy,
and the range of condtions in which it may be useful, will also
require further study.

General Consideration of Lysosome Dynamics

     Certain aspects of the dynamics of lysosomes, and of storage
diseases, provide a frame of reference for interpreting the findings in tissue specimens. As currently visualized, cellular vacuoles containing material ingested by phagocytosis or pinocytosis
(endocytosis), or portions of cytoplasm (autophagic vacuoles),
form, when fused with primary lysosomes, secondary lysosomes. The

acid hydrolases furnished by the primary lysosomes digest the carbohydrates, lipids, proteins or nucleoproteins contained in the
secondary lysosome, with addition of the products of endocytosed
substances to the metabolic pool of the cell, or with turn-over
of the constituents of autophagocytosed cell cytoplasm and
organelles. A lysosomal storage disease will occur when, for a
given substance or substances, there is deficiency of an appropriate hydrolase, the substance is sufficiently insoluble (or the
lysosomal membrane is impermeable) and there is no adequate alternative pathway of degradation. The degree of lysosomal storage
thus will depend on the amount of a given substance to be degraded
and on the amount of appropriate enzyme available, enzyme-deficiency
situations including circumstances where there is no normal lysosomal enzyme capable of degrading the material present (? true for
cystine in cystinosis, and for lipofuscin). Circumstances where
the supply of material to be processed appears to exceed normal
lysosomal enzyme capacity include Type 1 hyperlipoproteinemia,
where lack of the normal lipoprotein lipase of endothelium leads
to "overloading" of reticuloendothelial cells, with production of
foam-cells; similar overloading of normal enzyme capacities presumably occurs also in Types 3 and 5 hyperlipoproteinemia, at least,
and similar over supply of globosides may explain the Gaucher-like
cells found in the reticuloendothelial system in chronic myeloid
leukemia and in thalassemia[10]. Failure of lysosomal digestion
need not necessarily imply deficiency of an acid hydrolase, although
such deficiency has been demonstrated for a number of the diseases
listed in Table 1; for example, the failure of bacterial killing
and digestion by leukocytes in the chronic granulomatous diseases
is not the result of acid hydrolase deficiency [1,7]. The relation
of the metabolic defects in these diseases to the lipofuscin
accumulation in macrophages seen in septic granulomatosis is unclear, as is whether the source of the lipofuscin is bacterial or
not. Whether the accumulation and persistence of various micro-
organisms in macrophages in histoplasmosis, leprosy, Whipple's
disease, rhinoscleroma, granuloma inguinale, kala azar, etc., can
be considered the result of normal lack of an appropriate lysosomal
hydrolase by humans, whether the situation more nearly approximates
overloading of a normally limited enzyme capacity,   or other
possible explanations, is not clear.

Lipofuscin provides a good illustration of the above considerations. Considered a product of polymerization of peroxidized
unsaturated fatty acids, lipofuscin production is increased by
excessive ingestion of polyunsaturated fatty acids [5], by vitamin
E deficiency (especially common in malabsorbtion situations like
fibrocystic disease) and by excessive presence of iron (which
catalyzes the peroxidation process), as in hemochromatosis, thalassemia, etc. Increased lipofuscin in affected cells in Niemann-
Pick disease, hyperlipoproteinemia[5], etc. can be attributed to

the presence of excessive amounts of peroxidizable lipid, but the explanation for the excessive lipofuscin accumulation in the Jansky-Bielschowsky, Spielmeyer-Vogt and Kufs neural lipidoses is not known, in part because the extent of normal lysosomal capacity, if any, to digest lipofuscin is not known.

Relevant also to the capacity of certain cells to develop lysosomal storage disease is their inherent pace of formation of primary and secondary lysosomes. That macrophages normally have a high rate of lysosome formation is not surprising, and that storage lysosome accumulation should be greater in longer-lived than in short-lived cell types is also reasonable, but the apparently considerably greater production of lysosomes by nerve cells as compared to skeletal muscle fibers is not so easily understood since both are long-lived "fixed postmitotic" cell types. Perhaps the low rate of cytoplasmic turnover by autophagocytosis in skeletal muscle fibers reflects the necessity of physical integrity of cytoplasmic components for their proper function. The apparently higher rate of cytoplasmic turnover in neurons thus may indicate that persistent physical integrity of the cytoplasm is not necessary, or perhaps even not tolerable, for the proper functioning of neurons. The phenomenon of axonal flow may support the latter view.

Chemical - Ultrastructural Relationships in Lysosomal Storage Disease (the rigid, or 1/1, hypothesis)

That to a considerable extent one can reach the diagnosis of a specific lysosomal storage disease by chemical (or histochemical) demonstration of the stored material(s), by chemical demonstration of an enzyme abnormality, or by ultrastructural study of the storage organelle has been discussed above. That more than one material may accumulate in various cells in a lysosomal storage disease is well known; examples include the accumulation of lipid in neurons, of acid mucopolysaccharide in many cell types, and of glycoprotein in liver at least, in Hurler's disease[8], of ganglioside and mucopolysaccharide in generalized GM I gangliosidosis Type 1[18], of monoglycosyl ceramide and lactosyl ceramide in Gaucher's disease [14], etc. That the chemical material(s) stored in various cells in many of these diseases differ, that ultrastructurally different storage organelles can be found in various cell types in such disorders, and also that ultrastructurally different organelles can be found in the same or different cell types in diseases in which only one abnormal substance is known to date are presented in other papers in this symposium, and have been shown in previous papers in this symposium series [11,22]. If one proposes that there is actually a rigid or 1/1 relation between the chemical nature of a stored substance, and the ultrastructure of the corresponding storage lysosome, the occurence of ultrastructurally different organelles serves to alert the chemist to search for stored

materials as yet undemonstrated. This logical sequence actually
has been employed in the development of our understanding of generalized GM I gangliosidosis [18]. Similarly, the occurrence of
ultrastructurally different instances of a substance called by one
chemical term could provide notice that chemical difference actually
exist. Since the unsaturated fatty acids from which lipofuscin is
produced differ in chain length, degree of unsaturation, presence
of branching, etc., and since they may be attached to different
sphingosines, etc., it is not surprising that several ultrastructurally quite different forms of lipofuscin are known. Even when the
chemical term appears more precise (e.g., glucocerebroside, GM I
or GM II ganglioside, lactosyl ceramide[4], etc.), one must recall
that their constituent ceramides may differ in sphingosine or fatty
acid composition, or both. The rigid or 1/1 relation hypothesis
would seem to have enough predictive power, if valid, to merit
serious consideration, and possible exceptions in the literature
(e.g., similar membranous cytoplasmic bodies in GM I and GM II
gangliosidosis[20] may well merit more detailed study.

Fig. 19 - Testis of 8 9/12 year old male with Hurler's disease
(mucopolysaccharidosis 1) showing cytoplasmic vacuolo-granulation
of intertubular cells (H&E, X 515).

Fig. 20 - Testis of 11 month old male with Niemann-Pick disease,
showing massive interstitial infiltration by vacuolar histiocytes.
(H&E, X 515).

Fig. 21 - Electron micrograph of same specimen as Fig. 20 (autopsy
tissue originally fixed in formaldehyde), showing massive accumulation of membranous cytoplasmic bodies similar to those seen in
ganglioside storage diseases. (X 5,000).

Fig. 22 - Higher magnification of same specimen as Fig. 21, showing "rose flower" pattern of stored material. (X 30,000).

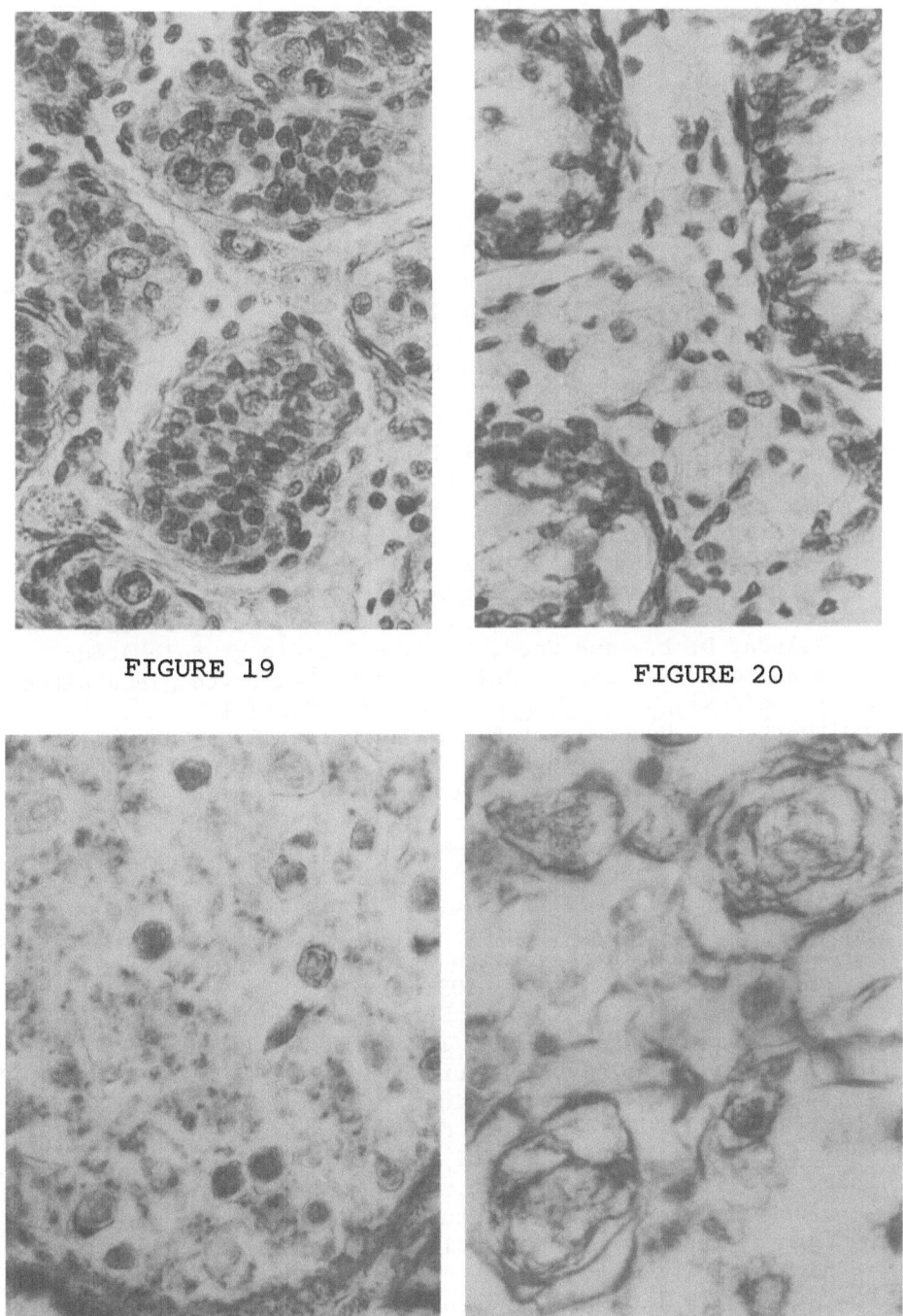

FIGURE 19   FIGURE 20

FIGURE 21   FIGURE 22

REFERENCES

1. Baehner, R. L. and Nathan, D. G. - Leukocyte Oxidase: defective
    activity in chronic granulomatous disease, Science 1967,
    155:835-836
2. Brett, E. M. and Berry, C. L. - Value of rectal biopsy in ped-
    iatric neurology: report of 165 biopsies, Brit. Med. J. 1967
    5:400-
3. Carson, M. J., Chadwick, D. L., Brubaker, C. A., Cleland, R. S.
    and Landing, B. H. - Thirteen boys with progressive septic
    granulomatosis, Pediatrics 1965, 35:405-412
4. Dawson, G. and Stein, A. O. - Lactosyl ceramidosis: catabolic
    enzyme defect of glycosphingolipid metabolism, Science 1970,
    170:556-558
5. Ferrans, V. J., Buja, L. M. Roberts, W. C. and Fredrickson,
    D. S. - The spleen in Type 1 hyperlipoproteinemia: histo-
    chemical, biochemical, microfluorometric and electron
    microscopic observations, Am. J. Path. 1971, 64:67-96
6. Guazzi, G. C., Martin, J. J., Philippart, M., Roels, H.,
    van der Eecken, H., Vrints, L., Delbeke, M. J. and Hooft, C.
    - Wolman's disease, European Neurology 1968, 1:334-362
7. Holmes, B., Park, B. H., Malawista, S. E., Quie, P. G.,
    Nelson, D. L., and Good, R. S. - Chronic granulomatous
    disease in females; a deficiency of leukocyte glutathione
    peroxidose, N. E. J. Med. 1970, 283:217-221
8. Hultberg,B., Ockerman, P-A and Dahlquist, A. - Gargoylism:
    hydrolysis of B-galactosides and tissue accumulation of
    galactose - and mannose - containing compounds, J. C. Inv.,
    1970, 49:216-224
9. Landing, B. H., Silverman, F. N., Craig, J. M., Jacoby, M. D.,
    Lahey, M. E. and Chadwick, D. L. - Familial neurovisceral
    lipidosis: an analysis of eight cases of a syndrome pre-
    viously reported as "Hurler-Variant," Pseudo-Hurler Disease"
    and "Tay-Sachs Disease with visceral involvement."
    Am. J. Dis. Child. 1964, 108:503-522
10. Lee, R. E. and Ellis, L. D. - The storage cells of chronic
    myelogenous leukemia, Lab. Invest. 1971, 24:261-264
11. Loeb, H., Jouniaux, G., Tondeur, M., Danis, P., Grégoire, P. E.
    and Wolff, P. - Etude clinique, biochimique et ultra-
    structurelle de la Maladie de Fabry chez l'enfant, Helv.
    Paediat. Acta. 1968, 23:269-286
12. Loeb, H., Tondeur, M., Toppet, M. and Cremer, N. - Clinical,
    biochemical and ultrastructural studies of an atypical
    form of mucopolysaccharidosis, Acta. Paediat. Scand. 1969,
    58:220-228
13. Lou, T. Y., Teplitz, G., and Thayer, W. R., Jr. - Ultra-
    structural morphogenesis of colonic PAS - positive macro-
    phages ("colonic histiocytosis"), Human Path. 1971, 2:421-
    440

14. Malmquist, E., Ivemark, B. I., Lindsten, J., Maunsbach, A. B. and Martensson, E. - Pathologic lysosomes and increased urinary glycosylceramide excretion in Fabry's disease. Studies on a family with evidence of linkage with the sex-linked blood group Xg, Lab. Invest. 1971, 25:1-14

15. Nakai, H. and Landing, B. H. - Suggested use of rectal biopsy in the diagnosis of neural lipidosis, Pediatrics 1960, 26:225-228

16. O'Brien, J. S., Stern, M. B., Landing, B. H., O'Brien, J. K. and Donnell, G. N. - Generalized gangliosidosis. Another inborn error of ganglioside metabolism? Amer. J. Dis. Child. 1956, 109:338-346

17. Rogers, S. and Berton, W. M. - Application of paper chromatography to some of the general problems of pathology, Lab. Invest. 1957,6:310-323

18. Scott, C. R., Lagunoff, D. and Trump, B. F. - Familial neurovisceral lipidosis, J. Pediat. 1967, 71:357-366

19. Seitelberger, F., Jacob, H. and Schnobel, R. - The myoclonic variant of cerebral lipidosis, in Inborn Disorders of Sphingolipid Metabolism, Proceedings of the Third International Symposium on the Cerebral Sphingolipidoses, Ed., S. M. Aronson and B. W. Volk. Pergamon Press 1967, pp. 43-74

20. Suzuki, K., Suzuki, K. and Kamoshita, S. - Chemical pathology of GM I - gangliosidosis (generalized gangliosidosis), J. Neuropath. Exp. Neurol. 1969, 28:25-73

21. Van Hoof, F., and Hers, H. G. - The abnormalities of lysosomal enzymes in mucopolysaccharidoses, Europ. J. Biochem. 1968, 7:34-44

22. Wallace, B. J. Lazarus, S. S. and Volk, B. W. - Electron microscopic and histochemical studies of viscera in lipidoses. Proceedings of the Third International Symposium on the Cerebral Sphingolipidoses, Ed., S. M. Aronson and B. W. Volk. Pergamon Press 1967, pp.43-74

LYSOSOMAL DISEASES AND FIBROBLAST CULTURES:

BIOCHEMICAL AND ELECTRON MICROSCOPIC OBSERVATIONS

George Hug, William K. Schubert and Shirley Soukup

The Children's Hospital Research Foundation, University of

Cincinnati College of Medicine, Cincinnati, Ohio 45229

Most lysosomal diseases are fatal, often after a protracted downhill course that is painfully apparent to patient, parents and physician. This interim report relates our attempts to treat such patients; and to find ultrastructural and biochemical markers in fibroblast cultures for the study of pathophysiology and treatment of lysosomal disease.

During the past eight years patients with the following lysosomal diseases have been seen in the Clinical Research Center of the Cincinnati Children's Hospital (number of patients are given in parenthesis): Type II glycogenosis (13); metachromatic leucodystrophy (3); Hurler syndrome (5); Tay-Sachs disease (2); Gaucher disease (1); Krabbe disease (2); Chediak-Higashi disease (2). These conditions were diagnosed by biochemical, and/or clinical and electron microscopic means as outlined in a recent review (1). For the present, we shall limit our comments to some observations on the first three of the conditions listed above.

TREATMENT OF PATIENTS

Type II Glycogenosis (GSD II)

The classical form of GSD II that becomes clinically apparent soon after birth and comprises the majority of cases is a fatal disease of infancy. There are, however, well documented cases of formes frustes of GSD II in adults (2). The ultrastructural abnormality of the disease, i.e. the membrane surrounded accumulation of lysosomal glycogen (the "abnormal lysosome") was found in the liver (3) as had been anticipated after the demonstration of deficient lysosomal acid α-glucosidase (4).

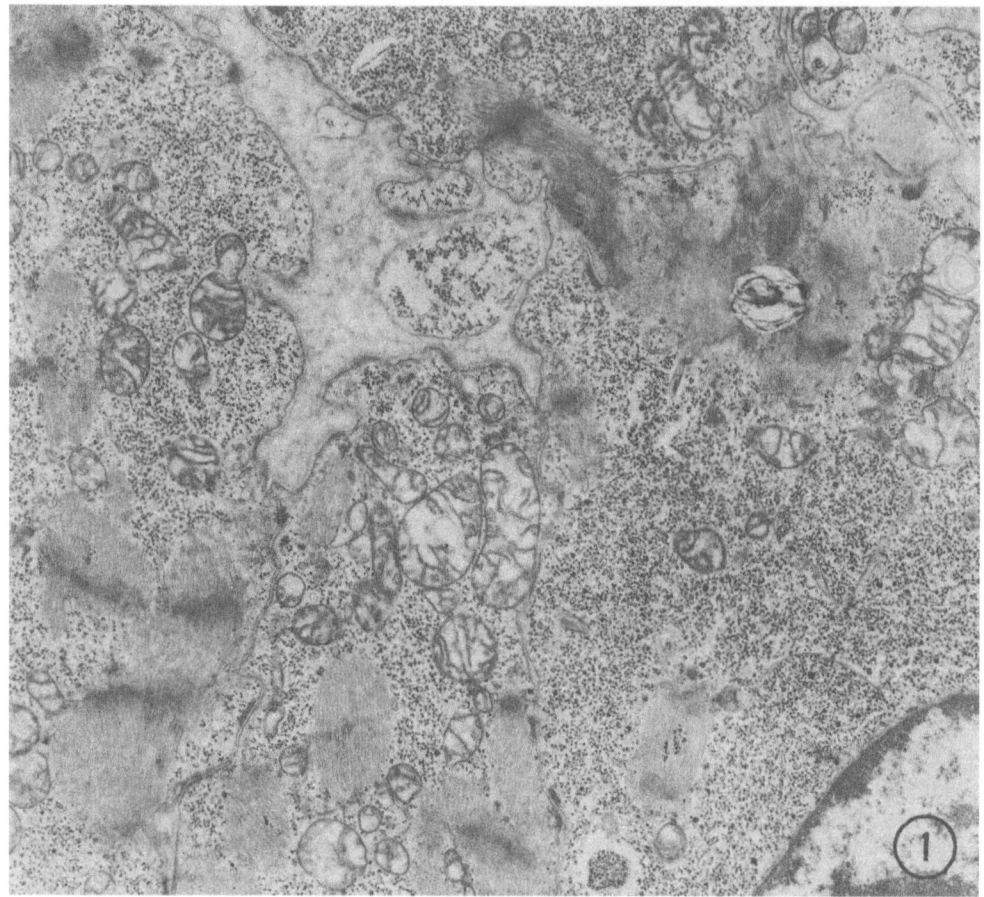

<u>Figure 1</u>: Fetal myocardium, Type II glycogenosis. Contractile
elements have disintegrated and are replaced by excessive
<u>cytoplasmic</u> glycogen. (X 10,000) (All sections in this report
have been stained with lead citrate for five minutes.)

However, on the basis of this <u>lysosomal</u> enzyme deficiency we
still do not understand the excessive accumulation of <u>cytoplasmic</u>
glycogen as observed in skeletal muscle (5) and in other tissues
of GSD II. For example, we found excessive cytoplasmic glycogen
in myocardium of a twenty week old fetus with GSD II (Figure 1).

Attempts at treatment of patients with GSD II have included
administration of epinephrine; or of glycogen degrading enzymes;
or of a variety of other agents.

Epinephrine administration and starvation in a patient with GSD II led to the depletion of cytoplasmic glycogen in liver but not muscle. The lysosomal glycogen was not mobilized (5).

Intravenous administration of glycogen degrading enzymes prepared from Aspergillus niger (7 cc daily of a solution containing 25 mg of protein per cc that formed 22 μm of glucose from glycogen per mg per minute at pH 4 and 37°C) to a patient with GSD II was followed, after 19 days of treatment, by the disappearance of lysosomal glycogen in the liver. The cytoplasmic glycogen was not mobilized (Figures 2,3) (6). A previous attempt by others with such treatment had been without this effect perhaps because of differences in route and duration of enzyme administration (3). The clinical improvement seen in the initial weeks of therapy was not sustained. After four months of enzyme treatment hypocomplementemic nephritis developed and treatment was stopped. One week later the child died of GSD II (7). Such immunological complications could be treated with immunosuppression. However, a prerequisite for successful treatment with enzyme administration is entry of the enzyme into cardiac and skeletal myocytes since children with GSD II die of respiratory and cardiac muscle failure. At autopsy, there was some evidence for enzymatic action in heart and skeletal muscle, although uptake of enzyme into myocytes had not been demonstrable during treatment (7). Finally, the conclusion that the hepatic lysosomal glycogen was mobilized by glycolytic enzymes in the Aspergillus extract is consistent with, but not proven by, the recovery of the enzymes from the liver.

We have treated one other patient with GSD II by infusion of highly purified, recrystallized human salivary amylase. There were no complications of treatment. Despite the recovery of high amylase activity from the liver, hepatic ultrastructure and glycogen concentration remained abnormal; and there was no clinical improvement. The lack of a hepatic effect might be explained by amylase inactivity at pH 4-5, or at the pH thought to prevail within lysosomes.

Other agents we used for treatment of GSD II included vitamin A, progesterone, tris(hydroxymethyl)aminomethane (Tris), hyperbaric oxygen and Trasylol ⓡ. These agents had been reported at one time or another, to be of potential use in treatment of lysosomal disease. In doses at the limit of tolerance, none has produced clinical, biochemical or ultrastructural benefit in GSD II.

Metachromatic Leucodystrophy (MLD)

An attempt at treatment of a patient with MLD was made by intravenous (and intrathecal) administration of beef brain

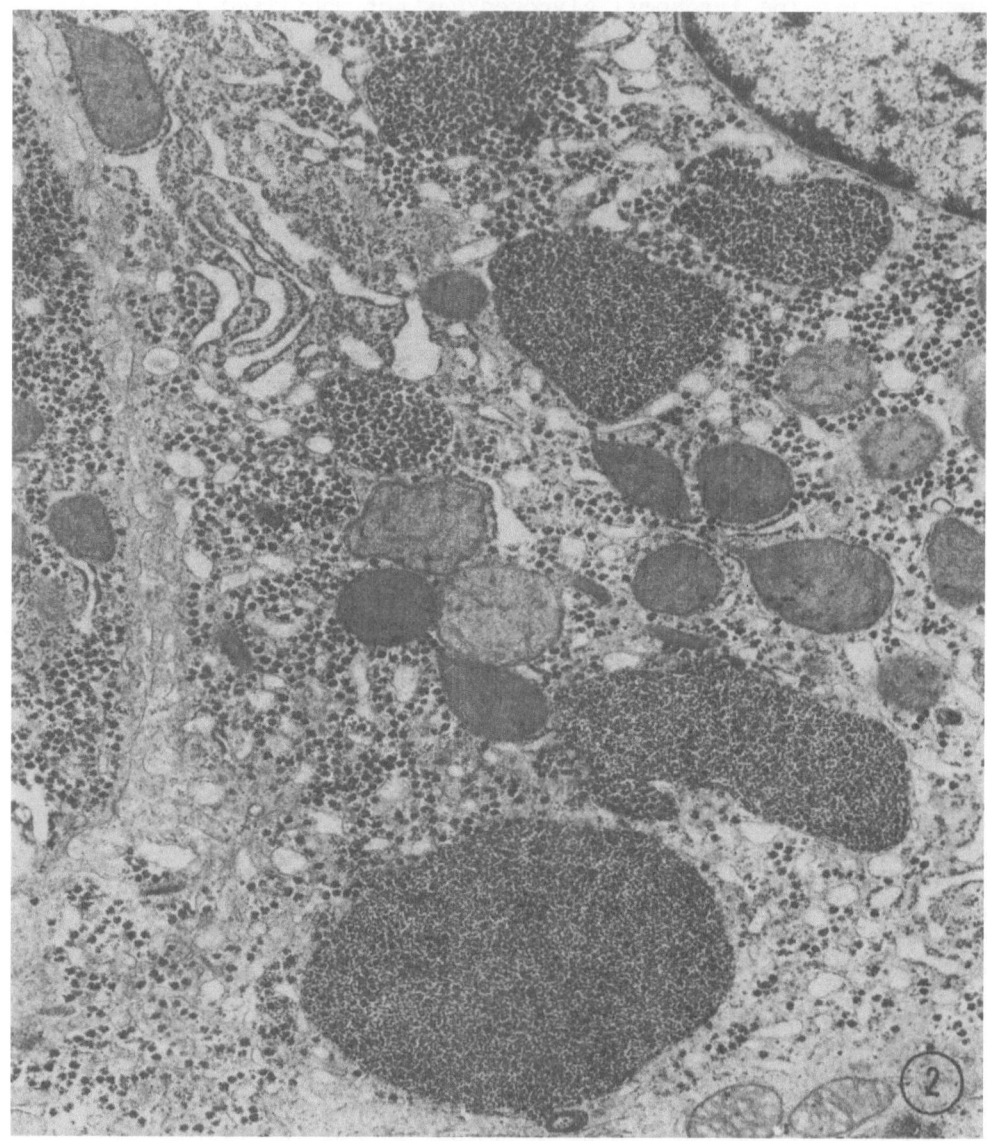

<u>Figure 2</u>: Type II glycogenosis; needle biopsy specimen of the
liver <u>before</u> infusion of Aspergillus niger extract shows numerous
"abnormal lysosomes" filled with lysosomal glycogen in every
hepatocyte. (X 10,000).

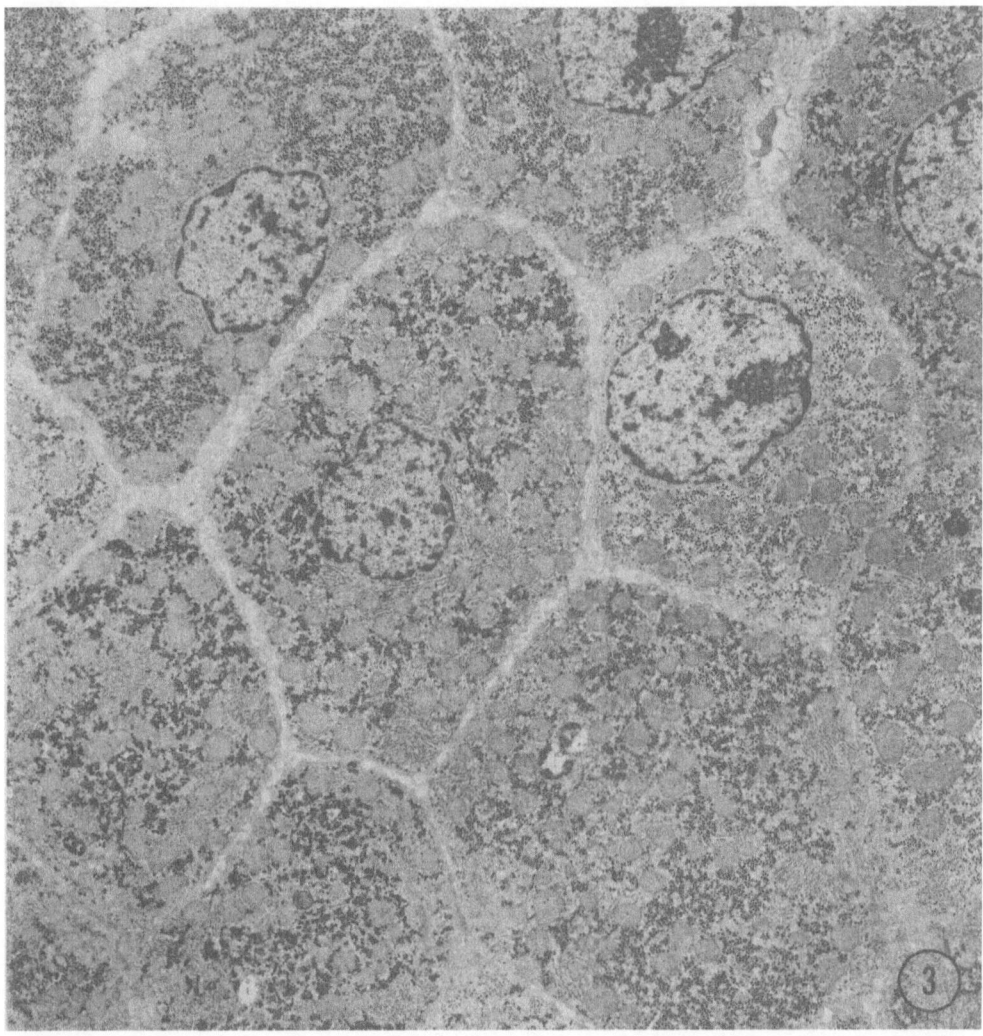

Figure 3: Type II glycogenosis; same patient as Figure 2. Needle biopsy specimen of liver after 19 days of infusion of Aspergillus niger extract. The glycogen filled abnormal lysosomes of the pre-infusion specimen have disappeared. (X 4,000)

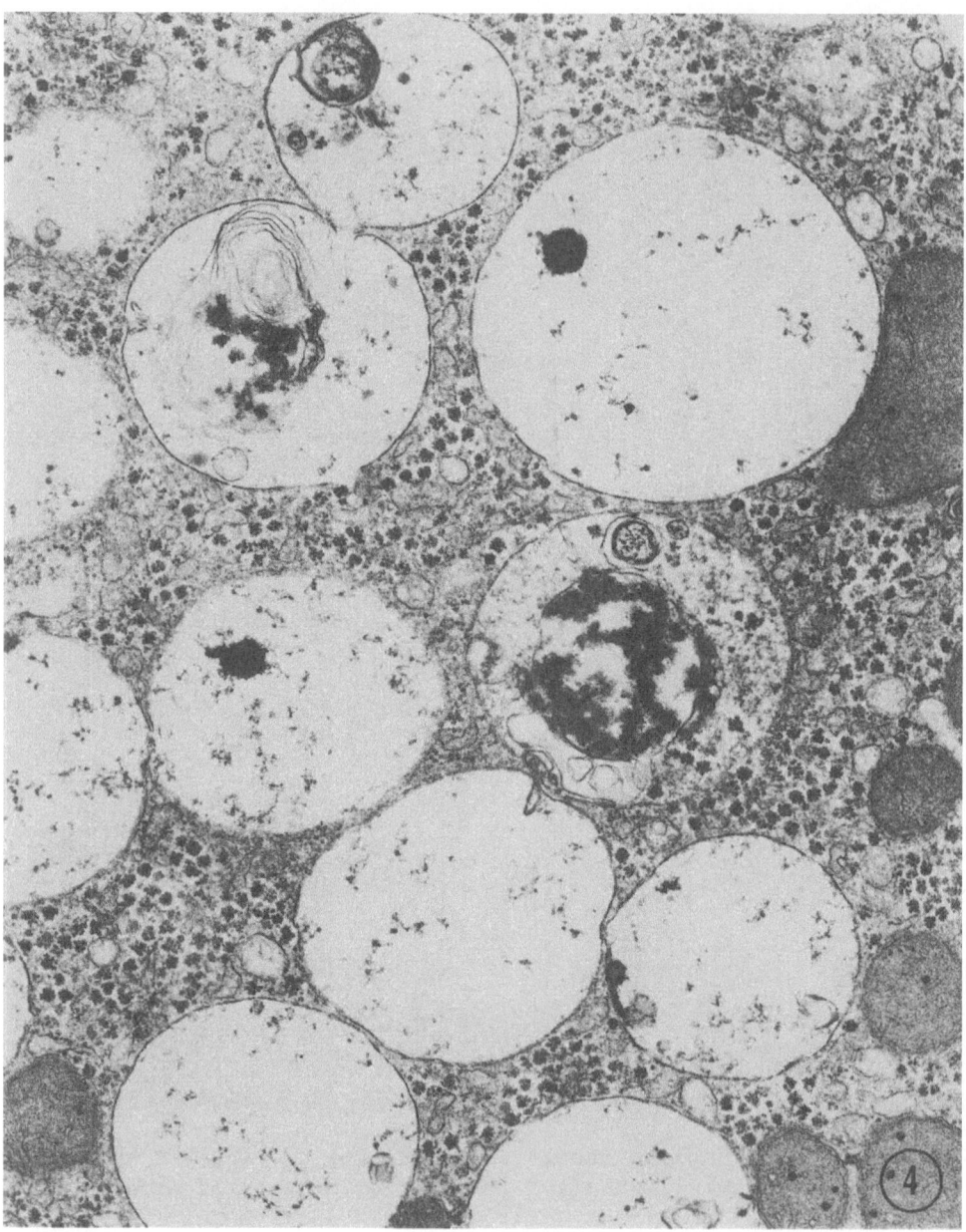

Figure 4: Needle biopsy specimen of liver in Hurler syndrome indicating the typical abnormal vacuoles that persist unchanged after clinically beneficial plasma infusion to the patient. (X 20,000)

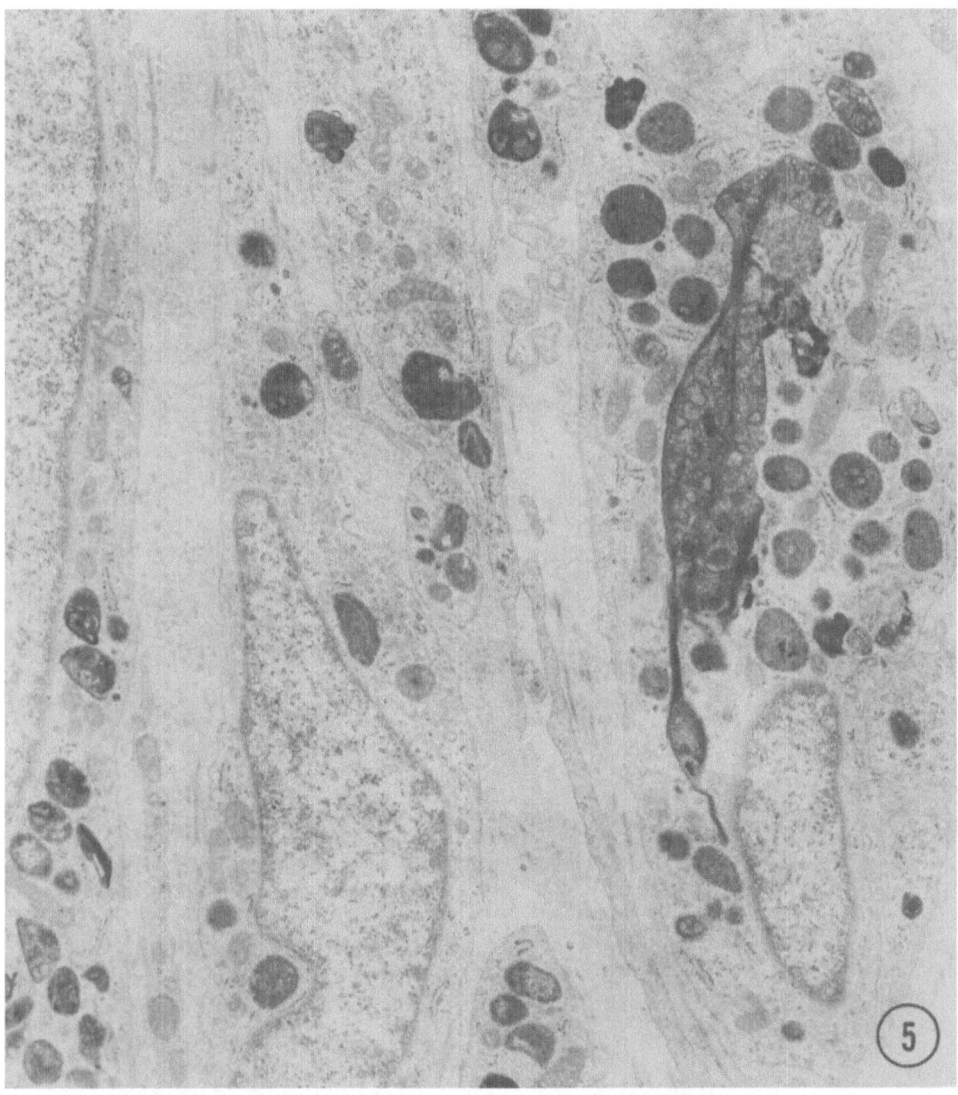

Figure 5: Metachromatic leucodystrophy; cultured fibroblasts.
Some of the dark inclusions look "suspicious." However, at this
magnification, only the single large, elongated body is
indicative of MLD, whereas inclusions like the smaller electron
dense bodies also occur in some normal control fibroblasts, and
in cultured fibroblasts of other lysosomal diseases. (X 10,000)

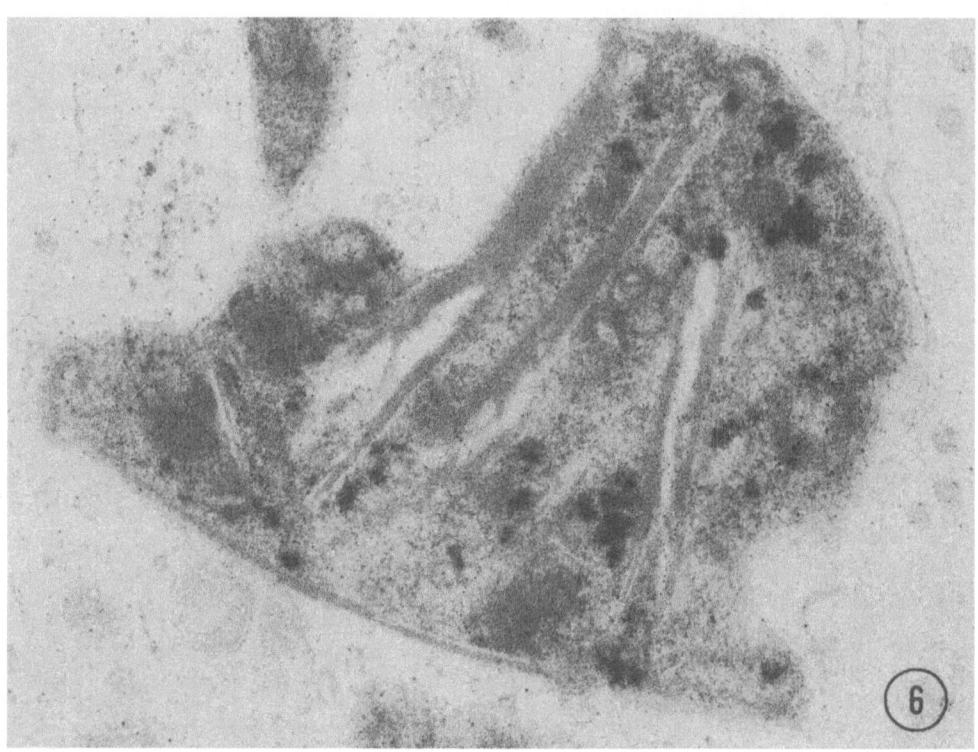

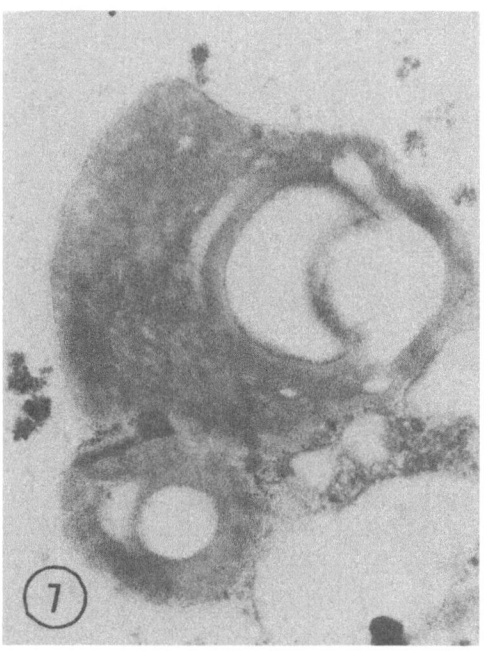

Figure 6: Inclusion body of
a cultured fibroblast in MLD
with the lamellar internal
organization also observed
in MLD inclusions of brain
and liver. (X 50,000)

Figure 7: Needle biopsy
specimen of liver in MLD.
Parallel and circular
lamellae make up an inclusion
of the kind seen abundantly
in hepatocytes of MLD.
(X 50,000)

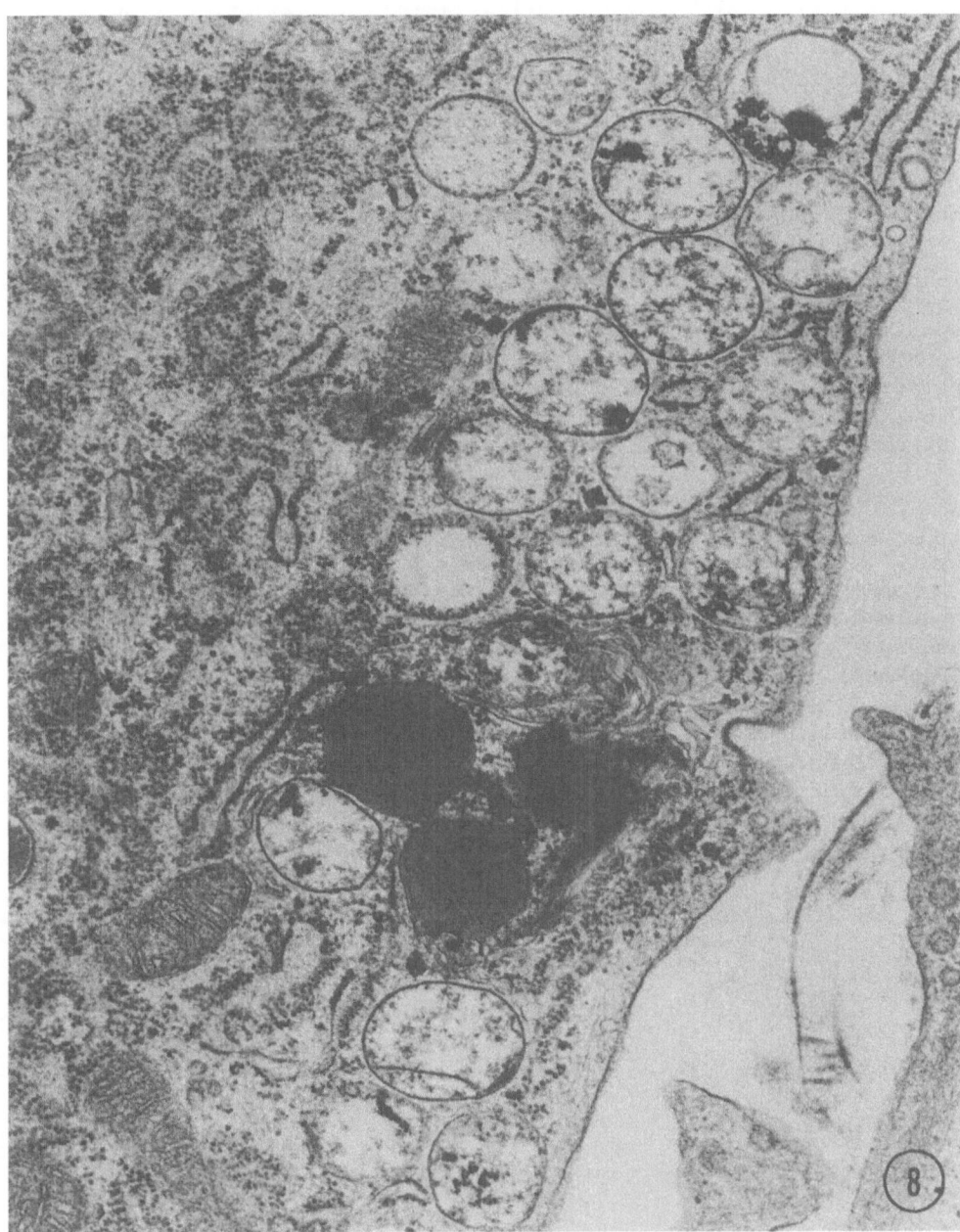

Figure 8: Hurler syndrome; cultured fibroblast with vacuoles similar to those seen in hepatocytes of such patients. In the center there are three normal lipid "droplets". (X 35,000)

arylsulfatase-A for 32 days (8). There were no immunological
complications. The infused enzyme could be recovered from liver,
but not brain. There was no clinical improvement nor was there
post-infusion disappearance of the lamellar residual bodies seen in
hepatocytes of patients with MLD (8,1) (Figure 7).

Hurler Syndrome

In patients with Hurler syndrome dramatic clinical improvement has recently been reported after infusion of human blood
plasma (9). Dr. Meinhard Robinow of Dayton, Ohio applied this
treatment to one of his patients on two occasions (each time with
clinical benefit). He provided us with hepatic needle biopsy
specimens before and after the second course of treatment. The
hepatocytes of the treated patient remained deficient in β-
galactosidase activity and contained the membrane surrounded
vacuoles that are typically found in hepatic specimens from
untreated patients with Hurler syndrome (Figure 4).

FIBROBLAST CULTURES

Skin fibroblast cultures of the patients were examined for
biochemical and electron microscopic markers. As others had
previously described (10,11,12,13), we found that the activity of
acid α-glucosidase or arylsulfatase-A was deficient in liver and
cultured fibroblasts of GSD II or MLD respectively, whereas β-
galactosidase was deficient in liver but not in fibroblasts of
Hurler syndrome. Homogenates of liver or cultured fibroblasts of
Hurler syndrome had markedly increased activity of hexosaminidase
(Table 1).

Table 1

Activities of Three Acid Hydrolases in Tissue Homogenates

	Fibroblasts		Liver	
	GSD II	Hurler	GSD II	Hurler
α-glucosidase	1	100	5	100
β-galactosidase	100	117	100	12
hexosaminidase	100	150	100	835

The figures represent mean values in percent of normal
(i.e. 100 signifies 100 % of normal).

On electron microscopy, some normal control fibroblast cultures contained numerous electron dense inclusions. They resembled unspecific residual bodies of hepatocytes. In part, the appearance of these inclusions was determined by culture conditions, but it also depended on the donor of the specimen. Cells grown from biopsy samples taken on six separate times at least one month apart from the same healthy volunteer contained such inclusions under culture conditions that produced no inclusions in growing cells from other controls. These "non-specific" inclusions could also be observed in cultured fibroblasts of individuals with lysosomal disease. These non-specific electron dense inclusions had only minimal internal organization. Fibroblast inclusions were considered indicative of a lysosomal disease when they resembled "abnormal lysosomes" observed in organs of patients with the same disease. For example, cultured fibroblasts of MLD (14) contained inclusions with stacks of circular and parallel lamellae that resembled those present in liver (1,8) and brain (8,15) of children with MLD (Figures 5,6,7).

Inclusions of the kind observed in hepatocytes of patients with Hurler syndrome were also found in cultured fibroblasts of the same patient (16) (Figures 4,8). We have found such "Hurler inclusions" less frequently in cultured fibroblasts of Gaucher disease, Tay-Sachs disease, GSD II and rarely of normal controls.

Fibroblast cultures have been established from eight of our patients with GSD II and have been maintained for up to eighteen passages. These cultures were deficient in acid α-glucosidase. The fibroblasts consistently contained many membrane surrounded accumulations of β-glycogen particles (17) (Figure 9). These "abnormal lysosomes" appeared identical to those seen in hepatocytes of children with GSD II (Figure 2) and they have not been encountered in cultured fibroblasts of controls or of other lysosomal diseases. The ease of recognition of these inclusions and their ubiquitous presence allowed the prenatal diagnosis of GSD II using electron microscopy of cultured and uncultured amniotic fluid cells. Direct electron microscopy of uncultured amniotic fluid cells provided the diagnosis within days after the amniocentesis (18,19).

The mechanism by which therapeutic agents, e.g. enzymes, might enter the lysosome was studied by adding colloidal gold to fibroblast cultures. Normal cultured fibroblasts as well as those affected with GSD II or Hurler syndrome were shown to pinocytose electron dense particles of colloidal gold. In the case of the diseased cultures, these particles were eventually deposited within the abnormal lysosomes (1,20).

This being a symposium on Tay-Sachs disease, I shall conclude by mentioning our results on polyacrylamide gel electrophoresis

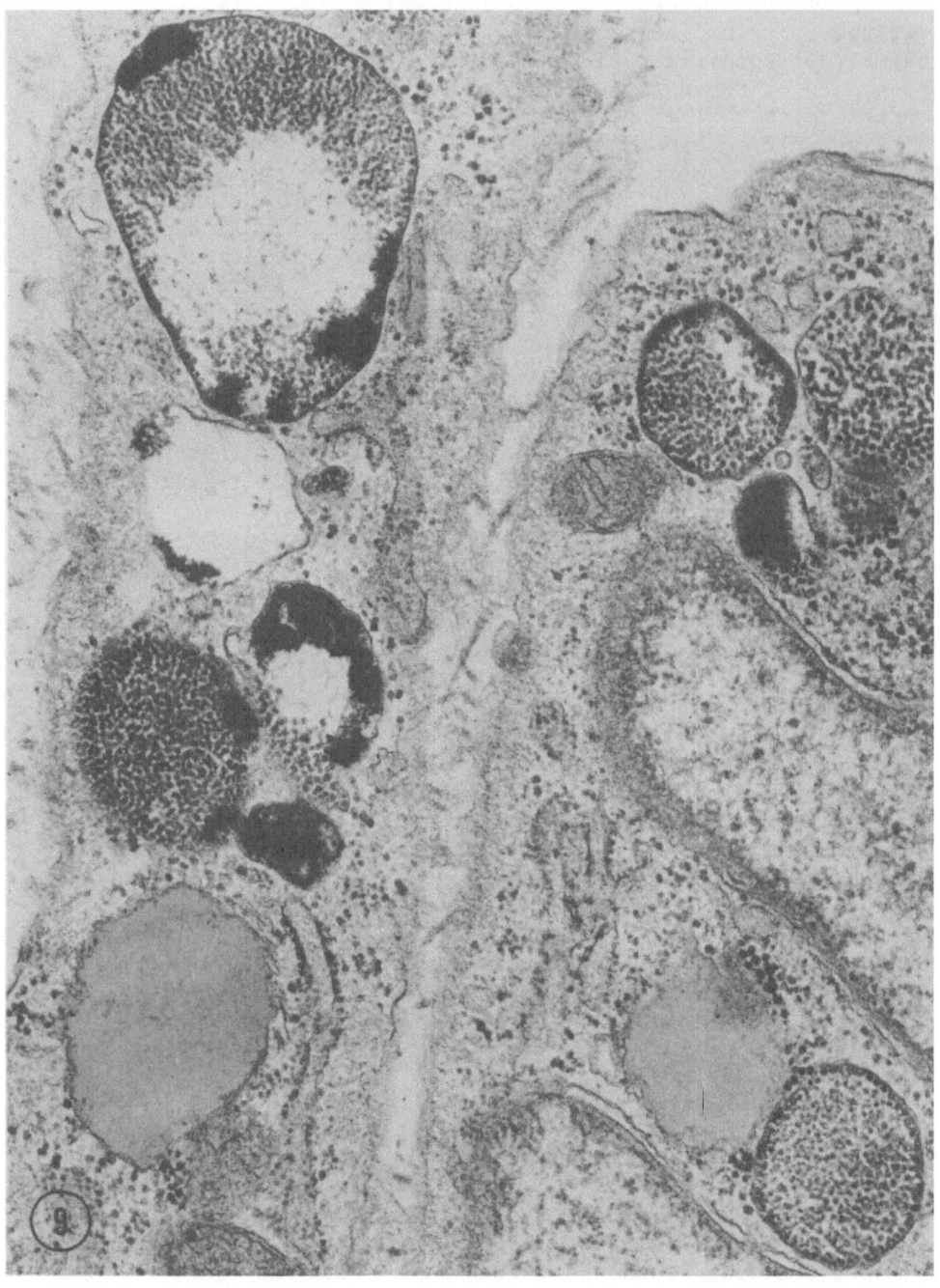

Figure 9: Type II glycogenosis; detail of cultured fibroblast with "abnormal lysosomes" as also observed in liver of GSD II, but not in solid tissues or fibroblast cultures of other lysosomal diseases or normal controls.   (X 40,000)

and on enzymatic analysis of fibroblast homogenates from two patients with Tay-Sachs disease. On electrophoresis, hexosaminidase band A was absent and hexosaminidase band B was present in both patients (a finding identical to that reported by others(21)). The B band was unusually broad in one of the patients on repeated analysis. On enzymatic analysis in the test tube, there was no statistical variation of total hexosaminidase activity measured at zero time or its components A and B measured after 3 or 4 hours of incubation at 50° C between normal controls and the two patients.

SUMMARY

Infusion of fungal α-glucosidase to one patient with GSD II resulted in the disappearance of the characteristic abnormal inclusions from hepatocytes and in temporary clinical improvement.

Infusion of plasma to one patient with Hurler syndrome, while clinically beneficial, did not change the abnormal hepatic inclusions.

Electron dense "non-specific" inclusions occurred in fibroblast cultures of normal controls and of lysosomal diseases.

In addition, fibroblast cultures of lysosomal disease contained "specific" inclusions similar to the ones observed in solid tissues of the disease in question.

There was overlap in the sense that inclusions typical of one lysosomal disease were detected infrequently in cultures of others, and rarely in cultures of normal controls.

However, such overlap was not observed in GSD II where the specific and easily recognizable inclusions occurred abundantly in cultures of GSD II but not of controls or other lysosomal diseases.

Characteristic inclusions in uncultured amniotic fluid cells provided the diagnosis of GSD II that was confirmed in the aborted fetus.

Cultured fibroblasts from GSD II as well as Hurler syndrome demonstrated entry of gold particles into the cell by pinocytosis with eventual deposit in abnormal lysosomes.

Measurements of hexosaminidase activity in fibroblast homogenates of two patients with Tay-Sachs disease indicated a component that resembled hexosaminidase A of normal controls with respect to amount and heat inactivation, but not with respect to electrophoretic mobility.

REFERENCES

1. Hug, G.: Non-bilirubin genetic disorders of the liver.
    International Academy of Pathology Monograph No. 13
    "The Liver" ed. by E.A. Gall, The Williams and Wilkins Co.
    Baltimore, Md.; 1972.

2. Engel, A.G.: Acid maltase deficiency in adults: Studies in
    four cases of a syndrome which may mimic muscular dystrophy
    or other myopathies. Brain 93:599, 1970.

3. Baudhuin, P., Hers, H.G., and Loeb, H.: An electron
    microscopic and biochemical study of Type II glycogenosis.
    Lab. Invest. 13:1139, 1964.

4. Hers, H.G.: Alpha-glucosidase deficiency in generalized
    glycogen storage disease (Pompe's disease). Biochem. J.
    86:11, 1963.

5. Hug, G., Garancis, J.C., Schubert, W.K., and Kaplan, S.:
    Glycogen storage disease, Types II, III, VIII, and IX.
    Amer. J. Dis. Child. 111:457, 1966.

6. Hug, G. and Schubert, W.K.: Lysosomes in Type II glycogenosis.
    Changes during administration of extract from Aspergillus
    niger. J. Cell Biol. 35:C1, 1967.

7. Hug, G., Schubert, W.K., and Chuck, G.: Type II Glycogenosis:
    Treatment with extract of Aspergillus niger. Clin. Res.
    16:345, 1968.

8. Greene, H.L., Hug, G., and Schubert, W.K.: Metachromatic
    leukodystrophy: Treatment with arylsulfatase-A. Arch.
    Neurol. 20:147, 1969.

9. Di Ferrante, N., Nichols, B.L., Donnelly, P.V., Neri, G.,
    Hrgovcic, R. and Berglund, R.K.: Induced degradation of
    glycosaminoglycans in Hurler's and Hunter's syndromes by
    plasma infusion. Proc. Nat. Acad. Sci. U.S.A. 68:303, 1971.

10. Porter, M.T., Fluharty, A.L., Kihara, H.: Metachromatic
    leukodystrophy: Arylsulfatase-A deficiency in skin
    fibroblast cultures. Proc. Nat. Acad. Sci. U.S.A. 62:887,
    1969.

11. Nitowsky, H.M. and Grumfeld, A.: Lysosomal alpha-glucosidase
    in Type II glycogenosis; activity in leucocytes and cell
    cultures in relation to genotype. J. Lab. Clin. Med. 69:
    472, 1967.

12. Ho, M.W. and O'Brien, J.S.: Hurler's syndrome: Deficiency of a specific beta galactosidase isoenzyme. Science 165:611, 1969.

13. Fluharty, A.L., Porter, M.T., Lassila, E.L., Trammell, J., Carrel, R.E. and Kihara, H.: Acid glycosidases in mucopolysaccharidoses' fibroblasts. Biochem. Med. 4:110, 1970.

14. Hug, G., Schubert, W.K., and Soukup, S.: Ultrastructure and deficient arylsulfatase-A in fibroblast cultures of metachromatic leucodystrophy. J. Pediat. 76:970, 1970.

15. Gregoire, A., Perier, O., and Dustin, P. Jr.: Metachromatic Leukodystrophy: An electron microscopic study. J. Neuropath. Exp. Neurol. 25:617, 1966.

16. Hug, G., Schubert, W.K., and Soukup, S.: Ultrastructure of fibroblast cultures, lymphocytes, and liver in mucopolysaccharidoses Types I, II, III, IV and VI. Proc. Electron Microscopy Society of America 28:204, 1970.

17. Hug, G., Schubert, W.K., and Soukup, S.: Ultrastructure and enzymatic deficiency of fibroblast cultures in Type II glycogenosis. Pediat. Res. 5:107, 1971.

18. Hug, G., Schubert, W.K., and Soukup, S.: Prenatal diagnosis of Type-II glycogenosis. Lancet 1:1002, 1970.

19. Hug, G., Schubert, W.K., and Soukup, S.: Type II glycogenosis: Ultrastructure of amniotic fluid cells. In: Antenatal diagnosis, ed. by A. Dorfman, The University of Chicago Press, Chicago, Ill., 1972.

20. Hug, G., Schubert, W.K., and Soukup, S.: Electron microscopic demonstration of colloidal gold uptake into abnormal lysosomes of cultured fibroblasts from patients with Hurler's syndrome and with Type II glycogenosis. Proc. Soc. Pediat. Res. 81:5, 1971.

21. Okada, S., Veath, M.L., Leroy, J., and O'Brien, J.S.: Ganglioside GM_2 storage diseases: Hexosaminidase deficiencies in cultured fibroblasts. Amer. J. Hum. Genet. 23:55, 1971.

ACKNOWLEDGEMENTS

We thank Mrs. Linda Walling, Mrs. Diane Clark and Mrs. Ruby Cole for their excellent assistance. Original work was supported by National Institutes of Health Grants AM 13903, HD 05221 and RR-123.

THE MORPHOGENESIS AND BIOCHEMICAL CHARACTERISTICS OF CEROID ISOLATED FROM CASES OF NEURONAL CEROID-LIPOFUSCINOSIS

Aristotle N. Siakotos, Hans H. Goebel, Vimalkumar Patel,
Itaru Watanabe and Wolfgang Zeman

Department of Pathology, Indiana University Medical
Center, Indianapolis, Indiana

INTRODUCTION

Two distinctly different groups of disorders have emerged from the
conditions generically classified as amaurotic familial idiocies.
One is characterized by grossly abnormal profiles for cerebral
sphingolipids, for example the G_{M1} and G_{M2} gangliosides. The other
group is composed of patients with normal sphingolipid profiles,
but with neuronal accumulation of lipopigments of the ceroid-lipo-
fuscin type. The sphingolipidoses have been shown by a number of
investigators to meet the classic concept of Hers (1965) for lysosomal diseases. This view has been repeatedly reinforced by continuing studies which show the lack or reduction of specific
hydrolases, resulting in the accumulation of biochemical compounds
which cannot be degraded to metabolically utilizable substances.
The concept of lysosomal diseases has led many investigators to
search for a single accumulating lipid or a deficient hydrolytic
enzyme unique to neuronal ceroid-lipofuscinoses. Since many of the
lysosomal disorders became better understood by the elucidation of
the chemical properties of a specific lipid, present in unphysio-
logically large quantities, the pronouncement by Donahue et al.
(1966) before this group, that the "chemical analysis of cytoplasmic lipopigment granules (from the brains of patients with
Batten's disease) will contribute little towards an understanding
of this disease" was decidedly unwise. Although it is correct,
that autofluorescent lipopigments lack chemical specificity and
result from a great variety of pathogenetic situations (Porta and
Hartroft, 1969), Donahue et al. (1966) failed to recognize the
distinct possibility, that certain repetitive patterns in the
chemical composition and ultrastructure of these residual bodies

may indicate a specific formative pathogenesis. On the strength
of this argument, we developed methods to isolate lipopigments in
pure preparations and the first results have proved already the
soundness of this concept. As it turned out, the previously held
concept of a close relationship between lipofuscin and ceroid had
to be abandoned and replaced by the theses that these classes of
lipopigment are distinctly different entities, albeit both represent residual bodies and both contain polymeric substances
(Siakotos et al., 1970).

At the present time, it appears safe to state that lipofuscins are
cross-linked polymers which accumulate in tertiary lysosomes or
residual bodies as a function of time and are therefore linked
closely to the aging process in mammals, whereas ceroids occur,
perhaps exclusively, in diseased and dysfunctional mammalian tissue.
Thus, in the non-gangliosidases that were formerly included in the
group of amaurotic idiocies, ceroids represent the predominating,
if not only, class of lipopigments.

The present communication concerns analytical data obtained on
pigment fractions isolated from various tissues which are discussed
in the light of current hypotheses on the pathogenesis of the
Batten syndrome or the neuronal ceroid-lipofuscinoses. The basic
method for isolating these two types of lipopigments, lipofuscin
and ceroid, from brain have been published (Siakotos et al., 1970).

RESULTS

Figure 1 depicts the fine structure of lipofuscins, or "age"
pigments, isolated from various normal human brains. At least 5
or 6 different morphological types have been observed; however,
such ultrastructural heterogeneity is not seen in pigments isolated
from heart and liver where only one or two species of lipofuscin
seem to be present. Our interpretation of the complexity in brain
is that the various species of lipofuscins are derived from the
large numbers of different neurons found in brain. Figure 2 shows
the predominant pigment fraction, a finely granular ceroid, isolated from the brain of an 11-year-old patient with Batten's disease
at low power. Figure 3 represents a minor but more dense fraction
obtained from the same patient. Figure 4 is a preparation of the
curvilinear type ceroid obtained from a 5-year-old patient with
neuronal ceroid-lipofuscinosis. Ceroid bodies from the brain of an
English Setter with neuronal ceroid-lipofuscinosis (Koppang, 1970)
are shown in Figure 5. As can be readily noted, the lipopigment
isolates obtained from brain tissue by these methods are pure.

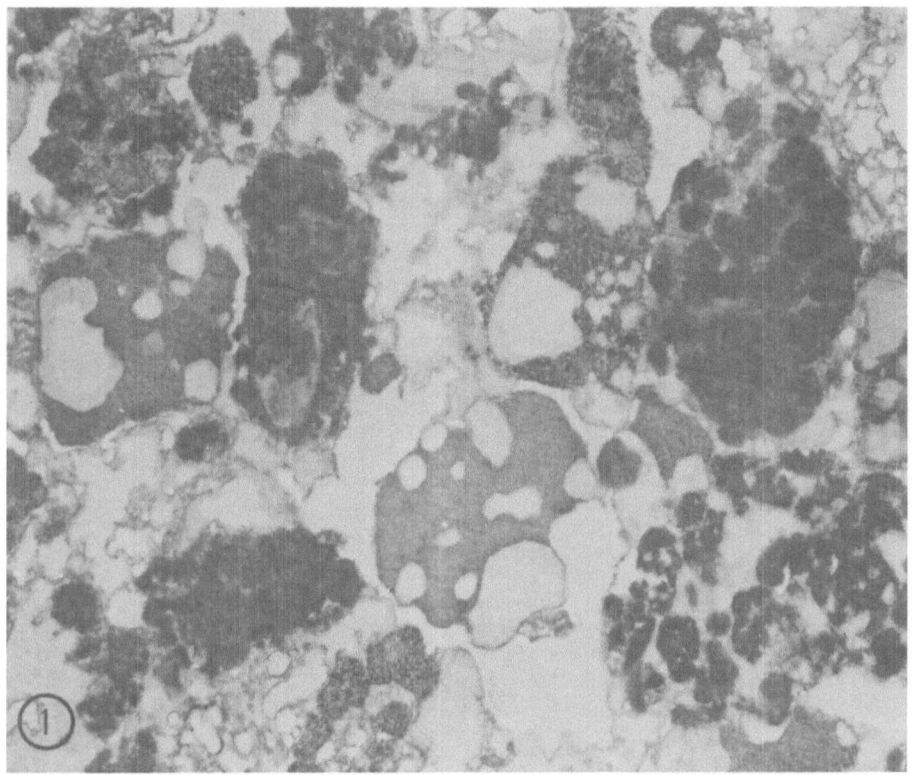

Figure 1.   Lipofuscin fraction from normal human brain.   X14,500.

The various classes of lipopigments are separated from each other
by their respective specific gravities as summarized in Table 1.
Significant differences are seen in the specific gravities of lipofuscins and ceroids from brain and other organs.   Although differences in density may vary from organ to organ, the specific
gravity of ceroids is quite consistent.   At this point several
important features affecting the density of these two classes of
lipopigments should be mentioned, one is the ability of salts to
alter the density of lipofuscin.   More striking is the ability of
chelating agents to dissolve ceroid.   Lipofuscins on the other hand
are stable to chelating or ion exchange agents.   Other differences
concern the cation composition of these two classes of lipopigments
(Table 2).   Brain ceroid from patients with neuronal ceroid-lipofuscinosis contains significantly higher concentrations of calcium,

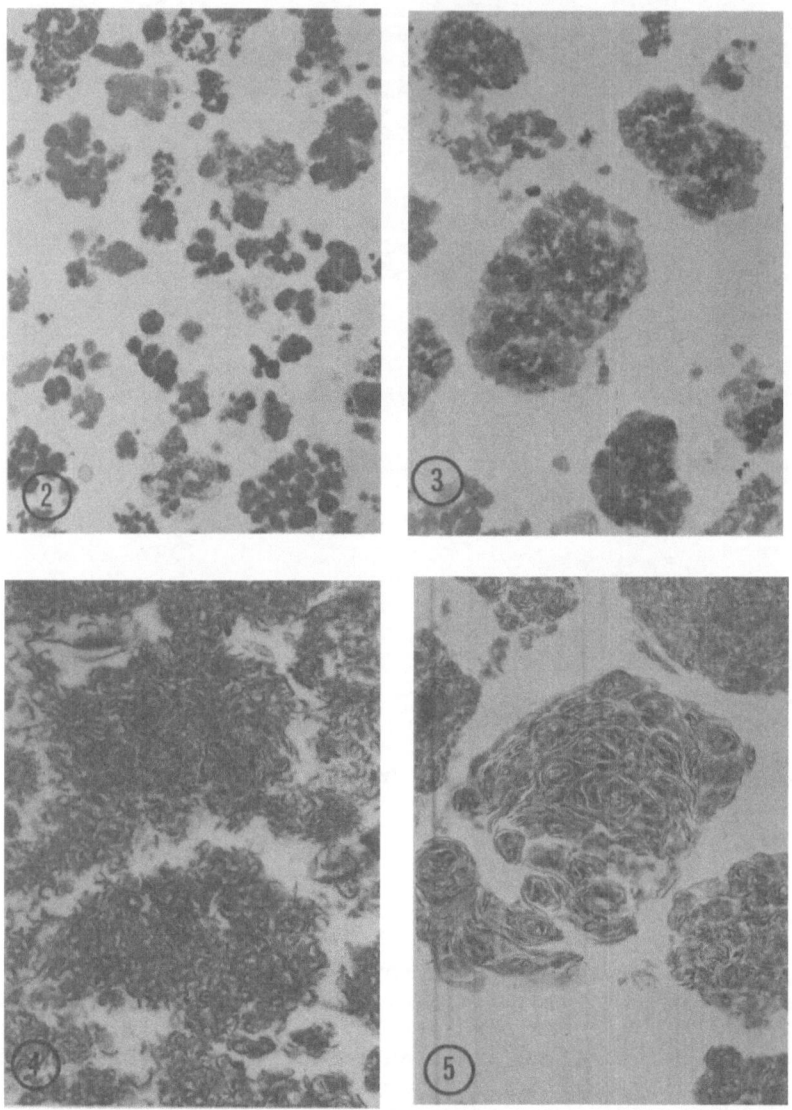

Figure 2. The major ceroid fraction from case 1 of neuronal
         ceroid-lipofuscinosis.   X13,000.

Figure 3. A minor ceroid fraction from case 1 of neuronal ceroid-
         lipofuscinosis.   X13,000.

Figure 4. Curvilinear ceroid from case 2 of neuronal ceroid-
         lipofuscinosis.   X30,000.

Figure 5. Ceroid bodies from the dog neuronal ceroid-lipofuscinosis.
         13,000.

Table 1.   LIPOPIGMENTS: CURRENT STATUS

Density	Brain, Normal	Brain, NCL	Heart, Normal	Liver, Normal	Liver, Cirrhotic
-1.00			very high "floating lipid"	very high (human) very low (animal) "floating lipid"	low to high "floating lipid"
1.00-1.05	.05 gm/Kg Lipofuscin	Trace Lipofuscin	Trace Lipofuscin	5-50 gm/Kg Lipofuscin	very low to high Lipofuscin
1.10-1.20	Trace Lipofuscin		1-50 gm/Kg Lipofuscin	Trace Lipofuscin	very low to high Lipofuscin
1.25-1.30		10-25 gm/Kg Ceroid			1-10 gm/Kg Ceroid

Table 2.   CATION COMPOSITION OF BRAIN LIPOPIGMENTS

	Cu	Mn	Ca	Fe	Zn	
Lipofuscin	20	1.3	240	300	400	ppm
Ceroid	70	2	960	1500	110	ppm

iron and copper, whereas lipofuscin exhibits a high level of zinc.

Enzymatic evidence for the lysosomal origin of both classes of lipopigments is shown in Table 3. On comparing lipofuscin and ceroid from brain, no real differences are seen in the specific activities of the various lysosomal hydrolases. Of special note is the high specific activity of cyclic 2,3 AMP phosphohydrolase, previously considered to be a marker enzyme for myelin.

Table 3.   Hydrolytic Enzymes in Lipopigments
                         Specific Activity/hr.

| Enzyme | Lipofuscin | | | Ceroid |
	Brain	Liver	Heart	Brain
Acid Phosphatase	5000	4500	420	6400
Cathepsin D	234	131	57	195
β-Galactosidase	230	170	120	253
β-Hexosaminidase	310	185	95	446
β-Glucosidase	420	24	4	-
α-Glucosidase	13	9	1.5	9
α-Mannosidase	9	7	0.7	-
α-Fucosidase	5	-	-	-
AMP-hydrolase	6200	525	350	3750

Pure preparations of isolated lipopigments obtained from brain and
other organs were extracted and purified, using the procedures of
Rouser et al., 1970, and of Siakotos and Rouser, 1965. Two-
dimensional thin-layer chromatograms of such preparations are given
in Figure 6.

The total lipid extract was passed through a Sephadex G-25 column
(Siakotos and Rouser, 1965) and resolved into two fractions: F_1,
the total lipids including "neutral" lipid polymers, and F_2, an
acidic fraction. The F_1 fractions of brain lipofuscin are shown
in 6A. Note the relative absence of native phospholipids and the
high concentration of polymeric material at the origin (P). The
F_1 fraction of ceroid isolated from a patient with alcoholic
cirrhosis is shown in 6B while the F_1 fraction from normal liver
lipofuscin is given in 6C. A high concentration of polymeric
material is observed at the origin (P) but only in the ceroid
preparation, whereas normal liver lipofuscin (6C) does not contain
significant amounts of polymers; on the other hand it contains a
high level of native phospholipids. The F_1 fraction of brain
ceroid (6D) isolated from the brain of a patient with neuronal
ceroid-lipofuscinosis also contains a relatively high concentration
of native phospholipids but a low concentration of polymers (P).
However, an examination of the F_2 fraction of brain ceroid (6E)
revealed a high concentration polymeric material at the origin (P).
The relative distribution of these polymeric materials in brain
lipopigments is shown in Table 4.

The lipofuscins appear to contain more "neutral" polymer in contrast to the ceroid preparation from case 1 (neuronal ceroid
lipofuscin). The "acidic" polymer fraction, F_2, is clearly in
higher concentration in the isolated brain ceroid.

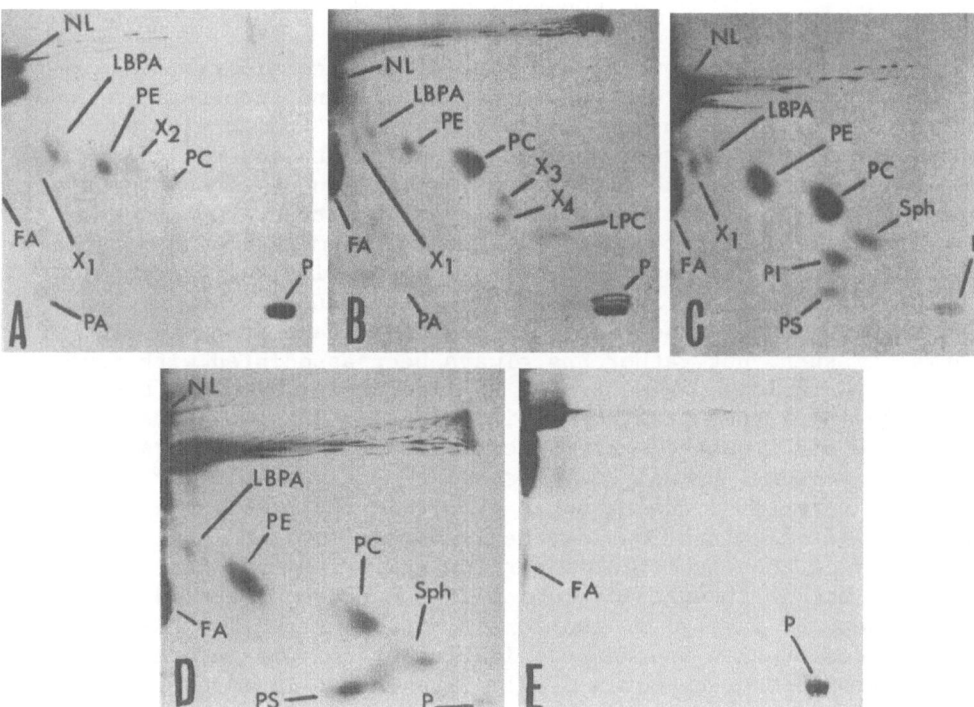

Figure 6. Polar lipids of lipofuscin and ceroid as separated by
two-dimensional thin-layer chromatography on silica gel, plain,
with 10% magnesium silicate and the solvent systems (a) 65/25/5
chloroform, methanol, 28% aqueous ammonia followed by (b)
3/4/1/1/0.5 chloroform, acetone, methanol, acetic acid and water
(Siakotos and Rouser, 1965). A. Brain lipofuscin. B. Ceroid from
cirrhotic liver. C. Normal liver lipofuscin. D. F_1, Brain ceroid
from case 1 (neuronal ceroid-lipofuscinosis). E. F_2, Acidic
polymer fraction from the same case. Abbreviations: NL, neutral
lipids; LBPA, lysobisphosphatidic acid; PE, phosphatidyl ethanolamine; PC, phosphatidyl choline; LPC, lysophosphatidyl choline;
PI, phosphatidyl inositol; PS, phosphatidyl serine; Sph, sphingomyelin; PA, phosphatidic acid; X_1–X_4, unknown compounds;
P, polymeric lipid.

Table 4.   Relative Distribution of Polymeric
                   Materials in Brain Lipopigments

	F_1	F_2
Lipofuscin	91.89%	8.11%
Ceroid	57.42%	42.58%

CONCLUSIONS

Porta and Hartroft (1969) have offered considerable histochemical evidence for distinguishing ceroid and lipofuscin on the
basis of solubility in organic solvents. Our studies with the
pure lipopigments showed that both lipopigments contain only
small insoluble residues and the major portion of these pigments
are soluble in solvent systems employed in extracting tissues
for lipids (Rouser, et al, 1970). The two pigments can be readily
distinguished on the basis of cation composition, with ceroid
containing significantly higher concentrations of iron, calcium,
and copper. In our studies ceroid has never been isolated from
normal tissues, but rather has always been associated with some
form of pathology, in contrast, to lipofuscin which has been
observed in tissues from normal individuals. The two pigments
cannot be distinguished enzymatically and since both contain
similar lysosomal hydrolases, lysosomes are probably involved
in their formation. The response of ceroid to chelating agents
implies that divalent ions may be important for the in vivo
stability of this subcellular particulate. With this fact in
mind the basic pathogenic process in the neuronal ceroid-lipofuscinoses may involve a disorder in cation metabolism, as well
as, an acceleration in the peroxidation of polyunsaturated fatty
acids, as proposed by Zeman (1971). The native lipid composition
of lipofuscin or ceroid does not seem to be remarkable except
that some pigments (brain lipofuscin) contain unusually low concentrations of native phospholipids. However, the lipofuscins
are characterized by a high concentration of a relatively nonpolar
lipid polymer, while the ceroids are unique in containing a high
concentration of an acidic lipid polymer. We propose that this
acidic lipid polymer is the "stored substance" in the neuronal
ceroid-lipofuscinoses.

REFERENCES

1. Donahue, S., W. Zeman, and I. Watanabe. Electron microscpic
   observations in Batten's disease. In Inborn Disorders of
   Sphingolipid Metabolism. Proceedings of the Third International Symposium on the Cerebral Sphingolipidoses. Pergamon
   Press, Oxford, England, 1966, pp. 3-22.

2. Hers, H. G., Inborn Lysosomal Diseases. Gastroent. 48: 625-633,
   (1965).

3. Koppang, N., Neuronal ceroid-lipofuscinosis in english setters.,
   J. Small Animal Pract. 10: 639-644 (1970).

4. Porta, E.A. and W.S. Hartroft, Lipid pigments in relation to aging and dietary factors (lipofuscins). In Pigments in Pathology, Ed. M. Wolman, Academic Press, N.Y.C., 1969, pp. 192-235.

5. Rouser, G., C. Kritchevsky, A.N. Siakotos, and A. Yamanoto, Lipid composition of the brain and its subcellular structures. In Neuropathology: Method and Diagnosis, Ed. C.G. Tedeschi. Little, Brown and Co., Boston, Mass., 1970, pp. 691-753.

6. Siakotos, A.N. and G. Rouser, Analytical separation of non-lipid water soluble substances and gangliosides. J. Am. Oil Chem. Soc., 42:913-919, 1965.

7. Siakotos, A.N., I. Watanabe, A. Saito, and S. Fleischer, Procedures for the isolation of two distinct lipopigments from human brain: lipofuscin and ceroid. Biochem. Med., 4: 361-375, 1970.

8. Zeman, W., The neuronal ceroid-lipofuscinosis -- Batten-Vogt syndrome: a model for human aging? Adv. in Geront. Res., 3:147-170, 1971.

Supported by PHS Grants NS 08639, NS 04907 and NS 09797. Dr. Patel is a special trainee under training USPS Grant NS 05450.

EFFECT OF CONDITIONS OF EXTRACTION ON THE

EXTRACTABILITY OF BRAIN GANGLIOSIDES

J. Folch-Pi, M.D.

McLean Hospital, Belmont, Mass. 02178 and

Harvard Medical School, Boston, Mass. 02115

It has been known for a long time that although gangliosides
are freely soluble in water, they cannot be extracted from brain
tissue, or from other tissues, by aqueous solutions, including 5%
trichloracetic acid. Their extraction requires the use of organic
solvents, mixtures of chloroform:methanol being the extracting
mixture that has gained the widest usage (1). It has been accepted implicitly that these particular requirements for extraction of gangliosides indicate that they are bound to other tissue
components, presumably proteins by ionic bonds through their
strong carboxylic group, and by nonpolar bonds through the ceramide end of the molecule. The nonpolar bonds would make gangliosides unextractable by aqueous solvents. On the other hand,
chloroform:methanol mixtures would dissociate the nonpolar bonds
and the ionic bonds would be dissociated by the tissue electrolytes present in the extract. The closest demonstration of the
occurrence of the ionic bonds has been provided by the work of
Spence and Wolfe (2) who found that when tissue electrolytes have
been removed by dialysis of the tissue homogenate, chloroform:
methanol fails to extract gangliosides, except in small amounts,
and that subsequent addition of KCl and or NaCl restores the extractability of gangliosides by chloroform:methanol.

In the course of the development of a procedure for the extraction of lipids from brain tissue by the use of biphasic mixtures of chloroform, methanol and water, it was found that when
chloroform and methanol are present in identical proportions,
both gangliosides and other lipids are extracted as completely as
in the classical method of extraction by chloroform:methanol 2:1,
v/v. However, when the proportion of chloroform in the system is

increased, with a corresponding decrease in the proportion of
methanol, the extraction of gangliosides becomes incomplete, and
at C:M, 3:1 or 4:1, v/v, only one-fifth, or less, of the gangliosides present are extracted, in spite of the fact that gangliosides are freely soluble in the extracting mixture used. This
decrease in extractability is particular to the gangliosides, the
extraction of other lipids being essentially complete at the
proportions mentioned.

The present paper reports the elaboration and extension of
this observation.

MATERIAL AND METHODS

Slaughterhouse bovine brains were transported to the laboratory under refrigeration, freed of their membranes and gray
matter obtained by gross dissection of the hemispheres. The tissue included a substantial amount of underlying white matter.
Hence more than gray matter, the tissue used represented "gray-
matter enriched" superficial portion of the hemisphere. The
lipid content of the tissue samples used was 9 to 10% wet weight,
which indicated a content of white matter of 25 to 30% by weight.

The gangliosides used in recovery experiments were prepared
by the modified method of Folch et al. (1), as described by
Quarles and Folch-Pi (3). No special effort was made to carry
the purification of gangliosides very far, because the effects
studied were those on gangliosides in presence of the whole
brain lipid mixture.

Extraction of tissue samples. - The tissue has been extracted either by the classical method of Folch et al. (1) or
by biphasic mixtures of chloroform, methanol and water.

In the extraction by the biphasic mixtures, the tissue (1g)
was homogenized for 2 m. with chloroform:methanol, 1:1, v/v
mixture (5 ml.) to which enough water had been added to bring
the concentration of water in the medium to 16.6%, by volume,
including the water contributed by the tissue. By centrifugation
at 2000 rpm for a few minutes, the homogenate is resolved into
an upper phase, a lower phase, and a tissue pad, which floats
at the interface. The upper phase represents about 43% and the
lower phase about 57% of the total liquid volume of the homogenate. The two phases and the tissue pad can be collected
separately without difficulty. The tissue pad, however, retains
about 1/6 of each of the two phases. If the separation of phases
is to be made quantitative, the tissue pad is resuspended in the
same chloroform:water:methanol mixture used originally, and,

after mixing, and centrifugation, the secondary upper and lower phases are collected separately and combined with the original phases. The procedure can be repeated if a more strictly quantitative collection of phases is desired.

Small variations in the proportion of water present appear to have no effect on the extraction process, provided the extracting mixture remains biphasic. Also the relative proportions of chloroform to methanol have been varied from C:M, 1:1 to C:M, 1:0, without requiring any departure from the procedure outlined above.

<u>Isolation of gangliosides</u>. - Gangliosides in the biphasic extract are isolated essentially as described in the classical method (1). The lower phase is washed four times in succession with "pure solvents upper phase" portions of about the same size as the original upper phase. The successive upper phases are combined and the combined solution is concentrated to about twice the volume of the starting tissue, and dialyzed against 100-fold its volume of distilled water at 4°, the outside water being changed twice a day for three days. The retentate is then collected, concentrated if necessary, and analyzed for sialic acid content.

When the extraction with biphasic mixtures is used, the "pure solvents upper phase" is prepared by mixing chloroform, methanol and water in the same proportions as in the extracting mixture, and collecting the upper phase of the resulting biphasic system.

<u>Estimation of combined sialic acid</u>. - Sialic acid has been estimated on the isolated gangliosides either by a modified form of the browning reaction (4) or by the Warren method (5).

The modified browning reaction is carried out in small glass stoppered tubes calibrated to 1 ml. To a 0.1 ml aqueous sample in the tube containing from 15 μg to 75 μg is added 0.05 mL of 60% $HClO_4$. The tube is stoppered, heated in a boiling water bath for exactly 10 m. and cooled in ice. The volume is made up to 1 ml. with n-propanol, the tube buzzed for 15 seconds to disperse the color, and then centrifuged for 10 m. at 800 rpm in an International Clinical Centrifuge (Model Cl) or equivalent. The optical densities of the solution are read at 475 mμ on a Beckman DU at 10 mm. light path, with a pin hole light source. The amounts of NANA in the samples are determined from a standard curve.

Extensive studies of the modified browning reaction have shown that few substances found in biological materials interfere to any significant extent. A mixture of desoxyribose

and tryptophan give a significant amount of color when present at
about the same concentration as sialic acid. Ascorbic acid which
by itself gives no color, increases the color produced by sialic
acid. No possible interference could have resulted from any of
these compounds in the particular experiments described in this
paper.

In the estimation of sialic acid by the Warren method, it
was found that the acid hydrolysis reduced by 17% the color given
by sialic acid standards. Hence the values obtained with the
Warren method for ganglioside NANA should be corrected by the
factor 100/83. This correction has not been used in this paper
because the values for NANA are important only relatively to
each other and not as absolute values.

RESULTS

Effect of varying the relative proportion of chloroform to
methanol in the extraction by biphasic systems on the amount of
ganglioside obtained from the tissue. - The gray matter enriched brain tissue was diced and ground gently, and 5 gram portions taken and homogenized with about 25 ml. of inmiscible mixtures of chloroform, methanol and water in various proportions.
By centrifugation each homogenate was resolved into an upper
phase, a lower phase and a tissue pad at the interface. The two
phases and the tissue pad were collected separately, and the
lower phase washed four times in succession with portions in
"pure solvents upper phase".

The original upper phase and the subsequent washings were
combined, taken to dryness, and the residue suspended in about
10 ml. of water. The suspension was dialyzed against 1 liter
of distilled water at $4°$, the outside water being changed twice
a day for 3 days. The retentate was then collected, concentrated
to 5 ml. and gangliosides estimated by the modified browning
reaction.   The result of this and similar experiments are given
in Table I. It can be seen that the amount of gangliosides extracted from comparable samples of tissues was markedly affected
by the relative proportion of chloroform to methanol in the
extracting mixture. At C:M, 1:1, v/v the amount of gangliosides
extracted was five-fold or larger the amount extracted at C:M,
3:1. In series III of extractions, the missing or unextracted
gangliosides were recovered from the corresponding tissue pads
by extraction by the classical method (1). In series I of extractions the tissue pads were left with the lower phase throughout the four successive washings with pure solvents upper phase.
This had little or no effect on the results obtained, showing
that the differences observed were not due to a mechanical

TABLE I

EXTRACTION OF BOVINE BRAIN GRAY MATTER WITH IMMISCIBLE
MIXTURES OF CHLOROFORM, METHANOL AND WATER

Effect of varying the proportions of chloroform and
methanol on the amount of gangliosides extracted.
Tissue to solvent mixture ratio 1:5

Composition of extracting mixtures			Gangliosides in extracts			Gangliosides extracted subsequently from tissue pads from III with CM 2:1
	v/v/v		Series			
			I	II	III	
C	M	W	mg./g. tissue			mg./g. tissue
2.5	2.5	1	3.4	3.2	3.6	0.46
3.0	2.0	1	3.0	2.55	3.2	0.46
3.33	1.66	1	2.15	2.15	2.6	1.30
3.75	1.25	1	0.90	0.44	0.55	2.64

occlusion of the gangliosides by the tissue pad. That these
differences did not reflect differences in solubility was shown
by the observation that gangliosides were freely soluble in all
biphasic systems used and, that in absence of tissue, samples of
gangliosides run through the procedure described were recovered
quantitatively.

In summary, the differences observed appeared to be due to
a specific ability of the tissue pad to retain gangliosides under
certain of the conditions used. The ganglioside samples obtained
by incomplete extraction and those recovered from the tissue
pads, gave similar patterns by thin layer chromatography. Hence
the retention by the tissue pads appeared to apply to all gangliosides, at least qualitatively.

In an extension of these observations, the effect of addition of salts to the tissue, and of further variation in the
relative proportion of chloroform to methanol was investigated.
Four samples of tissue rendered relatively homogeneous by dicing
and gentle grinding were extracted by homogenization, and handled
for isolation of gangliosides, under the conditions described
in Table II. It can be seen that the addition of salts did not
affect the extent of extraction of gangliosides, and that the
decrease in the amount of gangliosides extracted with increasing
proportion of chloroform, continued to the point that chloroform
alone with water extracted only 5% of the gangliosides from the
tissue. The gangliosides not extracted were recovered by subsequent extraction of the tissue pad by the classical method of Folch
et al. (1). Finally, at C:M 4:1, the extraction of lipids was
essentially the same as at C:M 1:1, with or without addition
of salts.

Recovery of exogenous gangliosides in the extraction by
biphasic systems. - Enough brain tissue was diced and ground
gently to yield two 15 g. samples of tissue. These were homogenized for 2 m. with 75 ml. C:M:water, 3.75: 1.25 v/v/v, the
tissue being assumed to contain 80% water in the computation of
the water to be added to the system. To one of the samples, 30
mg. of gangliosides, containing 5.1 mg. sialic acid, by Warren
estimation (uncorrected) had been added in aqueous solution prior
to homogenization. After centrifugation, the two phases and the
tissue pad were collected separately. The lower phases were
washed four times with "pure solvents upper phase", already described, and the respective washings and original upper phases
combined and processed for isolation of gangliosides. The tissue
pads were handled for isolation of gangliosides by the method of
Folch et al. (1). The various fractions obtained were then analyzed for ganglioside NANA by the Warren method (5).

TABLE II

EFFECT OF VARIATIONS IN SOLVENT COMPOSITION AND OF
ADDED ELECTROLYTES ON THE EXTRACTION OF GANGLIOSIDES
FROM BRAIN TISSUE BY CERTAIN BIPHASIC SYSTEMS

Exp. 70-I	I	II	III	IV
Weight of tissue sample	14 g.	14 g.	15 g.	15 g.
C:M, v/v	1:1	1:1	5:1	1:0
Vol. solvent	70 ml.	70 ml.	75 ml.	75 ml.
H_2O	7	-	7	7
°Aqueous elect.	-	7	-	-
Gangliosides in extract as µg NANA/g. tissue	242	229	36	11
Gangliosides in tissue pad as µg NANA/g. tissue	33	36	137	221
Total ganglioside NANA as µg/g. tissue	273	265	173	233
°°Total Lipids in extract as mg./g. tissue	95.5	100.5	96.0	56.5

°NaCl: 0.330 M; KCl: 0.570 M; $CaCl_2$: 0.012 M; $MgCl_2$: 0.025 M.

°°The values obtained have been increased by 1/6th to allow for
the portion of the extract left in the tissue pad. The difference between I and III on the one hand, and II on the other,
can most likely be accounted for by the presence of added salts
in II, which must have caused a greater compacting of the tissue pad and, hence a relatively greater collection of lower
phase.

The results obtained are given in Table III. They confirm
the results of Table I to the effect that the particular biphasic
mixture used extracted only about one-fifth of the gangliosides
in the tissue, and that the missing gangliosides are recovered
from the tissue pad by the classical method of ganglioside extraction. The results, however, show that the added gangliosides behave exactly the same as the endogenous gangliosides,
i.e., the tissue pad sequesters the added gangliosides to the
same extent to which it retains the endogenous gangliosides.

In addition the 97.5% recovery of added ganglioside NANA
shows that losses of gangliosides during the procedure followed
for their isolation are negligible.

Recovery of exogenous gangliosides added to bovine brain
tissue in aqueous medium. - To see if the sequestering of exogenous gangliosides by tissue components took place in aqueous
medium, i.e. in vitro conditions, 15 g. samples of diced and
gently ground tissue were homogenized for 2 m., one with 8-fold
its volume of 0.9% aqueous NaCl, and another with the same
solution containing 10 mg. of gangliosides. The homogenates
were separated by centrifugation at 3600 rpm into a supernatant
and a residue, the supernatant decanted, and the residue washed
twice with the saline solution. The combined supernatant and
washings and the washed residue were handled separately for isolation of gangliosides by the classical method of Folch et al.
(1), and the NANA content of the various final ganglioside
fractions estimated by the method of Warren (5).

The results are given in Table IV. They show that the bulk
of added gangliosides is recovered in the supernatant, i.e.,
if there is any sequestering of gangliosides by tissue residue
components it is to a much lesser degree than that found in
extraction by biphasic systems rich in chloroform. On the
other hand, the results fail to eliminate the possibility of
partial sequestering of gangliosides. Thus the recovery of
added gangliosides in the supernatant is only 69% of theory.
This leaves 31% of the gangliosides which must be accounted for
either by enzymatic destruction, or by partial sequestering.
Only further experimentation will permit the settling of this
important point.

DISCUSSION

The original observation in this experimental series was
obtained in the course of the routine development of a method
for the isolation of brain tissue lipids which had the advantage
over the classical method of being faster and representing a

TABLE III

RECOVERY OF EXOGENOUS GANGLIOSIDES IN THE EXTRACTION
OF BOVINE BRAIN TISSUE BY THE BIPHASIC SYSTEM
C: M: H_2O, 3.75: 1.25: 1.0, v/v/v

Exp. 69-XXIII	Extraction I µg/g. tissue	Extraction II µg/g. tissue
Gangliosides added as NANA	None	340
Gangliosides in extract as NANA	61[+](22.2%)	113 (18.6%)
Ganglioside in tissue pad as NANA	216[+](77.8%)	496 (81.4%)
Total ganglioside NANA recovered	277[+](100%)	609 (100%)

Recovery of added NANA   609 µg − 277 µg = 332 µg, i.e.
                                                97.5% recovery

---

[+] Values in parentheses express percentile distribution of
ganglioside NANA

TABLE IV

RECOVERY OF EXOGENOUS GANGLIOSIDES ADDED TO
BOVINE BRAIN TISSUE IN 0.9% AQUEOUS NaCl

Ext. 70-VII	Extraction I µg/g. tissue	Extraction II µg/g. tissue
Ganglioside NANA added	None	120
Ganglioside NANA in supernatant	12	95
Ganglioside NANA in tissue residue	215	239
Total Ganglioside NANA in homogenate	227	334

Recovery of added ganglioside NANA
   in homogenate: 334 - 227 = 107   NANA/g. tissue, i.e. 89%
                                          of theory
   in supernatant: 95 - 12 = 83   NANA/g. tissue, i.e. 69%
                                          of theory

marked saving in the amount of solvents used.

The partial extraction of gangliosides at high concentrations of chloroform could not be explained on a solubility basis, since gangliosides were found to be soluble in all the biphasic systems used. Hence it was first thought that the minimal extraction was due to an inability of the particular mixtures used to break the bonds which have generally been accepted as occurring between gangliosides and proteins, and which are responsible for the inextractability of gangliosides by aqueous solvents. The results of the recovery of added gangliosides put this idea in question, since it was found that the exogenous gangliosides were sequestered by the insoluble tissue components and that they behaved like the endogenous gangliosides. Instead the observed facts suggested that gangliosides were freed by the solvent medium, and then recaptured by some of the components in the tissue pad. The bond or bonds that were at the basis of the sequestering might or might not be identical with the bonds that originally held the gangliosides in the tissue. The final observations on the recovery of gangliosides added to the tissue in aqueous media gave somewhat equivocal results, in the sense that although there was no evidence of massive sequestering of exogenous gangliosides, there might well be a low rate sequestration. The incomplete recovery was specially difficult to interpret because it suggested that there was destruction of gangliosides by enzymatic action, an event that makes interpretation of balance experiments very uncertain.

Clearly the present experimental series is insufficient to provide answers to many of the questions that it raises and much more work will be required before the observations already made can be explained satisfactorily. A few facts appear established. They are that the sequestering of gangliosides is not due to differences in solubility in the different media used; that it is not due to mechanical occlusion since there is little difference in the yield of gangliosides whether the tissue pad is subjected to repeated washings with "pure solvents upper phase" or not, and that the gangliosides are sequestered through a bond or bonds that depend for their stability on certain conditions that prevail in a biphasic medium in which chloroform predominates. The nature of this bond or bonds is a matter of pure speculation. They are not only ionic bonds because the sequestering of the gangliosides is not affected either by the presence, or the absence of gangliosides. Thus, when the tissue pads are extracted with C:M, 2:1, in a single phase, by the classical method, the gangliosides are extracted quantitatively, in spite of the fact that the amount of salts present is well within the range at which Spence and Wolfe (2) have found that gangliosides have become unextractable to a major extent.

Purely as a working hypothesis, one can advance the idea
that these sequestering bonds are both ionic, through the
strong carboxyl group, and nonpolar through the ceramide end of
the molecule. Both of these bonds must be broken before the
gangliosides become extractable. In aqueous media it would be
the nonpolar bonds that would be responsible for the inextractability of gangliosides, since the ionic bonds would clearly be
broken by competition from other ions. In pure chloroform,
the opposite would hold true, and the ionic bonds would keep the
gangliosides inextractable. At the usual C:M, 2:1 extraction,
the medium would permit both the dissociation of the ionic bonds
by ionic competition, and the solvation of the nonpolar bonds by
the action of chloroform. In other words, gangliosides would be
extractable in media in the middle range of polarity values.
If this is accepted, it is worth drawing comparisons between the
polarity of the media as indicated by the value of the dielectric
constant, and the changes in extractability in extraction by
biphasic systems. It is seen that at C:M:water, 1:1:0.4, at
which the extraction of gangliosides is essentially complete,
the system consists of two phases of rather similar composition,
to wit:

	Chloroform:methanol:water v/v/v		
Total system	41.7%	41.7%	16.6%
Upper phase	29%	49.5%	21.5%
Lower phase	47%	39.5%	13.5%

Both phases contain substantial proportions of chloroform:
methanol and water, and their dielectric constant should fall in
the middle range of values from chloroform to water. On the
other hand, as the proportion of chloroform in the mixture increases, the composition of the upper phase changes towards a
simple water:methanol mixture, and the composition of the lower
phase approaches pure chloroform. Consequently, the value of
the dielectric constant of each phase shifts towards the higher
and lower ends of the range of values, to the obliteration of
the middle values. It is at those extreme values that the
sequestering of gangliosides occurs. Presumably the nonpolar
bonds would be placed in an effective polar medium, and the
ionic bonds would be in a nonpolar medium, in conditions which
would give to both of them maximal stability.

This speculation leaves unanswered the question of whether
the sequestering bonds are the same that hold gangliosides
bound in the living tissue. A priori one would think that they
are not, both because of their operation in chloroform:methanol
media, and because sequestering does not seem to operate in

in vitro physiological conditions, i.e. in tissue homogenate in
physiological saline. However, it is possible that the absence
of sequestering, or the only partial sequestering observed under
the latter conditions might be due to the presence of lipids,
which are bound to proteins by bonds similar to those that bind
gangliosides. In aqueous media, the sequestering of gangliosides
would be in competition with lipids, whereas in chloroform:methanol
media, the lipids would have been removed.

A final point to be made is that the extraction of gangliosides from tissues cannot be taken for granted unless there is
definite evidence that the extraction is complete. Of course
this point only need be established when a definite change in
the procedure of extraction is introduced. In that case it is
incumbent upon the experimenter to ascertain that gangliosides
are indeed completely extracted under the new conditions that are
being used.

SUMMARY

1. When brain tissue is extracted with immiscible mixtures
of chloroform:methanol and water, the extent of extraction of
gangliosides is substantially affected by the proportion of
chloroform to methanol in the extracting biphasic mixture. At
C:M, 1:1, v/v, the extraction of gangliosides appears to be essentially complete; with an increase in the proportion of
chloroform, the extraction soon becomes incomplete and at C:M,
3:1, only about one-fifth of the tissue gangliosides are extracted. By thin layer chromatography it appears that all
gangliosides are equally affected by the decreased efficiency of
the extraction process. The missing gangliosides are recovered
from the tissue pad. Extraction of lipids appears to be complete
at the proportions mentioned.

2. Recovery of exogenous gangliosides follows the same pattern as the extraction of endogenous gangliosides: the recovery
is complete when the extraction is complete. On the other hand,
at C:M, 3:1, about one-fifth of endogenous gangliosides are extracted, and only about one-fifth of added gangliosides are
recovered.

3. The observed decrease in efficiency of extraction cannot
be explained by differences in solubility of gangliosides in the
different mixtures, since gangliosides are soluble in all the
mixtures used, and, in absence of tissue, recovery of gangliosides submitted to the procedure of extraction and isolation is
quantitative. Instead it must be explained in terms of an active

sequestration of both endogenous and exogenous gangliosides by the tissue pad.

4. The composition of phases shows that maximal extraction is obtained by solvent mixtures, or phases, exhibiting values for dielectric constant in the middle of the range between the values for water and values for chloroform. Extraction is specially incomplete with extracting mixtures in which the dielectric constants of the two phases are shifted to the ends of the range, with obliteration of the values in the middle of the range.

REFERENCES

1. Folch-Pi, J., Lees, M. and Sloane Stanley, G.H., J. Biol. Chem., 226, 497 (1957).

2. Spence, M.W. and Wolfe, L.S., J. Neurochem., 14, 585 (1967).

3. Quarles, R. and Folch-Pi, J., J. Neurochem., 12, 543 (1965).

4. Folch, J., Arsove, S. and Meath, J.A., J. Biol. Chem., 191, 819 (1951).

5. Warren, L., J. Biol. Chem., 234, 1971 (1959).

GANGLIOSIDES OF CSF AND PLASMA: THEIR RELATION TO THE NERVOUS SYSTEM

R. W. Ledeen and R. K. Yu

Saul R. Korey Department of Neurology and Department of Biochemistry, Albert Einstein College of Medicine, Bronx, New York 10461

INTRODUCTION

The lipid composition of body fluids has become a subject of growing interest in the field of sphingolipidoses and related disorders ever since the recognition that lipid abnormalities which characterize these diseases are often manifested in one or more sueh fluids. CSF[1] has special significance in relation to neurological disorders and some evidence suggests that lipid alterations in this fluid may be correlated with certain categories of disease. Thus, on the basis of one survey Christensen and Matzke (1965) suggested that the ratio of cerebroside to lecithin provides an index of white matter destruction. A detailed study of CSF lipids in multiple sclerosis patients by Tourtellotte and Haerer (1969) revealed several lipids to be elevated above normal with cerebrosides showing the most characteristic increase. Hagberg and Svennerholm (1960) detected sulfatides in the CSF of patients with late infantile metachromatic leucodystrophy but did not quantify or compare them with normal levels.

Gangliosides within brain tissue undergo substantial alterations in pattern and level for all the gangliosidoses, and less pronounced secondary changes in a variety of other

---

[1]Abbreviations: CSF, cerebrospinal fluid; TLC, thin-layer chromatography, GLC, gas-liquid chromatography; NANA, N-acetylneuraminic acid; NGNA, N-glycolylneuraminic acid; CNS, central nervous system; ACD, acid-citrate-dextrose.

neurological disorders (Suzuki, 1967: Ledeen, et al. 1968a).
However it is not known to what extent these alterations are
reflected in the CSF. Bernheimer (1968) has studied one such
condition - Tay-Sachs disease - and found evidence of Tay-Sachs
ganglioside in the spinal fluid. He also reported the presence
of gangliosides in normal CSF (Bernheimer, 1969) with a TLC
pattern similar to that of normal brain.

In the hope of eventually examining other diseases from this
standpoint we have attempted to establish procedures for the
isolation and quantification of CSF gangliosides, taking into
account their very low concentration in this fluid. The present
report deals primarily with a description of the methodology
developed for this purpose. In addition to CSF analysis, the
general technique has been applied to isolation and assay of
blood plasma gangliosides of three species: human, rabbit and
bovine. Some preliminary experiments are described concerning
transport of gangliosides between blood, CSF and brain.

MATERIALS AND EQUIPMENT

Two sources of cerebrospinal fluid were employed: (1) a
large volume of ventricular fluid from a 5-year old male patient
with hydrocephalus due to cerebellar astrocytoma, and (2) a
pooled collection of lumbar fluid taken from a large number of
patients. The latter included samples from both neurologically
normal and abnormal patients, and each sample was established as
free of bacterial infection, visible sediment or color.   Prior
to freezing, the CSF was centrifuged at 300 x g for 15 minutes
to remove possible cellular material. Samples were obtained
through the kind cooperation of Drs. G. Szilagyi, N. Kovach,
and J. French.

Plasma was prepared from freshly drawn citrated blood by
centrifugation at 2500 x g for 30 minutes followed by
recentrifugation of the supernatant fluid at 8000 x g for
another 30 minutes, all at 10°C. The human plasma showed little
evidence of hemoglobin resulting from hemolysis but the bovine
and rabbit samples indicated some. Corrections were made for
the volumes of ACD[1] added.

Merck reagent grade chloroform and methanol were employed
for extraction and chromatography. In the final stages of
purification these solvents were distilled before use. TLC[1] was
performed with precoated silica gel G plates, 250 microns thick,
from Analtech, Inc. (Wilmington, Delaware). The plates were
freshly activated at 110° for 40 minutes. For GLC[1], a Hewlett-

Packard model 402 was employed with flame ionization detector
and helium carrier gas. GLC column packings, obtained from
Supelco, Inc. (Bellefonte, Pa.) were of two types: OV-1, 3%
on 100-120 chromosorb W HP, and OV-225, 3% on 100-120
supelcoport. Both were U-shaped columns, 6 ft. x 4 mm. Peak
areas were determined with an Infotronics CRS-100 electronic
integrator.

METHODS

CSF samples were treated with one-tenth volume of 0.5 M
EDTA (tetrasodium salt), dialyzed two days in the cold and
lyophilized to dryness in a round-bottom flask. Lipids were
extracted in the same flask by adding two ml water plus 40 ml
$CHCl_3$-CH_3OH (1:1) and stirring one hour. The mixture was
occasionally agitated in an ultrasonic bath, 100 watts (Heat
Systems Ultrasonics, Inc., Plainview, N.Y.) and finally
transferred to a centrifuge tube. After centrifugation at 300 x
g for 15 minutes in the cold, the supernatant fraction was
removed and filtered through a sintered glass funnel of medium
porosity. The round-bottom flask was rinsed with 20 ml
$CHCl_3$-CH_3OH (1:1) with the aid of sonication, transferred to the
same centrifuge tube and processed similarly. The rinsing
procedure was repeated and the combined filtrates were evaporated
to give a crude lipid extract. The defatted protein residue
(now entirely transferred to the centrifuge tube) was dried and
set aside for subsequent assay of protein-bound sialic acid.

The crude lipid extract usually contained a measurable
amount of protein despite the filtration, but this contaminant
was eliminated in subsequent steps. The dried sample in a 12 ml
centrifuge tube was suspended in 0.1 ml H_2O, treated with 8 ml
$CHCl_3$-CH_3OH (1:1), agitated well in an ultrasonic bath and
cooled in ice. The insoluble protein was removed by
centrifugation and combined with the main portion of defatted
residue while the supernatant fraction containing lipid was
refiltered. Any small amount of protein remaining in solution
was removed at a later stage by column chromatography (vide
infra). The sintered glass funnel used for filtration collected
a negligible portion of the total protein (most of it having
been sedimented on centrifugation) but the step was necessary
to preclude mechanical transfer of small protein particles to
the lipid fraction.

The lipid solution was adjusted to $CHCl_3$-CH_3OH (2:1) and
partitioned four times according to Folch, et al. (1957) with
omission of salt in the aqueous phase. This type of
partitioning was necessary to insure quantitative removal of

less-polar gangliosides from the lower phase but it suffered
from the disadvantage of allowing more contamination in the upper
phase. The following steps were designed to eliminate these
impurities. Combined upper phases were evaporated to dryness,
dissolved in 50 ml $CH_3OH-CHCl_3-H_2O$ (60:30:8) and added slowly to
a column containing 1.0 g of DEAE-sephadex (A-25; Pharmacia Fine
Chemicals, Inc.; Piscataway, N.J.). The resin had been
previously equilibrated overnight in an excess of $CH_3OH-CHCl_3-$
0.8 M sodium acetate (60:30:8), followed by thorough rinsing with
$CH_3OH-CHCl_3-H_2O$ (60:30:8). The column was packed in the latter
solvent and the resin washed with 100-200 ml of the same. After
application of the sample, the column was eluted with an
additional 50-100 ml of the same solvent to remove all uncharged
lipid contaminants. Gangliosides together with a small amount of
acidic lipid contaminants were eluted with 90 ml of $CH_3OH-CHCl_3-$
0.8 M sodium acetate (60:30:8). After evaporation to dryness,
the residue was warmed a few hours with three to five ml of 0.2 N
$NaOH-CH_3OH$, then transferred to a pre-washed dialysis bag by
rinsing with an excess of water. Dialysis for two days in the
cold was followed by lyophilization. The dried sample was
dissolved in 3 ml of $CHCl_3-CH_3OH$ (1:1) with the aid of
sonication, then treated with 7 ml $CHCl_3$ and applied to a one g
column of Unisil (200-325 mesh silicic acid) packed in $CHCl_3$.
Elution with 50 ml $CHCl_3-CH_3OH$ (85:15) removed additional lipid
contaminants which may have survived to this point, such as
sulfatides and free fatty acids. The ganglioside fraction was
then eluted in relatively pure form with 100 ml of distilled
$CHCl_3-CH_3OH$ (2:3).

The above procedure was employed for relatively large
volumes of CSF (50 ml or more) where the amount of ganglioside
was sufficiently large to preclude loss during dialysis. For
smaller volumes a simplified procedure was employed which
omitted the DEAE-sephadex column and subsequent dialysis. In
this case dialysis of original CSF was still performed as a
first (and essential) step without loss of ganglioside. (It is
possible that gangliosides of CSF are bound to lipoproteins, as
they appear to be in blood plasma (Marcus and Cass, 1969), and
this may explain their retention on dialysis of whole CSF. After
extraction, however, gangliosides were frequently lost during
dialysis if the concentration was below approximately 05 μg
sialic acid per 5 ml). Following $CHCl_3-CH_3OH$ extraction and
Folch-partitioning, the residue from combined upper phases was
applied directly to a one g Unisil column and eluted as
described. Although not as pure as samples prepared by the full
procedure, such material was sufficiently pure for reliable
sialic acid assay by GLC (vide infra).

The same basic procedure was employed for isolation of plasma gangliosides. An alternative procedure which led to essentially similar results was to extract the plasma directly with twenty volumes of $CHCl_3$-CH_3OH (1:1) followed by Folch-partitioning of the crude lipid extract. The combined upper phases were evaporated and then dialyzed (with EDTA) to remove excess salt before applying the sample to a DEAE-sephadex column. The latter was increased in size to 2.2 g DEAE-sephadex (since plasma contains more ganglioside than CSF) and the ganglioside fraction was eluted with 180 ml of CH_3OH-$CHCl_3$-0.8 M sodium acetate (60:30:8). Unisil chromatography was the final purification step, as above, with somewhat larger volumes of solvent being employed for elution.

The sialic acid content of CSF and plasma gangliosides was quantified by a GLC procedure described previously (Yu and Ledeen, 1970). Samples containing 0.2 - 3.0 µg sialic acid were dissolved in one ml of 0.05 N HCl-CH_3OH in a 10 ml tube with teflon-lined screw-cap and heated one hour at 80°C. This liberated most of the sialic acid in the form of methyl ketoside methyl ester. This product was analyzed by GLC as the trimethylsilyl ether derivative using phenyl N-acetyl-α-D-glucosaminide as internal standard. Most analyses were carried out with the OV-1 column while the OV-225 column was used to provide confirmatory data where necessary. Since the yield of NANA methyl ketoside methyl ester differs somewhat for different ganglioside structures and is always less than 100%, the quantification is based on empirical correlations (Yu and Ledeen, 1970). The method has proved sensitive and reliable for ganglioside preparations from diverse sources, provided these have been previously subjected to some type of purification.

Protein-bound sialic acid was assayed by a very similar procedure recently tested on several sialoglycoproteins (Yu and Ledeen, 1971). The defatted residue from CSF was treated with H_2O-CH_3OH (10:1) in a ratio of 6 ml per mg and sonicated to give a stable suspension. Aliquots containing approximately 300 µg protein were evaporated to dryness, treated with 2 ml 0.05 N HCl-CH_3OH and heated at 80°C for 1.5 hours. GLC analysis was performed in the same manner as for ganglioside sialic acid but quantification was based on a standard curve obtained with orosomucoid. Protein-bound sialic acid from human plasma was assayed in a similar manner after subjecting the defatted residue to dialysis.

RESULTS AND DISCUSSION

The presence of gangliosides in human cerebrospinal fluid was confirmed by GLC detection of sialic acid, sphingosine bases and fatty acids in the purified fraction. TLC visualization provided additional evidence that the material isolated was indeed ganglioside. Since the concentration of ganglioside was only a small fraction of the total bound sialic acid in CSF, it was important for accurate quantification to insure complete removal of the small quantity of protein which invariably solubilized along with lipid in the original $CHCl_3-CH_3OH$ extract. Experiments with several glycoproteins indicated that the precipitation procedure and final chromatography on Unisil accomplished this effectively, and this was confirmed by the minimal amount of sialic acid positive material seen at the TLC origin.

Quantitative Analyses

The GLC assay procedure enables measurement of submicrogram quantities of bound sialic acid and also permits differentiation of NANA and NGNA[1]. Since the methanolysis reaction is carried out under mild conditions each sialic acid retains its original N-acyl group, although O-acyl units are readily cleaved. Figure 1 indicates a representative chromatogram obtained from a mixture of ganglioside standards containing both types of sialic acid. NANA was the only species detected in the glycolipid and glycoprotein fractions of human CSF.

Analytical results for human CSF are presented in Table 1. Two different pooled samples of lumbar fluid were analyzed, the aliquot size being five ml and 10 ml, respectively. Analytical precision was comparable in the two groups, and the results demonstrate the feasibility of utilizing five ml of CSF for ganglioside assay. Smaller volumes (down to one ml) were also assayed with similar results but variability increased. The greater precision observed for the ventricular-hydrocephalus CSF probably resulted from the larger aliquots employed.

The data in Table 1 are intended to illustrate the potentials of the analytical method and cannot be used to infer true normal levels since the CSF included pathological material. However, the values for lumbar CSF are fairly close to the qualitative estimate given by Bernheimer (1969), and our own preliminary studies indicate that the values for normal subjects will not differ greatly from the above results. It should be further emphasized that no corrections have yet been made for recovery. The concentration of gangliosides in the ventricular fluid of the

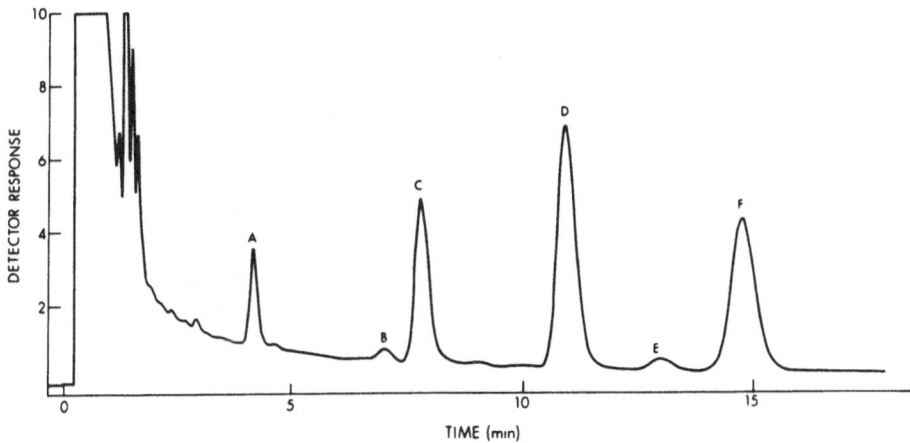

Fig. 1. GLC of sialic acids on OV-1 column. A mixture of hematoside-NANA and hematoside-NGNA was heated 1 hr at 80°C in 0.05 N methanolic HCl, and the products were converted to TMS derivatives. Column was run isothermally at 205°C. Peak identification: A, methoxyneuraminic acid methyl ester (deacylated product); B, α-NANA; C, β-NANA; D, internal standard; E, α-NGNA; F, β-NGNA. The terms "α-NANA", etc. refer to the methyl ketoside methyl esters of appropriate configuration.

hydrocephalus patient employed in this study was significantly lower than the pooled lumbar levels, but assay of normal ventricular CSF will be necessary to determine whether this lower value was due to its ventricular origin or some aspect of the disease.

Protein-bound sialic acid was found to be approximately 770 μg per 100 ml of human lumbar fluid and 885 μg for the ventricular-hydrocephalus sample. Ganglioside sialic acid thus comprises only a few percent of total sialic acid in CSF. It is interesting to note that a similar proportion exists in human

Table 1. Concentration of Gangliosides in Human CSF

Sources of CSF	Vol. Analyzed ml	Ganglioside NANA µg per 100 ml
lumbar	5	25.8
	5	27.2
	5	34.0
	5	29.8
		ave: 29.2
lumbar	10	29.6
	10	22.5
	10	14.1
		ave: 22.1
ventricular (hydrocephalus)	55	7.8
	55	8.3
	100	7.2
	100	7.0
		ave: 7.6

plasma where ganglioside sialic acid is less than one per cent of
the protein-bound level. Both fluids are quite dissimilar from
brain which has more lipid-bound than protein-bound NANA
(Brunngraber, 1969). An estimation of total CSF protein was
obtained from the weight of the defatted, dialyzed residue; this
was 98 mg per 100 ml for the lumbar sample and 97 mg for the
hydrocephalus.

Ganglioside concentrations in blood plasma of three species
are summarized in Table 2, together with the proportion of NGNA.
The identity of the latter sialic acid was verified by the use of
both OV-1 and OV-225 columns during GLC assay. Bovine plasma
gangliosides have approximately equal amounts of the two sialic
acids, resembling in this respect other bovine tissue (Ledeen,
et al. 1968b). The total ganglioside content of human and bovine
plasma were similar but that of rabbit was found to be
consistently lower in several determinations.

A comparison of ganglioside concentrations in various
tissues and fluids is given in Table 3. The values for brain
were determined previously (Yu and Ledeen, 1970) while the liver
value was obtained from Dr. K. Suzuki (personal communication).
Tissue densities of one were assumed in calculating concentration

Table 2. Ganglioside Content of Blood Plasma

Species	μmoles Sialic Acid per 100 ml	% NGNA
human	1.14	0.0
bovine	1.38	52.2
rabbit	0.24	1.1

per 100 ml. The CSF ganglioside level is quite low in relation
to plasma and the three tissues, especially when calculated on a
volume basis. We observed here a two-fold difference between
CSF and plasma gangliosides when related to dry weight, and this
may be compared with the finding of Tourtellotte (1959) that
several other lipids are twice as concentrated in plasma as CSF
when related to protein weight. The concentration of lipid-
bound sialic acid we have found in CSF is of the same magnitude
as the CSF concentrations of cerebroside (0.087 μmoles/100 ml)
reported by Nagai and Kanfer (1971) and total lipid phosphorus
(0.052 μmoles/100 ml) reported by Tourtellotte and Haerer (1969).

Table 3. Comparison of Ganglioside Concentrations

	μmoles sialic acid per:	
	g dry wt.	100 ml
gray matter	16.8	290
white matter	2.9	84
liver	1.1	22
plasma	0.12	1.14
CSF	0.06	0.07

Thin-Layer Patterns

A TLC comparison of CSF and brain gangliosides is shown in
Figure 2. A striking difference is evident between gangliosides
from the lumbar and ventricular (hydrocephalus) specimens, the
former resembling brain mixture to a large extent and the latter

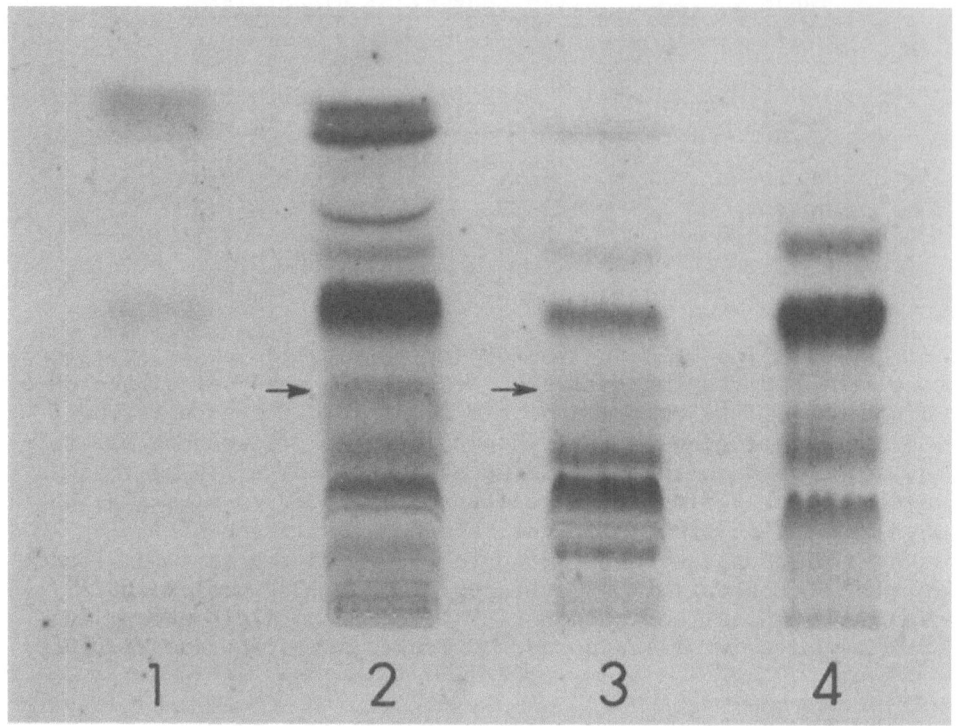

<u>Fig. 2.</u> TLC comparison of gangliosides from ventricular
(hydrocephalus) CSF (2), lumbar CSF (3) and bovine brain (4).
Channel (1) is hematoside standard. Silica gel G, 250 microns
thick; two ascending runs in $CHCl_3$-CH_3OH-2.5 N aq.NH_3 (60:40:9);
resorcinol spray. All bands are purple except those indicated
with arrow.

having considerably more hematoside[2]. (The hematoside band is
occasionally seen to split into two components, as shown in
figure 2. The cause is not known but has been postulated as due
to fatty acid chain length differences). Several of the CSF
bands appear to migrate parallel to brain fractions but structural

---

[2]The term "hematoside" is used here to designate gangliosides
which lack hexosamine. The principle form is lactosylceramide
bonded at the C_3-hydroxyl of galactose to one sialic acid. The
term "brain-type" gangliosides is used to designate slower
migrating species which contain hexosamine, regardless of tissue
origin.

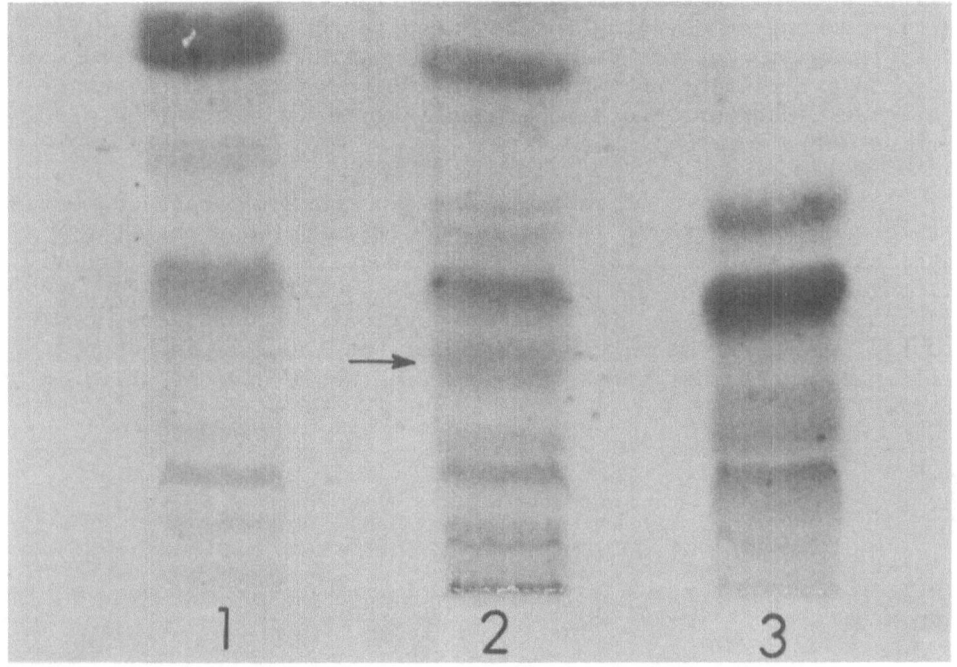

<u>Fig. 3.</u> TLC comparison of gangliosides from human plasma (1),
ventricular (hydrocephalus) CSF (2) and bovine brain (3).
Conditions same as fig. 2. All bands are purple except that
indicated with arrow.

comparisons have not yet been carried out. A consistent feature
is the presence of major bands in the CSF samples which migrate
behind the slowest brain fraction (trisialoganglioside) and this
suggests the presence of tetra- and/or pentasialogangliosides.
Such species occur in very low concentration in mammalian brain.

Figure 3 shows the same sample from hydrocephalus-
ventricular CSF, compared with gangliosides of brain[3] and human
plasma. The fastest moving of the plasma bands has been
identified as hematoside (Yu and Ledeen, 1971) and it is note-
worthy that this is abundant in both hydrocephalus-ventricular
CSF and plasma. A similar pattern was obtained for a second
hydrocephalus sample (not shown). Only a trace of hematoside,

[3]Although this sample of gangliosides was prepared from beef
brain its TLC pattern was not significantly different from that
of human brain gangliosides.

however, was visible in the lumbar CSF gangliosides (Fig. 2). The
yellow band indicated with an arrow in Figures 2 and 3 was consistently present in CSF gangliosides despite the extensive purification, though it has not been seen in mammalian brain gangliosides.
This could represent an unknown acidic glycosphingolipid lacking
sialic acid, but structural characterization has not yet been
carried out.

The TLC patterns of gangliosides from human, rabbit and bovine
plasma samples are shown in Figure 4. It is evident that the
ganglioside composition of this fluid is quite species dependent.
All three samples contained hematosides as well as brain-type
gangliosides, though in variable proportions. Hematosides accounted for approximately two-thirds of the total lipid-bound
sialic acid in human plasma, one-half in rabbit and one-third in
bovine plasma.

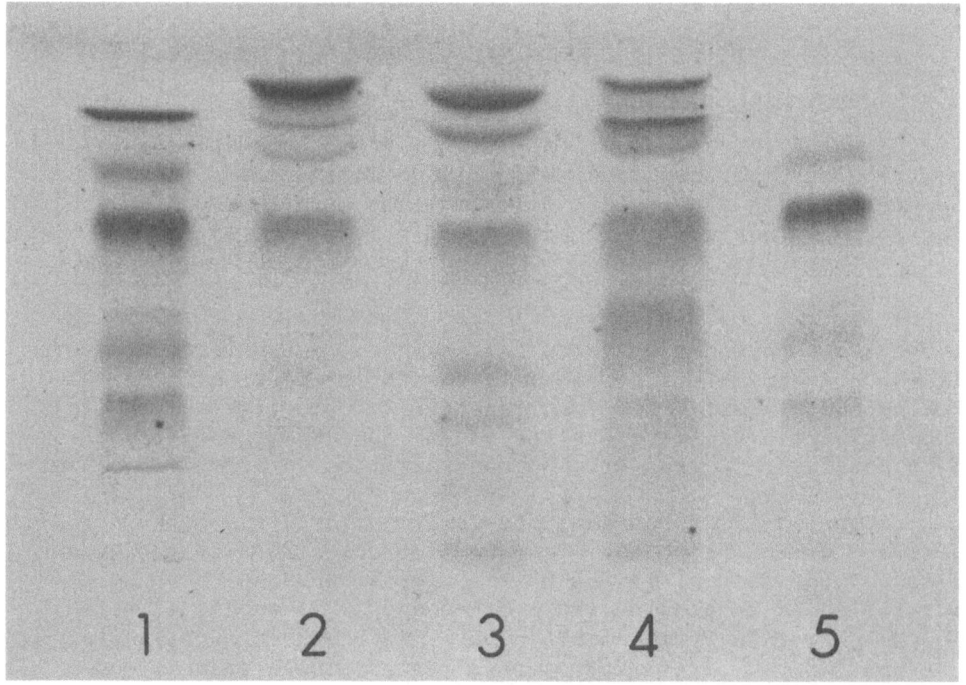

Fig. 4. TLC comparison of gangliosides from human plasma (2),
rabbit plasma (3), and bovine plasma (4). Channels (1) and (5)
are bovine brain galgliosides while (1) has Tay-Sachs ganglioside
in addition. Conditions same as Fig. 2.

Fatty Acids and Long-Chain Bases

Comparison of the above TLC patterns would suggest a plasma origin for the gangliosides of this sample of hydrocephalic CSF and a brain origin for at least a portion of the lumbar CSF gangliosides. Support for this hypothesis comes from the results of long-chain base analyses, summarized in table 4. The major C_{18} and C_{20} bases were sphingosine and 4-eicosasphingenine, respectively. Their ratios were determined by GLC assay of the aldehydes produced by periodate oxidation of the long-chain bases according to the method of Sweeley and Moscatelli (1959). The gangliosides were analyzed as a group without sub-fractionation. Since human plasma gangliosides contain virtually no C_{20}-sphingosine this base is a convenient marker for gangliosides of brain origin. These data indicate that lumbar CSF gangliosides include species from both plasma and brain with the former probably predominating. The fact that the ganglioside TLC pattern shows more resemblance to brain may indicate preferential uptake by the CSF of brain-type gangliosides from plasma; the latter contain little if any C_{20}-sphingosine. On the other hand, the low percentage of C_{20}-sphingosine in ventricular (hydrocephalus) CSF indicates that only a small proportion of this fluid's ganglioside came from brain tissue, the majority presumably arising from plasma.

Fatty acid analyses gave a qualitatively similar picture, as shown in table 5. All values refer to human specimens. Both lumbar and ventricular (hydrocephalus) gangliosides have stearate levels which are intermediate between those of brain (74%) and plasma (8-28%) gangliosides. The greatest contrast between lumbar and ventricular gangliosides was seen for the 24:0 and 24:1 values. Only the five major fatty acids are given in table 5.

Thus it is evident that gangliosides from the ventricular-hydrocephalus CSF differ both qualitatively and quantitatively from those of lumbar CSF. Further work will be needed to

Table 4. Long-Chain Base Composition of Gangliosides

	Ratio: C_{20}/C_{18}
brain (Sambasivarao and McCluer, 1964)	1.05
lumbar CSF	0.34
ventricular (hydrocephalus) CSF	0.08
plasma (human)	0.01

Table 5. Fatty Acid Composition of Gangliosides

| FATTY ACID | BRAIN | CSF | | PLASMA | |
		Lumbar	Ventricular (hydroceph.)	Brain Type	Hematoside
16:0	3.5	13.4	10.7	26.8	25.0
18:0	73.6	51.6	48.2	28.3	18.4
22:0	1.3	6.6	7.5	13.1	16.4
24:1	2.1	1.7	15.8	10.8	2.7
24:0	1.1	1.8	4.2	9.5	12.2

determine whether the hydrocephalic condition has caused a significant departure from the normal ganglioside pattern and concentration which prevails in the ventricles. The possibility exists in this condition of a breakdown in the blood-brain and/or blood-CSF barriers due to damage to ependyma and periventricular necrosis (Weller and Wisniewski, 1969).

No clear picture has yet emerged concerning the origin of CSF lipids. Although the percentage distribution of these lipids resembles that found in plasma (Tourtellotte, 1959), present evidence would discount the theory that lipids enter the CSF directly from the blood stream under normal conditions (Sastry and Stancer, 1968b; Tourtellotte and Haerer, 1969). The presence of triglycerides and cholesterol esters in normal CSF (Tourtellotte and Haerer, 1969) suggests at least some contribution from plasma since these lipids are not likely to have come from brain tissue. On the other hand, human CSF was recently shown (Nagai and Kanfer, 1971) to contain galactosyl-ceramide, the characteristic cerebroside of brain tissue, and virtually no glucosylceramide which is the principle cerebroside of human plasma (Vance and Sweeley, 1967). These previous findings and the present study support the concept that CSF lipids are derived from both brain and blood and there is the additional suggestion that brain lipids may be relatively more prominent in lumbar CSF than ventricular.

Ganglioside Transport

In order to assess the possibility of ganglioside transport between blood, brain and CSF compartments some preliminary experiments have been carried out in which labeled ganglioside was injected into blood and CSF of rabbits. The material employed was NGNA-hematoside and the sialic acid itself served as the label since NGNA is absent from rabbit brain gangliosides

(Yu and Ledeen, 1970) and comprises only one per cent of rabbit plasma ganglioside (table 2). Its estimation was carried out simultaneously with endogenous NANA by the GLC technique described above.

In the first experiment samples of NGNA-hematoside containing 150-200 µg NGNA were injected into the cisterna magna of each of two rabbits. The first rabbit was sacrificed after 100 minutes by exsanguination through heart, and the CSF and CNS[1] tissues were removed immediately after death. GLC analyses revealed that approximately 16-18% of the original NGNA-hematoside had gone into plasma while 11-13% remained in the CSF. The second rabbit was sacrificed 270 minutes after injection and in this case 15-17% of the original NGNA-hematoside was recovered in the plasma while 4-6% remained in the CSF. In neither of these two rabbits was any NGNA-hematoside detected in CNS tissue, the examined areas including cerebral cortex, midbrain and spinal cord. The unrecovered material could have been metabolized by visceral organs but its fate is not known with certainty.

In the second experiment NGNA-hematoside (1.04 mg NGNA) was injected intravenously into one rabbit which was sacrificed seven hours later by exsanguination. No NGNA-hematoside was detected in the brain tissue (analyzed as a whole) or the CSF while 10-12% of the injected sample was recovered in blood plasma.

These preliminary experiments indicate a certain barrier to transport of gangliosides from blood to CSF in the rabbit, although the limited data cannot be interpreted as indicating an absolute barrier in the rabbit. No data are yet available on this point for other species including man. The results here do indicate, however, the relative ease with which gangliosides migrate from CSF into blood, and this effect is very likely a general one involving the well-known mechanism of bulk-flow. The recent observation that Tay-Sachs ganglioside is elevated in the blood of Tay-Sachs patients (Sastry and Stancer, 1968a) might be retionalized in terms of this phenomenon, suggesting a CNS origin for such material. As mentioned previously, Tay-Sachs patients were also shown to have elevated Tay-Sachs ganglioside in their cerebrospinal fluid.

SUMMARY

Gangliosides have been isolated from human cerebrospinal fluid and purified with the aid of DEAE-sephadex and Unisil chromatography. GLC assay of sialic acid following methanolysis

gave average values of 22 μg and 29 μg ganglioside NANA per
100 ml for lumbar fluid and 7.6 μg for hydrocephalic-ventricular
CSF. In both cases the quantity of lipid-bound sialic acid was
a small fraction of total sialic acid, most of it being protein-
bound. The isolation procedure and GLC assay could be performed
with as little as one to two ml CSF.

TLC patterns indicated a close similarity between
gangliosides from the hydrocephalic-ventricular CSF and plasma,
while the lumbar sample was closer to the brain pattern. Fatty
acid and long-chain base analyses supported these relationships
and indicated that the lumbar CSF gangliosides contained
substantial contributions from both plasma and brain.

Gangliosides injected into CSF of rabbits moved rapidly into
plasma, only 4-6% remaining in the CSF after 4.5 hours.
Ganglioside migration from blood to CSF, on the other hand,
encountered a substantial barrier in the rabbit.

Gangliosides were isolated from human, bovine and rabbit
plasma and quantified by GLC. TLC revealed important species
differences but all three contained both hematosides and brain-
type gangliosides.

ACKNOWLEDGEMENTS

We wish to thank Dr. H. Wisniewski for his generous assistance
in the animal experiments and for his helpful suggestions throughout the course of this work.

This study was supported by grants NS 04834 and NS 03356
from the U. S. Public Health Service and the Marie L. Morgin
Memorial Grant for Research on Multiple Sclerosis (#669-A).
Figure 1 is reproduced with permission from the Journal of Lipid
Research.

REFERENCES

Bernheimer, H. (1968). Klin. Wschr. 46, 258.

Bernheimer, H. (1969). Klin. Wschr. 47, 227.

Brunngraber, E. (1969). In "Handbook of Neurochemistry" (A.
Lajtha, ed.), Plenum (New York), p. 223.

Christensen, L., and Matzke, J. (1965). Acta Neurol. Scand. 41,
445.

Folch, J., Lees, M., and Sloane-Stanley, G. (1957). J. Biol.
Chem. 226, 497.

Hagberg, B., and Svennerholm, L. (1960). Acta Paediat. Scand. 49, 690.

Ledeen, R., Salsman, K., and Cabrera, M. (1968a). J. Lipid Res. 9, 129.

Ledeen, R., Salsman, K., and Cabrera, M. (1968b). Biochemistry 7, 2287.

Marcus, D., and Cass, L. (1969). Science 164, 553.

Nagai, Y., and Kanfer, J. (1971). J. Lipid Res. 12, 143.

Sambasivarao, K., and McCluer, R. (1964). J. Lipid Res. 5, 103.

Sastry, P., and Stancer, H. (1968a). Clin. Chim. Acta 20, 487.

Sastry, P., and Stancer, H. (1968b). Clin. Chim. Acta 22, 301.

Suzuki, K. (1967). In "Inborn Disorders of Sphingolipid Metabolism" (S.M. Aronson and B.W. Volk, eds.), Pergamon Press, p. 215.

Sweeley, C., and Moscatelli, E. (1959). J. Lipid Res. 1, 40.

Tourtellotte, W. (1959). Neurol. 9, 375.

Tourtellotte, W., and Haerer, A. (1969). Arch. Neurol. 20, 605.

Vance, D., and Sweeley, C. (1967). J. Lipid Res. 8, 621.

Weller, R., and Wisniewski, H. (1969). Brain 92, 819.

Yu, R., and Ledeen, R. (1970). J. Lipid Res. 11, 506.

Yu, R., and Ledeen, R. (1971). In Preparation.

GANGLIOSIDE INNER ESTERS

Robert H. McCluer and James E. Evans

Eunice K. Shriver Center at the Walter E. Fernald

State School, Waltham, Massachusetts

The glycosphingolipids are derivatives of N-acylsphingosines (ceramide) to which a carbohydrate unit, composed of one or more glycosyl moieties, is bound glycosidically in a β linkage to the hydroxyl at carbon 1 of sphingosine. The gangliosides are glyco-sphingolipids which contain one or more sialic acid residues as one of the glycosyl moieties (1). Gangliosides occur in most organs and body fluids but their highest concentration is in the central nervous system. The brain gangliosides are primarily lo-cated in neuronal dendritic processes and different brain areas have significantly different complements of the various ganglio-sides. Analyses of subcellular fractions have revealed that the ganglioside content of nuclei, mitochondria and synaptic vesicles is low while microsomes and synaptic membranes contain the high-est amount of gangliosides. Thus gangliosides appear to be neuronal membrane components and perhaps participate in the com-plex molecular events at the synapse which are necessary for infor-mation processing. The combination of a large hydrophilic moiety with a strongly charged sialic acid and the hydrophobic ceramide portion suggest that gangliosides are membrane components which are suited for interaction with the microenvironment. It is pos-sible that interaction of gangliosides with cations could lead to changes in the molecule which would in turn produce changes in the properties of the synaptic membrane. Calcium has a pronounced effect on the solubility of gangliosides. Reactions which would alter the number of negative charges in a ganglioside molecule such as formation of an ester could conceivably play an important role in modification of synaptic membrane properties.

The detection of a neutral ganglioside in extracts of adrenal gland has prompted us to study the structure and properties of ganglioside inner esters (2).

EXPERIMENTAL

A preparation of bovine adrenal gland sialosylactosyllceramides (SLC) containing N-acetyl and N-glycolyl neuraminic acid was employed for these studies. It was first observed by TLC analysis, that storage of SLC in glacial acetic acid lead to the formation of a relatively non-polar resorcinol positive substance. This material was not retained by DEAE-cellulose and is referred to as neutral ganglioside (NG).

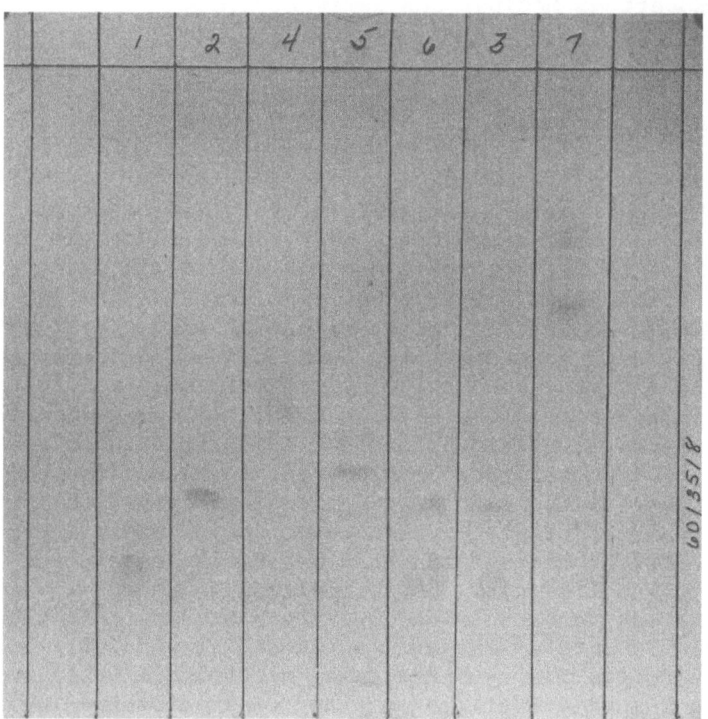

Fig. 1   TLC of sialosyllactosylceramides
(SLC) and inner esters.
An Analtech 250u thick silica G plate was employed. The
solvent used was C-M-H$_2$0 (60:35:8). Spots were demonstrated
with resorcinol reagent. Samples from left to right are:
(1)   N-glycolylneuraminosyllactosylceramide:
(2)   N-acetylneuraminosyllactosylceramide;
(4)   Neutral gangliosides (NG) formed from mixed SLC
      preparation;
(5)   NG treated with NH$_4$DH;
(6)   NG treated with Na$_2$CO$_3$;
(3)   mixed SLC preparation
(7)   galactosylceramide and lactosyl ceramide

The mixed SLC preparation was dissolved in glacial acetic acid and kept at room temperature. Aliquots were taken at various times and analyzed by TLC with C–M–H$_2$O (60:35:8) as the developing solvent. Neutral ganglioside was gradually formed so that after four days there was practically quantitative conversion of SLC into neutral ganglioside. The reaction mixture was lyophilized, the residue dissolved in C–M (2:1) and placed on a DEAE-cellulose (acetate) column. The neutral ganglioside was eluted with C–M (2:1) and remaining SLC was eluted with glacial acetic acid. The NG was reconverted to the parent SLC by treatment with 0.1N Na$_2$CO$_3$ at 60°C for 1 hr. To demonstrate aminolysis, the neutral ganglioside was dissolved in conc. NH$_4$OH, the solution evaporated to dryness, dissolved in C–M (2:1) and spotted. A compound with TLC mobility intermediate between NG and SLC was observed. These results are shown in Figure 1.

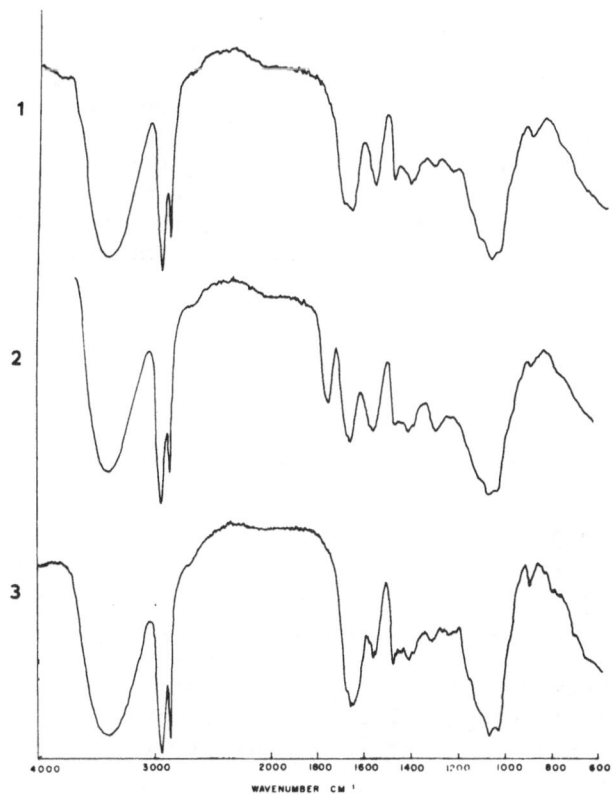

Fig. 2 IR spectra of (1) NG treated with NH$_4$OH, (2) NG and (3) SLC.
Samples were prepared in KBr pellets and spectra obtained with a Beckman IR-33 instrument.

One mole of ester per mole of sialic acid was detected with the hydroxamic acid method of Snyder and Stephens (3). Mannitol hexaacetate was used as an ester standard. The IR spectra of SLC, NG and ammonia treated NG are shown in Figure 2. NG shows the typical ester absorption at 1750 cm^{-1}, but the ammonia treated material shows no ester absorption and added absorption in the amide regions. These data suggest that NG is a lactone or ester and the ammonia treated material is SLC amide.

Examination of molecular models of sialic acid glycosides, as indicated by Yu and Ledeen (4) reveals that the carboxyl group in the α-D configuration is _trans_ to the hydroxyl group at carbons 4 and 7. Yu and Ledeen demonstrated that the $1 \rightarrow 7$ and $1 \rightarrow 4$ lactones can only form with the β anomer. The configuration of sialic acid in SLC is known to be α-D due to its susceptability to hydrolysis by neuraminidase. Thus the presence of a $1 \rightarrow 4$ or $1 \rightarrow 7$ lactone in NG sialic acid appears to be ruled out.

Examination of molecular models of SLC indicated that a lactone involving hydroxyl groups of carbons 8 or 9 was possible but unlikely. We therefore subjected the NG to oxidation with periodate which will lead to the production of formaldehyde if hydroxyl groups of carbons 8 and 9 are free. In order to insure the stability of inner ester during oxidation, NG was dissolved in glacial acetic acid made 0.1M with periodic acid and the formaldehyde found was assayed by the chromotropic acid method (5). Mannitol was used as a standard. One mole of formaldehyde per mole of sialic acid was formed from both SLC and NG. These data are presented in Table I and indicate that hydroxyl groups of carbons 8 and 9 of NG are free.

Table I
Periodate oxidation of SLC and SLC inner ester

Material Oxidized*	HCHO	Moles/mole	
	15 min.	2.5 hrs.	4.5 hrs.
SLC	0.94	1.04	1.02
Inner Ester	0.94	0.94	0.95
Mannitol	1.78	2.0	2.0

*Samples were dissolved in glacial acetic acid made 0.1M with periodic acid. Aliquots were removed at times indicated and formaldehyde measured by the chromotropic acid method.

The molecular models also revealed that formation of an inner ester with hydroxyl groups on either carbons 2 or 4 of the adjacent galactose was a likely reaction which would result in the formation of a 6-membered lactone ring.

In an attempt to obtain direct evidence for such a structure,
NG was subjected to permethylation with methyliodide in dimethylformamide with Ba(OH)$_2$ and BaO and also with AgO as catalysts.   In
each case only 2,3,6 tri-0-methyl glucose and 2,4,6 tri-0-methyl
galactose were detected as products by G$_{LC}$ after hydrolysis.
These results provide no evidence for substitution on the galactose
but presumably the ester bond is opened under the alkaline conditions
of methylation.

Further evidence for the formation of an inner ester involving
the galactose residue has been obtained with neuraminlactose.   Bovine colostrum neuraminlactose, as obtained from Sigma Chemical Co.
is a mixture of the sialosyl (2→3) galactosyl (1→4) glucose
and sialosyl (2→6) galactosyl (1→4) glucose.   These positional
isomers are easily distinguished on thin-layer plates developed
with propanol-water (6:2).   The neuraminlactose preparation was
incubated at room temperature for four days in glacial acetic acid
and then analyzed by TLC.   Only the sialosyl (2→3) galactosyl
(1→4) glucose formed an ester as shown in Figure 3.   These re---

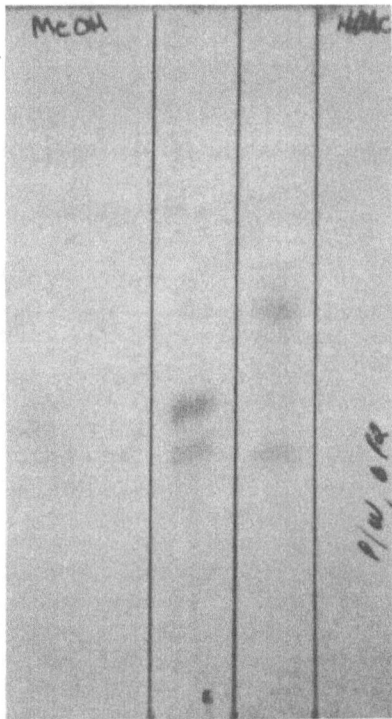

Fig. 3   TLC of glacial acetic acid-treated neuraminlactose.
Conditions employed as stated in Fig. 1: except the solvent
for TLC was propanol-H$_2$0 (6:2).   In the left lane is the
original neuraminlactose preparation: the sialosyl (2→3)
isomer is the upper sport and the (2→6) isomer is below.
The acetic acid treated material is on the right.

sults were confirmed with the individual compounds. Thus the formation of inner esters appears limited to sialic acid residues
bonded adjacent to a hydroxyl group. The proposed structure of
SLC inner ester is shown in Figure 4. Presumably the 1→4 ester
is just as likely to form as the 1→2 ester.

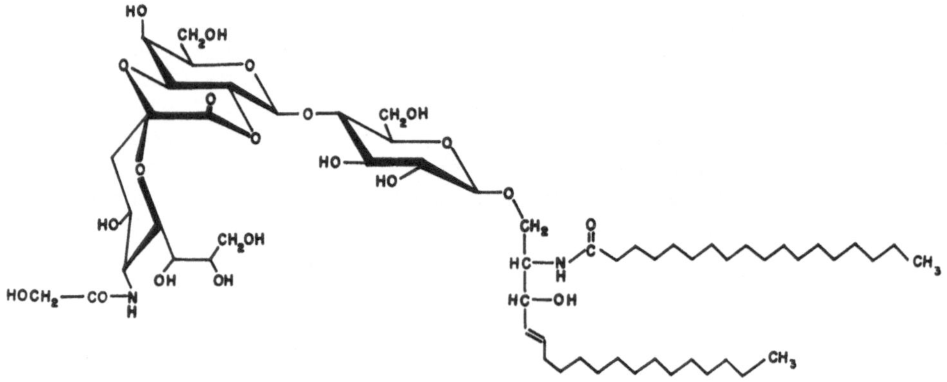

Fig. 4 N-glycolylneuraminosyllactosyl ceramide inner ester.

The ability of other gangliosides to form inner esters has
also been studied. Gangliosides G_{M2}, G_{M1}, G_{D1a}, G_{D1b} and G_{T1}
were incubated in glacial acetic acid for four days. Aliquots
of the acetic acid solutions were removed, lyophilized and residues
treated with Na_2CO_3 as stated above. Portions of the original
ganglioside solutions, acetic acid solutions and Na_2CO_3 treated
samples were spotted on TLC plates which were then developed in
C-M-H_2O (60:35:8). These results are shown in Figure 5.

Ganglioside G_{M1} and G_{M2} were shown to form small amounts of
neutral gangliosides under these conditions. This was demonstrated
by passage of the acetic acid treated samples over DEAE cellulose
and examination of the C-M (1:2) eluate by TLC. Gangliosides G_{D1a},
G_{D1b}, and G_{T1} were observed to form one, two and three products
respectively under these conditions. All of these products were
reconverted to their parent gangliosides by Na_2CO_3 which indicated
that cleavage of sialic acid residues did not produce these products. The two products formed from G_{D1b} were dissolved in C-M
(1:2) and placed on a small DEAE cellulose column. The top spot,

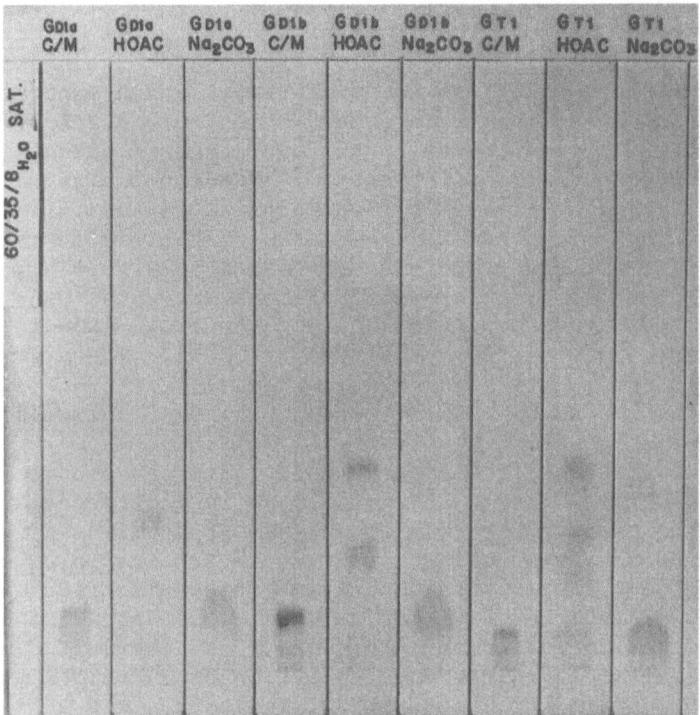

Fig. 5   TLC of ganglioside inner esters. Chromatographic
conditions as in Fig. 1. The samples were spotted from
chloroform-methanol (C/M) solutions, after treatment with
glacial acetic acid (HOAc), and subsequent treatment with
0.1 N Na_2CO_3.

G_{D1b} ester II, was eluted with C-M (2:1) whereas G_{D1b} ester I and
parent ganglioside were eluted with MeOH-acetic acid (1:1). The
ratio of ester groups to sialic acid residues in G_{D1b} ester II
was found to be unity. We thus conclude that G_{D1b} ester II is a
neutral compound in which both sialic acid residues are present
as inner esters. G_{D1b} ester I is assumed to have one sialic acid
residue in inner ester linkage. G_{D1b} esters I and II were shown
to be introconvertable upon further treatment with glacial acetic
acid. G_{D1a} also forms a neutral product. Thus all sialic acid
residues in the gangliosides will form inner ester bonds. Preliminary stability studies have shown that the inner esters are
stable at pH 6.0 for several hours in aqueous solution at room
temperature.

DISCUSSION

Wiegandt (6) has previously reported that gangliosides which contain a sialic acid residue in (2→8) linkage with another sialic acid residue will form an inner ester. Such esters are strictly analogous to that which occur in colominic acid (7) where the carboxyl groups are linked to the hydroxyls of carbons 7 or 9 of the neighboring sialic acid residue. These colominic acid esters are slowly cleaved at pH 8.0 at room temperature and will form in aqueous solutions at pH 2. We have shown that a sialic acid residue in brain gangliosides attached glycosidically to the 3 position of galactose is also capable of forming an ester bond with an adjacent hydroxyl group. Thus all of the brain ganglioside sialic acid residues can form inner ester bonds. These ganglioside inner esters are readily generated in glacial acetic acid and can be separted by TLC in C-M-H$_2$O systems and by DEAE cellulose columns for further analysis.

The fact that the sialic acid residues in gangliosides only occur in glycosidic linkage adjacent to hydroxyl groups may be related to the capacity of such structures to form inner esters. Although we do not have definitive evidence for the in vivo occurrence of any ganglioside esters, a sialosyllactosideceramide inner ester was isolated from adrenal gland (2) extracts, under conditions which do not normally produce this material. In 1964, Kuhn and Muldner (8) reported the isolation of a complex mucolipid from dog brain which contained gangliosides and exhibited properties of a polyester.

REFERENCES

1. H. Wiegandt, Angew. Chem. 7, 87 (1968).
2. J.E. Evans and R.H. McCluer, Fed. Proc. 30, 1133Abs (1971).
3. F. Snyder and N. Stephens, Biochim. Biophys. Acta 34, 244 (1959).
4. R.K. Yu and R. Ledeen, J. Biol. Chem. 244, 1306 (1969).
5. J.C. Speck in "Methods in Carbohydrate Chemistry" Vol. I, Ed. by Whistler and Wolfrom, Academic Press, N.Y. 1962, p. 441.
6. H. Wiegandt, Rev. Physiol. Biochem. Expt'l. Pharm. 57, 190 (1966).
7. E. McGuire and S.B. Binkley, Biochemistry 3, 247 (1964).
8. R. Kuhn and H. Muldner, Naturwissenschaften 51, 635 (1964).

HUMAN BRAIN LIPID COMPOSITION CHANGES WITH AGE AND ALTERATIONS IN

SOME PATHOLOGICAL STATES: A NEW METHOD OF GRAPHIC ANALYSIS

George Rouser and Gene Kritchevsky

City of Hope National Medical Center

Duarte, California 91010

ABSTRACT

A method is presented with which abnormalities of brain lipid composition can be disclosed and defined precisely. The total amount of lipid is first compared to that of normal brain by plotting values as percentage of the fresh weight against age and noting whether or not values are within the normal range. Abnormal proportions of lipid classes are disclosed by plotting values for each lipid class against the value for total phospholipid. This method of comparison to normal can be used with biopsy samples weighing only a few milligrams, although precise comparison to normal individuals on age plots is possible only with representative samples of whole brain and is thus limited to postmortem examinations. Results obtained with data from 17 cases of metabolic disorders are presented. In Tay-Sachs disease, GM_1 gangliosidosis, Niemann-Pick disease, and metachromatic leukodystrophy, total lipid is lower than normal, the percentages of all sphingolipids are generally increased, the percentage of phosphatidyl choline is decreased and the percentages of phosphatidyl ethanolamine, phosphatidyl serine, and phosphatidyl inositol are normal. A similar pattern of change was found in the brain of one phenylketonuria patient which in addition was found to have an elevated triglyceride level. In Farber's disease, cerebroside and sulfatide percentages were above normal and accumulation of a ceramide polyhexoside was noted. In Alzheimer's disease, a small reduction in the percentages of phosphatidyl ethanolamine was found. In one unclassfied case, only one abnormality, an elevation of minor acidic phospholipids, was apparent in brain and spleen. No distinct abnormalities were detected in acute infantile or chronic Gaucher's diseases, paranoid schizophrenia, mental depression, or an unclassified case with neurological

problems. The findings are discussed and the probability of Farber's
disease being a disorder of ceramide polyhexoside degradation is
emphasized.

INTRODUCTION

The lipid composition of blood and tissues is abnormal in many
pathological states. The cause of some of the abnormalities is an
alteration in the amount of an enzyme of lipid metabolism, whereas
in other cases lipid changes clearly are secondary to primary
changes in the levels of enzymes of carbohydrate or amino acid
metabolism or other metabolic pathways. When changes are large,
they are relatively easy to define as abnormal. Thus, abnormally
high levels of blood cholesterol and triglyceride are well known,
and the hyperlipoproteinemias have been divided into five major
categories by Fredrickson (1). Large tissue deposits of various
sphingolipids have been demonstrated. Some of these were recognized
before the development of chromatographic methods. Thus far, abnormally high tissue levels of phospholipids, glycolipids, and fatty
acids have been linked to specific degradative enzyme deficiencies
for sphingolipids (2,3) and phytanic acid (4). Enzyme deficiencies
for other lipids are to be expected and it is also important to
determine whether or not changes in lipid metabolism in brain,
even though of a secondary nature, are directly related to neuropathology.

Studies in this laboratory have proceeded in three distinct
but overlapping phases. In the first phase, accurate and precise
methods of lipid analysis were developed. In the second, data
were collected. The third period is characterized by development
and application of new methods of data analysis. Our major objectives were to define accurately and precisely the lipid composition of normal human brain and other major organs so that even
subtle differences in pathological states could be defined with
certainty. Similar studies were undertaken with other animal
species because experimental models for human disease are needed.

Two problems were encountered in the course of the work that
made a large number of samples essential. One was the large change
in human brain lipid composition with age. These changes appear to
take place throughout life. The other was the wide normal range of
variability. In this report, we describe the changes with age of
normal human brain, define the normal range of variation, demonstrate the relationships among the lipid classes of normal brain,
and present data illustrating that it is now possible to determine
whether or not there are abnormalities in lipid class levels in
pathological states using a piece of brain tissue weighing only a
few milligrams from any region of brain.

METHODS

Two types of brain samples were used. Changes with age are precisely definable only with representative samples of whole brains.
Such samples were obtained by cutting the brain in half longitudi-
nally and grinding to a uniform paste by passage through a meat
grinder four or five times. Small samples from different regions of
brain were also studied. An electric cork borer was used to provide
cores of the desired size from frozen brains. Small samples were
ground under liquid nitrogen to a uniform powder in a mortar. Portions of the homogeneous samples were extracted by grinding in a
Waring blender (large samples) or glass homogenizer (small samples)
with chloroform/methanol 2/1 (twice), chloroform/methanol 1/2
(once), and then chloroform/methanol/concentrated aqueous ammonia
7/1/5 (v/v/%) as previously described (5,6). Solvent was removed
(6) and the lipid taken up in chloroform/methanol 19/1 about 80%
saturated with water, applied to a Sephadex G-25 column, and
fractions eluted as previously described (5,7). The first fraction
from Sephadex is composed of lipids other than gangliosides. Fraction
one is free of water-soluble, low-molecular weight contaminants and
contains no more than 1-2% by weight protein. The second fraction
contains gangliosides with some protein. The third fraction contains
the nonlipid contaminants.

Molar amounts of phospholipids were determined by phosphorus
analysis after separation of lipid classes by two-dimensional thin
layer chromatography (8,9). Cerebroside and sulfatide were separated
from phospholipids by one-dimensional thin layer chromatography with
chloroform/methanol/water 65/25/4, the spots were located by spraying with water, dried, aspirated from the plate, and the molar
amounts determined by the hydrolytic trinitrobenzenesulfonic acid
procedure (10). Cholesterol was separated from other lipids by
one-dimensional thin layer chromatography with chloroform/methanol
98/2, spots aspirated into tubes, cholesterol extracted into 4 ml
of hexane after addition of 2 ml of water and 2 ml of ethanol, and
the molar amount of cholesterol determined in a 2 ml aliquot of the
hexane extract by the zinc chloride-acetyl chloride method (11).
Phospholipid determinations were done in quadruplicate. At least
8 determination of cerebroside, sulfatide and cholesterol were
needed to obtain data of comparable accuracy and precision.

Graphic analysis was accomplished as previously described (12,
13). Lipid class values (millimoles per 100 gm fresh weight) were
plotted against age or other lipid values on 16 x 20 inch graph
paper.

Brain samples from two cases of Tay-Sachs disease, one case of
infantile and two cases of juvenile Niemann-Pick disease, two cases
of acute infantile and one of chronic Gaucher's disease, and one
case of metachromatic leukodystrophy were provided by Dr. A. Knudson.

Tissue from Farber's disease was provided by Dr. Hugo Moser, from
Alzheimer's disease by Dr. Charles Altschuler, from GM_1 gangliosidosis by Dr. George Amromin, from paranoid schizophrenia and
mental depression by Dr. John Stevens, and from phenylketonuria by
Dr. Frank Yatsu. Two incompletely characterized forms of neuropathology (XP_1 and XP_2) were provided by Dr. Herbert Ichinose and
Dr. Kenneth Swaiman, respectively.

RESULTS

The lipid composition of normal human brain changes throughout
life (12-16). The changes can be defined graphically by plotting
lipid values for representative samples of whole brain against age.
The changes with age in total lipid content as percentage of the
fresh weight of normal human brain are shown in Figure 1. Three
periods are recognizable. The first period is one of rapid increase
of total lipid. In the second, total lipid increases slowly, and
in the third, total lipid declines. Although the changes may be
exponential in nature, segments can be divided into straight line
periods and similar results are obtained using arithmetic, semi-
logarithmic, or logarithmic paper.

Total lipid may be below normal or normal in metabolic disorders (Fig. 1). Total lipid content as percentage of the fresh
weight of brain is in the normal range in acute infantile and
chronic Gaucher's diseases, Alzheimer's disease, and some incompletely characterized forms of neuropathology such as case XP_2, as
well as patients classified as paranoid schizophrenic or depressive.
Total lipid is greatly reduced in Tay-Sachs disease, GM_1 gangliosidosis, metachromatic leukodystrophy, and infantile and juvenile
Niemann-Pick diseases.

When the total lipid content of brain is lower than normal on
the total lipid vs. age plot, the amounts of all or most of the
lipid classes will also be below normal when plotted as a function
of age. Thus, plots of lipid class values against age are difficult
to use for definition of abnormalities in the relative proportions
of lipid classes. Abnormal proportions (relative amounts) of the
lipid classes are clearly disclosed, however, by plotting lipid
class values against total phospholipid regardless of the total
lipid content.

The relationships among the polar lipid classes of normal
human brain that are disclosed by plotting values for representative samples of whole brain at different ages are the same as those
obtained by plotting values for samples from different regions of
the same adult brain (12,13). The relationships can thus be shown
with samples from different regions of adult brains (Fig. 2). The
good fit of lines to points demonstrates that both analytical and
biological variability are small. The values for the regions of two

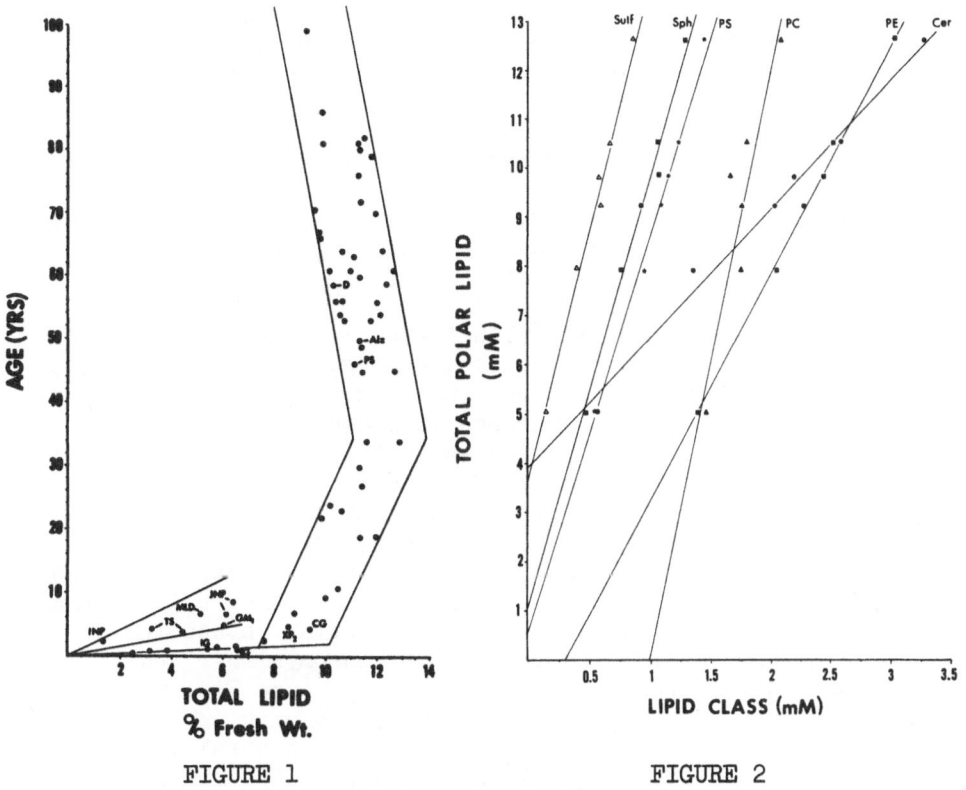

FIGURE 1

FIGURE 2

Fig. 1. <u>Plot of normal human brain total lipid (as percentage of
the fresh weight) against conceptual age in years.</u> Normal values
are not labeled. Values from metabolic disorders are designated as:
TS, Tay-Sachs disease; GM_1, GM_1 gangliosidosis; INP, infantile
Niemann-Pick disease; JNP, juvenile Niemann-Pick disease; MLD, metachromatic leukodystrophy; IG, acute infantile Gaucher's disease;
CG, chronic (juvenile) Gaucher's disease; Alz, Alzheimer's disease;
PS, paranoid schizophrenia; D, mental depression; XP, unclassified
disorder.

Fig. 2. <u>Plot of values (millimoles per 100 gm fresh weight) for
different lipid classes against total polar lipid</u> of different
regions of a normal human brain. Abbreviations: Sulf, sulfatide;
Sph, sphingomyelin; PS, phosphatidyl serine; PC, phosphatidyl
choline; PE, phosphatidyl ethanolamine; Cer, cerebroside. Note
that the values make straight lines, some of which have intercepts
on the vertical axis (percentage of component increases as total
lipid increases) and others with intercepts on the horizontal axis
(percentage of the component decreases as total lipid increases).

different brains are the same except that sphingomyelin is lower in
one. As total lipid rises, the molar percentages of cerebroside,
sulfatide, and sphingomyelin increase and the percentages of phosphatidyl choline and phosphatidyl ethanolamine decrease. Thus,
galactolipids and sphingomyelin replace phosphatidyl choline and
phosphatidyl ethanolamine. The exact nature of the substitution is
disclosed by plotting sums of values for lipid classes, i.e. values
for those that increase are added to those that decrease and plotted
against total polar lipid (12,13). The lipid classes that substitute for each other are determined by observing which sums give
straight lines passing through the origin.

Three lipid class sums give lines passing through the origin
(Fig. 3). The plots demonstrate that, during normal development,
cerebroside and sphingomyelin substitute for phosphatidyl choline,
and sulfatide substitutes for phosphatidyl ethanolamine. Also
acidic phospholipids substitute for each other. When cholesterol
values for representative samples of whole brain are plotted
against total polar lipid, straight lines passing through the
origin are obtained. Thus, cholesterol does not appear to engage
in substitution with polar lipid. In human brain there are three
polar lipid substitution groups. When data for other animal organs
were evaluated (12) it was found that phosphatidyl ethanolamine can
substitute for phosphatidyl choline and sphingomyelin. Thus, there
are only two general organ substitution groups (see Fig. 3). Group
I is composed of phosphatidyl choline, sphingomyelin, phosphatidyl
ethanolamine, sulfatide, cerebroside, and other neutral glycolipids.
Group II is composed of the acidic phospholipids (phosphatidyl
serine, phosphatidyl inositol, diphosphatidyl glycerol, and miscellaneous minor acidic phospholipids). As shown in Fig. 3, the
values for representative samples of whole brain from different
individuals form the same lines obtained with samples from different regions of one brain.

The results obtained for lipid classes of normal human brain
plotted against millimoles of total polar lipid or total lipid (as
percentage of the fresh weight) are summarized as equations for
lines defining the ranges, means, and subgroups in Tables I and II.
Abnormal proportions of lipid classes are not always detected when
lipid class values for abnormal states are plotted against total
polar lipid or total lipid because changes in one lipid class may
be counterbalanced by changes in another and cause values that are
in fact abnormal to fall within the normal range. In contrast,
abnormalities are clearly defined by plotting lipid class values
against total phospholipid.

The normal range was determined for each lipid class as shown
for phosphatidyl ethanolamine in Fig. 4. The spread of phosphatidyl
ethanolamine values is small and samples from different regions of

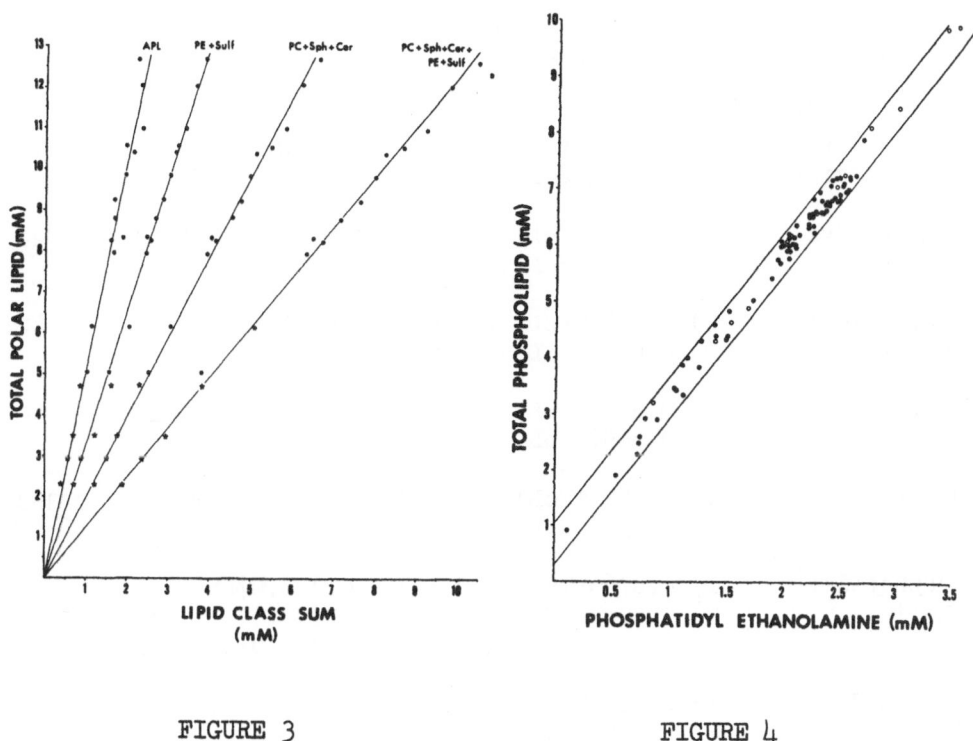

FIGURE 3   FIGURE 4

Fig. 3. <u>Plot of values (millimoles per 100 gm fresh weight) for
sums of lipid classes against total polar lipid</u> of different regions of 2 normal human brains (solid circles) and representative
samples from 4 whole brains (stars). Abbreviations as for Fig. 2
and in addition APL, acidic phospholipid. See text for comments.

Fig. 4. <u>Plot of values (millimoles per 100 gm fresh weight) for
phosphatidyl ethanolamine against total phospholipid</u> of normal
human brain to show the method used to find normal ranges. Solid
circles are values from representative samples of 52 different
whole brains and open circles are values from different regions
of 4 brains. Note that all values form a narrow range and that
values from whole brain and different regions of brain fall into
the same range. See text for further comments.

Table I

Ranges and Subgroup Lines for Lipid
Classes on Total Polar Lipid Plots[*]

Lipid Class	Range Lines	Mean Values and Subgroups
Phosphatidyl ethanolamine	1) 0.216(TPoL) + 0.138 2) 0.216(TPoL) + 0.407	M) 0.216(TPoL) + 0.274
Phosphatidyl serine	1) 0.119(TPoL) − 0.111 2) 0.119(TPoL) + 0.060	M) 0.119(TPoL) − 0.020
Phosphatidyl inositol	1) 0.014(TPoL) + 0.005 2) 0.014(TPoL) + 0.079	M) 0.014(TPoL) + 0.041
Cerebroside	1) 0.386(TPoL) − 1.702 2) 0.399(TPoL) − 1.502	M) 0.371(TPoL) − 1.440
Sulfatide	1) 0.099(TPoL) − 0.490 2) 0.099(TPoL) − 0.233	M) 0.099(TPoL) − 0.360
Phosphatidyl choline	1) 0.0765(TPoL)+ 0.964 2) 0.0765(TPoL)+ 1.403	G1) 0.0765(TPoL)+ 1.072 G2) 0.0765(TPoL)+ 1.180 G3) 0.0765(TPoL)+ 1.304
Sphingomyelin	1) 0.114(TPoL) − 0.319 2) 0.114(TPoL) − 0.067	G1) 0.114(TPoL) − 0.268 G2) 0.114(TPoL) − 0.199 G3) 0.114(TPoL) − 0.129
Ganglioside	Up to 4.44 mM TPoL 0.0363(TPoL) − 0.003 From 4.44 mM TPoL 0.0100(TPoL) + 0.202	
Substitution group I	1) 0.848(TPoL) 2) 0.756(TPoL)	G1) 0.838(TPoL) G2) 0.812(TPoL) G3) 0.786(TPoL)
Substitution group II	1) 0.139(TPoL) 2) 0.237(TPoL)	G1) 0.162(TPoL) G2) 0.188(TPoL) G3) 0.214(TPoL)

[*]Values as millimoles/100 gm fresh weight of tissues. Total polar lipid is the sum of the molar amounts of total phospholipid, cerebroside, and sulfatide. M is the mean value for lipid classes with one line only; G1, G2, and G3 are the three subgroups that differ in the amounts of the particular lipid class.

Table II

Ranges and Subgroup Lines for Lipid
Classes on Total Lipid Plots[*]

Lipid Class	Range Lines	Subgroups
Total Phospho- lipid	1) 0.452(TL) + 1.030 2) 0.452(TL) + 2.310	1) 0.452(TL) + 1.240 2) 0.452(TL) + 1.680 3) 0.452(TL) + 2.055
Phosphatidyl ethanolamine	1) 0.169(TL) + 0.256 2) 0.169(TL) + 0.704	1) 0.169(TL) + 0.325 2) 0.169(TL) + 0.467 3) 0.169(TL) + 0.604
Phosphatidyl serine	1) 0.689(TL) + 0.098 2) 0.689(TL) + 0.448	1) 0.689(TL) + 0.158 2) 0.689(TL) + 0.267 3) 0.689(TL) + 0.381
Phosphatidyl inositol	1) 0.0078(TL) + 0.023 2) 0.0078(TL) + 0.113	1) 0.0078(TL) + 0.004 2) 0.0078(TL) + 0.071 3) 0.0078(TL) + 0.096
Cerebroside	1) 0.271(TL) − 1.332 2) 0.271(TL) − 0.570	1) 0.271(TL) − 1.160 2) 0.271(TL) − 0.941 3) 0.271(TL) − 0.728
Sulfatide	1) 0.0728(TL) − 0.474 2) 0.0728(TL) − 0.104	1) 0.0728(TL) − 0.399 2) 0.0728(TL) − 0.285 3) 0.0728(TL) − 0.166
Phosphatidyl choline	1) 0.0515(TL) + 1.103 2) 0.0515(TL) + 1.582	1) 0.0515(TL) + 1.180 2) 0.0515(TL) + 1.347 3) 0.0515(TL) + 1.512
Sphingomyelin	1) 0.0855(TL) − 0.251 2) 0.0855(TL) − 0.014	1) 0.0855(TL) − 0.200 2) 0.0855(TL) − 0.130 3) 0.0855(TL) − 0.043
Cholesterol	1) 0.493(TL) 2) 0.717(TL)	1) 0.520(TL) 2) 0.607(TL) 3) 0.680(TL)
Substitution group I	1) 0.607(TL) 2) 0.780(TL)	1) 0.639(TL) 2) 0.693(TL) 3) 0.742(TL)
Substitution group II	1) 0.128(TL) 2) 0.184(TL)	1) 0.139(TL) 2) 0.155(TL) 3) 0.171(TL)

[*]Total lipid as percentage of the fresh weight and determined from
the weight of Sephadex fraction 1 which excludes gangliosides.
Lipid class values as millimoles/100 gm fresh weight.

adult brains fall in the same range as those for representative
samples of whole brain at different ages. There is very little
biological or analytical variability in this case. All plots
except that for total ganglioside (Fig. 5) give lines without a
turn upward or downward (12,13).

The normal ranges for the lipid classes and findings in abnormal states are shown in Figs. 6-16. The findings are summarized
in Table III. The amounts of phosphatidyl ethanolamine, phosphatidyl serine, and phosphatidyl inositol are in or very near the
normal range in all abnormal states. In most cases, the relative
amounts of cerebroside, sulfatide, and sphingomyelin are increased
in the sphingolipidoses regardless of which sphingolipid accumulates
to the greatest extent and the percentage of phosphatidyl choline
is reduced. Patients with the least deviation from normal of
total lipid content show the least deviation from normal of lipid
class distribution. The changes in phenylketonuria resemble those
in the sphingolipidoses, but the abnormalities are even greater
and a large increase in the amount of triglyceride is apparent by
thin layer chromatography. Cerebroside and sulfatide percentages
are above normal in Farber's disease, and accumulation of a
ceramide polyhexoside is apparent by thin layer chromatography.
No distinct abnormalities were apparent in Alzheimer's disease,
acute infantile and chronic (juvenile) Gaucher's diseases, paranoid
schizophrenia, mental depression, or the incompletely characterized
case XP_1. One of the unclassified patients (XP_2) with a normal
total lipid had only one lipid class percentage abnormality, a high
level of residual acidic phospholipids (total acidic phospholipid
minus phosphatidyl serine and phosphatidyl inositol).

                                DISCUSSION

The earliest analyses of normal human brain cerebral cortex
and white matter showed that, compared to grey matter, white matter
contains a greater percentage of galactolipid and sphingolipid and
a lower percentage of phosphatidyl choline. It was concluded that
myelin contains more galactolipid and sphingomyelin than other membranes in brain and this has since been confirmed by analysis of
purified myelin preparations. Several laboratories studied changes
with age of normal human brain lipids by analysis of grey and white
matter samples and found the changes to be confined to about the
first year of life (14-21). Subsequent study of the changes with
age (fetal life to 98 years) using representative samples of 13
whole brains disclosed that lipid changes occur throughout life
(22-24). When the number of samples in the series was increased,
it became apparent that the total lipid content and lipid class
composition of brains from individuals of the same age can be
different (12,13).

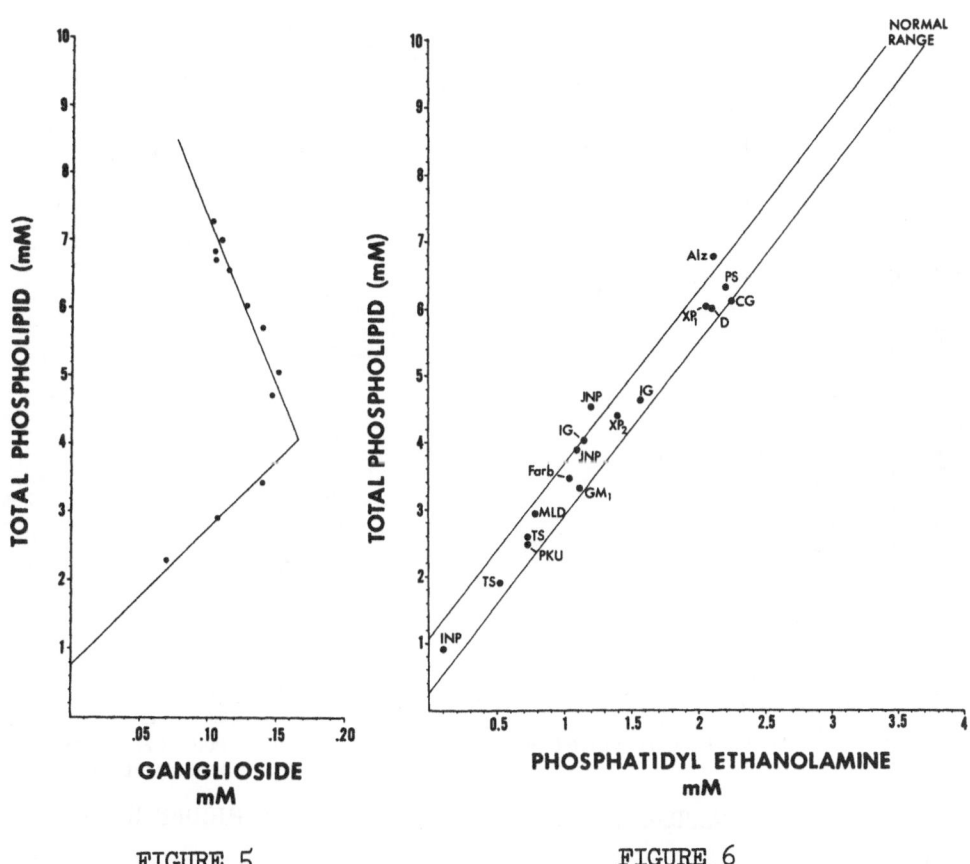

FIGURE 5   FIGURE 6

Fig. 5. <u>Plot of normal human brain values (millimoles per 100 gm</u>
<u>fresh weight) for total ganglioside against total phospholipid.</u>
Total ganglioside first increases and then decreases in contrast
to all other lipid classes that have the relationships shown in
Fig. 2.

Fig. 6. <u>Plot of values (millimoles per 100 gm fresh weight) of</u>
<u>phosphatidyl ethanolamine against total phospholipid</u> obtained
from brains of persons with metabolic disorders with the normal
range defined. Abbreviations are given in the legend of Fig. 1.
Note that all values are essentially normal. See text for further comments.

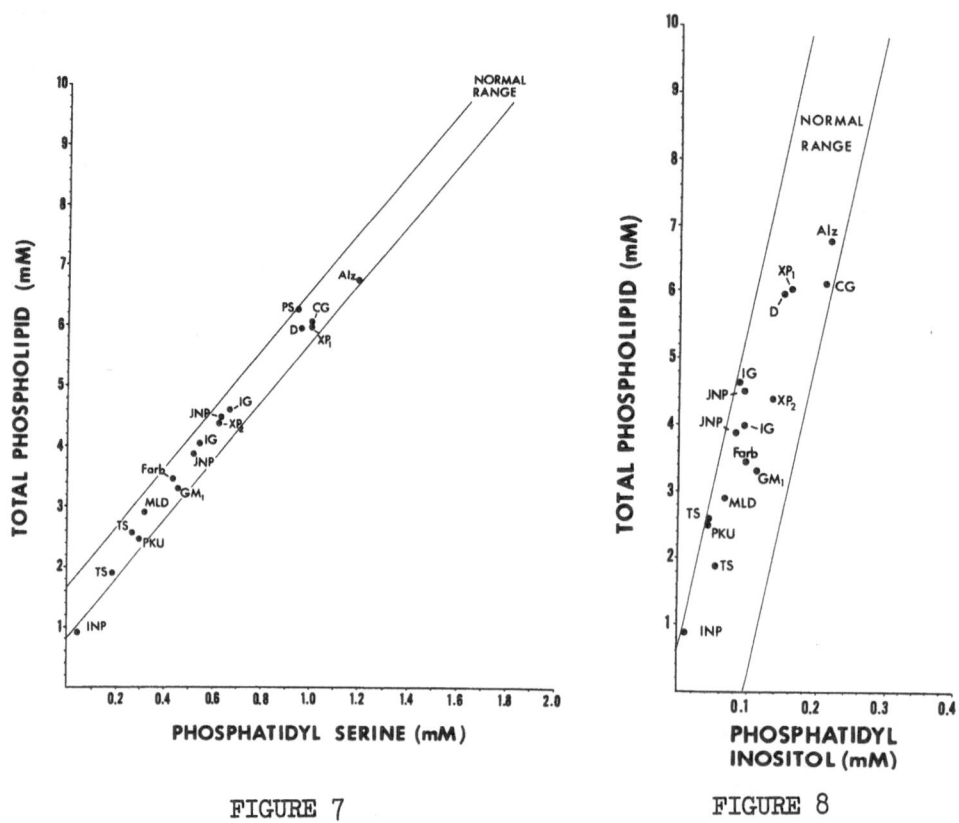

FIGURE 7   FIGURE 8

Fig. 7. <u>Plot of values (millimoles per 100 gm fresh weight) of phosphatidyl serine against total phospholipid</u> obtained from brains of persons with metabolic disorders with the normal range defined. Abbreviations are given in the legend to Fig. 1. Note that all values are essentially normal. See text for additional comments.

Fig. 8. <u>Plot of values (millimoles per 100 gm fresh weight) of phosphatidyl inositol against total phospholipid</u> obtained from brains of persons with metabolic disorders with the normal range defined. Abbreviations are given in the legend to Fig. 1. See text for comments.

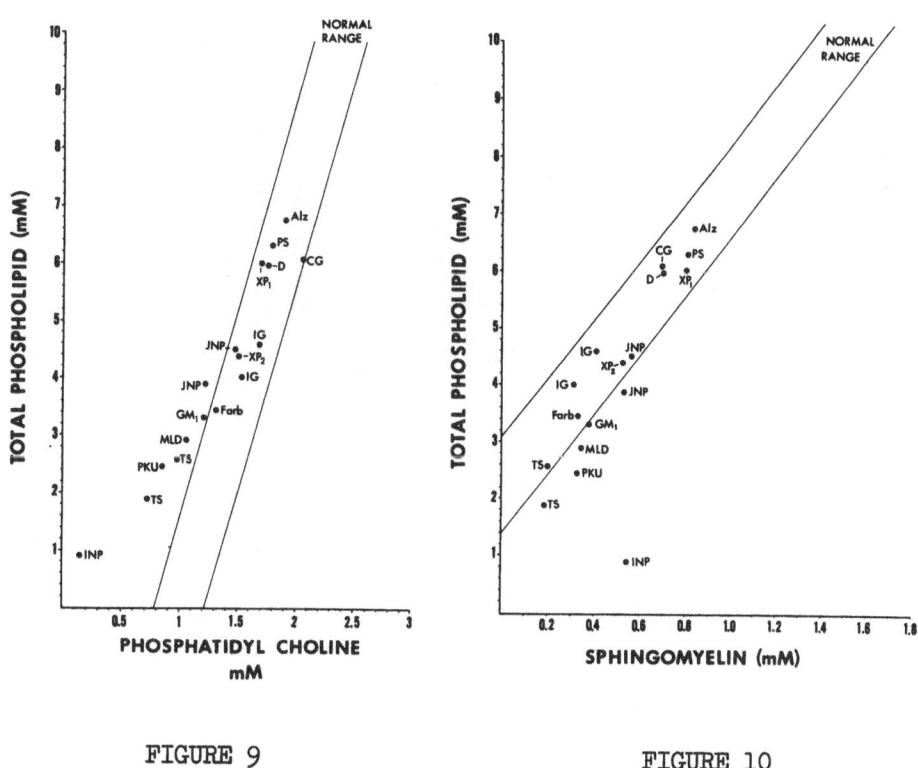

FIGURE 9   FIGURE 10

Fig. 9. Plot of values (millimoles per 100 gm fresh weight) of
phosphatidyl choline against total phospholipid obtained from
brains of persons with metabolic disorders with the normal range
defined. Abbreviations are given in the legend to Fig. 1. Note
that values for sphingolipid disorders are generally low. See
text for additional comments.

Fig. 10. Plot of values (millimoles per 100 gm fresh weight) of
sphingomyelin against total phospholipid obtained from brains of
persons with metabolic disorders with the normal range defined.
Abbreviations are given in the legend to Fig. 1. See text for
comments.

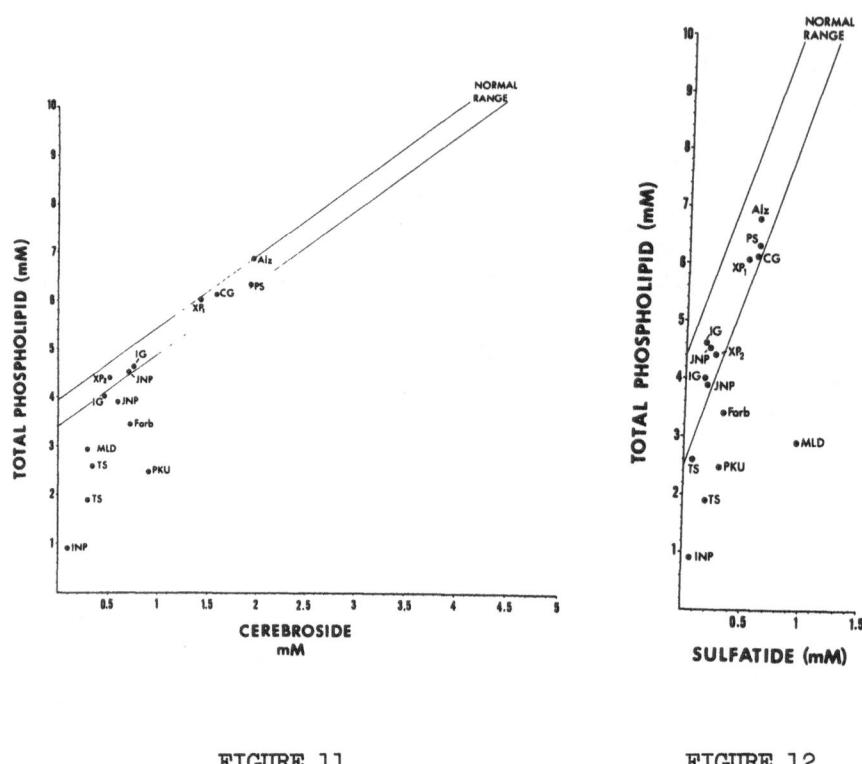

FIGURE 11   FIGURE 12

Fig. 11. <u>Plot of values (millimoles per 100 gm fresh weight) of
cerebroside against total phospholipid</u> obtained from brains of
persons with metabolic disorders with the normal range defined.
Abbreviations are given in the legend to Fig. 1. Note in particular the large increase of cerebroside in phenylketonuria. See
text for additional comments.

Fig. 12. <u>Plot of values (millimoles per 100 gm fresh weight) of
sulfatide against total phospholipid</u> obtained from brains of
persons with metabolic disorders with the normal range defined.
Abbreviations are given in the legend to Fig. 1. Note that values
for the sphingolipid disorders, phenylketonuria and Farber's
disease are above normal.

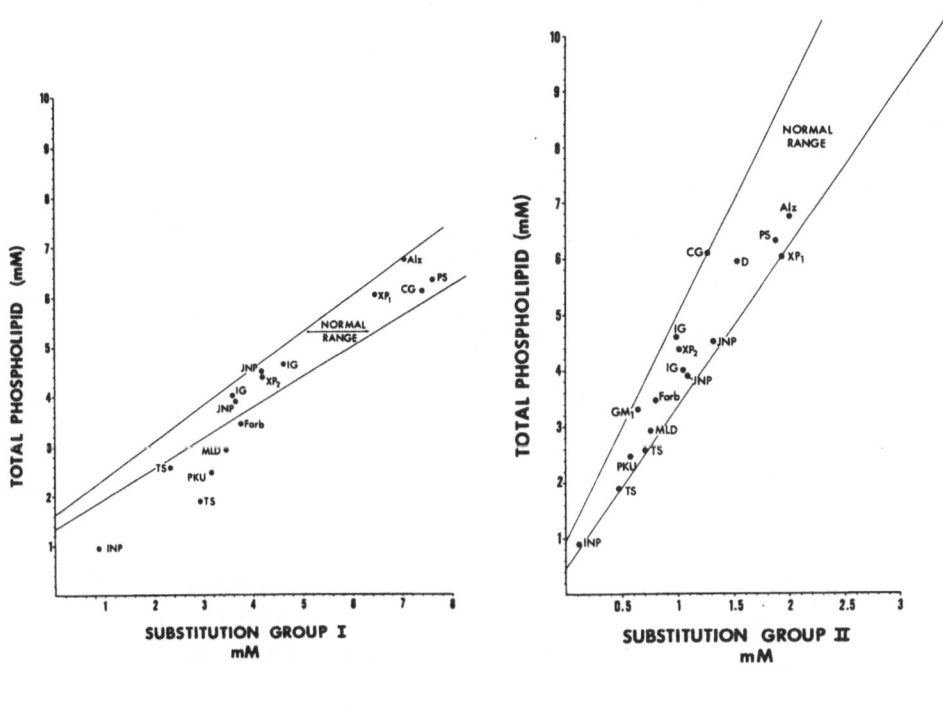

FIGURE 13   FIGURE 14

Fig. 13. <u>Plot of values (millimoles per 100 gm fresh weight) of</u>
<u>substitution group I against total phospholipid</u> obtained from
brains of persons with metabolic disorders with the normal range
defined. Abbreviations are given in the legend to Fig. 1. Note
that most values are in or only slightly outside the normal range.
See text for additional comments.

Fig. 14. <u>Plot of values (millimoles per 100 gm fresh weight) of</u>
<u>substitution group II against total phospholipid</u> obtained from
brains of persons with metabolic disorders with the normal range
defined. Abbreviations are given in the legend to Fig. 1. See
text for comments.

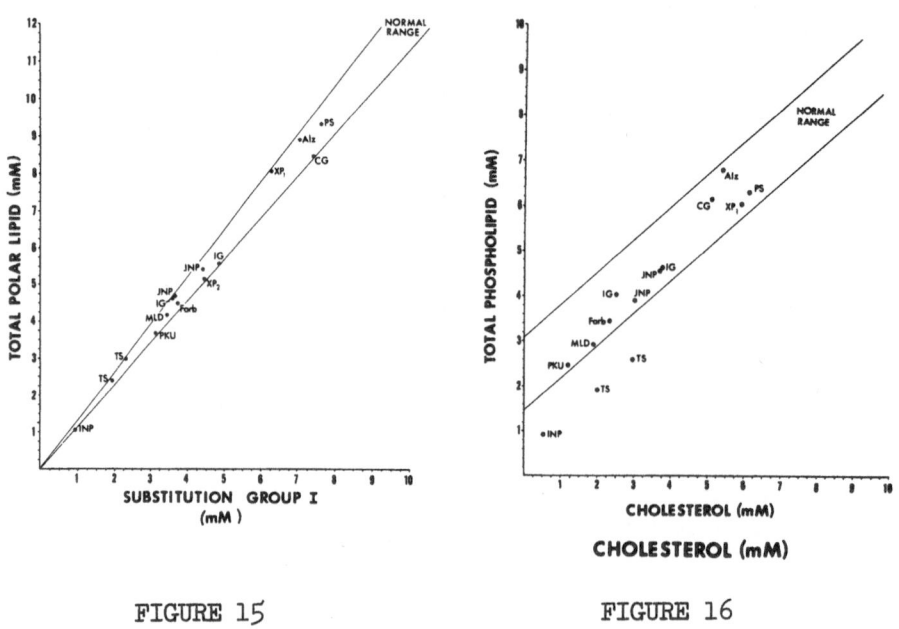

FIGURE 15   FIGURE 16

Fig. 15. <u>Plot of values (millimoles per 100 gm fresh weight) of
substitution group I against total polar lipid</u> obtained from brains
of persons with metabolic disorders with the normal range defined.
Abbreviations are given in the legend to Fig. 1. See text for
comments.

Fig. 16. <u>Plot of values (millimoles per 100 gm fresh weight) of
cholesterol against total phospholipid</u> obtained from brains of
persons with metabolic disorders with the normal range defined.
Abbreviations are given in the legend to Fig. 1. A distinct
elevation is clear for Tay-Sachs disease. See text for additional comments.

TABLE III

SUMMARY OF FINDINGS FOR LIPID CLASS

DISTRIBUTION IN PATHOLOGICAL STATES*

Case	TL/Age	PC	Sph	Cer	Sulf	G	PE	PS	PI	RAPL	SG I	SG II	Chol
1. PS	N	N	N	N	N	N	N	N	N	N	N	N	(+)
2. D	N	N	N	N	N	N	N	N	N	N	N	N	(+)
3. CG	N	N	N	(+)	N	N	N	N	N	N	N	N	N
4. IG-1	N	N	(-)	N	N	N	N	(-)	N	N	N	N	N
5. IG-1	N	N	N	N	(-)	N	(-)	(-)	N	(+)	N	N	N
6. Alz	N	N	N	N	N	N	N	(+)	N	N	N	(+)	(+)
7. XP-1	ND	ND	N	H	H	H	N	N	N	N	N	N	H
8. TS-1	L	L	(+)	H	H	H	N	N	N	N	N	N	H
9. TS-2	L	L	(+)	H	H	H	N	N	N	N	N	N	(+)
10. GM1	L	L	H	H	H	H	(-)	N	(-)	(+)	N	N	H
11. INP	L	L	H	(+)	N	H	N	N	(-)	(+)	N	N	N
12. JNP-1	L	N	(+)	N	(+)	(+)	N	N	N	N	N	N	N
13. JNP-2	L	L	H	N	H	H	N	N	N	N	N	N	N
14. MLD	L	L	H	H	H	H	N	N	N	N	N	N	(+)
15. PKU	ND	L	N	N	N	H	N	N	N	N	N	N	(+)
16. XP-2	N	N	N	H	H	H	N	N	N	H	N	(+)	N
17. Farb	ND	N	N	H	H	H	N	N	N	N	N	N	N

*Abbreviations for cases as in the legend for Fig. 1, also Farb, Farber's disease; PKU, phenylketonuria. Lipid class abbreviations as in the legend for Fig. 2, also Chol, cholesterol; G, total ganglioside; and RAPL, residual acidic phospholipids (substitution group II minus phosphatidyl serine and phosphatidyl inositol). N, normal; (+), slightly above normal; (-), slightly below normal; H, high; L, low; ND, not determined. The most significant deviations from normal are made more apparent by their inclusion in rectangles.

      The large range of individual variability makes precise defi-
nition of normal human brain changes with age difficult because
fitting of range lines and lines through points on graphs cannot
be done unambiguously unless data are available for a large number
of samples. The most recently published equations (13) appear to
be reasonably accurate, although more precise definition will be
possible when more data are available.

      Precise definition of the relationships of each lipid class to
total lipid, total polar lipid, total phospholipid, and other lipid
classes has been attempted only recently (12,13). Three major
difficulties were encountered. One was how to proceed with graphic
analysis. Another was the finding that, because of individual
variations, a large number of samples was necessary. In addition,
analytical errors were detected that arose from mistakes of the
analyst rather than the relatively small random fluctuations of
the methods when properly applied. The lipid class relationships
reported in this communication differ in some respects from those
previously published (12,13) and represent steady progress in over-
coming each of the major difficulties noted above. The larger
number of normal samples available at present (52 whole brain values
for most lipid classes and values for 15 samples from different
regions of 4 brains) make the extent of individual variations more
apparent. Two methods were used for detection of errors outside
of the range of variation of the methods used. First, samples
were selected at random and values were redetermined. Second, samples showing values that appeared to be higher or lower than most
of the samples when examined by graphic analysis were analyzed
again.

      The best current analysis of the data indicates that, within
the range of experimental error, only one line is obtained when
values for phosphatidyl ethanolamine, phosphatidyl serine, phosphatidyl inositol, cerebroside, and sulfatide are plotted against
total phospholipid or total polar lipid. The range for phosphatidyl
choline, sphingomyelin, and cholesterol is outside of the range of
analytical variability. This suggests that biological variation
is responsible for the broad range. Normal human whole brain
values give the impression of a continuum for phosphatidyl choline
and sphingomyelin (25). However, a definite clustering of points
about the central region and the two outer regions of the range of
values is seen on cholesterol plots (25), and thus, three separate
groups are indicated for cholesterol. Samples from different
regions of one brain can be used to determine whether or not values
may wander around within the entire range of normal values. As
indicated in Figs. 2, 3, 9, 10, and 16, values for different
regions of one brain do not fall throughout the entire range of
phosphatidyl choline, sphingomyelin, and cholesterol values.
Rather, they form straight lines restricted either to the central
or outer parts of the range of values. This indicates that there

are at least three different and reproducible biological subgroups.
These subgroups are indicated by the three lines within the range
lines in Figs. 10-12 and 14-16. The large ranges for all lipid
classes on plots against total lipid appear to arise from the
existence of at least 3 subgroups (Table II).

The large elevations in brain of ganglioside in Tay-Sachs disease and sphingomyelin in Niemann-Pick disease as well as the elevation of cerebroside in organs in Gaucher's disease were recognized
even before chromatographic techniques were available. In the absence
of such large increases in the relative amount of one lipid class,
most investigators have not been able to distinguish abnormalities of
brain development with normal lipid class distribution from those in
which the lipid class distribution is abnormal. The nature of the
brain lipid changes in disease can be defined very precisely with
accurate data obtained by the analytical methods now available and
the method of data analysis presented in this report.

The lipid composition of brain in chronic Gaucher's disease
appears to be normal in every respect. This is not surprising
since there is no prominent neurological abnormality. The failure
to find any distinct abnormality of brain polar lipids in the acute
infantile form of Gaucher's disease in which functional abnormalities of the nervous system are present is, however, somewhat unexpected. Our findings confirm our earlier report (26) but differ
from those of Banker et al. (27). The differences are explainable
by use of better methods for lipid analysis and an improved means
of comparison to normal values in our studies. In our studies, no
distinct abnormalities of brain lipid class distribution were observed in any case with total phospholipid at or above 4.5 millimoles
per 100 gm fresh weight. It is apparent that brain lipids may not
be altered appreciably by enzyme changes that produce large changes
in other organs or blood plasma. Abnormalities of lipid metabolism
may thus be detected in some cases only by analysis of blood and
organs other than brain.

The sphingolipid disorders in which a large increase in one
sphingolipid is found show a common pattern of change. Regardless
of which sphingolipid accumulates, the amounts of the other
sphingolipids are increased. Patients with the smallest increases
of the lipid for which there is an enzyme deficiency may show little
or no increase of the other sphingolipids. The increase of sphingolipids is balanced by a decrease of phosphatidyl choline. The
relative amounts of phosphatidyl ethanolamine, phosphatidyl serine,
and phosphatidyl inositol are normal. Thus, failure to degrade any
one sphingolipid leads to replacement of phosphatidyl choline by
sphingolipids. The present findings are in agreement with those in
our earlier report (26). Brain polar lipid changes in phenylketonuria are similar to those found in the sphingolipid disorders. In
addition, an increase in triglyceride is apparent. The latter change

indicates that brain degeneration with release of fatty acids was
more rapid than oxidation or loss of fatty acids to blood. The
increased levels of sphingolipids in the sphingolipidoses and
phenylketonuria can be explained by slower degradation of sphingolipids than phosphatidyl choline during brain degeneration. This
interpretation is in keeping with isotope studies that have shown
sphingolipids to turn over more slowly than phosphatidyl choline.
We conclude that the brain lipid changes in phenylketonuria are
the result of degeneration caused in some unknown manner by the
abnormality of phenylalanine metabolism.

Brain lipid changes in Farber's lipogranulomatosis are rather
similar to those seen in the classical sphingolipid disorders. A
definite increase of ceramide polyhexoside and ganglioside is apparent and the relative amounts of cerebroside and sulfatide are
above normal. Studies of other organs have indicated accumulation
of both glycolipid and polysaccharide (see review of the literature
in ref. 28). Lipid analysis by older methods indicated accumulation
of sphingomyelin, ganglioside, and neutral glycolipid in organs
other than brain with a large elevation of ceramide that did not
arise from a deficiency of ceramidase (28). Based upon these
findings, Prensky et al. (28) concluded that Farber's disease is a
lipidosis. Clausen and Rampini (29) studied brain and liver lipids
in Farber's disease and noted in particular an elevation of ganglioside and a ceramide polyhexoside with a glucose to galactosamine
ratio of 4/1.

The Farber's disease tissues investigated by Prensky et al. (28)
have been examined in our laboratory, although the data have not
been published. The data confirm and extend previous findings. A
very polar ceramide polyhexoside with chromatographic mobility
similar to that of red cell globoside was found in above normal
amounts in brain, liver, lung, and kidney. The large elevation
of ceramide reported by Prensky et al. (28) was confirmed by
two-dimensional thin layer chromatography. Free fatty acid was
also increased as was sphingomyelin, particularly in kidney. There
was a striking decrease of phosphatidyl ethanolamine without
accumulation of lysophosphatidyl ethanolamine in liver, lung, and
kidney (but not in brain). The data suggest that the disorder
arises from a deficiency of a degradative enzyme acting upon the
ceramide polyhexoside. The accumulation of ganglioside does not
appear to arise from a failure to degrade ganglioside since a
normal distribution of ganglioside types was found (28). The
increase of ganglioside, ceramide, sphingomyelin, and free fatty
acid as well as the decrease in phosphatidyl ethanolamine are
probably secondary changes. It is to be noted that large secondary
changes are found in Niemann-Pick disease in which lysobisphosphatidic acid accumulates in liver and spleen (30). It appears that
Farber's disease is similar to GM_1 gangliosidosis in which there

is polysaccharide accumulation with both lipid and polysaccharide changes probably arising from the same enzyme deficiency. It seems probable that the conclusion derived from analysis of all lipid classes in organs from Farber's disease will prove to be as accurate as those drawn previously for Tay-Sachs disease, Gaucher's disease, metachromatic leukodystrophy, and Niemann-Pick disease (31-33) and since confirmed by enzyme assay.

Total lipid was in the normal range on the age plots for case XP_2. All major lipid class levels were normal, but the miscellaneous minor acidic phospholipids (residual acidic lipids) were elevated. This suggests a deficiency of a phospholipase with specificity for acidic phospholipids. This is also suggested by our finding that, in spleen, lysobisphosphatidic acid is increased to about 4.5% of the total phospholipid. Abnormal lipid deposits in spleen were apparent histologically. The significance of these changes is uncertain, however, because lysobisphosphatidic acid is increased in Niemann-Pick disease (30), and a large accumulation (up to 27% of the total phospholipid) has been associated with the administration of a drug (34, 35).

It is important to note that graphic analysis can be used to determine whether or not lipid class proportions are normal when a few milligrams of tissue from any region of the brain is available from biopsy or autopsy. Since our method for determination of phospholipids is quite sensitive, as little as 100 nanograms of lipid phosphorus (2.5 µg of phospholipid) is adequate for one accurate determination of the amounts of phosphatidyl choline, phosphatidyl ethanolamine, sphingomyelin, phosphatidyl serine, and phosphatidyl inositol. This can be done with as little as 100 µg of total lipid obtainable on the average from about 1 mg of tissue. Slightly larger samples make possible evaluation of cholesterol, cerebroside, and sulfatide levels as well. Quadruplicate determination of all phospholipid classes including minor components, cholesterol, cerebroside, and sulfatide can be performed accurately and conveniently with lipid from 15-50 milligrams of tissue.

ACKNOWLEDGEMENTS

This work was supported in part by U.S. Public Health Service Grants NS 01847 and NS 06237 from the National Institute of Neurological Diseases and Stroke.

REFERENCES

(1) Fredrickson, D.S., and Lees, R.S. in The Metabolic Basis of Inherited Disease, 2nd Ed. (Eds. J.B. Stanbury, J.B. Wyngaarden, and D.S. Fredrickson), Blakiston Div., McGraw-Hill Book Co., 429-485 (1966).

(2) Brady, R.O. Chem. Phys. Lipids 5: 261 (1970).

(3) O'Brien, J.S., Okada, S., Ho, M.W., Fillerup, D.L., Veath, M.L., and Adams, K. Fed. Proc. 30: 956 (1971).

(4) Steinberg, D., Herndon, J.H.,Jr., Uhlendorf, B.W., Avigan, J., Mize, C.E., and Fales, H.M. J. Clin. Invest. 46: 1120 (1967).

(5) Rouser, G., Simon, G., and Kritchevsky, G. Lipids 4: 599 (1969).

(6) Rouser, G., Kritchevsky, G., Heller, D., and Lieber, E. J. Amer. Oil Chemists' Soc. 40: 425 (1963).

(7) Siakotos, A.N. and Rouser, G. J. Amer. Oil Chemists' Soc. 42: 913 (1965).

(8) Rouser, G., Siakotos, A.N., and Fleischer, S. Lipids 1: 85 (1966).

(9) Rouser, G., Fleischer, S., and Yamamoto, A. Lipids 5: 294 (1970).

(10) Yamamoto, A., and Rouser, G. Lipids 5: 442 (1970).

(11) Hanel, H.K., and Dam, H. Acta Chem. Scand. 9: 677 (1955).

(12) Rouser, G., Yamamoto, A., and Kritchevsky, G. Arch. Int. Med. 127: 1105 (1971).

(13) Rouser, G., Yamamoto, A., and Kritchevsky, G. in Advances in Exp. Med. & Biol., Vol. 14: Chemistry and Brain Development (Eds. R. Paoletti and A.N. Davison), Plenum Press, 91-109 (1971).

(14) Cumings, J.N., Goodwin, H., Woodward, E.M., and Curzon, G. J. Neurochem. 2: 289 (1958).

(15) O'Brien, J.S., Fillerup, D.L., and Mead, J.F. J. Lipid Res. 5: 109 (1964).

(16) O'Brien, J.S., and Sampson, E.L. J. Lipid Res. 6: 537 (1965).

(17) Ställberg-Stenhagen, S. and Svennerholm, L. J. Lipid Res. 6: 146 (1965).

(18) Menkes, J.H., Philippart, M., and Concone, M.C. J. Lipid Res. 7: 479 (1966).

(19) Fillerup, D.L., and Mead, J.F. Lipids 2: 295 (1967).

(20) Svennerholm, L. J. Lipid Res. 9: 570 (1968).

(21) Svennerholm, L., and Ställberg-Stenhagen, S. J. Lipid Res. 9: 215 (1968).

(22) Rouser, G., and Yamamoto, A. Lipids 3: 284 (1968).

(23) Rouser, G., and Yamamoto, A. in Handbook of Neurochemistry, Vol. I (Ed. A. Lajtha), Plenum Press, 121-169 (1969).

(24) Rouser, G., Kritchevsky, G., Siakotos, A., and Yamamoto, A. in Neuropathology: Methods and Diagnosis (Ed. C.G. Tedeschi) Little Brown & Co., 691-752 (1970).

(25) Rouser, G., Kritchevsky, G., Yamamoto, A., and Baxter, C.F. in Advances in Lipid Research (Eds. R. Paoletti and D. Kritchevsky), Academic Press (in press)

(26) Rouser, G., Kritchevsky, G., Galli, C., Yamamoto, A., and Knudson, A. in Inborn Disorders of Sphingolipid Metabolism (Eds. S.M. Aronson and B.W. Volk), Pergamon Press, 303-316 (1967).

(27) Banker, B.Q., Miller, J.Q., and Crocker, A.C. in Cerebral Sphingolipidoses (Eds. S.M. Aronson and B.W. Volk), Academic Press, 73-99 (1962).

(28) Prensky, A.L., Ferreira, G., Carr, S., and Moser, H.W. Proc. Soc. Exper. Biol. Med. 126: 725 (1967).

(29) Clausen, J., and Rampini, S. Acta Neurol. Scand. 46: 313 (1970).

(30) Rouser, G., Kritchevsky, G., Yamamoto, A., Knudson, A., and Simon, G. Lipids 3: 287 (1968).

(31) Rouser, G., Galli, C., and Kritchevsky, G. J. Amer. Oil Chemists' Soc. 42: 404 (1965).

(32) Rouser, G., Feldman, G., and Galli, C. J. Am. Oil Chemists' Soc. 42: 411 (1965).

(33) Rouser, G., Kritchevsky, G., and Galli, C. J. Amer. Oil Chemists' Soc. 42: 412 (1965).

(34) Yamamoto, A., Adachi, S., Ishibe, T., Shinji, Y., Kaki-Uchi, Y., Seki, K.I., and Kitani, T. Lipids 5: 566 (1970).

(35) Yamamoto, A., Adachi, S., Kitani, T., Shinji, Y., Seki, K., Nasu, T., and Nishikawa, M. J. Biochem. 69: 613 (1971)

BRAIN GLYCOPROTEINS AND INTER-CELL RECOGNITION:

TAY-SACHS' DISEASE AND INTRANEURONAL RECOGNITION

Samuel Bogoch, M.D., Ph.D.

Boston University School of Medicine

Foundation for Research on the Nervous System and

Dreyfus Medical Foundation

INTRODUCTION

In earlier work we demonstrated that the carbohydrate abnormality in Tay-Sachs' Disease was not confined to the brain gangliosides, but that there was in addition a generalized increase in glycoprotein hexose and hexosamine (4). One glycoprotein fraction, 10B, was found to be markedly increased in concentration. It was noted that this might be a function of the marked gliosis, since there was other evidence that 10B is a glial constituent. In that report, the information functions of the brain glycoproteins was proposed, and in related studies (summarized in reference 1) the general function of brain glycoproteins in intercell recognition was proposed ("Sign-Post" Theory).

In the present report, the hypothesis is advanced that Tay-Sachs' Disease is a disorder of intraneuronal recognition, and two types of further evidence in support of the "Sign-Post" theory are summarized:

1. Expression: changes occur in both the concentration of, and radioactive exchange of the carbohydrates in glycoproteins of the training as compared to resting brain.

2. Regression: changes in the structure of the carbohydrate moieties of the brain glycoproteins occur with the loss of higher cell functions. These changes in the case of glial tumors appear to result in the "unmasking" of certain antigenic sites

of 10B, permitting immunofluorescent labeling of their cells or origin by specific 10B antisera. That the unmasking of 10B occurs only in actively dividing astrocytic glia at the growing edge of glial brain tumors suggests that this is an index of malignant change. Malignant change is characterized by the loss of such higher information functions as specific recognition, contact and position of cells. That these changes in brain glycoproteins can be observed in the glycoproteins of the intact brain of mice at some distance from the glial tumor implanted subcutaneously on their backs, as reported here, suggests the existence of a Distance Factor (DF) which may be responsible for the induction of precancerous or early cancerous change in normal cells.

In the discussion, the overgrowth of membranes in Tay-Sachs' Disease is compared to the overgrowth of cells in tumors.

SUMMARY OF RECENT STUDIES ON BRAIN GLYCOPROTEIN 10B

Brain glycoprotein 10B was first isolated from normal brain tissue and from brain tumors in 1964. 10B was also isolated from a brain tumor of the ependymoma-glioma type grown subcutaneously in mouse (1), from normal cat hippocampus and caudate nuclei (1), from normal mouse brain, normal pigeon brain, and from subcellular fractions of guinea pig brain (1). 10B is structurally distinguished from microtubule protein (7), S100 protein (8), antigen α (9), and the alkylated brain protein (10). Antisera prepared to brain 10B did not react with proteins of other organs or serum.

10B was found to be concentrated six to nine fold in glial brain tumors (1). In addition it was shown to be increased in concentration in Tay-Sachs' Disease brain in the presence of marked gliosis (4). It was found to be concentrated in glial tumor cells grown in tissue culture (1), and in the outer membranous fractions ("ghosts") of lysates of these glial tumor cells (1). These observations together led to the impression that 10B is a glial constituent. This assumption is clearly supported by the immunochemical data herein reviewed.

10B was shown to increase in concentration in normal pigeon brain during operant conditioning (1, 2). ^{14}C-Glucose was rapidly and markedly incorporated into the carbohydrates of 10B during training (1, 2, 5). The increase in 10B concentration was followed days later by a return to normal levels of 10B and a concomitant increase in the concentration of the associated brain glycoprotein 11A (1). For this reason, and because of the structural similarities later demonstrated between 10B and 11A, the possibility that 10B is a biosynthetic precursor of 11A has been considered (2).

PREPARATION OF 10B

Normal brain or brain tumor tissue is dissected free of meninges and gross blood, and homogenized in 0.005M phosphate buffer, pH 7, in the ratio of 1 gram of tissue to 100ml. of buffer. For samples under 0.5g, the Potter Elvejham homogenizer is used and for samples greater in size than 0.5g., the Waring blender is used. Specimens are extracted in the cold room in pre-cooled homogenizers. The first extraction is over a three minute period. The homogenate is centrifuged at 80,000 for 30 minutes in a Beckman Model L ultracentrifuge. The supernate is decanted, the residue rehomogenized with a further equal volume of phosphate buffer, centrifuged again, and the second supernate combined with the first. The extraction of the residue is repeated with fresh buffer until less than 50 micrograms of protein is extracted from the residue. For most specimens this is accomplished in 4 or 5 homogenizations. The soluble proteins thus obtained are combined (extract A), dialyzed at 4° C for four hours against 4 liters 0.005M phosphate buffer, with constant magnetic stirring of the dialyzate, then concentrated approximately ten-fold by perevaporation to a final volume of dialysand of around 15ml. This dialysand is dialyzed once more against 4 liters of phosphate buffer a 4^0C with stirring. On completion, the volume of the dialysand is noted, an aliquot is taken for total protein analysis, and the balance is fractionated in the cold room on a DEAE cellulose (Cellex D) column, 2.5 x 11.0 centimeters, which has been equilibrated with 0.005M sodium phosphate buffer. Stepwise eluting solvent changes are made according to the schedule previously given (ref. 1, see pg. 123) such that solution 1 begins with tube 1, solution 2 with tube 88, solution 3 with tube 98, solution 4 with tube 144, solution 5 with tube 155 and solution 6 with tube 187. Solution 7, which begins with 212, provides groups 10B and 11A, and finally 0.3% Triton X-100 is begun with tube 260, to elute groups 11B, 12 and 13. Folin-Lowry protein determinations are made on each tube (1). The total protein in all of the groups thus obtained provides the final yield of protein, in milligram per gram of original weight of brain or tumor tissue. The 10B thus isolated can be rechromatographed on a fresh column of Cellex-D, with the same solvents, with no essential loss.

Table 1
AMINO ACID COMPOSITION OF BRAIN PROTEINS 10 B1 AND 10 B11
(Residues per 1000 residues)

	10 B1		10 B11	
	Pigeon	Human Tumor	Pigeon	Human Tumor
Glu	129.5	136.8	132.9	139.6
Asp	103.2	102.5	98.7	109.0
Leu	87.7	95.2	85.2	97.9
Ala	87.0	95.7	92.9	99.0
Gly	78.9	73.1	76.8	72.6
Lys	72.2	70.9	80.7	70.3
Ser	66.1	65.4	55.5	65.0
Val	61.4	51.8	63.2	51.0
Threo	52.6	54.8	51.0	54.9
Arg	48.6	51.3	59.4	52.3
Isoleu	43.8	29.5	43.2	28.3
Pro	41.8	41.7	43.2	47.8
Phe	33.0	36.8	31.8	36.4
Tyr	26.3	26.9	22.6	24.5
His	25.0	26.9	24.5	27.6
Cysteic	23.6	17.1	25.8	10.2
Meth (+cys)	19.6	14.6	12.9	13.3

Table 2
CARBOHYDRATE COMPOSITION OF PIGEON BRAIN GLYCOPROTEINS
10 B1, 10 B11 and 11A, as % of Protein (2)

Hexose	11.1	16.7	10.9
Hexosamine	16.2	17.9	4.6
Neuraminic Acid	0.6	1.0	0

PROPERTIES OF 10 B

10 B differs from microtubule protein (7) in its amino acid composition (Table 1), solubility at acidic pH (3 to 4), and insolubility at neutral and alkaline pH, and in that 10 B contains much more carbohydrate (Table 2) than microtubule protein.

10B differs from S100 protein (8) in several ways:

1. Its amino acid composition is quite different (Table 1);
2. Its carbohydrate content is high, whereas carbohydrate constituents are absent from S100;
3. Immunologically, 10B and S100 are completely distinct (2);
4. S100 appears to be cytoplasmic, whereas 10B appears to be predominately membranous in localization (1, 11);

10B differs also in its amino acid composition from antigen α (9).

HYDROLYSIS OF GLYCOPROTEINS, ION-EXCHANGE COLUMN CHROMATOGRAPHY AND THIN-LAYER CHROMATOGRAPHY OF CONSTITUENT HEXOSE AND HEXOSAMINE.

The methods described here will be more fully presented elsewhere (25). Each glycoprotein was hydrolyzed under nitrogen in a sealed glass tube with 2N HCl (50 mg. in 10ml.) for five hours at 100°C and after cooling evaporated to dryness in a small erlenmeyer flask in an evacuated desiccator over NaOH sticks and concentrated H_2SO_4. Excess of HCl was removed by evaporating the hydrolyzate three times, a little water being added before each evaporation. The hydrolyzate was filtered, extracted two times with a chloroform, dried and kept under vacuum in a dessicator until constant weight was reached. The sample was fractionated by column chromatography. The column, having an internal diameter of 15mm. and a length of 40mm, was made of a pyrex glass tube with fitted teflon stopcock which facilitated adjustment of the flow rate, a sealed-in coarse porosity fitted disc, and a spherical reservoir at the top of the column with a connection for N_2 pressure. The column was coated inside with one percent dimethyldichlorsilane in benzene to minimize zone deformation and prepared with cation exchange resin (H+) 100-200 mesh of AG-50W-X12 (14cm. high) on the bottom, and with an ion-retardation desalting resin 50-100 mesh AG-11A8 (6-7cm. high) on the top. (Absorbents and dimethyldichlorosilane from Bio-Rad Laboratories). The AG-50W-X12 was slurried first with water and all entrained air removed by placing the slurry under nitrogen gas pressure and dearating until bubbling ceased and slurry settled to 14cm. in height above the sintered disc. After the absorbent bed formed, AG-11A8 was slurried under the N_2 pressure to 6cm. in height. The column was washed with several volumes of water, using approximately the same flow rate that will be used for the elution. Control of temperature, eluent concentration, and quality of exchanger (column must not be allowed to become dry) are required. The column was operated under mild N_2 pressure at 25°C. After eluting the water to the top of the bed level the hydrolyzate sample was added to the top of the bed using a capillary pipette, then was washed carefully into the top of the bed with a small amount of water. Neutral sugars were washed from the column with water in the first eluate; water, (0.5ml./min. flow rate), collected in 10ml. fractions (50-60ml. total). Amino sugars were eluted in the second eluate 0.3N HCl (35-45ml. total), and amino acids were eluted in the third eluate 3N HCl (30-40ml. total).

One dimensional, two-step thin layer chromatography was performed on MN300-Cellulose thin-layer plate developed in following two step solvent system:
    1. Butanol-Pyridine-Acetic Acid-Water (60:45:4:30 v/v/v/v/) (26).
    2. Ethyl Acetate-Isopropanol-Pyridine-Water (70:30:20:20 v/v/v/v/) (27).

All solvents were redistilled prior to use. The thin-layer chromatographic analysis was performed on glass plates which must be very clean (fat free). A slurry was prepared from NM300 cellulose powder (Macherey and Nagel, Duren, W. Germany) as follows:

15g of cellulose powder was pre-washed in solvent mixture of Ethyl Alcohol: Carbon Tetrachloride: Water (6:3:1v/v/v/) to remove a brownish impurity . The prewashed powder was mixed with the use of a magnetic stirrer in 90ml. of deonized water. The plates were allowed to stand for 4 to 6 hours at room temperature before they were oven dried and then activated by heating for 30 minutes at 60°C and stored in a dessicator until used, and they were prepared freshly each time just prior to chromatography. The chromatographic plates were irrigated at 23°C in the ascending direction with solvent system 1 for 3.5 hours, then after 15 minutes drying, with solvent system 2 for 1.30 minutes in the same ascending direction. In the first solvent system, the developing was stopped when the solvent front had reached the top edge of the plate and in the second solvent system 0.5cm. before the first solvent front. After the second development, the plates were left inside the hood until the solvent had evaporated.

After the plates were air dried, the spots localized by

spraying with 0. 2 percent tetrazolium blue in 10 percent NaOH (40:60) for neutral and amino sugars, and 0. 5 percent ninhydrin in acetone for detection of amino acids.

R_f values obtained for sugars follow:

L - Rhamnose---------0. 74
D - Ribose-----------0. 68
D - Xylose-----------0. 62
D - Mannose----------0. 58
D - Glucose----------0. 52
D - Galactose--------0. 47
D - Mannosamine------0. 41
D - Glucosamine------0. 38
D - Galactosamine----0. 33

INCORPORATION OF ^{14}C-GLUCOSE INTO TRAINING AND RESTING PIGEON BRAIN 10B AND OTHER GLYCOPROTEINS

Glucose labelled in the first carbon was injected intravenously into pigeons at rest. They were then allowed to rest, or to engage in a training procedure for varying periods of time before sacrifice in a dry ice-acetone bath. The brain glycoproteins were extracted and separated as previously described (1, 2). Figure 1 summarizes the findings.

At rest for thirty minutes, only slight incorporation was observed in groups 2, 3 and 11B. Much more incorporation was observed at only 10 minutes of training.

Furthermore, the nature of the most actively labelled groups was a function of time. Thus while at 10 minutes training, groups 1, 10A and 10B were most prominently labelled. At 20 minutes, groups 10A. 10B and 10B2, 11B 12 and 13 were most active. At 60 minutes, groups 1 and 2 were active, a gether with groups 7, 11A and 11B. The fact that groups 1 and 2 are associated with the lateral dendritic processes (1), and that 10B proteins are associated with astrocytic glia, indicate that the sequential activity of glycoproteins of different cellular organelles as well as of different cell types (glia and neurones) will require further individual examination.

What is clear is that there is an extremely active turnover of carbohydrates in the brain glycoproteins of training pigeons, and that much of this activity occurs within minutes. We had previously noted (1, 2) that these changes occured earlier

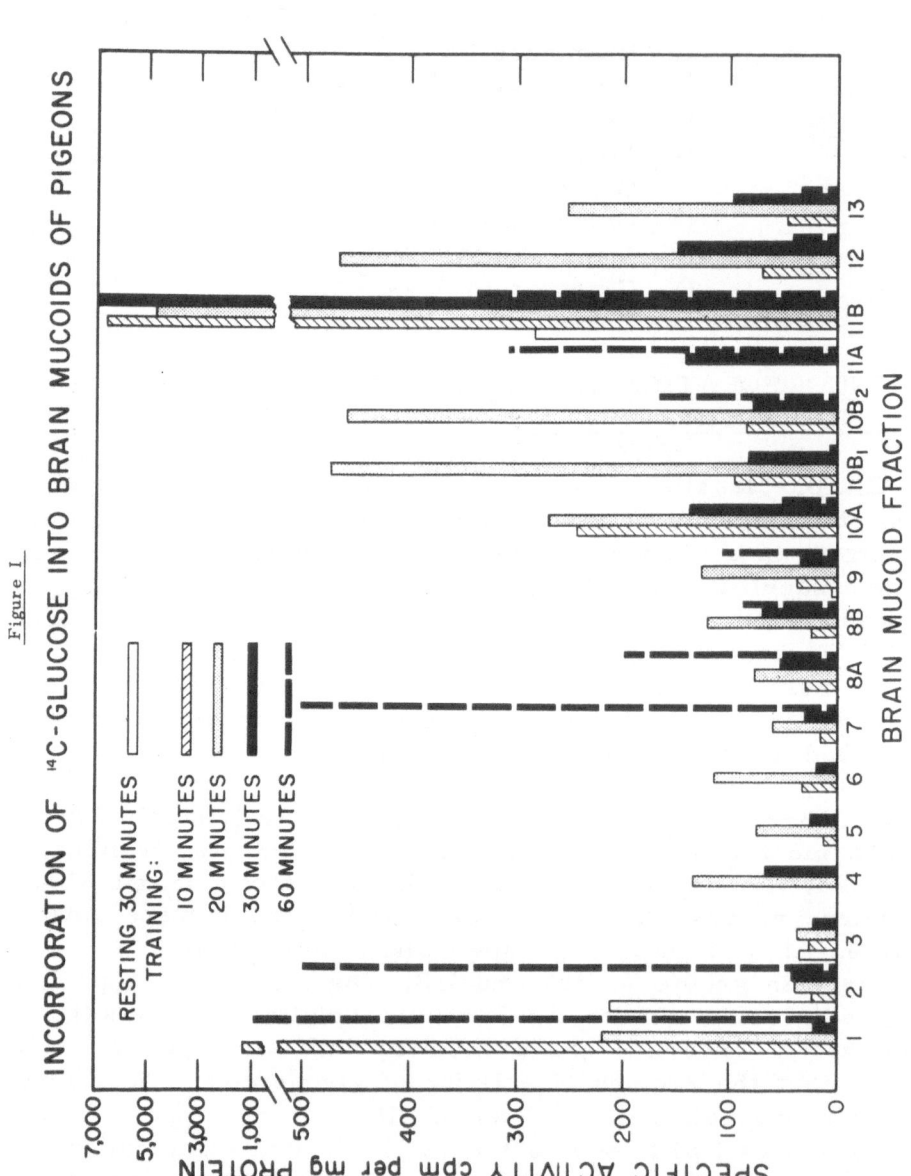

Figure I

INCORPORATION OF ¹⁴C-GLUCOSE INTO BRAIN MUCOIDS OF PIGEONS

than those times usually examined in such studies, and the present data confirms the importance of examining discrete and short time periods in relation where possible to specific glycoproteins and specific cell fractions.

CONCENTRATION OF CONSTITUENT HEXOSE OF BRAIN AND TUMOR 10B AND OTHER GLYCOPROTEINS

It was noted earlier that brain glycoprotein 10B concentration is increased in human brain glial tumors and that its protein-bound hexose is reduced (ref. 1, pg. 150). In the subsequent analysis of specimens of human brain tumors and of surrounding brain tissue for the concentration and type of of glycoprotein present, the total protein-bound hexose in the tumor itself, 2.7%, was less than that in surrounding glial capsule, 6.2% or in the outside normal cortical tissue, 5.1%.

In cases where the demarcation of tumor from surrounding tissue was not as clear as that above, and the degree of infiltration of normal tissue by tumor cells was variable, it was difficult to impossible to carry out this type of comparative analysis. Edema and hemorrage in the surrounding tissue also militate against such study.

To avoid this problem, ependymoma-glioma tumors previously grown in C3H mice, were transferred to subcutaneous sites on the back of the mouse, in doses of 5 to 20mg./mouse to permit analysis of the tumor as well as the brain of the same mouse, free of local pathology. The tumors were grown for two weeks, the mice being kept in individual cages to avoid canabalism and to keep track of the volume of fluid intake. The mice received diphenylhydantoin (DPH) or its solvent alone in their drinking water, of which the volume consumed daily was recorded. DPH has been shown previously to increase brain free glucose and glycogen (15, 16, 17) and to counteract anoxia (see ref. 18). The mice were sacrificed, and tumors and brains from groups of six mice were each pooled and extracted for total glycoproteins.

In tumor-bearing animals, total brain protein-bound hexose (Table 3) and hexose in isolated brain glycoprotein 10B (Table 4) were observed to be greater in concentration in DPH-treated than in non-treated mice. In normal mouse brain, (non-tumor-bearing) the concentration of total brain protein hexose has not constantly been observed to increase with DPH, but under certain conditions to decrease or to remain unchanged (13).

Table 3

TOTAL HEXOSE BOUND TO ALL PROTEIN GROUPS OF
MOUSE BRAIN, AS % OF PROTEIN

	No DPH	With DPH
Brain, control	4. 6, 5. 5	7. 9, 8. 0
Brain, in "tumor-bearer"	2. 6, 2. 3	6. 8, 7. 0

Table 4

HEXOSE BOUND IN GLYCOPROTEIN 10B OF MOUSE
BRAIN, AS % OF PROTEIN

	No DPH	With DPH
Brain, control	5. 4	4. 8
Brain, in "tumor-bearer"	3. 7	10. 5

STEPWISE HYDROLYSIS AND IDENTIFICATION OF
CONSTITUENT CARBOHYDRATES OF BRAIN AND
GLIAL TUMOR GLYCOPROTEINS

The total glycoproteins were hydrolysed by means of a stepwise acidic procedure previously described (2). The liberated sugar residues were isolated by dialysis at each hydrolytic step and separated from the amino acids and salts by means of the two phase column chromatography procedure earlier described. The separated sugars and amino acids were then studies by thin layer chromatography as earlier described.

The results are summarized in Table. 5. There were several differences: 1. A fast-running sugar with R_f of Rhamnose was observed only in the DPH-treated tumor glycoproteins. 2. An amino sugar with the R_f of mannosamine was prominently released in the DPH-treated tumor but was questionable or absent in the non-DPH treated tumor. 3. Two sugars with the mobility of oligosaccharides, labeled Oligosaccharide 1 and 2 in Table 5, were released prominently in the DPH-treated group. but were absent in the non-DPH treated tumor. 4. In DPH-treated brain, the glycoproteins demonstrated the preponderance of galactose; whereas galactose did not appear to be present or was present in trace amounts only, as a readily released sugar in non-DPH treated material.

Subtler differences observed which may merit further consideration in future studies are as follows: with DPH treatment, galactosamine appears to be preponderant over glucosamine, whereas in the non-DPH treated tumors the reverse holds, that is, glucosamine appears to be preponderant over galactosamine. These differences in sugars as demonstrated by thin layer chromatography are now being investigated by gas chromatographic methods.

Table 5

CONSTITUENT CARBOHYDRATES OF THE ISOLATED GLYCOPROTEINS OF

| | PIGEON BRAIN | | | GLIAL TUMOR | |
	10B1	10BII	11A	No DPH	With DPH
Rhamnose (?)	+	+			+
Fucose (ribose)	+	+		+	+
Xylose	+	+			
Mannose	+	+	+	+	+
Glucose	+	+	+	+	+
Galactose	+	+	+	+	+
Mannosamine (?)	+	+			+
Glucosamine		+		+	+
Galactosamine	+	+		+	+
Oligosaccharide 1	+				+
Oligosaccharide 2	+				+

IMMUNOLOGICAL STUDIES OF 10B: SPECIFICITY FOR REACTIVE ASTROCYTES

Utilizing an antiserum to 10B, prepared in rabbits, it has been possible to show that at highest dilutions immunofluorescence occurs only in the astrocytic glia, and exclusively in 'reactive astrocytes', both in astrocytomas and in glioblastoma multiforme (14)(Figure 2). No staining of frankly neoplastic cells, of normal glia, or of ganglion cells occured.

These observations are in agreement with earlier data, cited in the introduction, indicating that 10B is a glial constituent. That it is accessible to fluorescent staining, that is, to combination with specific antiserum in situ only when in a 'reactive' or dividing cell suggests that either its structure is altered in this state, and/or that it has become "unmasked" by the removal of some blocking cell constituent or group, which would normally not permit applied 10B antibody to contact the 10B antigen and react with it. The implications of such a change in cell constituent reactivity in relation to the development of the malignant process will be taken up in the discussion.

From a practical point of view, both with regard to diagnostic and therapeutic potential, it became of interest to determine how specific the antiserum is to a particular 10B which is isolated from a given human or animal brain tumor. To this end we have begun to extract and purify 10B from each specimen of human brain tumor, and from each specimen of surrounding more or less normal brain tissue, and separately to prepare antisera to these 10B antigens.

After concentration of 10B antigen in solution at 0.1 - 0.2 mg/ml there is some precipitation of 10B. Only the soluble supernate is injected, after Folin-Lowry protein determination. The first injection is with complete Freund's adjuvant, into the foot pads; intravenous booster is given 10 days later; intramuscular injection in complete Freund's adjuvant is given two weeks later. Rabbit sera were tested on Ochterlony double diffusion for the degree of antibody formation.

Table 6 records the data obtained to date. Each reactive line is denoted a or b, and its intensity graded + or +++. It may be seen that without cross-absorption or other purification of either antisera or antigens, there is some indication of specificity and some of cross-reactivity. Cross absorption and other purification steps are now in progress for both antigen and antibody. It is important to note that the ability of isolated antigen and antibody to combine in a gel or in solution without impediment is quite a different matter from reaction of antibody with in situ cellular 10B antigen. Thus 10B antigen is available in reactive astrocytic glia to combination with 10B antibody, but it is unavailable for such combination in non-reactive astrocytes.

Table 6

CROSS REACTIONS BETWEEN 10B ANTIGENS AND THEIR
ANTISERA ISOLATED a) FROM HUMAN GLIAL TUMORS
AND b) FROM SURROUNDING "NORMAL" BRAIN TISSUE

ANTIBODY TO:

10B Antigen From:	I. J. "Normal"	I. J. Tumor	J. C. "Normal"	J. C. Tumor
I. J. "Normal"	a+	a+	-	-
I. J. Tumor	a++	a+++	a++ b++	-
J. C. "Normal"	-	a++	a+++ b+	a++
J. C. Tumor	-	a+	a+++	a+++

Figure 2

IMMUNOFLUORESCENT STAINING OF REACTIVE ASTROCYTES
IN GLIOBLASTOMA: PRODUCED WITH ANTISERUM TO BRAIN
GLYCOPROTEIN 10B (14).

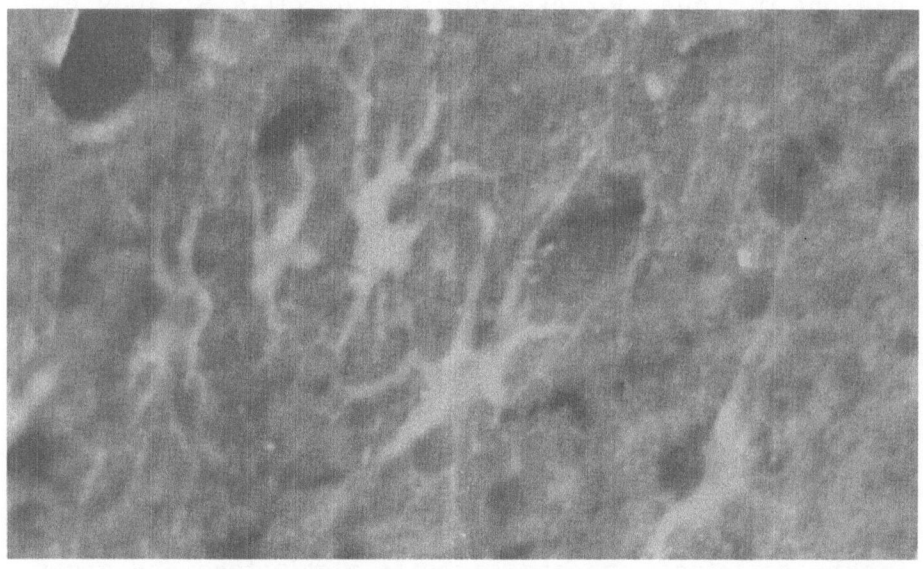

DISCUSSION

I.   SIGN-POST THEORY OF BRAIN CIRCUITRY

The activity here demonstrated of rapid exchange of hexose macromolecular carbohydrates in brain is compatible with the theory that these molecules are operating in transmission functions in the nervous system.

I have previously proposed (1, 2) that the glycoproteins of the nervous system are involved in cell recognition, contact and position functions and that these properties are responsible for the stable intercell circuitry necessary for information handling and storage by the nervous system. That is, the glycoproteins determine which nerve cells grow together in contact during development to permit transmission, as well as the facility of transmission at a given synaptic junction throughout life.

"A single carbohydrate end group might determine whether or not transmission of an impulse is facilitated between neuron A and B. Consider that on the presynaptic membrane belonging to neuron A there is a glycoprotein, glycoprotein A^1, whose carbohydrate end group can be of two types, which determine whether contact is or is not taking place with the postsynaptic membrane belonging to neurone B. Thus, for example, glycoprotein A^1 may exist with its end group a galactosamine residue, but with the postsynaptic membrane B possessing the specific receptor B^1 (possibly, but not necessarily, also a glycoprotein) specific only for a galactose residue. In the "resting" state, A^1 does not combine with B^1 and no synaptic contact results. Thus, although transmission is possible between A and B, it may not occur, or it may occur without facilitation. To state it another way, the threshold for transmission between neurons A and B may be an inverse function of the amount of physical contact between the membranes of A and B: the more contact, the lower the threshold.

A synthetic mechanism, a galactose transferase here taken as only one example, could be present at or in A, which could upon the proper stimulus attach a galactose residue to the galactosamine end group of A^1, thus changing the galactosamine end group to a galactose end group for A^1. This galactose end group of A^1 would combine immediately with receptor B^1, ionically or covalently, the contact between A and B would be increased, the threshold lowered, and transmission between A and B facilitated. It is possible that the "proper stimulus" for attachment of galactose is the passage of an excitatory impulse of sufficient intensity through A. The question of whether A can fire B will depend upon (1) whether the synthetic reaction necessary to attach the correct end group on A^1 is at hand and immediately available, or if repressed, is able to be derepressed; and (2) whether the receptor B^1 is at hand to react with A^1 galactose. These paired configurations might be laid down with complete or relative specificity by genetic coding mechanisms and realized in the morphogenesis of the nervous system. Thus the chemical specificities of A and B which allow them to grow together in synaptic contact in the first place would be the same specificities determining their contact and the transmission of an impulse between them throughout the life of the organism.

The influence of experience would enter in terms of (1) The frequency of stimuli, or strength of stimuli, or both, passing through A causing it to fire B. That is, the potential to synthesize A^1-galactose may require the activation by strong and/or repeated stimulation. (2) The competitive pathways available. That is, neuron A could transmit to neuron C, A to D, A to E etc. All might be programmed genetically as possibilities, then a combined selection-instruction mechanism brought to bear by experience to determine which pathway is selected, or which alternative pathways are preferred, and their order of preference. A DNA-specified repression-derepression type of induction requiring experiential input for activation could well be invoked for the A^1-galactose transferase reaction. The potential of the system may be quite extensive, as genetically programmed, but each component would require experiential realization in order to perform. That is, the degree of depression in each instance would be a direct function of experiential input.

For A^1-galactose, it might be necessary to substitute A^1-(glycosaminoglycan)$_n$-galactose, "n" representing the number of residues actually required to bridge the synaptic cleft so that the molecule A^1 may reach B^1.

Even greater complexity and selectivity could be

achieved by having more than one specific glycoprotein and receptor present per synapse, thus A^1, A^2, A^3, A^n and B^1, B^2, B^3, and B^n.

Chemical coding of information in the brain would thus be visualized as a specific set of instructions determining whether, and under what conditions, each neuron will fire any other accessible neuron. The actual information coded in glycoprotein A^1 could be no more than that required to define whether or not B^1 would be contacted. The mucoids would thus act as switching mechanisms, "sign-posts" which route transmission. The mucoids would thus be the chemical basis of the make-break mechanisms of the brain's circuitry, the chemical basis of the establishment of the cluster of specific circuits which constitute a memory trace. They might also underlie specificities of contact between glia and neurons."

The experimental evidence in support of this "Sign-Post" theory, summarized in the above references, has included the fact that a change in the structure and function of the brain glycoproteins should accompany both the expression of and the regression of these higher nervous system functions. Evidence for chemical accompaniments of the expression of these functions has been summarized in the above references. The regression of function, as observed in the mental deficiency accompanying certain inborn errors of metabolism, such as Tay-Sachs' disease is associated with glycoprotein pathology (14).

II. INVERSE RELATIONSHIP OF MUCOID-CONTACT FUNC- TIONS AND DNA REPLICATION

Search for the chemical expression of higher information functions of brain cells has led in addition to findings of structural changes in the same molecules upon regression of these higher functions, in brain tumors. The antisera which we have obtained to a brain tumor cell antigen 10B have possible application to both diagnosis and therapy of brain tumors. Thus since only the 10B of reactive astrocytes will combine with injected 10B antisera, it may be possible to outline radioactively a brain tumor for active viewing on screens, or photography for permanent record. Further, if the 10B antibody injected is coupled with chemically or radioactively toxic compounds, or with such compounds which can be activated by chemical or physical means, destruction of cells in the brain tumor area can be much more selective in sparing normal cells than hitherto possible. In addition, if circulating antibody to brain tumor antigen 10B can be detected in human serum, a further diagnostic procedure may become available.

The growth of ependymoma-glioma tumors subcutaneously in the mouse provides the opportunity to study a brain tumor growing outside the nervous system, and at the same time to study the chemistry of the essentially normal brain (and other organs) in the same animal able to be influenced by the subcutaneously growing brain tumor. The decrease in protein-bound hexose of brain under these conditions suggests the influence of a diffusable factor from the distant brain tumor. As pointed out in the introduction, this factor may be responsible for the induction of a precancerous or early cancerous change in normal cells.

The concentration of total protein-bound hexose in brain under the influence of distant tumor is in agreement with the data obtained for human brain tumors. It is also in general agreement with the previous observations that the concentration of protein-bound hexose in brain is greater: (a) the more complex the anatomical structure of the brain, (b) the more ordered the chemical structure, as in membranes opposed to cytoplasmic cell constituents, and (c) the more complex or active the functional state of the animal (1, 2). Thus, the greater the "experiential" or environmental informational content or activity of a given structure of function, the greater the concentration of protein-bound hexose. The training brain cell, with relatively high experiential informational content, contains more protein-bound hexose (1). The tumor cell, with relatively low experiential informational content, but high 'genetic' (mitotic) activity, contains less protein-bound hexose.

This relationship may be generalized to the proposition that I have made that when DNA and cell replication functions are stimulated, as in tumors, normal mucoid biosynthesis is inhibited (19). During normal morphogenesis of brain, DNA and cell division would be more active at one stage, and mucoid biosynthesis for specific interneuronal connections would be more active at another stage (1).

This postulated inverse relationship of mucoid-contact functions to DNA replication could account for the cessation of

DNA synthesis in retinal ganglion cells observed to be correlated with the time of specification of their central connections
(20). The theory would also be consistent with the reported
relationship of malignancy to loss of contact inhibition (21),
if contact recognition is indeed a function of mucoids. This
cell surface difference in malignancy has been related to the
presence of an agglutinin with specificity for the N-acetylglucosamine determinant (22). If nucleic acid bases, uridine and
cytidine, were available either for nucleic acid synthesis or
for transferase activity for mucoid synthesis, but not for both
simultaneously, then a control mechanism would be at hand
for determining which of the two cell functions--replication
or contact positioning--occured.

III. TAY-SACHS' DISEASE:A FAILURE OF INTRACELLULAR RECOGNITION ?

The abnormal intracellular accumulation of membranous
material raises a question about the basic defect in Tay-Sachs'
Disease. This is demonstrated 1) morphologically, by the excess rolled-up membranous bodies (23) lying in cytoplasm
or in lysosomes, and 2) chemically, by our findings, that not
just lipid-bound carbohydrate but protein-bound carbohydrate
glycoprotein (4), which are membranous constituents,are abnormally increased .

All of our studies point to the idea that macromolecular
carbohydrate constituents form the molecular basis for recogn-
tion phenomena in cells. One consequence of the failure of
recognition mechanisms as in normal contact inhibition is the
failure to shut off DNA and cell replication when the space
for cells has been used up.

It is here proposed that Tay-Sachs' Disease represents
another disorder of recognition mechanism. Thus if the membrane production continues,and the membranes for whatever
reason are not used, then the accumulation of these membranes
should be recognized by the cell and should signal a turn-off
of membrane production. Just as the growth of cancer cells
does not successfully signal a turn-off of DNA replication, the
non-use of membranes in Tay-Sachs' disease fails to signal
a turn-off of membrane production.

If the membrane never gets to its ultimate destination in

the cell, it would not be able to set off the signal that delivery and placement have been accomplished, so that production, which may be at a normal rate, continues, and membranes spiral up in the cytoplasm.

A manufactured cell organelle may not be placed correctly because: 1) It has a defect in its terminal carbohydrate structure which prevents normal contact and recognition functions to occur. 2) Its structure is normal, but the transport, delivery and placement, and turnoff systems are impaired.

The transport mechanism appears to be intact at least to the extent that intact external neuronal membranes are produced. It is the turn-off mechanism for synthesis of new membranes which is impaired, just as the turn-off mechanism for cell division is impaired in cancer.

In this sense, Tay-Sachs' disease can be thought of as a cancer of membranes just as tumors are cancers of whole cells. In tumor there is a failure of intercellular recognition; in Tay-Sachs' disease there is a failure of intracellular recognition. In tumors, cells accumulate; in Tay-Sachs' disease, membranes accumulate.

SUMMARY

1. The isolation and properties of brain glycoprotein 10B are described. 10B is increased in concentration in glial tumors in humans and animals, but its hexose content is reduced.

2. Specific antibodies to 10B have been prepared. The in situ 10B antigen is only available for staining by antibody immunofluroescence when the astrocytic glia are in the "reactive" state as when with glial brain tumors.

3. When ependymoma-glioma tumors are grown subcutaneously in the mouse at a distance from the brain of the animal, changes in the brain glycoproteins can be detected, suggesting the presence of a Distance Factor (DF) which may be responsible for the induction of cancerous changes in distant cells. Individual 10B antigens are now being isolated from individual human brain tumor and surrounding tissue specimens, and antisera prepared to test the diagnostic and therapeutic potential of the availability of specific antibody to this specific brain tumor cell antigen.

4. 10B concentration is increased during one phase of training in the pigeon. ^{14}C-Glucose is incorporated more rapidly into 10B during training than during resting. During one hour of training, 10B and other brain glycoproteins are labelled at different times.

5. Carbohydrate moieties of glycoproteins of brain cells and tumor cells have been isolated and compared by thin-layer chromotography.

6. The "Sign-Post" theory (1) of brain glycoprotein function is supported. In addition recent evidence has led to the extension of the concept to the proposal that mucoid biosynthesis is inversely related to DNA replication. That is, DNA and cell division are inhibited during cell positioning and the formation of inter-cell contacts (the proposed glycoprotein Sign-Post 'experiential' function), and mucoid biosynthesis is inhibited when DNA and cell division are active.

7. The proposal is made that just as there is a failure of inter cellular recognition in tumors with consequent accumulation of cells, there is in Tay-Sachs' disease a failure of intra-cellular recognition with consequent accumulation of membranes.

REFERENCES

1. BOGOCH, S., The Biochemistry of Memory; With An Inquiry Into the Function of the Brain Mucoids. Oxford University Press, New York, London, 1968.

2. BOGOCH, S. Glycoproteins of The Brain of the Training Pigeon: In: Symposium on Protein Metabolism of the Nervous System. Lajtha, A., Ed., Plenum Press, 1969, p. 555.

3. BOGOCH, S., Quantitative Studies of Brain Proteins in Disorders of the Nervous System and In Learning. In: Eighth International Congress of Neurology, International Congress Series, Constans, J. P., Gibberd, F. B. and Junze, K., Eds. Amsterdam: Excerpta Medical Foundation, 1965, p. 139.

4. BOGOCH, S. and BELVAL, P. Brain Proteins in the Sphingolipidoses: Tay-Sachs' Disease Protein. In: Inborn Disorders of Sphingolipid Metabolism. Proceedings of the Third International Symposium on the Cerebral Sphingo-lipidoses. Aronson, S. and Volk, B. W., Eds. New York: Pergamon Press, 1966, p. 273.

5. BOGOCH, S., SACKS, W., SWEET, W. H., KORSH, G. and BELVAL, P. C. Structure of, and Incorporation of (^{14}C) Glucose Into Isolated Protein and Carbohydrate Macro-molecules of Brain Subcellular Membranous Components in Resting, Training and Tumor Brain Tissue. In: Protides of the Biological Fluids. Proceedings of the Fifteenth Colloquium, Bruges, 1966. Peeters, H., Ed., New York Elsevier Publishing Company, 1968, p. 129.

6. BOGOCH, S., Proteins. In Handbook of Neurochemistry, Vol. 1, Lajtha, A., Ed. Plenum Press, 1969, p. 75.

7. WEISENBERG, R. C., BORISY, G. G., and TAYLOR, E. W. Biochemistry $\underline{1}$, 4466, 1968.

8. MOORE, B. W. and McGREGOR, D., J. Biol. Chem. $\underline{240}$, 1647, 1965.

9. BENNETT, G. S. and EDELMAN, G. M., J. Biol. Chem. $\underline{243}$, 6234, 1968.

10. FALXA, M. L. and GILL, T. J. Arch. Biochem. and Biophys. $\underline{135}$, 194, 1969.

11. QUAMINA, A., and BOGOCH, S., Subcellular Fractionation of Glycoproteins and Mucoids of Human and Rat Brain. In: Protides of the Biological Fluids. Proceedings of the Thirteenth Colloquium, Bruges, 1965. Peeters, H., Ed., New York, Elsevier, 1966, p. 211

12. BOGOCH, S., RAJAM, P. C. and BELVAL, P. C. Nature $\underline{204}$, 73, 1964.

13. BOGOCH, S. , BOGOCH, E. , KORSH, G. and DAS, B. R.
     unpublished results.

14. BENDA, P. , MORI, T. and SWEET, W. H.   J. Neurosurg. 33,
     281-286, 1970.

15. WOODBURY, D. M. , TIMIRAS, P. S. and VERNADAKIS, A.
     Modification of Adrenocortical Function Centrally Acting
     Drugs and the Influence of Such Modification on the Central
     Response to these Drugs. In Hormones, Brain Function and
     Behavior. H. Hoagland, Ed. , Academic, 1957, p. 38.

16. BRODDLE, W. D. , and NELSON, S. R.   Fed. Proc. 27, 751,
     1968.

17. HUTCHINS, D. A. and ROGERS, K. J.   Brit. J. Pharmacol.
     39, 9, 1970.

18. BOGOCH, S. , and DREYFUS, J. J. The Broad Range of Use
     of Diphenylhydantoin : Bibliography and Review. Dreyfus
     Medical Foundation, New York, 1970.

19. BOGOCH, S. , Inverse Relationship Between Cell Replication
     and Macromolecular Carbohydrate Concentration: A Distance
     Factor (DF) in Brain Tumors. Abstracts, Third Internation-
     al Meeting of the International Society for Neurochemistry,
     Budapest, July 5 - 9, 1971.

20. JACOBSON, M. , Develop. Biol. 17, 219, 1968.

21. STOKER, M. , and RUBIN, H. , Nature 215, 171, 1967.

22. BURGER, M. M. , and GOLDBERG, A. R. Proc. Natnl. Acad.
     Sci. U. S. 57, 359, 1967.

23. KOREY, S. and TERRY, R. D. J. Neuropath. Exp. Neurol.
     22, 2, 1963.

24. BOGOCH, S. , Brain Glycoprotein 10B: Further Evidence on
     the "Sign-Post" Role of Brain Glycoproteins in Cell Recog-
     nition, Its Change in Brain Tumor, and the Presence of a
     'Distance Factor'. In Proteins of the Nervous System.
     I. Morgan, Ed. Plenum Press, in press.

25. BOGOCH, S. and KORSH, G. Methods for Hydrolysis of Glycoproteins, Ion-exchange Column Chromatography and Thin-layer Chromotography of Constituent Hexose and Hexosamines. to be published

26. ESSER, K., J. Chromatog., 18, 414, 1965.

27. GUNTER, H., and SCHWEIGER, A. J. Chromatog., 17, 602, 1965.

A FAST MOVING PROTEIN IN TAY-SACHS DISEASE

Denise Karcher, A. Lowenthal and W. Zeman

Fondation Born-Bunge, Berchem-Antwerpen, Belgium

Indiana University School of Medicine, Indianapolis, Ind.

INTRODUCTION

In 1968 Adriaenssen et al.[1] demonstrated a hitherto unknown hydrosoluble protein in the forebrain of two patients with Tay-Sachs disease and suggested that it might represent a disease-specific substance. Later on, Zeman et al. (1970)[13] showed that this protein was not present in the brains of all patients with Tay-Sachs disease although the resolution of their techniques was probably not sufficient to detect concentrations of less than 10% of the total of hydrosoluble proteins. Nevertheless, these authors established a direct relationship between the brain weights of patients with Tay-Sachs disease and the relative concentration of the unusual protein, indicating a possible relationship with the edema that, according to Aronson and Volk (1962),[2] accounts for the megalobarencephaly of Tay-Sachs disease.

Karcher et al. (1970)[7] purified the protein by column chromatography and performed a series of experiments with the isolated substance. These studies revealed the protein from Tay-Sachs brains to be very similar to a particular hydrosoluble protein which was extracted from functionally normal spinal cords and from a variety of normal and diseased brains (Chamoles et al., 1970).[5] Karcher et al. (1970)[7] named the substance α-albumin because it exhibits a relative mobility in agar gel from 0.900 to 0.920 in relation to 1.000 for serum albumin and thus migrates between albumin and α-globulin. The relative mobilities were calculated on the basis of a standard solution run in parallel with the specimen. Furthermore, using double diffusion procedures, they observed a precipitation pattern which suggested an antigenic

parentage with serum albumin. However, the amino acid residues
of human serum albumin and α-albumin isolated from the brains of
patients with Tay-Sachs disease and from normal human spinal cords,
were markedly different. The most perplexing findings were obtained
with relation to the molecular weight of α-albumin which from the
elution volume of the sephadex column was calculated to be in the
range of 600,000, whereas ultracentrifugal analysis produced a
sedimentation constant of 3.8 at 20° C, indicating a molecular
weight between 35,000 and 40,000. A similar value was calculated
from the amino acid composition of hydrolysates, taking a micro-
molar value of 0.05 for histidine as unity.

This uncertainty, together with the distinct possibility that
the antigenic parentage between α-albumin and serum albumin was
the result of a contamination of the former by the latter, prompted
us to perform further isolation experiments, employing gel filtration and preparative isoelectric focusing and to study α-albumin
with the help of a specific antiserum.

MATERIALS AND METHODS

A. For the present experiments we used the following sera and
    antisera:

    1. Anti-α-albumin rabbit antiserum was prepared by Wellcome
        Reagents Ltd. from purified α-albumin isolated as reported
        by Karcher et al. (1970).[7]

    2. Commercial rabbit anti-human serum albumin (Behringwerke).

    3. Human serum albumin (Calbiochem).

    4. Aqueous extracts from human tissues of various proveniences
        either purified for α-albumin or native, prepared as de-
        scribed by Karcher et al. (1970) under materials and
        methods A.[7]

    5. Various human sera served as controls.

B. The following procedures were employed.

    1. Standard agar gel electrophoresis after Wieme[12] as a rapid
        screening procedure for α-albumin.

    2. Electroimmunodiffusion after Krøll[8,9] for the identifica-
        tion and quantitation of α-albumin.

    3. Isoelectric focusing on preparative columns (LKB) for the
        purification of α-albumin.

4. Thin-layer isoelectric focusing[3] modified by Delmotte (1971)[6] for identification of α-albumin.

5. Two-dimensional electroimmunodiffusion after Laurell[10,11]. In this procedure, our working conditions were as follows: the sample is introduced into a well in agarose and horizontally electrophoresed at 70 volts for 90 minutes on a one inch gel strip placed at the edge of a 7.5 x 7.5 cm glass plate. Thereafter the remainder of the plate is covered with agarose which contains antiserum in a ratio of .3 ml to 6.7 ml agarose. The whole plate is now electrophoresed at a 90° angle so as to move the separated proteins into the antiserum-containing gel at 20 volts for 16 hours.

6. The modification of this method by Axelsen and Svendsen[4] introduces--following the horizontal electrophoresis--a second gel strip neighboring and parallel to the first one, that contains another sample which may or may not be related to the first; the remainder of the plate is covered with agarose which contains the antiserum; the second or vertical electrophoresis is then performed. The course of the precipitation line will clarify the relationship of the two samples.

RESULTS

α-Albumin in Tay-Sachs Disease

An LKB Isoelectric Focusing Column with a total volume of 110 ml, charged with a sucrose gradient, ampholytes of pH 3 to 6 and total aqueous extract from the brain of a patient with Tay-Sachs disease, known to contain α-albumin, was eluted after 50 hours at 660 volts. Collecting approximately 2 ml per tube, a total of 54 fractions was obtained and pooled as shown in Fig. 1. As revealed by agar gel electrophoresis, the α-albumin collected in tubes 15 to 22, corresponds to a pH from 5.64 to 4.89. Albumin has an isoelectric point of 4.9. Tubes 15 and 16 with a pH of 5.64 and 5.46, respectively, were pooled and identified as fraction F. Tubes 17 and 18 with a pH of 5.33 and 5.21, respectively, were pooled and identified as fraction G. Tubes 19 and 20 with a pH of 5.12 and 5.07, respectively, were pooled and identified as fraction H, and tubes 21 and 22 with a pH of 5.00 and 4.89 were pooled and identified as fraction I.

These 4 fractions, as well as a total extract of spinal cord containing α-albumin, the total brain extract that was introduced into the column, and an aqueous extract of the patient's kidney were applied in punched holes in an agarose gel strip

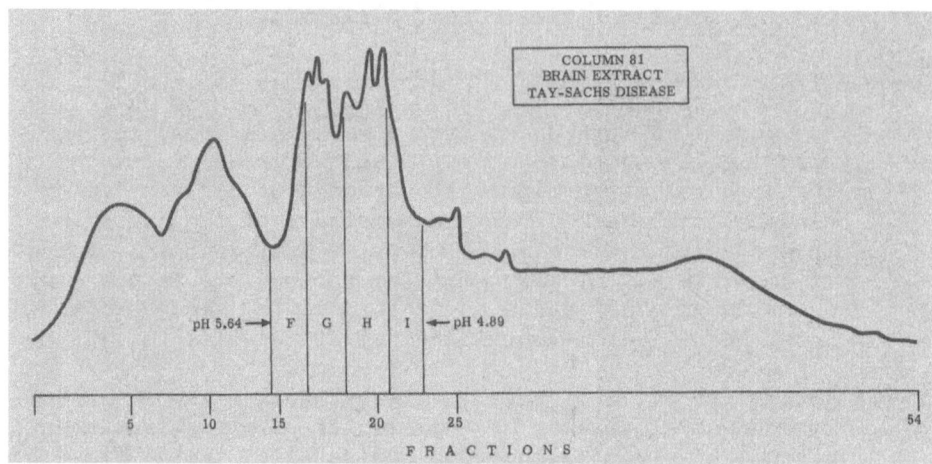

Fig. 1. Elution curve of LKB isoelectric focusing column charged
   with ampholytes pH 3.0 to 6.0 and an aqueous extract of brain
   tissue from a patient with Tay-Sachs disease. The fractions
   which contain α-albumin are identified from F to I.

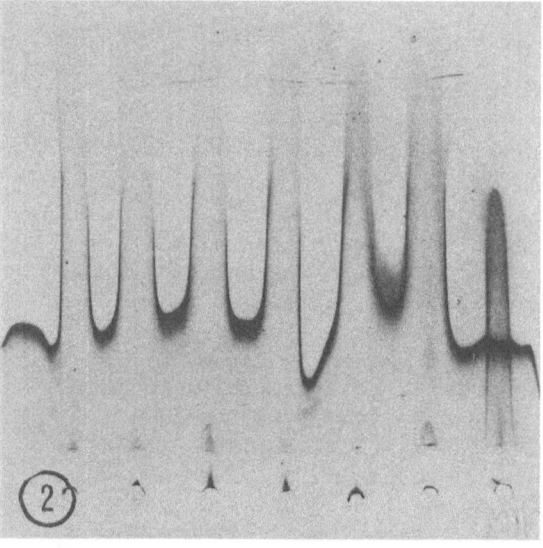

Fig. 2. Electroimmuno-
   diffusion after Krøll.
   The basal gel strip contains 20λ of spinal cord
   extract with α-albumin and
   the upper gel .3 ml of
   anti- α-albumin. Wells
   from left to right:
   spinal cord extract;
   fractions I; H; G; F;
   extract from brain of
   patient with Tay-Sachs
   disease; kidney extract
   from same patient.

containing 20 λ of spinal cord extract with α-albumin, and then
electrophoresed into agarose containing rabbit anti- α-albumin,
following the method of Krøll (Fig. 2). The spinal cord and
brain extracts as well as the pooled isoelectrically focused
fractions of the same brain extract produce one continuous precipitation line which excludes the kidney extract, indicating
that this organ does not contain α-albumin.

Thin-layer isoelectric focusing, a visual illustration of
the isoelectric focusing column, resolves α-albumins from spinal
cord extracts into distinct zones which have the same position
for extracts from different specimens (Fig. 3) but are slightly
shifted to the cathode in comparison with the column fractions.
Serum albumin is far towards the anode and is therefore not
demonstrated in this preparation.

CATHODE   ANODE

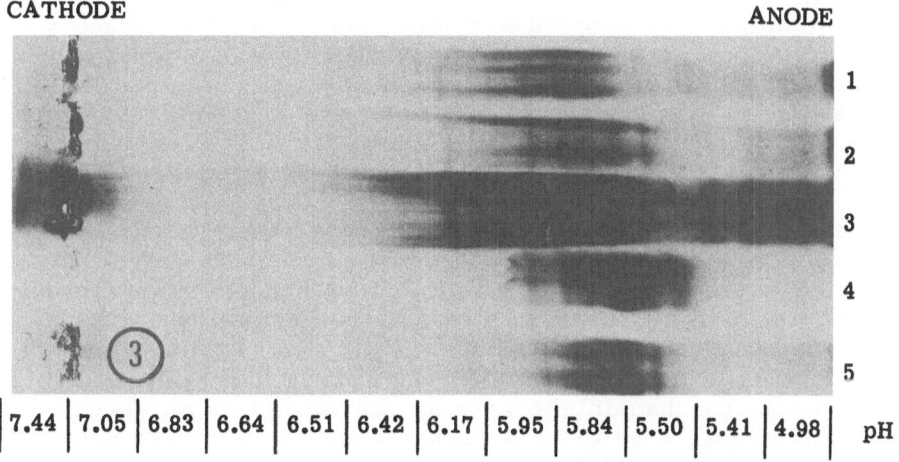

| 7.44 | 7.05 | 6.83 | 6.64 | 6.51 | 6.42 | 6.17 | 5.95 | 5.84 | 5.50 | 5.41 | 4.98 | pH |

Fig. 3. Thin-layer electrofocusing of various spinal cord extracts
   in ampholytes with a pH from 5 to 8. 1) Pooled extracts,
   2) spinal cord, 3) another spinal cord, 4) α-albumin isolated
   on sephadex G 100 column, 5) α-albumin isolated by immuno-
   adsorbence.

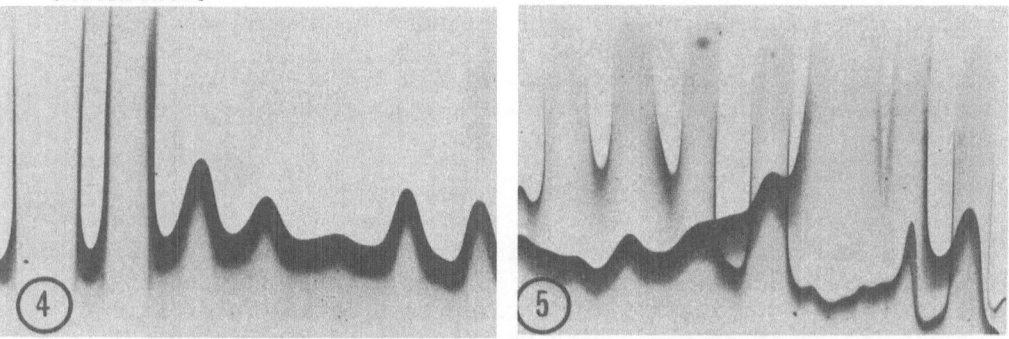

Fig. 4. Electroimmunodiffusion after Krøll. Bottom strip contains
   20 λ human serum albumin 1 mg/ml. The top gel contains .3 ml of
   anti-albumin. Left to right: 2 mg/ml albumin; 1 mg/ml albumin;
   spinal cord extract; fractions I; G; H; Tay-Sachs brain extract.

Fig. 5. Electroimmunodiffusion after Krøll. Bottom strip contains
   spinal cord extract and albumin, top layer anti-α-albumin and
   anti-albumin. Left to right: isolated α-albumin; fractions I; G; H;
   Tay-Sachs spinal fluid, albumin 1 mg/ml; Tay-Sachs brain extract.

Tay-Sachs α-Albumin Different from Serum Albumin

Further evidence for the difference between human serum albumin and human α-albumin is obtained by electrophoresing samples of both proteins together applied to a gel with commercial albumin, into agarose containing rabbit anti-human serum albumin (Fig. 4). The two "rockets" on the left are produced by the reaction of 2 mg and 1 mg/ml of serum albumin (Calbiochem), respectively, whereas subsequent holes were charged with equal amounts of an aqueous extract of spinal cord,[3] fractions taken off the isofocusing column and total extract from the brain of a patient with Tay-Sachs disease. This experiment suggests some degree of contamination of the α-albumins with serum albumin which is lowest in fraction G and greatest in the spinal cord extract.

The conclusion which springs from these observations, namely that α-albumin and serum albumin are not related to each other and that our previous suggestion to that effect was due to a contamination of α-albumin with serum albumin, is further strengthened by the experiment shown in Fig. 5.

The wells punched in the agarose containing human serum albumin and spinal cord with α-albumin were charged with equal quantities of various α-albumin preparations, spinal fluid from a patient with Tay-Sachs disease and serum albumin. These samples were electrophoresed into agarose containing both, anti-α-albumin and anti-serum albumin. Two continuous precipitation lines are produced, one by α-albumin of the spinal cord with four peaks on the left and one on the right, and the other due to the interaction of the human serum albumin included in the agarose strip with anti-albumin which includes the albumin and the spinal fluid sample. Thus, it appears that spinal fluid does not contain α-albumin, even if it is present in high concentrations in the brain.

Spinal Cord α-Albumin

The same theme is presented in Fig. 6 with the only difference, that the α-albumin from which the isoelectrically focused fractions (wells 1 to 4) originated, was derived from spinal cord extract (well 6) which is compared with the extract of another spinal cord sample (well 7) and with serum albumin in well 5. Vertical electrophoresis was into agarose containing both, anti-α-albumin and anti-human serum albumin. The precipitation lines are more distinct in this preparation than in Fig. 5 where albumin was present in large amounts in the concentrated cerebrospinal fluid, causing the precipitation arc to become murky.

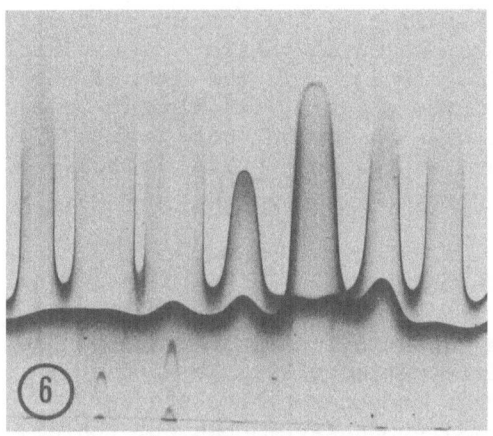 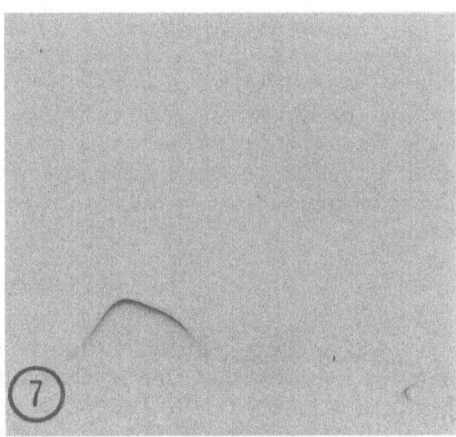

Fig. 6. Electroimmunodiffusion after Krøll. The bottom gel contains spinal cord extract and serum albumin. The top gel contains anti- α-albumin and anti-serum albumin. Wells from left to
right: isolated α-albumin: 3 fractions of spinal cord α-albumin
isoelectrically focused; albumin 1 mg/ml; spinal cord extract.

Fig. 7. Twodimensional electrophoresis after Laurell. Brain
extract from patient with Tay-Sachs disease was electrophoresed
in bottom gel, the upper gel contains anti-serum albumin.

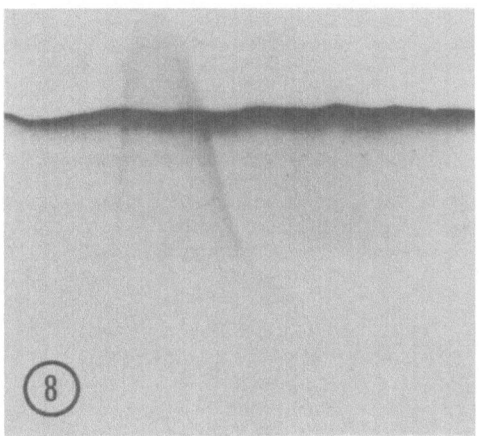 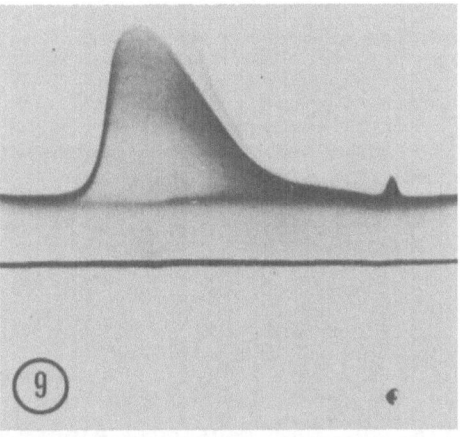

Fig. 8. Twodimensional electrophoresis, modification of Axelsen.
Normal serum was electrophoresed in bottom gel. Intermediate gel
contains spinal cord extract with α-albumin. Upper gel contains
anti- α-albumin.

Fig. 9. Twodimensional electrophoresis, as Fig. 8. Bottom gel:
electrophoresed isolated α-albumin from spinal cord, intermediate
gel:extract from another spinal cord; top gel:.3 ml of anti-
serum albumin and of anti- α-albumin.

All these experiments show a baseline either of albumin or of
α-albumin, the protein which is included in the agarose base strip.
Furthermore, since the α-albumin is introduced in the form of total
spinal cord extract which also includes albumin, the albumin baseline is not perfectly straight, because the spinal cord extract
adds albumin to that already present in the base strip in those
experiments where both, spinal cord extract and serum albumin, are
used.

Impurities in the Antisera

While Figs. 5 and 6 suggest a neat distinction of albumin and
α-albumin, aqueous brain extract from patients with Tay-Sachs
disease are contaminated with albumin as shown by the standard
Laurell[10] technique (Fig. 7). Normal human serum does not contain
α-albumin (Fig. 8); however, the rabbit anti-α-albumin is not
absolutely specific as also shown by Fig. 8. In this experiment,
the modification of Axelsen[4] was employed, normal serum was
electrophoresed and the intermediate strip contained spinal cord
extract with α-albumin. This reacted with the anti-α-albumin in
a relatively straight precipitation line, but the antiserum also
precipitates with an unknown serum protein in the form of an arc.

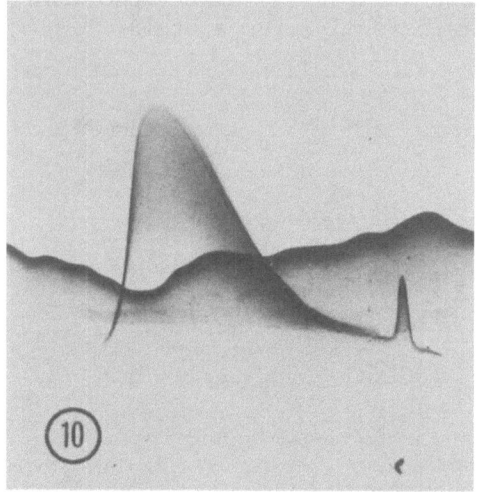 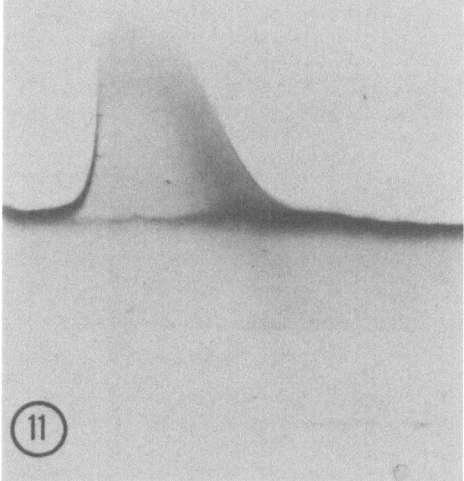

Fig. 10. Twodimensional electrophoresis, modification of Axelsen.
  Bottom gel: isolated α-albumin from spinal cord. Intermediate
  gel: albumin. Upper gel: .3 ml of anti-serum albumin and of
  anti-α-albumin.

Fig. 11. Twodimensional electrophoresis, as Fig. 10. Lower gel:
  brain extract from patient with Tay-Sachs disease. Intermediate
  gel: spinal cord extract. Upper gel: anti-α-albumin.

Of greatest significance is the fact that isolated α-albumin
from two different spinal cord extracts react in the same precipitation arc, and that neither precipitates with anti-albumin
as shown in Fig. 9, which was obtained by the Axelsen modification.
The precipitation lines are parallel, the first due to albumin
present in the spinal cord (straight dark line), the second due to
α-albumin forms a continuous line with the arc produced by the
isolated α-albumin. In a slightly modified experiment, isolated
anti- α -albumin was electrophoresed horizontally and the intermediate gel contained albumin. The additional gel contained both
anti- α -albumin and anti-serum albumin which produced two distinct
intersecting precipitation lines (Fig. 10).

Tay-Sachs α-Albumin Identical with Spinal Cord α-Albumin
and α-Albumin from Brains with SSPE

The identity of α-albumin from the brain of a patient with
Tay-Sachs disease and from a normal spinal cord is documented in
Fig. 11. One single precipitation arc in the characteristic
position of the α-albumin peak is produced and if this is compared
with Fig. 10, it becomes obvious that α-albumins of different
provenience are closely related to each but not to serum-albumin.

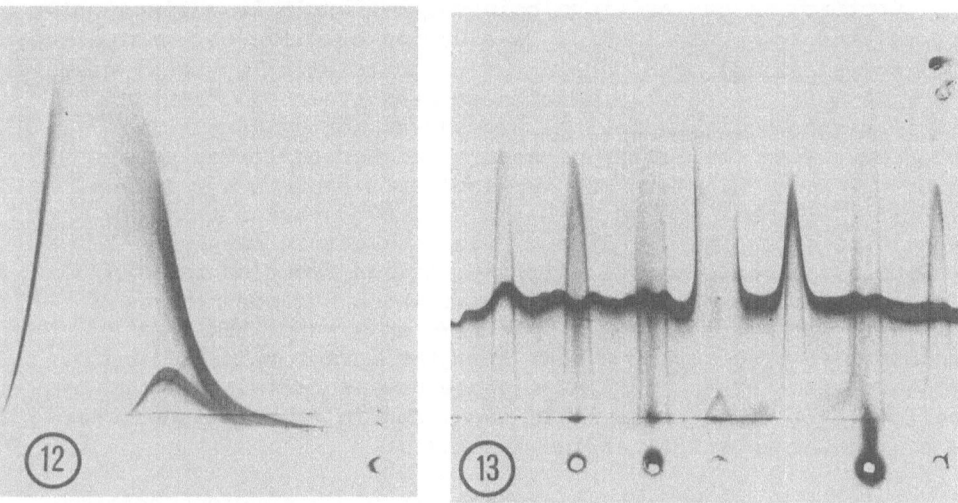

Fig. 12. Twodimensional electrophoresis after Laurell. Bottom
gel: extract from white matter of patient with SSPE. Upper gel:
anti-α-albumin.

Fig. 13. Modified electroimmunodiffusion after Krøll. Lower gel:
spinal cord extract with α-albumin. Upper gel: anti-α-albumin.
The wells were charged with tissue extracts from patient with
Tay-Sachs disease. From left to right: lung; pancreas; spleen;
brain; testis; liver; heart.

This statement can be extended so as to include α-albumin contained
in the brain of a patient with SSPE (Fig. 12). This experiment
demonstrated again the previously mentioned fact that the anti-
α-albumin antiserum is not absolutely pure but precipitates other,
unidentified proteins.

Considering that Tay-Sachs disease is a genetically controlled
disorder in which each cell suffers from the same metabolic defect,
it seems justified to entertain the possibility that α-albumin may
occur in tissues other than brain and spinal cord despite the fact,
that the presence of α-albumin is not restricted to Tay-Sachs
disease. We have therefore examined tissue extracts for the
presence of α-albumin, using a more sensitive modification of the
Krøll procedure, in which the application strip also contains
α-albumin (Fig. 13). No evidence for the presence of α-albumin
was obtained for tissues other than brain (well 4) which of course
was expected and curiously for testicle (well 5). Thus, it appears
that α-albumin is highly specific for brain and spinal cord but it
does not occur in demonstrable quantities in other tissues.

CONCLUSION

Contrary to our previous opinion, α-albumin is antigenically
not related to serum albumin. α-albumins of different provenience,
from normal spinal cord, brains of patients with Tay-Sachs disease
and with SSPE are closely related to each other and cannot be
distinguished by immunological procedures nor by isoelectric
focusing. With the latter procedure, either performed on a
column or on a thin layer of acrylamide, α-albumin has an isoelectric point between pH 5.64 and pH 4.89, whereas that of
albumin is around 4.9. Although the isoelectric range of
α-albumin is broad, each arbitarily defined fraction reacted
with anti-α-albumin in an identical fashion but did not precipitate with anti-serum albumin. It came as a surprise, that
α-albumin is practically absent from the cerebrospinal fluid of
patients with Tay-Sachs disease whose brains contain high concentrations. It is not present in serum and in other tissues, perhaps with the exception of the testicles.

While the present experiments confirm our previous observations on the existence of a hydrosoluble protein, present in
normal spinal cord and the brain of a patient with Tay-Sachs
disease and other disorders, that migrates in agarose to a
position between albumin and α-globulin, the new experiments
have not only not shed any new light on the genesis of this protein but rather tend to invalidate a previously entertained, somewhat attractive hypothesis. In view of our previous findings[5,7,13]
we were tempted to suggest that α-albumin may be nothing more than

a partly digested, perhaps aggregated or polymerized, serum-
albumin that has leaked through the cerebrospinal capillaries
into the tissue and been acted upon by the lysosomal cathepsins D
and E. This hypothesis seemed to explain the enormous quantities
of this protein in megalobaric brains of patients with Tay-Sachs
disease and in the spinal cords (Chamoles et al., 1970). In the
light of the now disproven antigenic parentage between albumin
and α-albumin this assumption has lost much of its luster. At the
present time, it is not clear whether further studies short of
amino acid sequencing will unravel the origin of α-albumin,
although an effort to localize α-albumin in brain tissue with the
help of immunofluorescence appears worthwhile.

SUMMARY

α-albumin is a protein that is isoelectrically focused at a
pH from 5.64 to 4.89. In this range it displays several peaks
which are again demonstrable upon thin-layer isoelectric focusing.
Despite this apparent heterogeneity, all fractions react identically
with a rabbit anti-α-albumin antiserum. Using a variety of modifications of twodimensional immunoelectrodiffusion and immunoelectrophoresis, no antigenic relationship between α-albumin and
serum-albumin has been found whereas α-albumins of different
provenience, such as from normal human spinal cords, from the
brains of patients with Tay-Sachs disease and with SSPE, all react
similarly with anti-α-albumin and are not precipitated by anti-
albumin.

These studies have further clarified the nature of α-albumin
but have not contributed to an understanding of its formative
pathogenesis. That these proteins occur predominantly, if not
exclusively, in brain and spinal cord and are particularly rich in
megalobaric brains of patients with Tay-Sachs disease suggests a
relationship to edema. That the protein does apparently not exist
in other edematous tissues could be explained by the fact that
neither brain nor spinal cord are endowed with lymphatics which
subserve the function of returning extravasated plasma proteins to
the blood.

REFERENCES

1. Adriaenssens, K., A. Lowenthal, D. Karcher, Y. Mardens, and
       M. Van Sande: Biochemical screening methods for brain
       biopsies. Some results of lipid, protein and amino-acid
       determinations. Path. europ. 3: 468-473, 1968.

2.   Aronson, S. M. and B. W. Volk: Pathogenesis of white matter
     changes in Tay-Sachs disease. In: Cerebral Sphingolipidoses,
     S. M. Aronson and B. W. Volk (Eds.), Academic Press, New
     York, 1962, pp. 15-28.

3.   Awdeh, Z. L., A. R. Williamson, and B. A. Askonas: Isoelectric
     focusing in polyacrylamide gel and its application to immuno-
     globulins. Nature 219: 66-67, 1968.

4.   Axelsen, N. H. and P. J. Svendsen: Human candida precipitens
     characterized by a modified antigen antibody crossed
     electrophoresis. Protides of the Biological Fluids
     19th Annual Colloquium, April - May 1971. H. Peeters (Eds.).
     To be published by Pergamon Press.

5.   Chamoles, N., D. Karcher, W. Zeman and A. Lowenthal: Studies
     on α-albumin in nervous tissue. II. Topographical distri-
     bution in normal tissue. Brain Res. 17: 315-324, 1970.

6.   Delmotte, P.: Gel isoelectric focusing of cerebrospinal
     fluid proteins: A potential diagnostic tool. Z. klin.
     Chem. u. klin. Biochem. 9: 334-336, 1971.

7.   Karcher, D., W. Zeman, A. Lowenthal, and N. Chamoles: Studies
     on α-albumin in nervous tissue. I. Biochemical investiga-
     tions. Brain Res. 17: 307-314, 1970.

8.   Krøll, J.: On the immunoelectrophoretical identification and
     quantitation of serum proteins. Scand. J. clin. Lab.
     Invest. 22: 79-81, 1968.

9.   Krøll, J. and R. Thambiah: Quantitative estimation of electro-
     phoretically heterogeneous proteins by electrophoresis in
     antibody-containing agarose gel. Protides of the Biological
     Fluids, Vol. 17, Elsevier Publishing Co., Amsterdam, 1970,
     pp. 533-536.

10. Laurell, C. B.: Antigen-antibody crossed electrophoresis.
     Analyt. Biochem. 10: 358-361, 1965.

11. Laurell, C. B.: Quantitative estimation of proteins by
     electrophoresis in antibody-containing agarose gel.
     Protides of the Biological Fluids, Vol. 14, Elsevier
     Publishing Co., Amsterdam, 1966, pp. 499-502.

12. Wieme, R. J. Agar Gel Electrophoresis. Elsevier Publishing
     Co., Amsterdam, 1965, 425 pp.

13. Zeman, W., D. Karcher, N. Chamoles, and A. Lowenthal:
     Studies on α-albumin in nervous tissue. III. Observations
     on pathological specimens. Brain Res. 17: 325-334, 1970.

EFFECT OF AMINO ACID IMBALANCE ON POLYRIBOSOME PROFILES AND PROTEIN SYNTHESIS IN FETAL CEREBRAL CORTEX

Paul W. K. Wong and Parvin Justice

The Infants' Aid Perinatal Research
Laboratories, Mount Sinai Hospital,
the Chicago Medical School, and the
Department of Pediatrics, Stritch
School of Medicine, Loyola University
of Chicago, Illinois, U.S.A.

Numerous "inborn errors" of amino acid metabolism have been described (15,22). Most of these are associated with clinical disease of varying severity. For example, while maple syrup urine disease is usually rapidly fatal (14) phenylketonuria is competible with relative longevity (10). In most instances, the inherited metabolic block in the amino acid(s) involved has been well defined. However, the pathogensis of the various clinical syndromes is less well delineated.

Our interest in the study of protein synthesis in fetal brain complicated by maternal amino acid imbalance has been stimulated by the following observations from various investigators:(a) The concentration of amino acids has been demonstrated to affect protein synthesis in the brain (18). Specific amino acids also influence the rate of synthesis. For instance, incorporation of amino acids by brain slices decreases when various acidic amino acids are added to the incubation medium (17). On the other hand, y-aminobutyric acid and glycine have been demonstrated to stimulate radioactive leucine incorporation in a cell-free system (4). (b) It has been observed that the concentrations of amino acids are generally higher in the fetal than in the maternal blood during pregnancy (8). Since many "inborn errors" of amino acid metabolism are associated with specific amino acid increase in the blood and

the tissues of these patients, it may be assumed that
a similar or even greater increase may occur in the
fetuses of affected mothers. (c) Non-phenylketonuric
newborns of untreated phenylketonuric mothers have
been observed repeatedly to suffer from intrauterine
growth retardation (9). Patients with untreated
phenylketonuria have been found to have reduced brain
weight (1). Newborn rats given excessive amounts of
phenylalanine, tyrosine, methionine, leucine, isoleucine,
valine or histidine have reduced brain weight(6).

These observations suggest that imbalance of
various amino acids during pregnancy may adversely
affect the protein synthesizing capacity of the rapidly
growing fetal brain. This paper reports some observations in our studies of the fetal brain under the
influence of induced maternal amino acid imbalance.

MATERIALS AND METHODS

Hotlzman rats were kept in a dark room with
controlled light-and-darkness cycle. After a mating
period of 4 hours, vaginal smears were examined for
sperms to determine the day of conception. The sperm-
positive females were segregated and maintained on
Purina rat chow. On the 20th day of gestation , normal
saline (NaCl 0.85% w/v), or 1g/kg of body weight of one
of the following L-amino acids in an isotonic solution
was given intravenously to the pregnant rats: threonine,
serine, glutamic acid, proline, glycine, alanine, valine,
cysteine, methionine, isoleucine, leucine, phenylalanine, ornithine, lysine, histidine, arginine and 0.5
g/kg of trytophan.

One hour after injection, the fetuses were delivered by caesarean section under ether anesthesia.
Immediately after decapitation, their cerebral cortices
were obtained by dissection and washed with cold buffer
(0.05M Tris-HCl, pH 7.4, 0.25 M Sucrose, 0.025 M KCl,
0.012 M MgCl2)(19). Cortical tissues from multiple
fetuses of the same litter were dried with filter
paper, pooled and homogenized in 4 volumes of the same
buffer by the method of Siegel et al. (19). The
homogenate was centrifuged at 12,000 g for 30 minutes
at 4°C to remove mitochondria and cell debris. One ml
of the cytoplasmic supernatant (corresponding to 0.2
g wet weight) was layered on 26 ml of a 12-35% (w/w)
linear sucrose gradient in the same buffer. After

centrifugation in a Spinco 25.1 rotor at 25,000 rpm
for 2 hours at 4°C, polysome profile was monitored at
260 mμ using a recording spectrophotometer and a perpex
peristaltic pump to maintain a steady flow.   After
absorbancy measurement, fractions from the effluent
were collected for electromicroscopy by the method of
Oppenheim et al.(16).

    The capacity of the "polysomal" fractions to carry
out protein synthesis was evaluated by in vitro amino
acid incorporation according to the method of Zomzely
et al.(29).   For this purpose "polysomal" fractions
containing both ribosomes and microsomes were obtained
from post-mitochondrial supernatant by centrifugation
at 105,000 g for 2 hours.   Cell-free synthesis was
assessed using uniformly labelled L-C^{14} leucine.   The
same preparation of pH-5 enzyme in a ratio of 2 parts
enzyme protein to 1 part of "polysomal" protein was
used for each set of experiments.   0.025 mg of "polysomal"
protein was used in each incubation; and the incubation
mixture of Zomzely et al.(29) was proportionally
scaled down. The incubation was terminated at appropriate
time by immersing the incubation mixture into an ice
bath and adding buffer containing 3 mg of carrier L-
leucine.   The mixtures were centrifuged at 105,000 g
for 90 minutes.   The pellet was dissolved in 1 N
potassium hydroxide.   Aliquots were taken for protein
determination by the method of Lowry et al.(11).   The
remaining solution was precipitated with 10% TCA.   The
precipitate was collected and its radioactivity was
counted by the method of Tewari and Baxter(23).

    Amino acid content of maternal plasma and fetal
cerebral cortex was determined by a modification of
the method of Spackman et al.(21) using a Jeolco
autoanalyser.   Plasma and brain trytophan was determined
by the method of Denckla and Dewey(7).

                          RESULTS

    Typical polyribosome profiles from cerebral
cortices of fetal rats after saline injection
(control) to the mother rats are shown in figures 1
and 2.   They are identical to those from fetuses whose
mother has not been injected with saline.   These
profiles show primarily large aggregates of ribosomes;
and in agreement with the observations of other
investigators, there is a relatively small number of
monomers and dimers.

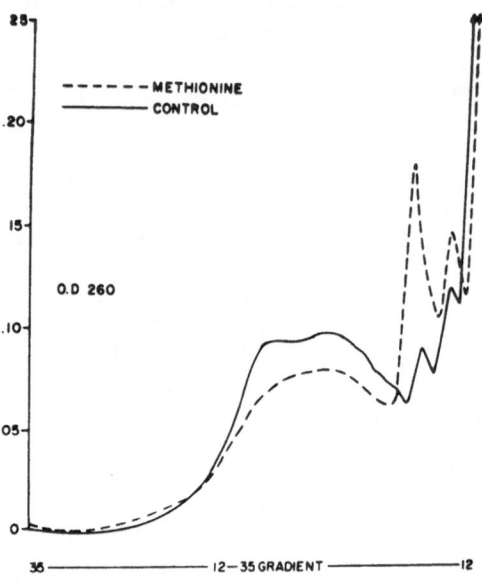

Figure 1.

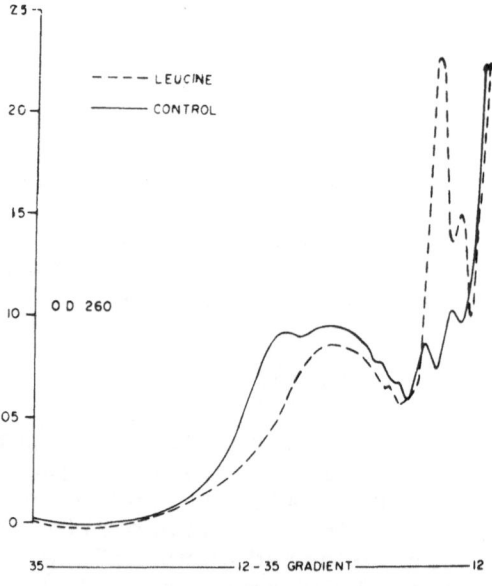

Figure 2.

Similarly, the polyribosome profiles from fetal cerebral cortices treated with threonine, serine, glutamic acid, proline, glycine, alanine, ornithine, lysine, histidine and arginine are essentially the same as the controls.

Injection of 1 g/kg of body weight of valine, cysteine, methionine, isoleucine, leucine, phenylalanine and 0.5 g/kg of trytophan result in disaggregation of polyribosomes and the appearance of increased number of monomers and dimers in fetal cerebral cortices. Figures 1 and 2 show typical polyribosome profiles from fetal cerebral cortices treated with methionine and leucine respectively. Profiles from fetal cortices treated with valine, cysteine, isoleucine, phenylalanine and trytophan are similar.

After absorbance measurement, fractions collected from the corresponding peaks were examined by electron-microscopy. This confirmed the nature of polymer, dimer and monomer peaks.

Table I shows the amino acid concentrations in maternal plasma and fetal cerebral cortices in the control, methionine-treated and leucine-treated animals. It is seen that in both cases, maternal hyperamino-acidemia is associated with increased concentration of the corresponding amino acid in the fetal brain. In addition, significant variations in other amino acids are observed. There is no consistant pattern in these changes. (Amino acids without significant changes are not listed).

After the injection of glutamic acid, alanine and ornithine to the mother rats, there is only a small increase of the corresponding amino acids in the fetal brain. The polyribosome profiles from the fetal cerebral cortices of these animals are normal. On the other hand, after the injection of glycine, proline, and threonine to the mother rats, there is a 2 to 4 fold increase in the corresponding amino acids in the fetal brain. There is no obvious disaggregation of the polyribosomes from the cerebral cortices of these animals.

After injection of methionine, leucine, valine, phenylalanine, trytophan and cysteine to the mother rats, there is a 10 to 40 fold increase of the corresponding amino acids in the fetal brain. Polyribosome

TABLE I

Amino Acid Concentration in Maternal Plasma and Fetal Cerebral Cortex

	Plasma (µmole/ml)			Cerebral Cortex (µmole/g)		
	Control**	Methionine* Treated	Leucine** Treated	Control***	Methionine* Treated	Leucine* Treated
Asp	0.008	0.014	0.005	1.222	2.040	1.540
Glu	0.210	0.163	0.210	3.829	5.350	5.564
Gly	0.146	0.115	0.100	0.526	1.003	0.686
Ala	0.594	0.517	0.338	1.140	1.740	2.078
Met	0.057	5.666	0.024	0.077	4.310	0.008
Isoleu	0.087	0.031	0.036	0.050	0.056	0.007
Leu	0.148	0.056	2.110	0.117	0.098	1.031
Tyr	0.059	0.026	0.063	0.124	0.081	0.041
yABA	–	–	–	0.354	0.497	0.330
Lys	0.845	0.790	0.606	0.327	0.513	0.297
Val	0.184	0.077	0.058	0.134	0.210	0.032

*n = 3, **n = 5, *** n = 10.

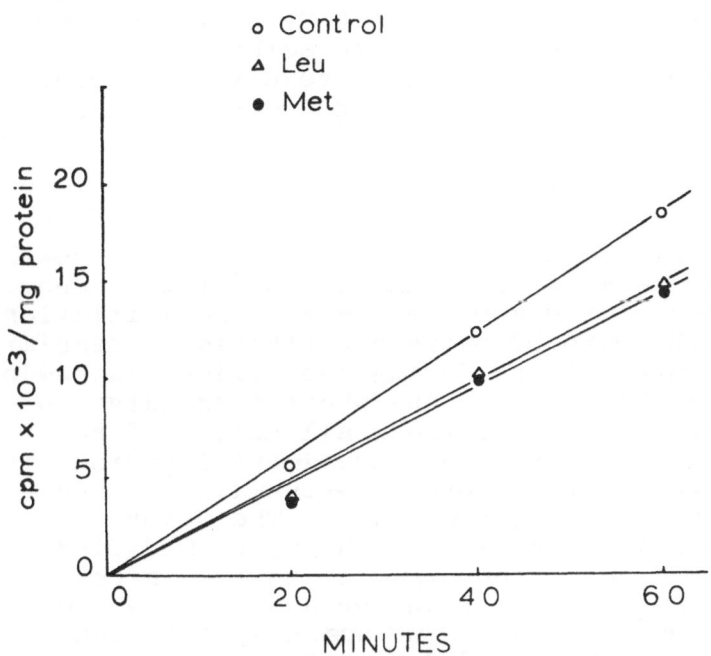

Figure 3.

Incorporation of L-C^{14} leucine into TCA precipitable protein is expressed as cpm per mg of "polysomal" protein. Each point represents the mean of 6 determinations for the controls and 3 determinations for the methionine and leucine treated animals. Other sets of identical experiments, using different preparations of pH-5 enzyme, show the same results.

profiles from these fetal cerebral cortices show
significant disaggregation. However, injection of
histidine to the mother rats results in a 30 fold increase in the fetal brain, there is no obvious
disaggregation of the polyribosomes.

Figure 3 shows the radioactivity of L-C^{14} leucine
incorporated into TCA precipitable protein by "polysomal" fractions from fetal cerebral cortices treated
with saline (control), methionine and leucine. It is
seen that there is a decrease in L-C^{14} leucine incorporation in preparations from both methionine and
leucine treated animals. Similar results are observed
in the phenylalanine and trytophan treated animals.

DISCUSSION

Cellular replication, differentiation and growth
are intimately related to transcription of the genome
and translation of the gene products. The initiation,
cessation or the rate of protein synthesis is regulated
by molecular interactions during the various phases of
the cell cycle(13). Due to the short term nature of
our experiments and due to the small number of replicat-
ing cells existing within the experimental period, it
may be suggested that our experiments mainly affect
the protein synthesizing mechanism. The major
components of this mechanism which may be modified by
the experimental conditions are (a) the 70S ribosomes,
(b) messenger RNA and (c) transfer RNA. Since the
same preparation of pH-5 enzyme was used for each set
of experiments, the observed differences in the control
and experimental conditions may be the result of
changes in the 70S ribosomes, the messenger RNA or both.

It has been observed that the rate of amino acid
incorporation into protein in vitro is correlated with
the degree of polysomal aggregation (5,20). In addition,
it has been demonstrated that the amount of polysomal
aggregation is influenced by the supply of amino acids.
Polysomal aggregation and the polysomal regulation of
the rate of protein synthesis have been generally
considered to be the physiological regulator of protein synthesis in vivo(2,28). The mechanism by which
amino acid concentrations regulate polysomal aggregation is unknown.

Our experiments demonstrate that injection of
valine, cysteine, methionine, isoleucine, leucine,

phenylalanine and trytophan to pregnant rats result in increased concentration of the corresponding amino acids in the fetal brain. This is associated with disaggregation of polyribosomes and decreased in vitro amino acid incorporation. Various mechanisms may be suggested to account for the disaggregation of the polyribosomes:(a) The changes accompanying the disturbed amino acid content in the fetal brain may result in degradation of RNA by ribonuclease. It has been observed that intracellular ribonuclease probably does not exist in a free form. It is mostly bound by ribonuclease-inhibitor, some of which is attached to ribosomes(24,25). Increased activity of the inhibitor in the polyribosomes has been correlated with increased rate of protein synthesis(12). It may be suggested, therefore, that the changes in the fetal brain induced by certain amino acid excess may lead to the dissociation of the binding between RNAase and the inhibitor. The inactive RNAase is then converted to an active form.(b) The changes in the fetal brain accompanying certain amino acid excess may result in conformational alterations in the ribosomal protein, leading to dissociation of mRNA and the ribosomes.(c) It is also possible that certain amino acid excess in the fetal brain may result in reduced synthesis of RNA. This in turn may lead to incomplete assembly of the ribosomal structural protein to precursor RNA.

The lack of similar effect of threonine, serine, glutamic acid, proline, glycine, alanine, ornithine, lysine, histidine and arginine on polyribosomal aggregation in the fetal brain may be due to a dosage-related phenomenon or due to the specific structure of the amino acids.

Although the time and the rate of neuronal replication and growth in the fetal brain vary in different species (26,27) and although the physiological significance of our in vitro experiments has to be tested in vivo, nonetheless, it may be postulated that any significant reduction in the capacity of protein synthesis in the developing brain for an extended period of time is potentially detrimental. Imbalance of amino acids during human pregnancies secondary to either inborn errors of metabolism or environmental factors may be regarded as undesirable for optimal fetal growth.

REFERENCES

(1) Alvord, E. C., Stevenson, L. O., Vogel, E. S. and
Egle, R. L.: Neuropathological findings in phenyl-
pyruvic oligophrenia (phenyl-ketonuria). J.
Neuropath. Exp. Neurol. 9, 298 (1950).

(2) Aoki, K. and Seigel, F.L.: Hyperphenylalaninemia:
disaggregation of brain polyribosomes in young
rats. Science 168, 129 (1970).

(3) Baglia, B. S., Pronczuk, A. W. and Munro, H. N.:
Regulation of polysome aggregation in cell-free
system through amino acid supply. J. Mole. Biol.
34, 199 (1968).

(4) Baxter, C. F.and Tewari, S.: Regulation by amino
acids of protein synthesis from immature rat brain:
stimulatory effect of y-aminobutyric acid and
glycine in Protein Metabolism of the Nervous
System. Lajtha, A. (editor), New York, Plenum
Press (1970) Page 439.

(5) Brener, C. B. and Florini, A. J.: Amino acid
incorporation into protein by cell-free system
from rat skeletal muscle. IV. Biochemistry 4,
1544 (1965).

(6) Chase, H. P. and O'Brien, D.: Effect of excess
phenyalanine and of other amino acids on brain
development in the infant rats. Pediat. Res. 4,
96 (1970).

(7) Denckla, W. D. and Dewey, H. K.: The determination
of trytophan in plasma, liver and urine. J. Lab.
Clin. Med. 69, 160 (1967).

(8) Ghadimi, H. and Pecora, P.: Free amino acids of
cord plasma as compared with maternal plasma
during pregnancy. Pediatrics 33, 500 (1964$_a$).

(9) Hsia, D. Y. Y.: Phenylketonuria: clinical, genetic
and biochemical aspects. Warsaw Congress Proceedings of the International Association for
Scientific Study of Mental Deficiency. (in press)

(10) Lang, K.: Die phenylpyruvische oligophrenie.
Ergebn, inn. Med. u. Kinderh. 6, 78 (1955).

(11) Lowry, O. H., Rosebrough, N. J., Farr, A. L. and Randall, R. J.: Protein measurement with Folin phenol reagent. J. Biol. Chem. 193, 365 (1951).

(12) Majumdar,C., Tsukada, K. and Liberman. I.: Liver protein synthesis after partial hepatectomy and acute stress. J. Biol. Chem 242,700 (1967).

(13) Medredev, Zh A.: Protein Biosynthesis and Problems of Heredity. Development and Ageing. Edinburgh, Oliver and Boyd (1966).

(14) Menkes, J. H., Hurst, P. L. and Craig, J. M.: A new syndrome: progressive familial cerebral dysfunction with an unusual urine substance Pediatrics 14, 462 (1954).

(15) Nyhan, W. L. (editor): Amino Acid Metabolism and Genetic Variation, New York, McGraw-Hill Book Company (1967).

(16) Oppenheim, J., Scheinbuks, J., Biava, C. and Marcus, L.: Polyribosomes in azotabacter vinelandii. Biochem. Biophys. Acta. 161, 386 (1968).

(17) Orrego, F. and Lipmann, F.: Protein synthesis in brain slices. J. Biol. Chem. 242, 665 (1967).

(18) Roberts, S. and Morelos, B. S.: Regulation of Cerebral metabolism of amino acid. J. Neurochem. 12, 373 (1965).

(19) Siegel, F. L. Aoki, K. and Colwell, R. E.: Polyribosome disaggregation and cell-free protein synthesis in preparation from cortex of hyperphenylalaninemic rats. J. Neurochem. 18, 537 (1970).

(20) Sox, H. C. and Hoagland, M. C.: Functional alteration in liver polysomes associated with starvation and refeeding. J. Molec. Biol. 20, 113 (1966).

(21) Spackman, D. H., Stein, W. H. and Moore, S.: Automatic recording apparatus for use in chromatography of amino acids. Analytical Chem. 30, 1190 (1958).

(22) Stanbury, J. B., Wyngaarden, J. B. and
      Fredrickson, D. S. (editors): The Metabolic
      Basis of Inherited Diseases. New York, McGraw-
      Hill Book Company (1966), pages 258-420.

(23) Tewari, S. and Baxter, C. F.: Stimulatory effect
      of y-aminobutyric acid upon amino acid incorpor-
      ation into protein by a ribosomal system from
      immature rat brain. J. Neurochem. 16, 171
      (1969).

(24) Tsukada, J., Majumdar, C. and Lieberman. I.:
      Liver polyribosomes and phospholipase A.
      Biochem. Biophys. Res. Commun. 25, 181 (1966).

(25) Utosunomiya, T. and Roth, J. S.: Studies on
      the function of intracellular ribonucleases.
      J. Cell. Biol. 29, 395 (1966).

(26) Winick, N.: Changes in nucleic acid and protein
      content of human brain during growth, Pediat.
      Res. 2, 352 (1968).

(27) Winick, M. and Noble, A.: Quantitative changes
      in DNA, RNA and protein during prenatal and
      postnatal growth in rats. Develop. Biol. 12,
      451 (1965).

(28) Wunner, E. H., Bell, J. and Munro, H. N.: The
      effect of feeding with a trytophan-free amino
      acid mixture on rat liver polysomes and
      ribosomal ribonucleic acid. Biochem. J. 101,
      417 (1966).

(29) Zomzely, C. E., Roberts, S. and Rapoport, D.:
      Regulation of cerebral metabolism of amino
      acids. J. Neurochem. 11, 567 (1964).

ACKNOWLEDGEMENT

This study was aided by a grant from the National
Foundation-March of Dimes. The authors would like to
thank Dr. D.Y.Y. Hsia for his encouragement and support;
and E. Emans and N. Becker for their technical assistance.

PURIFICATION AND PROPERTIES OF TWO SPHINGOLIPID HYDROLASES

Howard R. Sloan, Jan L. Breslow, Donald S. Fredrickson

Molecular Disease Branch

National Heart and Lung Institute

INTRODUCTION

Our understanding of the lipid storage disorders has progressed dramatically since 1881 when Warren Tay, a British opthalmologist, described a cherry-red macular degeneration in the fundus of an infant with marked weakness of the trunk and limbs (1). This patient was the first reported case of Tay-Sachs disease. In the 90 years that have followed, there has been a delineation of a large number of inherited metabolic disorders characterized by the accumulation within tissues of large amounts of lipids.

Progress in the understanding of inherited metabolic diseases has, in general, evolved through several identifiable stages. Meticulous description of the clinical signs and symptoms is frequently the first step toward the detailed understanding of a metabolic disease. The second step is the identification and chemical characterization of the substance, or substances, that are stored in the tissues of the patients. The demonstration of the metabolic, i.e. the enzymatic, defect that results in the accumulation of the specific substance is the third step.

Our knowledge of the sphingolipidoses has now advanced to the point where the enzymatic defect has been established in all of the major ones, and each can now be diagnosed with certainty by chemical and enzymatic analyses. It is also possible to perform an amniocentesis in pregnancies at risk for one of these disorders and to cultivate fibroblasts derived from the amniotic fluid cells. Specific enzymatic analyses performed on cultured fetal cells permit a definitive intrauterine diagnosis and if the enzymatic assay indicates an affected fetus, the pregnancy may be terminated.

We are now entering the fourth stage of our understanding of the lipid storage disorders. This is the discovery of the precise molecular nature of each defect, a step that depends upon the purification of the normal enzyme whose mutant counterpart is responsible for a given disease. Detailed study of the normal enzyme may enable us to delineate properties of the abnormal enzyme, which may explain deficiency or absence of its activity. From this will come the ability to determine whether an abnormal phenotype is the expression of a failure to produce normal amounts of a given sphingolipid hydrolase or to the production of a protein that is defective.

In our previous attempts to purify human liver sphingomyelinase, we have employed many of the classical methods of protein purification. These have included: differential centrifugation, freezing and thawing, extraction with detergent, ammonium sulfate fractionation, acetone and ethanol fractionation, gel chromatography, and ion exchange chromatography. With these methods we have achieved significant purification of human liver sphingomyelinase; we have, however, never obtained a pure enzyme preparation. In the liver, sphingomyelinase is located in the lysosomal portion of the cell (2) and is brought into solution with considerable difficulty. For this study we have used urine as a plentiful source of apparently soluble sphingolipid hydrolases. To the classical methods of protein purification we have added the new technique of specific affinity chromatography as a means for improved purification of the sphingolipid hydrolases.

METHODS

Source of Material

Twenty-four hour urine collections were obtained from normal individuals and stored at 4°C until processed further.

Preparation of Affinity Labeled Sepharoses

Succinylated sepharose was prepared according to the method of Cuatrecases (3). Sepharose was first reacted with cyanogen

AGAROSE AFFINITY CHROMATOGRAPHY

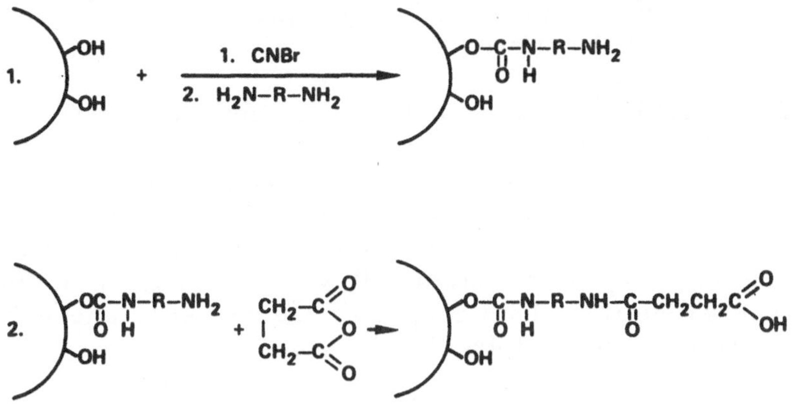

Fig. 1. Schematic representation of the preparation of succinyl-. ated sepharose. Semicircles in this and later figures represent beads of sepharose.

bromide and then with a diamine. Amino-sepharose was converted to the carboxyl form by reaction with succinc anhydride (Fig. 1).

Sphingosine-containing ligands were prepared by partial acid or basic hydrolysis of the corresponding sphingolipid. Psycho-sine sulfate was purchased from Pierce Chemical Company and was also prepared from sulfatide (Pierce) by butanolic-potassium hydroxide hydrolysis followed by treatment with sulphuric acid (4). Sphingosylphosphorylcholine was prepared from sphingomyelin by hydrolysis in butanolic-hydrochloric acid (5). Glucosyl ceramide was isolated from the liver of a patient with Gaucher's disease and converted to glucosyl sphingosine (psychosine) by hydrolysis with butanolic-potassium hydroxide (4). These ligands were purified by chromatography on columns of silicic acid. The ligands were coupled to the succinylated sepharose in aqueous solution employ-ing 1-ethyl-3-(3-dimethylaminopropyl) carbodiimide as described by Cuatrecasas (3).

p-Nitrocatechol sulfate (Sigma) was reduced with hydrogen over platinum to the corresponding amino compound. Sepharose 4B was activated by treatment with cyanogen bromide and coupled to 6-aminohexanoic acid; the water soluble carbodiimide procedure of Cuatrecases (3) was employed to couple this substituted sepharose with p-aminocatechol sulfate.

p-Nitro phenyl phosphorylcholine was prepared according to the method of Chesebro (6) and was reduced to the corresponding amino compound with hydrogen over platinum. The p-amino compound was then converted to p-diazonium phenyl phosphorylcholine by treatment with sodium nitrite in aqueous dilute hydrochloric acid. The resulting p-diazonium salt was then coupled to glycyl-tyrosyl-sepharose (6). This coupling occurred spontaneously upon mixing the two reagents at 4°C for 24 hours.

Before the application of enzyme preparations the affinity labeled sepharoses were thoroughly washed with buffer to remove all of the uncoupled ligands. The substituted sepharoses may be stored for extended periods of time at 4°C.

Purification of Arylsulfatase A

Urine was adjusted to pH 5.7 by the addition of 1.0 M sodium acetate and was filtered through glass fibre filter paper (Reeve Angel Grade 934AH) to remove debris (7). Ammonium sulfate was then added to a final concentration of 50%; the solution was stirred for one-half hour and then kept at 4°C without further stirring for two additional hours. The precipitate was collected by filtration and was solubilized in 0.1 M sodium acetate buffer pH 5.7. The enzyme solution was then subjected to a two-step acetone fractionation between 0 and 33%, and 33 to 67% (V:V). The bulk of the enzymatic activity was found in the 33-67% fraction and this material was then processed further. For the purification of arylsulfatase A, the material obtained by the acetone fractionation was applied to a small column of psychosine sulfate sepharose (Fig. 2). The column was washed with large amounts of 0.1 M sodium acetate pH 5.7 and the enzymatic activity was finally eluted with 0.1% Triton X-100 (W:V) in 0.1 M sodium acetate buffer, pH 5.7. Fractions with enzyme activity were pooled and applied to a 10 x 1500 mm column of Sephadex G-200 (Pharmacia). Those fractions with the greatest enzyme activity were pooled and concentrated to a small volume by filtration through a Diaflo membrane (Amicon). The concentrated

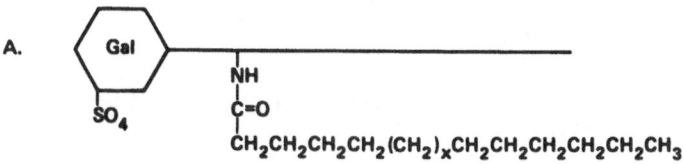

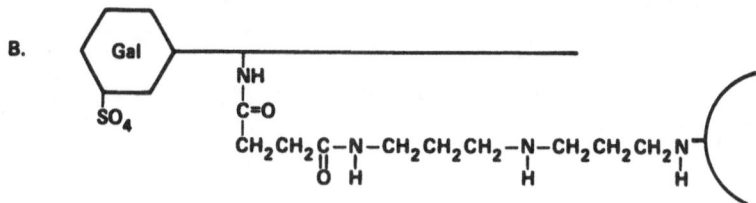

Fig. 2. (A) Schematic representation of sulfatide, and (B) Schematic representation of psychosine sulfate sepharose. Note the marked similarity between the two structures.

enzyme preparation was then subjected to preparative polyacrylamide gel electrophoresis in a Canalco apparatus employing the standard Ornstein-Davis system (8, 9). The eluting buffer was pumped at a rate of 50 ml per hour and 5 ml fractions were collected.

Purification of Sphingomyelinase

The purification of sphingomyelinase from human urine employs the same ammonium sulfate and acetone fractionation as described above for arylsulfatase A. The 33 to 67% acetone fraction was, however, applied to a column of sphingosylphosphorylcholine sepharose (Fig. 3). The sphingomyelinase activity was eluted from this column with 0.1% Triton X-100 (W:V) in 0.1 M sodium cacodylate, pH 6.1. Fractions with enzyme activity were

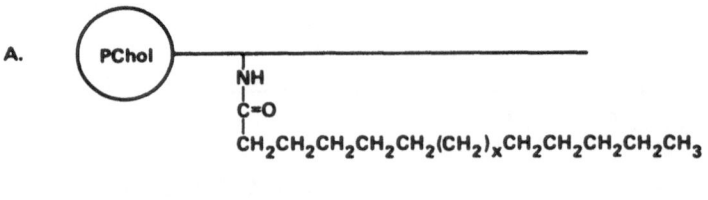

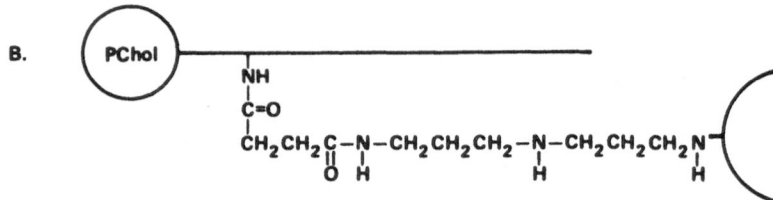

Fig. 3. (A) Schematic representation of sphingomyelin, and (B) Schematic representation of sphingosylphosphorylcholine sepharose. Note the marked similarity between the two structures.

pooled and concentrated by Diaflo membrane filtration and applied to a 12 x 420 mm Sephadex G-200 column which had been equilibrated with 0.1 M sodium cacodylate buffer pH 6.1.

Enzyme Assays

Arylsulfatase A activity was assayed as described by Baum (10). Sulfatide-35S and sphingomyelin-$[CH_3-^{14}C]$ were biosynthesized and purified as described previously (11, 12). The assays for sulfatide sulfatase activity and for sphingomyelinase activity were performed by methods that have been previously described (11, 12).

RESULTS

Arylsulfatase A

The five step purification scheme developed for arylsulfatase
A results in the preparation of an apparently pure enzyme (Fig. 4).

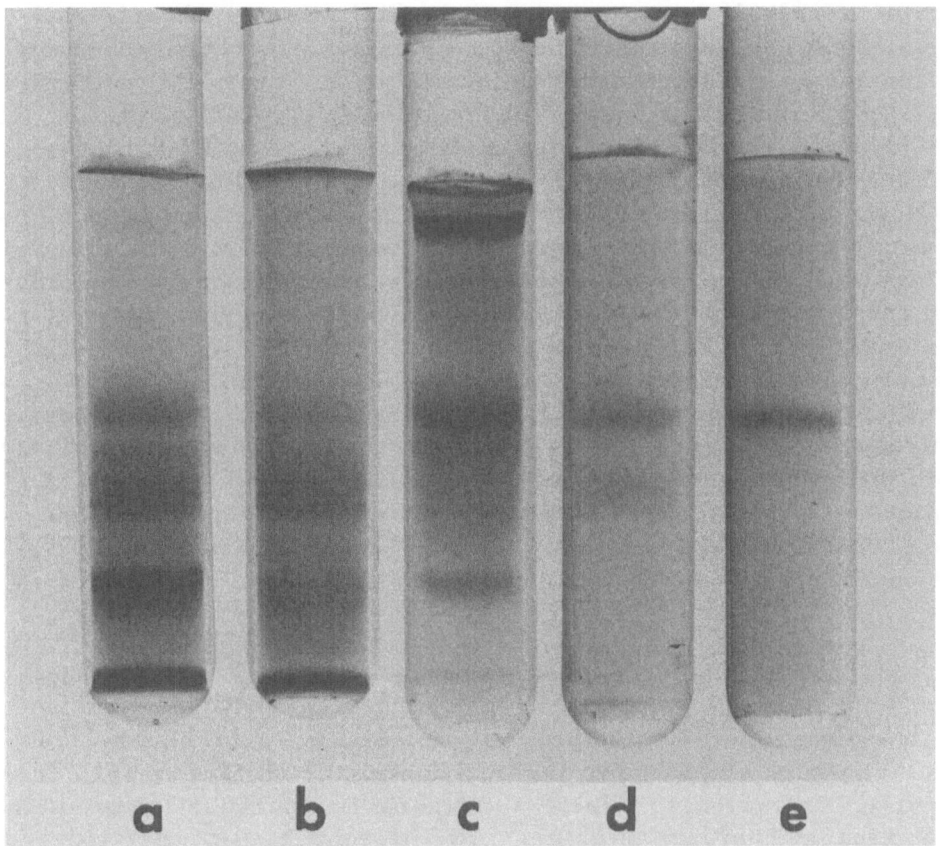

Fig. 4. Analytical polyacrylamide gels of arylsulfatase A at five
stages of purification. Following: (a) Ammonium sulfate precipitation, (b) acetone fractionation, (c) affinity chromatography,
(d) Sephadex G-200 chromatography, and (e) preparative polyacrylamide gel electrophoresis.

The ammonium sulfate precipitation serves primarily as an enzyme concentration step with some increase in the specific activity of the preparation (Fig. 4a). The fractionation with acetone effects a significant delipidation of the enzyme. This was confirmed by chromatography performed on thin-layer plates of silica gel G before and following the acetone procedure (13). Although the acetone fractionation did not produce a significant increase in specific enzyme activity (Fig. 4b), it was essential for further purification of the enzyme. Arylsulfatase A has a great affinity for psychosine sulfate sepharose. Attempts to elute the enzymatic activity with high concentrations of salt (sodium acetate, pH 5.7 up to 4M) extremes of pH (pH 3 and pH 10), and with the substrate, p-nitrocatechol sulfate (0.01 M), were essentially unsuccessful. At pH 10 (10^{-4} M NaOH) a very small amount (10%) of activity could be eluted; 0.1 M NaCl or 0.1 M buffer at pH 10 did not, however, elute the enzyme. Attempts to elute the enzymatic activity with 0.01 M sodium decyl sulfate resulted in complete inactivation of the enzyme. The only agent that was able to effect complete elution of arylsulfatase A was the non-ionic detergent Triton X-100. Dilute solutions (0.01%) did not remove the enzymatic activity from the column; 0.05% solutions eluted approximately 25% of the activity. A 0.1% concentration of Triton X-100 removed 100% of the enzymatic activity from the column in a very small volume of solution (Fig. 4c). Comparable results were obtained employing columns of arylsulfate sepharose. The enzymatic activity could only be eluted with Triton X-100.

Sphingomyelinase

The ammonium sulfate precipitation and the acetone fractionation that were employed in the purification of arylsulfatase A from human urine were also effective in the partial purification of sphingomyelinase from human urine. The protein that precipitated from the urine at 67% acetone concentration was collected by centrifugation and resuspended in 0.1 M sodium cacodylate buffer pH 6.1. The soluble enzymatic activity was then applied to a small column of sphingosyl phosphorylcholine sepharose; the column was washed thoroughly with 0.1 M sodium cacodylate, pH 6.1. Sphingomyelinase activity could not be eluted from the affinity column by the procedures usually employed in affinity chromatography, i.e., concentrations of salt up to 4M, buffers at pH 2 and pH 12, and solutions of known inhibitors of the enzyme (phosphate and phosphorylcholine). Aqueous dispersions of

sphingomyelin and sphingosyl phosphorylcholine were also not effective. As in the case of arylsulfatase A activity, sphingomyelinase
activity was eluted quantitatively from the column by 0. 1% Triton
X-100 in 0. 1 M sodium cacodylate, pH 6. 1. Comparable results
were obtained employing columns of aryl phosphorylcholine sepharose. Fractions with enzymatic activity were pooled and applied
to a Sephadex G-200 column; the enzymatic activity eluted in the
void volume. Polyacrylamide gel electrophoresis using the standard Ornstein-Davis (8, 9) system indicates that this fraction is
contaminated with at least two other proteins.

DISCUSSION

The analytical polyacrylamide gels shown in Figure 4 illustrate
that the 5 step method described in this paper for the purification
of arylsulfatase A from human urine yields an apparently pure protein. The yield is approximately 10% of the starting arylsulfatase
A activity. An acetone fractionation step was essential for complete purification of arylsulfatase A, indicating that, in the urine,
the enzyme is probably closely associated with lipid. Lipid interactions may be responsible for the aggregation of arylsulfatase
A or its complexing with other proteins.

The appearance of sphingomyelinase activity in the void volume
of a Sephadex G-200 column indicates that this enzyme is also
likely aggregated in polymeric form or is associated with a significant amount of other lysosomal membrane proteins. Further
treatment with dissociating agents such as sodium cholate may be
required to disaggregate the protein into smaller but still active
units.

Triton X-100 had a unique capacity to dislodge arylsulfatase A
and sphingomyelinase from sepharose bound psychosine sulfate
and sphingosylphosphorylcholine. This implies that hydrophobic
bonding is important in the interaction of these two enzymes with
the affinity labeled sepharose. It seems unlikely, however, that
hydrophobic interactions account solely for the high affinity of
these enzymes for the substituted sepharose, for arylsulfatase A
also binds tightly to aryl sulfate sepharose, a substituted sepharose
with only a very small segment of methylene groups. The failure
of salt in high concentration and buffers of extremely high or low
pH to elute much of the enzymatic activities would indicate that
ion exchange is probably not a major factor in the binding of these

proteins to the substituted sepharoses. Noting that 10% of the aryl-sulfatase A activity could be eluted at pH 10, however, we suspect that ionic forces do play some role in the binding of the sphingolipid hydrolases to the affinity columns.

It should be possible to extend affinity chromatography as employed here to isolation of others of the hydrolases involved in different sphingolipidoses. Glucosyl sphingosine sepharose and galactosyl sphingosine sepharose may prove to be useful reagents for the preparation of pure glucocerebrosidase and galactocerebrosidase, respectively. It also seems possible that galactosyl galactosyl glucosyl sphingosine can be coupled to succinylated sepharose and that this material may prove useful for the preparation of the α-galactosidase that is present in diminished activity in Fabry's disease. Attempts to synthesize ganglioside derivatives of sepharose may be less successful. The hydrolytic procedures that are used to cleave the fatty acid moieties from the gangliosides would probably also remove sialic acid. The fatty acid could be removed from the asialo-gangliosides and the resulting amine coupled to succinylated sepharose, producing a substituted sepharose that might be sufficiently similar to the gangliosides to bind the ganglioside hydrolases.

The strong interaction of arylsulfatase A with psychosine sulfate sepharose and of sphingomyelinase with sphingosyl phosphorylcholine sepharose does not prevent these proteins from exhibiting some enzymatic activity. This could be demonstrated by incubating either of the sepharose-bound enzymes with the appropriate substrate. Thus there may be dissociation-association reactions between the hydrolase and the substituted sepharose which briefly free the active site of the enzyme. It is at least equally possible that there is more than one active site on each bound enzyme molecule.

The fact that these sphingolipid hydrolases are active even when tightly associated with affinity labeled sepharose suggests a possible role for such complexes in the treatment of disorders characterized by the deficient activity of a specific sphingolipid hydrolase. It has recently been suggested that infusion of plasma may be useful in the therapy of Fabry's disease (14). It is believed that the infusion of plasma provides significant amounts of α-galactosidase and that this enzyme affects a reduction of the plasma levels of trihexosyl ceramide in the recipient. If α-galactosidase can be purified to a degree and then tightly associated with substituted sepharose it may be possible to produce a column by which trihexosyl ceramide could be selectively removed from the plasma of a patient with Fabry's disease; the patient's plasma could then be reinfused. This form of plasmapheresis would be cumbersome therapy, but would have the advantage of infusion of only isologous plasma.

Sphingolipid hydrolases associated with affinity labeled sepharoses satisfy the properties that have been suggested by Brady as desirable for therapy with enzymes encapsulated in a bio-degradable microspherule (15). Such complexes could be administered parenterally, and possibly taken up by the reticulo-endothelial system, hopefully followed by proper intracellular localization of the enzyme. It seems unlikely, however, that this process could result in the entry of sphingolipid hydrolases into the central nervous system where they are probably most acutely needed in most of the sphingolipidoses with cerebral manifestations.

ACKNOWLEDGMENTS

The authors are grateful to Mrs. Barbara Davis and Mr. Stephen Demosky for expert technical assistance.

REFERENCES

1. Tay, W., Trans. Ophthal. Soc. U.K., 1, 155 (1881).
2. Weinreb, N. J., Brady, R. O. and Tappel, A. L., Biochim. Biophys. Acta 159, 141 (1968).
3. Cuatrecasas, P., J. Biol. Chem. 245, 3059 (1970).
4. Carter, H. E. and Fujino, Y., J. Biol. Chem. 221, 879 (1956).
5. Kaller, H., Biochem. Zeitschrift 334, 451 (1961).
6. Chesebro, B. W., Personal Communication.
7. Breslow, J. L. and Sloan, H. R., in review.
8. Ornstein, L., Ann. N. Y. Acad. Sci. 121, 321 (1964).
9. Davis, B. J., Ann. N. Y. Acad. Sci. 121, 404 (1964).
10. Baum, H., Dodgson, K. S. and Spencer, B., Clin. Chim. Acta 4, 453 (1959).
11. Sloan, H. R., Chem. Phys. Lipids 5, 250 (1970).
12. Sloan, H. R., Uhlendorf, B. W., Kanger, J. N., Brady, R. O., and Fredrickson, D. S., Biochem. Biophys. Res. Commun. 34, 582 (1969).

13.   Kwiterovich, P. O., Sloan, H. R. and Fredrickson, D. S.,
      J. Lipid Res. 11, 322 (1970).
14.   Mapes, C. A., Anderson, R. L., Sweeley, C. C., Desnick,
      R. J. and Krivit, W., Science 169, 987 (1970).
15.   Brady, R. O., Bulletin of the New York Academy of Medicine
      47, 173 (1971).

DEFICIENCY OF SPECIFIC PROTEINS IN THE INBORN ERRORS OF MUCOPOLYSACCHARIDE METABOLISM

Elizabeth F. Neufeld, Robert W. Barton, Michael Cantz,
Jeffery G. Derge,[+] Clara W. Hall, Hans Kresse and James F. Scott

National Institute of Arthritis and Metabolic Diseases,
National Institutes of Health, Bethesda, Maryland 20014

This paper will summarize recent studies on the nature and function of those proteins which are deficient in the mucopolysaccharidoses.

Fibroblasts cultured from the skin of patients with the Hurler syndrome and related disorders, have an abnormal metabolism of sulfated mucopolysaccharide (MPS), as do the patients themselves. The abnormality is manifested as increased storage of MPS (usually dermatan sulfate) which can be detected by staining with histochemical dyes (1) or by chemical analysis (2); if $^{35}SO_4$ is used as marker, the abnormality is seen in the form of increased accumulation and lengthened turnover time of radioactive intracellular MPS (3).

The abnormal metabolism can be restored to normal ("corrected") if two genetically distinct lines of fibroblasts are mixed with each other (4) or if medium preincubated with one cell line is subsequently applied to the other (5). Such cross-correction experiments show that the abnormal metabolism is a consequence of the lack of some genotype-specific factor. This view of mucopolysaccharidoses as deficiency diseases is consistent with the recessive mode of their inheritance.

[+]Fellow of the National Cystic Fibrosis Research Foundation.
*International Postdoctoral Research Fellow of the U. S. Public Health Service.

TABLE I: Biochemical Classification of Mucopolysaccharidoses

Disorder	Deficiency	Reference
I, Hurler	Specific factor	5, 7
II, Hunter	Specific factor	5
III, Sanfilippo	Specific factor A or Specific factor B	8
IV, Morquio	Not studied	
V, Scheie	Same as Hurler	7, 9
VI, Maroteaux-Lamy	Specific	10

In the last two years, we have shown the existence of five distinct protein factors. The biochemical classification of mucopolysaccharidoses based on factor deficiency is in rather good agreement with the clinical classification of McKusick (6), as seen in Table I. The major differences are, on the one hand, biochemical heterogeneity within the Sanfilippo syndrome; and on the other, deficiency of the same protein in two clinically different disorders, the Scheie and Hurler syndromes. (The latter means that the Scheie and Hurler mutations affect the same protein, perhaps in allelic fashion; it does not imply that they are identical.) We fully expect that further research will uncover more biochemical heterogeneity, as has already been suggested (11).

Progress in the purification of the factor proteins has been made possible by their occurrence in normal human urine in relatively high specific activity. Typically, normal adult male urine contains, per mg of urinary protein: 40 units of Hunter factor and of both Sanfilippo factors, 5 units of Hurler factor and one unit of Maroteaux-Lamy factor. A factor unit is that amount which gives half-maximal correction in the appropriate cells. Urinary factors, like those in fibroblast secretions, are genotype-specific (12).

All five factors are precipitable from urine with 70% ammonium sulfate; a convenient subsequent purification step is gel filtration on Sephadex G-200. The apparent molecular weights of the factors, obtained on a calibrated column, are shown in Fig. 1.

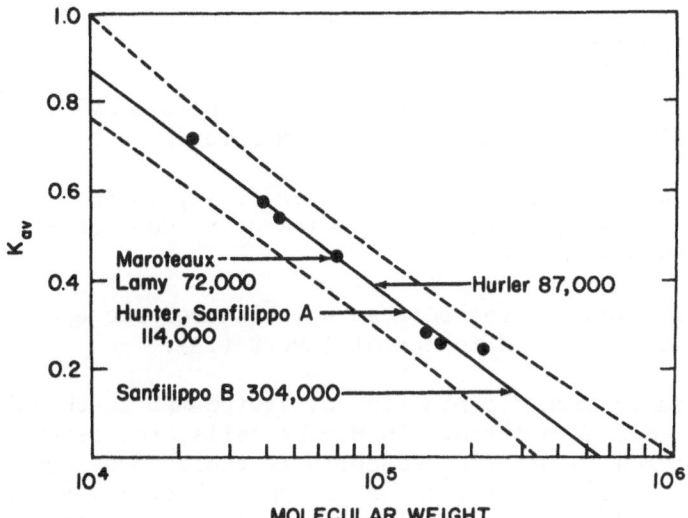

Fig. 1. Molecular weight estimates for five factors, obtained by chromatography on Sephadex G-200. ---- 95% confidence limits for the line. For standards used in calibration, see reference 7.

To date, three factors have been purified further: the Hurler, Hunter and Sanfilippo A factors. A summary of the three purifications is shown in Table II. The purified preparations were specific:

TABLE II: Purification of Factors

Factor	Steps	Purifi-cation	Estimated purity	Ref.
Hurler	Sephadex G-200 Carboxymethylcellulose Hydroxylapatite	1000	10%	7
Hunter	Sephadex G-200 Antialbumin sepharose Polyacrylamide gel electrophoresis	120	?	13
Sanfilippo A	Sephadex G-200 Carboxymethylcellulose Hydroxylapatite Polyacrylamide gel electrophoresis	850	40%	14

Hunter factor effected correction only in Hunter cells,
Sanfilippo A factor in Sanfilippo A cells, and Hurler factor, as
expected, in Hurler and Scheie cells.

The factors accelerate degradation of sulfated MPS in
recipient cells. This could be shown in several ways:

1) In chase experiments with Hunter cells, there is increased
disappearance of stored MPS, accompanied by an equivalent increase
in degradation products (5).

2) Degradation of proteoglycan administered exogenously to
Hunter cells is increased to normal levels (13).

3) Molecular size distribution of stored MPS is changed
toward a more normal pattern. In Hurler cells, the relatively
larger MPS stored in uncorrected cells is replaced by smaller
species (7). Paradoxically, in Sanfilippo cells, a very small
species is stored in uncorrected cells; upon correction, there
appears a more heterogenous mixture which includes larger molecules (14). This can be explained by postulating that the catabolism of the small molecular species is rate-limiting in uncorrected
Sanfilippo A cells, and that the factor specifically assists in
the breakdown of that species.

In spite of their catabolic function, the factors could not
be identified with known lysosomal enzymes. β-Galactosidase, a
deficiency of which had been proposed as causal in the mucopolysaccharidoses (e.g., 15-19), was not present in the purified
Hurler, Hunter and Sanfilippo A factors.

If the factors are degradative enzymes, their natural substrate
should be the MPS accumulated in uncorrected cells. On this hypothesis, we extracted $^{35}SO_4$-MPS from Hurler, Hunter and Sanfilippo
A fibroblasts, and incubated each one with the respective factor.
This approach was successful in the case of the Sanfilippo A
system. The factor released inorganic sulfate from the MPS, tentatively identified as heparan sulfate (14). The experiment suggests
that the Sanfilippo A factor may be a heparan sulfate sulfatase;
the absence of such an enzyme would explain the urinary excretion
of heparan sulfate by Sanfilippo patients.

The analogous experiments proved negative in the case of the
Hurler and Hunter factors, implying that these are not sulfatases.
We are presently labeling the MPS in the carbohydrate chain to
test the possibility that they are glycosidases.

It is obvious that our task of assigning an enzymatic function
to the factors would be much simpler if there existed a well

worked-out system for the catabolism of dermatan sulfate and heparan sulfate. It is generally believed that these MPS are degraded by a combination of sulfatases, endoglycosidases (such as hyaluronidase) and exoglycosidases, such as N-acetylhexosaminidases (β for dermatan sulfate and α for heparan sulfate), β-glucuronidase and the recently discovered L-iduronidase (20). The basis of this belief, however, is analogy with the chondroitin sulfates rather than experimental verification. Preliminary experiments using a rabbit lysosomal system suggest a requirement for the linkage region for initiating the chain of events that eventually leads to desulfation of dermatan sulfate (21). This would require a pathway more complicated than the proposed assortment of hydrolases.

Finally, the hypothesis of factors as catabolic enzymes is reinforced by two model systems. Fibroblasts from metachromatic leukodystrophy patients, deficient in arylsulfatase A, accumulate exogenously supplied cerebroside sulfate (22); this abnormal accumulation can be reduced to normal levels by the administration of partially purified arylsulfatase A (23, 24).

The second model system is that of fibroblasts from a patient with an atypical mucopolysaccharidosis. The cells lack β-glucuronidase and accumulate sulfated MPS; bovine β-glucuronidase serves as a corrective factor for the anomalous MPS metabolism (25).

CONCLUSION

Correction of mucopolysaccharidosis fibroblasts can be viewed as reconstitution of a catabolic pathway interrupted by the malfunction of one enzyme. When the normal enzyme enters the cell, presumably by pinocytosis, the block is relieved and mucopolysaccharide is degraded at a normal rate.

The ease with which correction occurs in fibroblasts encourages thoughts of therapy for patients. Enzyme replacement for lysosomal disorders was proposed as early as 1964 (26), and a few attempts have been made in the intervening years (27-29). The more promising ones are the recent infusions of plasma and leukocytes into Hurler and Hunter patients (30, 31). Our approach will be to use purified factor. Purification on an appropriately large scale promises to be tedious and expensive, but we are optimistic for the outcome.

REFERENCES

1. B. S. Danes and A. G. Bearn. Hurler's syndrome: a genetic study in cell culture. J. Exp. Med. 123, 1-16 (1966).

2. R. Matalon and A. Dorfman. Acid mucopolysaccharides in cultured human fibroblasts. Lancet 2, 838-841 (1969).

3. J. C. Fratantoni, C. W. Hall and E. F. Neufeld. The defect in Hurler's and Hunter's syndromes: faulty degradation of mucopolysaccharide. Proc. Nat. Acad. Sci. U. S. <u>60</u>, 699-706 (1968).

4. J. C. Fratantoni, C. W. Hall and E. F. Neufeld. Hurler and Hunter syndromes: mutual correction of the defect in cultured fibroblasts. Science <u>162</u>, 570-572 (1968).

5. J. C. Fratantoni, C. W. Hall and E. F. Neufeld. The defect in Hurler and Hunter syndromes, II. Deficiency of specific factors involved in mucopolysaccharide metabolism. Proc. Nat. Acad. Sci. U. S. <u>64</u>, 360-366 (1969).

6. V. A. McKusick. The Mucopolysaccharidoses, <u>in</u> "Heritable Disorders of Connective Tissue," pp. 325-399, C. V. Mosby, St. Louis (1966).

7. R. W. Barton and E. F. Neufeld. J. Biol. Chem. <u>in press</u>.

8. H. Kresse, U. Wiesmann, M. Cantz, C. W. Hall and E. F. Neufeld. Biochemical heterogeneity of the Sanfilippo syndrome: preliminary characterization of two deficient factors. Biochem. Biophys. Res. Communs. <u>42</u>, 892-898 (1971).

9. U. Wiesmann and E. F. Neufeld. Scheie and Hurler syndromes: apparent identity of the biochemical defect. Science <u>169</u>, 72-74 (1970).

10. R. W. Barton and E. F. Neufeld. A distinct biochemical deficit in the Maroteaux-Lamy syndrome (mucopolysaccharidosis VI). J. Ped. <u>in press</u>.

11. B. S. Danes and A. G. Bearn. Correction of cellular metachromasia in cultured fibroblasts in several inherited mucopolysaccharidoses. Proc. Nat. Acad. Sci. U. S. <u>67</u>, 357-364 (1970).

12. E. F. Neufeld and M. Cantz. Corrective factors for inborn errors of mucopolysaccharide metabolism. Ann. N. Y. Acad. Sci. <u>179</u>, 580-587 (1971).

13. M. Cantz, A. Chrambach and E. F. Neufeld. <u>in preparation</u>.

14. H. Kresse and E. F. Neufeld. <u>in preparation</u>.

15. F. van Hoof and H. G. Hers. The abnormalities of lysosomal enzymes in mucopolysaccharidoses. Eur. J. Biochem. <u>7</u>, 34-44 (1968).

16. P. A. Öckerman. Acid hydrolases in skin and plasma in gargoylism. Deficiency of β-galactosidase in skin. Clin. Chim. Acta 20, 1-6 (1968).

17. E. Gerich. Hunter's syndrome, β-Galactosidase deficiency in skin. N. Engl. J. Med. 280, 338-343 (1969).

18. M. MacBrinn, S. Okada, M. Woolacott, V. Patel, M. W. Ho, A. L. Tappel and J. S. O'Brien. β-Galactosidase deficiency in the Hurler syndrome. N. Engl. J. Med. 281, 338-343 (1969).

19. M. W. Ho and J. S. O'Brien. Hurler's syndrome: deficiency of a specific β-galactosidase isoenzyme. Science 165, 611-613 (1969).

20. R. Matalon, J. A. Cifonelli and A. Dorfman. L-Iduronidase in cultured human fibroblasts and liver. Biochem. Biophys. Res. Communs. 42, 340-345 (1971).

21. J. Derge and E. F. Neufeld. in preparation.

22. M. T. Porter, A. L. Fluharty, S. E. Harris and H. Kihara. The accumulation of cerebroside sulfates by fibroblasts in cultures from patients with late infantile metachromatic leukodystrophy. Arch. Biochem. Biophys. 138, 646-652 (1970).

23. M. T. Porter, A. L. Fluharty and H. Kihara. Correction of abnormal cerebroside sulfate metabolism in cultured metachromatic leukodystrophy fibroblasts. Science 172, 1263-1265 (1971).

24. U. N. Wiesmann, E. E. Rossi and N. W. Herschkowitz. Treatment of metachromatic leukodystrophy in fibroblasts by enzyme replacement. N. Engl. J. Med. 284, 672 (1971).

25. C. W. Hall, M. Cantz and E. F. Neufeld. in preparation.

26. P. Baudhuin, H. G. Hers and H. Loeb. An electron microscopic and biochemical study of type II glycogenosis. Lab. Invest. 13, 1139-1152 (1964).

27. G. Hug and W. K. Schubert. Lysosomes in type II glycogenosis. J. Cell Biol. 35, C1 (1967).

28. H. L. Greene, G. Hug and W. K. Schubert. Metachromatic leukodystrophy. Treatment with arylsulfatase A. Arch. Neurol. 20, 147-153 (1969).

29. C. A. Mapes, R. L. Anderson, C. C. Sweeley, R. J. Desnick
     and W. Krivit. Enzyme replacement in Fabry's disease, an
     inborn error of metabolism. Science 169, 987-989 (1970).

30. N. DiFerrante, B. L. Nichols, P. V. Donnelly, G. Neri,
     R. Hrgovcic and R. K. Berglund. Induced degradation of
     glycosaminoglycans in Hurler's and Hunter's syndromes by
     plasma infusion. Proc. Nat. Acad. Sci. U. S. 68, 303-307
     (1971).

31. A. G. Knudson, Jr., N. DiFerrante and J. E. Curtis. Effect
     of leucocyte transfusion in a child with type II mucopoly-
     saccharidosis. Proc. Nat. Acad. Sci. U. S. 68, 1738-
     1741 (1971).

THE DEGRADATION OF ACID MUCOPOLYSACCHARIDES

AND THE MUCOPOLYSACCHARIDOSES[1]

Albert Dorfman, Reuben Matalon*, J. Anthony Cifonelli,

Jerry Thompson and Glyn Dawson*

Departments of Pediatrics and Biochemistry, Joseph P.
Kennedy, Jr., Mental Retardation Research Center and
La Rabida-University of Chicago Institute, University of
Chicago

Since the original clinical descriptions by Hunter (18) and Hurler (19), a vast literature has appeared which is concerned with a group of genetic diseases characterized by the accumulation in tissues and excretion in urine of acid mucopolysaccharides. These studies have been reviewed by McKusick (28) and Dorfman and Matalon (11,12). The term mucopoly-saccharidoses was originally suggested by Brante (1) who discovered that the storage material present in livers of Hurler patients contained the characteristic components of acid mucopolysaccharides. Subsequently, Dorfman and Lorincz (10) showed that heparan sulfate and dermatan sulfate were excreted in large quantities in the urine of patients with Hurler's syndrome. The basis of accumulation of acid mucopoly-saccharides in these diseases has been subject to much speculation. The discovery by Van Hoof and Hers (31) of distended lysosomes in livers of patients with Hurler's disease and the demonstration by Neufeld and co-workers (4,15,16,17,22,29,32) of the existence of "corrective factors"

[1] Original investigations reported in this paper were supported by USPHS Grant Nos. AM-05996, HD-04583, RR-00305, the National Cystic Fibrosis Research Foundation and the Chicago and Illinois Heart Associations.

* Joseph P. Kennedy, Jr. Scholar

has strongly indicated the probability that these diseases result from deficiency of lysosomal acid hydrolases. However, in contrast to the lipid storage diseases, limited knowledge is available concerning the specific enzymic defects of the mucopolysaccharidoses. To some extent this is due to inadequate information regarding the normal catabolic pathways of these compounds and lack of knowledge concerning the detailed structure of the accumulated polysaccharides.

Table 1 summarizes the glycoside and sulfate linkages known to occur in mammalian connective tissue mucopolysaccharides and glycosphingo-lipids. Experience with G_{M1} gangliodidoses suggests that certain hydrolases may be involved in degradation of both glycosphingolipids and mucopolysaccharides or glycoproteins.

The linkages that are indicated are reasonably well established although a number of important problems remain to be solved:

1) The linkage of hyaluronic acid to protein in mammalian tissues is uncertain.
2) The existence of a branched structure in heparin and heparan sulfate is still uncertain.
3) The structures of keratan sulfates I and II are not fully established.

Although hydrolases for almost all of the linkages are known, the pathways of degradation of mucopolysaccharides are not clear. Several considerations complicate the elucidation of these pathways. Some of these may be enumerated as follows:

1) Sulfated mucopolysaccharides are known to be covalently linked to protein. Whether degradation of polysaccharide chain occurs before or after proteolysis is unknown.
2) Most mucopolysaccharides contain O- and N-sulfate groups. Since certain glycosidases do not appear to act on non-reducing terminal sulfated monosaccharides, the action of particular glycosidases may depend on prior sulfatase action. The number and specificity of sulfatases involved in mucopolysaccharide degradation is unclear.
3) Mucopolysaccharides are partly degraded by endoglycosidases such as hyaluronidase. The relationship of the action of exoglycosidases to that of endoglycosidases is not clear.
4) The distribution of lysosomal hydrolases may vary from tissue to tissue resulting in different pathways of degradation in different tissues.

TABLE 1 <u>LINKAGES</u> <u>OF</u> <u>GLYCOSAMINOGLYCANS</u> <u>AND</u> <u>GLYCOLIPIDS</u>

Linkages	Compounds
β -GlcNAc	HA, KSI, KSII
β -GalNAc	Ch-4-SO_4, Ch-6-SO_4, KSII (?), GL-4, G_{Ml}
α -GlcNAc	Hep Hep-SO_4
β -GlcUA	HA, Ch-4-SO_4, Ch-6-SO_4, D-SO_4, Hep, Hep-SO_4
α -L-IdUA	Hep, Hep-SO_4, D-SO_4
β -GlcNAc-Asp	KSI
GalNAc-Ser Thre	KSII
β -Glc	GL-4, G_{Ml}
β -Gal	Ch-4-SO_4, Ch-6-SO_4, Hep, Hep-SO_4, D-SO_4, KSI, KSII, GL-4, G_{Ml}, GL-lb
α -Gal	GL-4
α -Man	KSI, KSII
β -Xyl	Ch-4-SO_4, Ch-6-SO_4, D-SO_4, Hep, Hep-SO_4
α -Fuc	KSI, KSII
α -NANA	KSI, KSII, G_{Ml}
GalNAc-O-SO_4	Ch-4-SO_4, Ch-6-SO_4, D-SO_4
GlcNAc-O-SO_4	KSI, KSII, Hep, Hep-SO_4
Gal-O-SO_4	KSI, KSII, GL-lb
IdUA-O-SO_4	Hep, Hep-SO_4, D-SO_4
GlcN-SO_4	Hep, Hep-SO_4

Abbreviations: HA, hyaluronic acid; Ch-4-SO_4, chondroitin-4-sulfate; Ch-6-SO_4, chondroitin-6-SO_4; Hep, heparin; Hep-SO_4, heparan sulfate; KSI, corneal keratan sulfate; KSII, cartilage keratan sulfate; GL-4 GalNAc-β -(1→3)-Gal-α -(1→4)-Gal-β -(1→4)-Glc-Ceramide, G_{Ml} according to Svennerholm nomenclature.

5) Various forms of hydrolases (e.g. hexosaminidase A and B) may differ in substrate specificity.

The linkages summarized in Table 1 indicate that a relatively large number of hydrolases are required for complete degradation of

acid mucopolysaccharides and glycosphingolipids. Not included are the
peptide linkages present in the protein portions of the proteoglycans.

In the case of the lipid storage diseases, identification of the enzyme
defect has usually been preceded by determination of the chemical structure
of the stored substance. Such an approach has not yet been extensively
applied to the study of the mucopolysaccharidoses.

Knecht, Cifonelli and Dorfman (21) studied the chemical nature of
heparan sulfate present in liver and spleen and excreted in the urine of
Hurler's disease and Sanfilippo's disease. Both in tissues and urine, the
heparan sulfate was found to be of amall molecular weight in confirmation
of the earlier studies of Brown (3). Whereas heparan sulfate isolated
from aorta had a molecular weight of 24,000 to 29,000, the material
isolated from both Hurler's and Sanfilippo's patients was heterogeneous
with a molecular weight less than 5,500. Chromatography on Dowex
1 Cl$^-$ resulted in two distinct fractions differing in sulfate content. The
high sulfate fraction contained little or no N-acetylhexosamine, amino
acids, galactose, or xylose but had a high content of N-sulfate. In contrast
the low sulfate fraction contained N-acetylhexosamine and serine,
galactose and xylose in a ratio of 1:2:1.

When the dermatan sulfate excreted by a Hurler patient was examined,
a somewhat similar pattern was observed. Dermatan sulfate isolated
from Hurler urine was of lower molecular weight and more polydisperse
than that isolated from skin (9). These findings led to the conclusion that
both the storage and excreted materials in mucopolysaccharidoses were
partially degraded.

A pathway of partial degradation of dermatan sulfate was suggested
by the discovery of Fransson and Rodén (13) that dermatan sulfate is a
hybrid polysaccharide containing both L-iduronic acid and D-glucuronic
acid. Testicular hyaluronidase (or other mammalian hyaluronidases) is
an endoglycosidase which cleaves β-N-acetylhexosamindo-D-glucuronic
acid bonds, and hydrolyzes such linkages when they occur in dermatan
sulfate. Fransson, Sjöberg and Dorfman (14) found that the predominant
non-reducing terminal group of the oligosaccharides isolated from Hurler
urine are O-sulfated N-acetylgalactosamine residues. These results are
consistent with the possibility that the oligosaccharides found in Hurler
urines result from the cleavage of dermatan sulfate by hyaluronidase
followed by removal of non-reducing terminal glucuronic acid residues
by β-glucuronidase. It is possible that further degradation may not
occur because of failure of β-hexosaminidase to act on sulfated non-
reducing terminal groups. Whether this results from an absence of a

specific sulfatase in Hurler's disease or failure of the normal sulfatase
to act on hyaluronidase degraded products is not clear.

The nature of the heparan sulfate fragments suggests a similar pathway
but no endoglycosidase is known which acts on the presumed α-N-acetyl-
glucosaminidic linkages of heparan sulfate.   Mammalian hyaluronidases
would not be expected to cleave heparan sulfate unless it contains hitherto
unrecognized β-N-acetylglycosaminidic bonds.

When it was later established that skin fibroblasts cultured from Hurler
patients accumulated dermatan sulfate (25), it became of interest to
examine the molecular size of the dermatan sulfate isolated from Hurler
fibroblasts (26).   In contrast to that obtained from urine, fibroblast
dermatan sulfate was found to be of molecular weight comparable to that
isolated from normal skin.   Treatment of the fibroblast material by
testicular hyaluronidase resulted in degradation to fragments comparable
in size to those isolated from urine.   These data suggest that the
catabolism of dermatan sulfate is different in fibroblasts from that in
liver and spleen.

Since fibroblasts are probably the physiological site of synthesis of
dermatan sulfate, and this compound accumulates in cultured Hurler fibroblasts (25) a study was initiated to elucidate the pathway of degradation
of mucopolysaccharides in fibroblasts.   Normal liver, normal cultured
skin fibroblasts and cultured Hurler fibroblasts were extracted at pH 4. 5.
When hyaluronidase activity was determined in such extracts by the
sensitive viscosity method using hyaluronic acid as substrate (8), reduction
of viscosity by liver extracts was readily demonstrated, but little or no
reduction of viscosity by extracts of either Hurler or normal fibroblasts
was found.   Mixing of liver and fibroblast extracts showed no inhibition
of liver hyaluronidase activity (27).

In order to determine whether dermatan sulfate is degraded by
fibroblasts, labeled dermatan sulfate was prepared by incubating Hurler
fibroblasts with $^{35}SO_4$.   The labeled dermatan sulfate, isolated from such
cultures, was added to cultures of both normal and Hurler fibroblasts.
After incubation, preparations derived from both cells and medium were
separately chromatographed on Sephadex G-25.   It was readily
demonstrated that a portion of the label was present in a retarded peak
which migrated as inorganic sulfate on high voltage electrophoresis.

When hyaluronic acid-^{14}C and dermatan sulfate-^{14}C were added to
normal and Hurler fibroblast cultures, evidence for only minimal
degradation was obtained.

Since mucopolysaccharides are synthesized as protein complexes, complete degradation requires the action of proteases as well as glycosidases and sulfatases. Whether proteolysis precedes or follows glycosidase and sulfatase action is unknown. In order to test degradation of a proteoglycan by fibroblasts, ^{3}H-labeled chondroitin sulfate-proteoglycan was prepared by incubation of minced chick femoral epiphyses with acetate-[3]H. This material was incubated with pH 4. 5-extracts of normal and Hurler fibroblasts and normal liver. The reaction products were subjected to gel filtration on Sephadex G-100. The radioactive products of the incubation mixtures containing the liver extracts were eluted in fractions expected to contain tetra-, hexa-, and octasaccharides while the incubation mixtures containing either normal or Hurler fibroblast extracts showed no radioactivity in these fractions but did contain a small amount of radioactivity in more retarded fractions. When these more retarded fractions were recovered and rechromatographed on Sephadex G-25, they appeared to be mono-or disaccharides.

These results suggested that the pathway of catabolism of acid mucopolysaccharides in fibroblasts may involve the stepwise removal of monosaccharide units by acid hydrolases. The data of Neufeld and co-workers (4, 15,16,17,22,29,32) suggest that Hurler, Hunter, Sanfilippo I, Sanfilippo II and Morateaux-Lamy syndromes would each result from the deficiency of a different enzyme (or subunit) involved in the degradation of heparan sulfate and dermatan sulfate. A number of studies of hydrolase levels in serum, liver and fibroblasts in mucopolysaccharidoses have been published. These have been reviewed in detail elsewhere (12). No conclusive evidence has yet appeared demonstrating the absence of a particular hydrolase in any of the mucopolysaccharidoses.

Because heparan sulfate and dermatan sulfate accumulate in Hurler's disease and these compounds share an α-L-iduronic acid linkage, a search was made for α-L-iduronidase (6,24). Since no synthetic glycoside of L-iduronic acid was available, a natural substrate was prepared. Dermatan sulfate was desulfated by the procedure of Kantor and Schubert (20). Freshly prepared acetyl chloride in methanol (0. 3 ml acetyl chloride in 100 ml methanol) was added to 100 mg of dermatan sulfate. The mixture was stirred for 16 hr at 27°C, the precipitate allowed to settle, washed three times with methanol, dried and used as the substrate. In order to make a maximum number of non-reducing terminal L-iduronic acid groups available, assays for L-iduronidase were carried out in the presence of testicular hyaluronidase and liver β-glucuronidase. Since all extracts tested contained large amounts of β-hexosaminidase, this enzyme was not added. Enzyme extracts were prepared from 2-3 week old fibroblast cultures containing 1. 4 to 1. 6 x

10^7 cells per 100 mm plate. Cells were removed from the dishes with a rubber policeman, suspended in 0.05 $\underline{N}$ acetate buffer pH 4.5, containing 0.15 $\underline{N}$ NaCl; and disrupted with a Dounce glass homogenizer. Human livers were obtained at autopsy and kept frozen until used. Extracts were prepared by homogenization of 2 gm of liver in 5 ml of acetate buffer, pH 4.5 containing 0.15M NaCl, the homogenates were centrifuged at 600 xg for 10 minutes and the supernatant fractions were used as enzyme preparations. Enzyme concentrations were adjusted to 10 mg of protein per ml for fibroblasts, and 15 mg of protein per ml for liver. Leukocytes were separated by a modification of the dextran separation method (30). Twenty ml of blood were collected in oxalate containing tubes, 4 ml of 6% solution of Dextran 70 in 0.15$\underline{N}$ NaCl was then added. The mixture was allowed to settle for 1 hr at 37°C and then centrifuged at 60 xg for 10 minutes. The supernatant fraction containing the leukocytes was separated and centrifuged at 200 xg for another 10 minutes. The pellet containing the leukocytes was washed once with 0.15$\underline{N}$ NaCl. The leukocytes were sonicated in 1 ml of acetate-NaCl buffer for 30 seconds, centrifuged at 600 xg and the supernatant solution was used as a source of enzyme.

Each incubation mixture contained 10 mg of the desulfated dermatan sulfate substrate, 5 ml of enzyme extract, 3500 NF units of testicular hyaluronidase (Sigma type VI) and 10,000 Fishman units of β-glucuronidase (Sigma type B-3). Controls were prepared by boiling enzyme extracts for 2 min at pH 6.5, and re-adjusting the pH to 4.5 before addition of substrate, hyaluronidase and β-glucuronidase. After 36 hours of incubation at 37°C, the mixtures were centrifuged at 10,000 xg, chromatographed on Sephadex G-25 columns (superfine, 100 x 0.6 cm) using H_2O as eluent. The included fractions were pooled, desalted over Dowex 50, H^+ and adjusted to pH 2.0 with Dowex 3, $CO_3^=$. The solution was further adjusted to pH 6.8 with sodium carbonate and applied to a column of Dowex 1, acetate (200-400 mesh, 1 x 8 cm). The uronic acid fraction was eluted with 3.0 $\underline{M}$ acetic acid, and the eluate was concentrated and chromatographed on Whatman No. 1 paper, using tertiary amyl alcohol-isopropyl alcohol-water (4:1:1.5) or ethyl acetate-acetic acid-water (3:1:3). Spots were visualized with a silver reagent.

On paper chromatography the results illustrated in Fig. 1 were obtained. Incubation of extracts of liver and normal fibroblasts resulted in the release of a substance which migrated at the same rate as does L-idurone. Under the conditions of chromatography, L-iduronic acid is converted to L-idurone. A much less prominent spot was obtained as a result of incubation of the substrate with extracts of Hurler fibroblasts. In a separate experiment the release of L-idurone by extracts of normal leukocytes was demonstrated. Repetition of this experiment on a

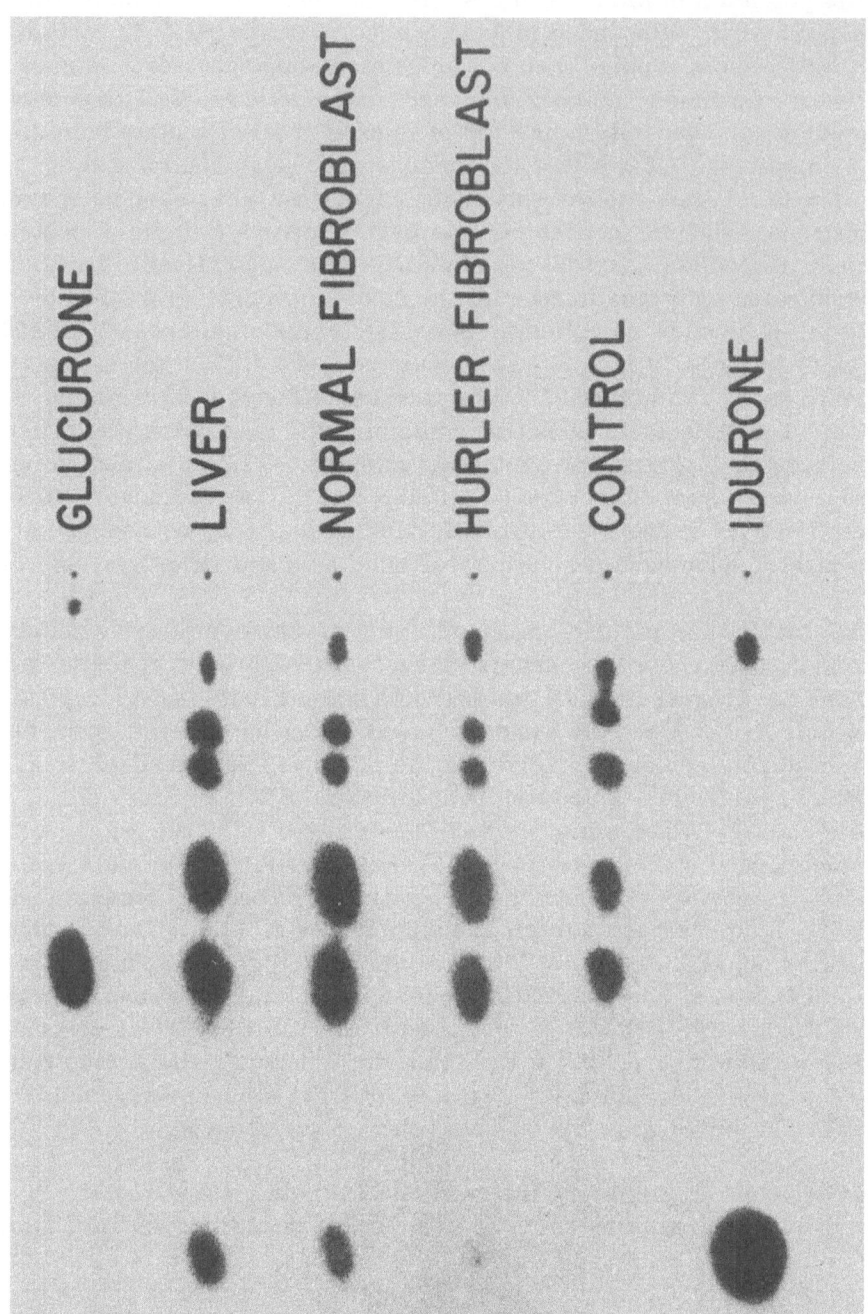

Fig. 1 Paper chromatogram of purified incubation mixtures utilizing desulfated dermatan sulfate as substrate. Control contains heated enzyme extract.

preparative scale permitted the elution of idurone which was analyzed by the orcinol (2) and carbazole (7) methods. The analyses given in Table 2 are consistent with those characteristic of L-idurone. The L-idurone was further identified by gas-liquid chromatography in the following manner. To the uronic acid-containing material eluted from paper, mannitol was added as an internal standard (0.02 μmoles). The trimethylsilyl derivative was prepared by reacting the mixture with 20 μl of pyridine-trimethylchlorosilane-hexamethyldisilazane (10:2:2) at room temperature for 10 minutes. Gas chromatography was carried out on a Hewlett-Packard unit-model 402 using a 6 ft glass column (1/8 in. I.D.) packed with 3% OV-1 on Supelcoport (100-120 mesh) and flame ionization detector. Samples (2 μl) were temperature programmed from 160°C to 200°C at 2°C per minute.

Since the desulfated dermatan sulfate is a poorly characterized substrate, an attempt was made to prepare a simpler more easily defined substrate. It has been previously shown by Cifonelli (5) that treatment of heparin with nitrous acid results in conversion of N-sulfated glucosamine residues to 2,5-anhydromannose with concomittant cleavage of the adjacent glycosidic bond. As a result, the product of this reaction contains the disaccharide, 4-0-α-L-iduronido-2,5-anhydromannose.

Since heparin contains sulfate groups in three different positions, glucosamine-O-SO$_4$, iduronic acid-O-SO$_4$ and glucosamine-N-SO$_4$ and may contain β-D-glucuronic as well as α-L-iduronic linkages the disaccharide obtained by this procedure may not be homogeneous. Further work is in progress to adequately characterize this substrate.

Crude heparin (20 gm. Wilson Laboratories) was hydrolyzed for 2 hr in a boiling water bath with 200 ml 1.0 N HCl, then cooled to 60°-70°C and the free sulfate was precipitated with barium acetate. The barium sulfate

TABLE 2 <u>ANALYSES</u> <u>OF</u> <u>IDURONOLACTONE</u> <u>ISOLATED</u> <u>AFTER</u> <u>PREPARATIVE</u> <u>PAPER</u> <u>CHROMATOGRAPHY</u>

Source	Uronic Acid		C/O
	Carbazole	Orcinol	
	μg	μg	
Liver	30	126	0.24
Normal Fibroblasts	24	54	0.42
Standard Iduronic Acid	36	168	0.22

was removed by centrifugation; sodium nitrite and water (30 gm of $NaNO_2$ and 500 ml of water) were added to the 200 ml of supernatant solution containing the desulfated heparin and HCl. The mixture was cooled to room temperature and allowed to react for 1 hr with occasional mixing, and neutralized with NaOH. The solution was desalted on a column of Dowex 50 H^+, the effluent containing the disaccharide was chromatographed on Sephadex G-25, and the retarded fractions containing the disaccharide were pooled and concentrated. The disaccharide was precipitated with 6 volumes of ethanol.

The disaccharide was incubated for 36 hr at $38^\circ C$ with extracts of Hurler and normal fibroblasts. Samples were purified as indicated above except that following elution from the Dowex 50, H^+ the material was passed over a column of Norit (30-80 mesh) and the uronic acid-containing material was eluted with 15% ethanol. After concentration, chromatography on paper showed results similar to those obtained with desulfated dermatan sulfate as substrate. L-idurone was released by extracts of normal liver and cultured skin fibroblasts and to a lesser extent by extracts of Hurler fibroblasts. These samples were also analyzed by gas-liquid chromatography. The results shown in Fig. 2 once again demonstrated the presence of L-idurone in incubation mixtures. Reaction mixtures containing extracts of Hurler fibroblasts show much smaller amounts than those containing extracts of normal fibroblasts. Preliminary quantitation on comparable incubation mixtures of a number of fibroblast preparations gave the values shown in Table 3.

TABLE 3 <u>RELEASE OF L-IDURONE BY FIBROBLAST EXTRACTS</u>

	μmoles	μmoles/mg protein/48 hr
Normal	0.049	15.0
Hunter	0.035	8.0
Sanfilippo	0.029	5.8
Hurler	0.005	<1.8

Substrate was disaccharide prepared by mild acid hydrolysis and nitrous acid treatment of heparin.

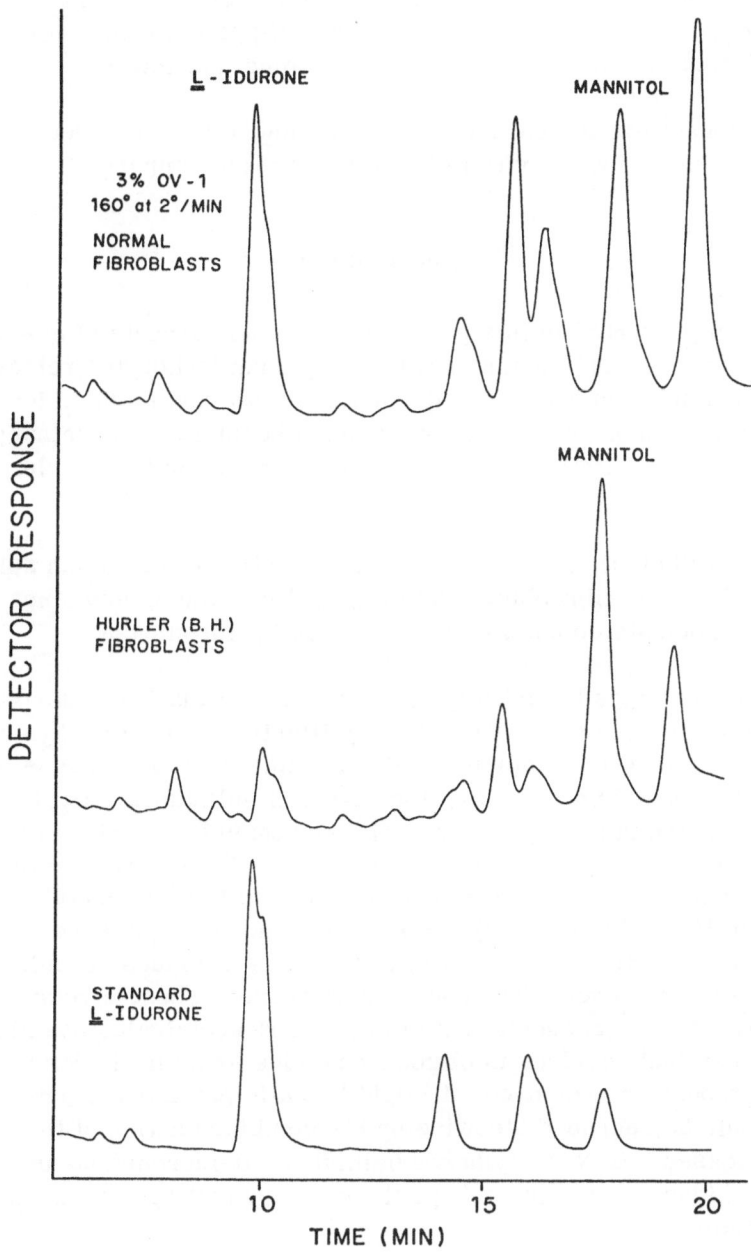

Fig. 2 Gas liquid chromatograms of purified enzyme extracts utilizing disaccharide preparation from heparan.

The marked decrease in Hurler's fibroblasts is obvious. In contrast extracts of fibroblasts from Hunter and Sanfilippo's disease were comparable in activity to normal although somewhat lower.

More recent studies on liver extracts show a markedly decreased iduronidase releasing activity in Hurler tissue as compared to normal.

DISCUSSION

The data presented in this paper indicate that extracts of cultured human skin fibroblasts, human liver, and human leukocytes release free L-iduronic acid from desulfated dermatan sulfate and from an iduronic acid-containing disaccharide prepared from heparin. Preliminary results indicate a marked diminution of this activity in extracts of Hurler fibroblasts.

It seems likely that the pathway of degradation of dermatan sulfate may be different in fibroblasts from that of liver and spleen since cultured fibroblasts do not appear to contain hyaluronidase.

Fig. 3 illustrates the possible pathway of degradation of dermatan sulfate by known enzymes. The pathway illustrated involves hyaluronidase. It is as yet difficult to completely delineate this pathway because of the absence of information regarding the action of sulfatases. Hyaluronidase acts on dermatan sulfate to produce oligosaccharides which contain non-reducing terminal β-glucuronic acid residues. These are readily removed by β-glucuronidase resulting in non-reducing sulfated N-acetylgalactosamine residues in Hurler's urine (14). Since known hexosaminidases do not appear to act on sulfated N-acetylgalactosamine residues, if sulfate groups are not removed, degradation may cease. These circumstances may account for the accumulation of sulfated N-acetylgalactosamine non-reducing terminal residues in oligosaccharides found in Hurler urine. If sulfate groups are removed, it might be anticipated that dermatan sulfate would be degraded stepwise by the combined action of the exoglycosidases, β-N-acetylhexosaminidase, α-iduronidase and β-glucuronidase. This is perhaps the primary pathway of degradation in fibroblasts.

The situation is further complicated by the recent discovery of Lindahl and Alexelson (23) that L-iduronic acid groups are sulfated. Further studies will be necessary to determine whether this sulfate group must be released by a specific sulfatase before L-iduronic acid may be released by L-iduronidase. Absence either of such a sulfatase or

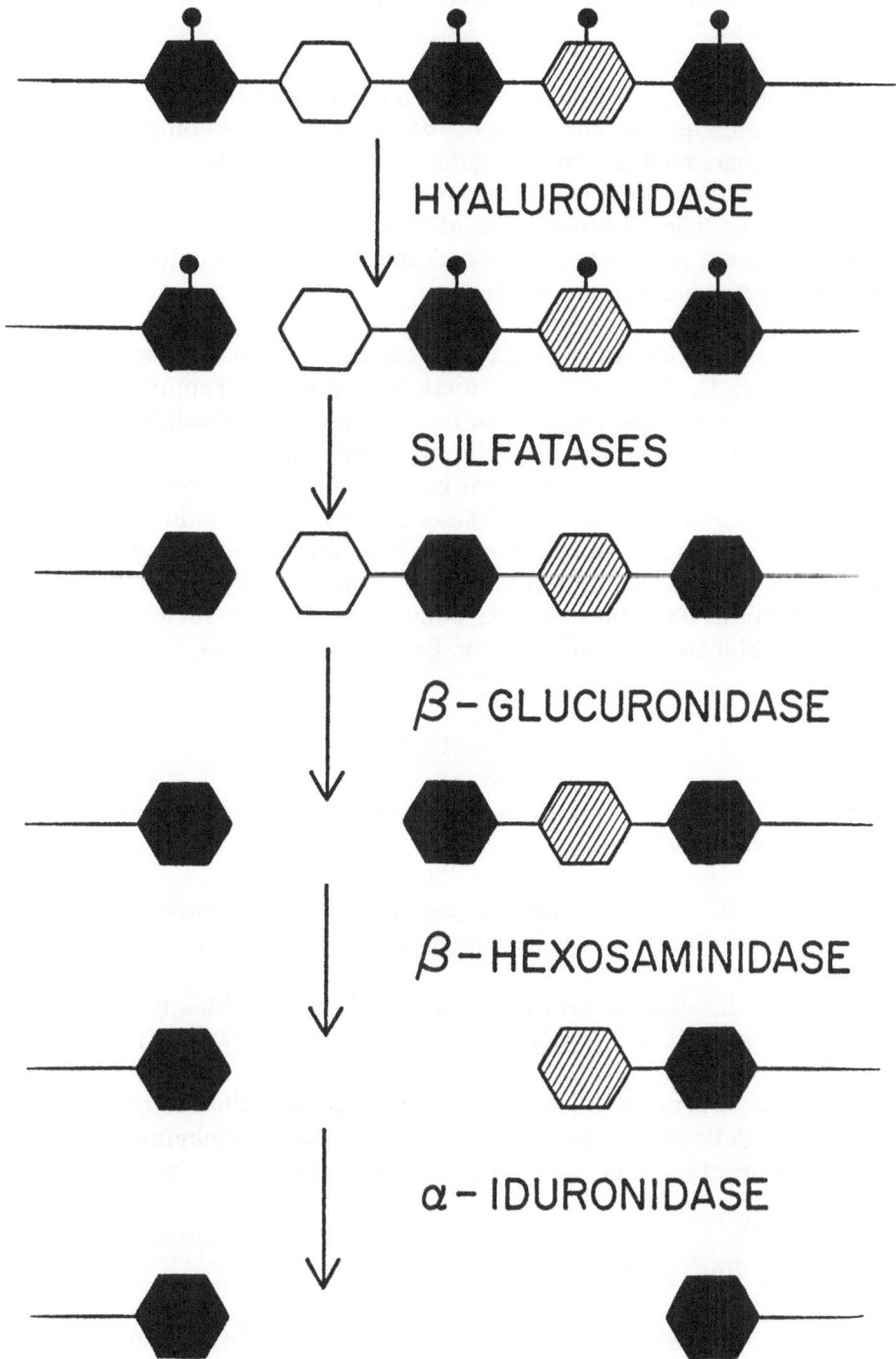

Fig. 3 Degradation of dermatan sulfate.

L-iduronidase would prevent degradation of both heparan sulfate and dermatan sulfate.

The summary of linkages present in mucopolysaccharides and glycolipids indicates that complete degradation of these compounds requires the concerted action of a number of hydrolases. This perhaps accounts for the large number of separate storage diseases that have been described. The diminished L-iduronic acid-releasing activity in Hurler fibroblasts may account for storage of dermatan sulfate and heparan sulfate in Hurler's disease.

Whereas these results strongly suggest that L-iduronidase activity is diminished in Hurler's disease, further studies are required with more rigorously characterized substrates to determine the possible role of sulfatases in the release of idurone. Since the amount of L-iduronic acid released is small, it is possible that both the desulfated dermatan sulfate and the disaccharide contain small amounts of iduronic acid groups that are sulfated. Release of idurone may depend on the activity of specific sulfatases in the extract. Further studies are needed to determine the nature of the defect in other closely related syndromes such as Hunter's, Sanfilippo's, Maroteaux-Lamy's, and Scheie's syndrome.

REFERENCES

1. Brante, G. Gargoylism: A mucopolysaccharidosis. Scand. J. Clin. Lab. Invest. 4: 43 (1952).

2. Brown, A. H. Determination of pentose in the presence of large quantities of glucose. Arch. Biochem. 11: 269 (1946).

3. Brown, D. H. Tissue storage of mucopolysaccharides in Hurler Pfaundler's disease. Proc. Nat. Acad. Sci. 43:783 (1957).

4. Cantz, M., Chrambach, A. and Neufeld, E. F. Characterization of the factor deficient in the Hunter syndrome by polyacrylamide gel electrophoresis. Biochem. Biophys. Res. Commun. 39: 936 (1970).

5. Cifonelli, J. A. Reaction of heparitin sulfate with nitrous acid. Carbohyd. Res. 8: 233 (1968).

6. Cifonelli, J. A., Matalon, R. and Dorfman, A. L-iduronidase in human tissues, urine and cultured fibroblasts. Fed. Proc. 30: 1207 (1971).

7. Dische, Z. A new specific color reaction of hexuronic acids.
    J. Biol. Chem. 167: 189 (1947).

8. Dorfman, A. The kinetics of the enzymatic hydrolysis of hyaluronic
    acid. J. Biol. Chem. 172: 377 (1948).

9. Dorfman, A. Metabolism of acid mucopolysaccharides. Biophys. J.
    4: 155 (1964).

10. Dorfman, A. and Lorincz, A. E. Occurrence of urinary acid
    mucopolysaccharides in the Hurler syndrome. Proc. Nat. Acad.
    Sci. 43: 443 (1957).

11. Dorfman, A. and Matalon, R. The Hurler and Hunter syndromes.
    Am. J. Med. 47: 691 (1969).

12. Dorfman, A. and Matalon, R. The mucopolysaccharidoses. In:
    The Metabolic Basis of Inherited Diseases, J. B. Stanbury, J. B.
    Wyngaarden and D. S. Frederickson (Eds.), 3rd Edition, New York,
    McGraw Hill, in press.

13. Fransson, L.-A. and Rodén, L. Structure of dermatan sulfate. I.
    Degradation by testicular hyaluronidase. J. Biol. Chem. 242: 4161
    (1967).

14. Fransson, L.-Å., Sjöberg, I., and Dorfman, A. In Preparation.

15. Fratantoni, J. C., Hall, C. W. and Neufeld, E. F. The defect in
    Hurler's and Hunter's syndromes: Faulty degradation of mucopoly-
    saccharide. Proc. Nat. Acad. Sci. 60: 699 (1968).

16. Fratantoni, J. C., Hall, C. W. and Neufeld, E. F. Hurler and
    Hunter syndromes: Mutual correction of the defect in cultured
    fibroblasts. Sci. 162: 570 (1968).

17. Fratantoni, J. C., Hall, C. W. and Neufeld, E. F. The defect in
    Hurler and Hunter syndromes. II. Deficiency of specific factors
    involved in mucopolysaccharide degradation. Proc. Nat. Acad.
    Sci. 64: 360 (1969).

18. Hunter, C. A rare disease in two brothers. Proc. Roy. Soc. Med.
    10: 104 (1917).

19. Hurler, G. Über einen typ multipler abartungen, vorwiegend am
    skelettsystem. Z. Kinderheilk. 24: 220 (1919).

20. Kantor, G. T. and Schubert, M.   A method for the desulfation of chondroitin sulfate.   J. Am. Chem. Soc. 79: 152 (1957).

21. Knecht, J. , Cifonelli, J. A. and Dorfman, A.   Structural studies on heparitin sulfate of normal and Hurler tissues.   J. Biol. Chem. 242: 4652 (1967).

22. Kresse, H. , Wiesmann, U. , Cantz, M. , Hall, C. W. and Neufeld, E. F.   Biochemical heterogeneity of the Sanfilippo syndrome: Preliminary characterization of two deficient factors.   Biochem. Biophys. Res. Commun. 42: 892 (1971).

23. Lindahl, U. and Axelsson, O.   Identification of iduronic acid as the major sulfated uronic acid of heparin.   J. Biol. Chem. 246: 74 (1970).

24. Matalon, R. , Cifonelli, J. A. and Dorfman, A.   L-iduronidase in cultured human fibroblasts and liver.   Biochem. Biophys. Res. Commun. 42: 340 (1971).

25. Matalon, R. and Dorfman, A.   Hurler's syndrome: Biosynthesis of acid mucopolysaccharides in tissue culture.   Proc. Nat. Acad. Sci. 56: 1310 (1966).

26. Matalon, R. and Dorfman, A.   The structure of acid mucopoly-saccharides produced by Hurler fibroblasts in tissue culture.   Proc. Nat. Acad. Sci. 60: 179 (1968).

27. Matalon, R. and Dorfman, A.   Unpublished data.

28. McKusick, V. A.   Heritable Disorders of Connective Tissue, 3rd Ed. , St. Louis, Mosby, 1966.

29. Neufeld, E.F. and Cantz, M.J.   Corrective factors for inborn errors of metabolism.   Ann. N.Y. Acad. Sci. 179: 580 (1971).

30. Rabinowitz, Y.   Separation of lymphocytes, polymorphonuclear leukocytes and monocytes on glass columns, including tissue culture observations.   Blood 23: 811 (1964).

31. Van Hoof, F. and Hers. H. G.   The ultrastructures of hepatic cells in Hurler's disease (gargoylism).   Comp. Rend. Acad. Sci. 259: 1281 (1964).

32. Weismann, U. and Neufeld, E. F.   Scheie and Hurler syndromes: Apparent identity of the biochemical defect.   Sci. 169: 72 (1970).

THE MUCOPOLYSACCHARIDOSES AS LYSOSOMAL DISEASES[*]

F. Van Hoof and H. G. Hers

Laboratoire de Chimie Physiologique

Université de Louvain, Louvain, Belgium

In this paper, we briefly summarize the evidence
that has accumulated during the recent years indicating
that the diseases known as mucopolysaccharidoses are due
to the primary defect of one acid hydrolase normally
present in lysosomes. We also report some original observations concerning the ultrastructure and the enzymatic activity of the tissues in this group of disorders.

The concept of inborn lysosomal diseases (4)

The intracellular degradation of many complex molecules occurs through their enzymatic hydrolysis inside
of vacuoles belonging to the lysosomal system. This process allows the digestion of most proteins, nucleic
acids, complex lipids and mucopolysaccharides. These
molecules may originate from the cell itself through
autophagy or may have been taken up by the cell from
the surrounding medium by endocytosis.
The defect of one lysosomal hydrolase will therefore lead to the intralysosomal deposition of all complex molecules that normally require the missing enzyme
for their degradation. As digestive enzymes are usually
specific for one type of linkage and not for a given
substrate, the material that will accumulate maybe highly heterogenous. For instance the defect of one glycosidase may cause the storage of various derivatives of mu-

[*]Supported by the Belgian FRSM and by NIH Grant AM-9235.

copolysaccharides, glycolipids and glycoprotein that have in common to bear the same osidic moiety with the required α or β configuration. All the osidic units that
are external to the metabolic block as well as the pep-
tidic moiety of the proteoglycans would have disappeared.

Electron microscopy reveals the enlargement of the
lysosomes and in some cases the nature of the depot material.

As a rule the enzyme deficiency affects most tissues
of the body but the amount of material stored may vary
to a large extent from tissue to tissue according to
their normal rate of synthesis and breakdown and to the
endocytis potentiality of each type of cell.

Delimitation of mucopolysaccharidoses

Strictly speaking, a mucopolysaccharidosis is a
storage disease in which the material in excess is made
exclusively of mucopolysaccharides. It is doubtful that
any of the known human pathological conditions corresponds to this definition. First, it appears that the
polysaccharides which are stored in the tissues of patients or excreted in their urine are partially degraded. A more careful denomination for this material would
for instance be "dermatan sulfate-like" or "heparan sulfate-like polysaccharides". Secondly, there is, in most
of these disorders, some chemical (see for instance 7,
22, 25) or morphological (see Table I) evidence for the
simultaneous storage of complex lipids. This is the reason why Hurler's syndrome had initially been considered
as a lipidosis. The terms "lipomucopolysaccharidosis"
or "mucolipidosis" would more adequately designate these
storage diseases.

We will therefore include in the group of the so-
called mucopolysaccharidoses not only the classical types I to VI of McKusick's classification (13) but also
G_{M1}-gangliosidosis, fucosidosis, mucosulfatidosis and the
lipomucopolysaccharidosis described by Spranger et al.
(21).

G_{M1}-gangliosidosis was initially known as pseudo
Hurler disease (6); it is clear that the storage of G_{M1}-
ganglioside in the brain is only one feature of that disorder whereas the liver accumulates galactose rich polysaccharides (23).

The term fucosidosis, on the contrary is non ambi-
guous since it does not impose any limitation to the number and to the chemical structures of the fucosides that
might accumulate in tissues as a result of the absence
of α-fucosidase. Fucose residues are mostly found in gly-

coproteins and in some sphingolipids, but are also present in keratan sulfate (14), a mucopolysaccharide that
contains no uronic acid.

The mucosulfatidosis is also called metachromatic
leucodystrophy variant or trisulfatase deficiency (2).
Patients with this disorder have an high level of glycosaminoglycans in their liver (15) and, as shown below,
the ultrastructure of the hepatocytes is very similar
to that seen in Hurler's disease.

Lipomucopolysaccharidosis is a clinical condition
resembling Hurler's syndrome but usually without muco-
polysacchariduria (11, 21). In the liver of the patients,
the activity of β-galactosidase is 3 to 12 times the
normal mean value (30) and the electron microscope reveals the presence of osmiophilic droplets inside of
large vacuoles, otherwise similar to those seen in Hurler's syndrome (11, 21).

I cell disease is another ill-defined pathological
condition with clinical resemblance to the Hurler's
disease and in which cultured fibroblasts display dark
cytoplasmic inclusions in phase contrast microscopy (9).
In liver, brain spleen and kidney of two cases we found
a normal amount of mucopolysaccharides. The ultrastructure of the liver is also very different from that in
Hurler's disease (Fig. 9).

The morphological evidence

We have shown in 1964 that the liver of patients
with Hurler syndrome contain no normal dense bodies but,
instead, a great number of very large vacuoles that are
lysosomes overloaded with mucopolysaccharides (27).
These vacuoles are indeed metachromatic in light microscopy. On this basis, we had proposed that the mucopolysaccharidoses could be considered as inborn lysosomal
diseases. Since that time, other tissues from patients
afflicted by various forms of mucopolysaccharidoses have
been examined with the electron microscope. Some of these observations are summarized in Table I. In nearly all
tissues that have been examined there is some kind of
lysosomal hypertrophy and overloading, giving rise to
three main types of vacuoles : A) Vacuoles containing a
finely granular material and remnants of the dense body
matrix. These vacuoles were presumably filled with some
kind of mucopolysaccharides which stain poorly with osmium or were extracted by the fixation procedure. This
would explain why some of them have a nearly empty appearance (Fig. 1). B) Vacuoles filled with lamellar inclusions that indicate the presence of polar lipids, na-

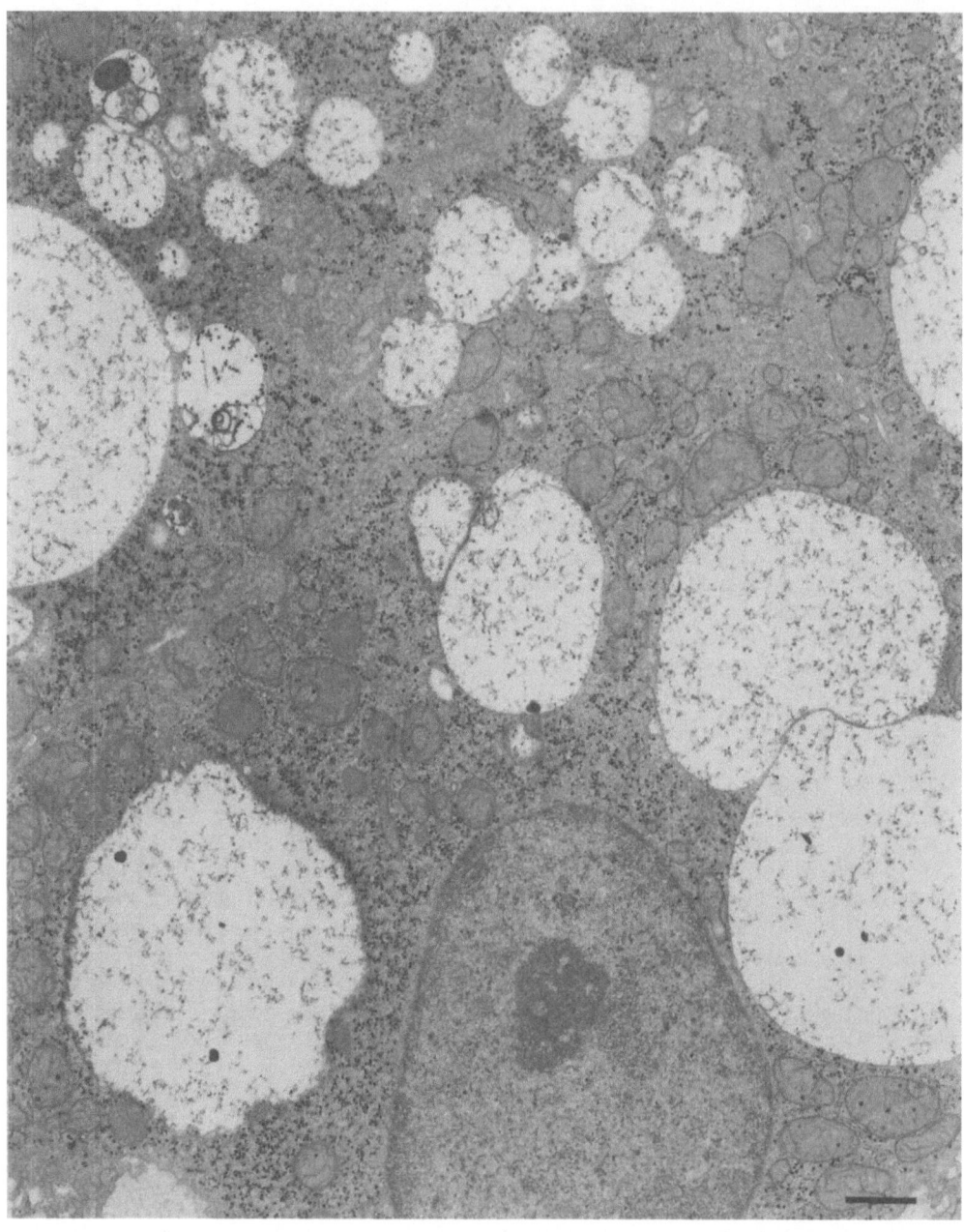

Fig. 1. Vacuoles of type A in hepatocytes of a patient with type I mucopolysaccharidosis.The line indicates the scale of one micron.

ULTRASTRUCTURAL FINDINGS IN MUCOPOLYSACCHARIDOSIS

| | LIVER | | BRAIN | | ENDO-THELIAL CELLS | FIBROBLASTS |
	Hepatocytes	Kupffer cells	Neurons	Glial cells		
TYPE I, II and III	A++ (27, Fig. 1)	A+ (27)	B (1)	A+ (1)	A+ (1)	A++ (5)
TYPE IV	A+− (26)	A (26)	−	−	A (19, 26)	A (19)
TYPE V	−	−	−	−	−	−
TYPE VI	A+− (Fig. 3)	A (Fig. 3)	−	−	A	A
G$_{M1}$-GANGLIOSIDOSIS	A++ (29)	A++ (29, Figs 6-7)	B (20)	C (20)	A+	A+
FUCOSIDOSIS	A, B, C (29)	A, C	A (10)	A,B,C (10)	A,B,C (10)	A, B, C (Fig.5)
MUCOSULFATIDOSIS	A++ (Fig. 4)	A+	−	−	−	A
LIPOMUCOPOLYSACCHARIDOSIS (Gal+)	■A (11, 21)	A (11, 21)	−	−	−	■A (Fig. 8)

A, B and C indicate the type of vacuoles as explained in text. The number of crosses indicate their size or abundance.
The numbers, in parentheses, refer to the bibliographic list.
■ These clear vacuoles contain also osmiophilic droplets.

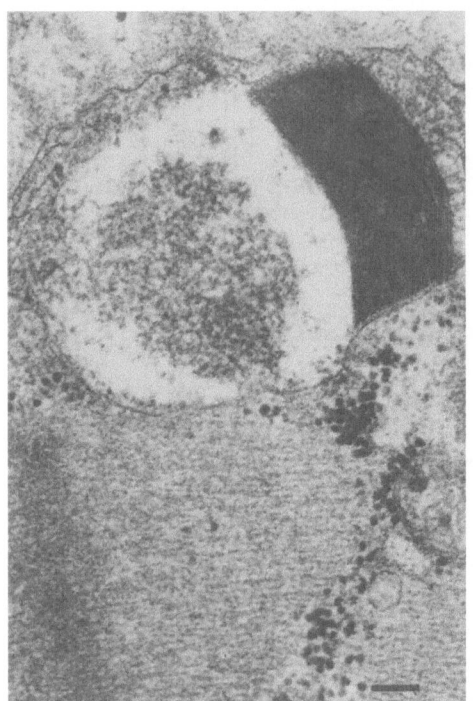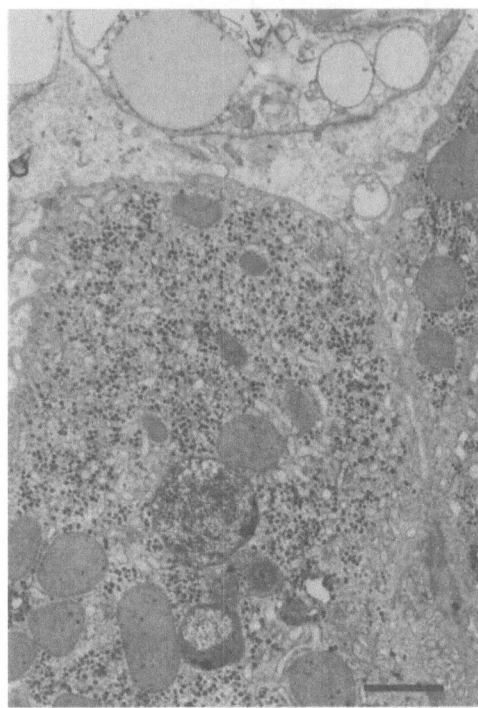

Fig. 2. Vacuole of type C in the skeletal muscle of
the same patient as in Fig. 1. The line indicates the
scale of 0.1 micron.

Fig. 3. Part of a Kupffer cell (top) and of hepatocytes in type VI mucopolysaccharidosis. The vacuoles were of type A with variability in the intensity of staining. The vacuoles were more abundant in Kupffer cells
than in the hepatocytes. The line indicates the scale
of 1 micron.

mely glycolipids; typical vacuoles of this type are the
zebra bodies. C) Vacuoles in which both types of storage
occur simultaneously to a various extent (Fig. 2).
    Vacuoles of type A are mostly found in visceral or-
gans and leucocytes and they can be extremely large (up
to 20 μ). Their presence in the liver is of great diagnostic value in cases suspected of mucopolysaccharidosis (Fig. 1). The similar ultrastructural appearance of
the liver in several forms of the disease, including
G_{M1}-gangliosidosis and mucosulfatidosis (Fig. 4), is ve-

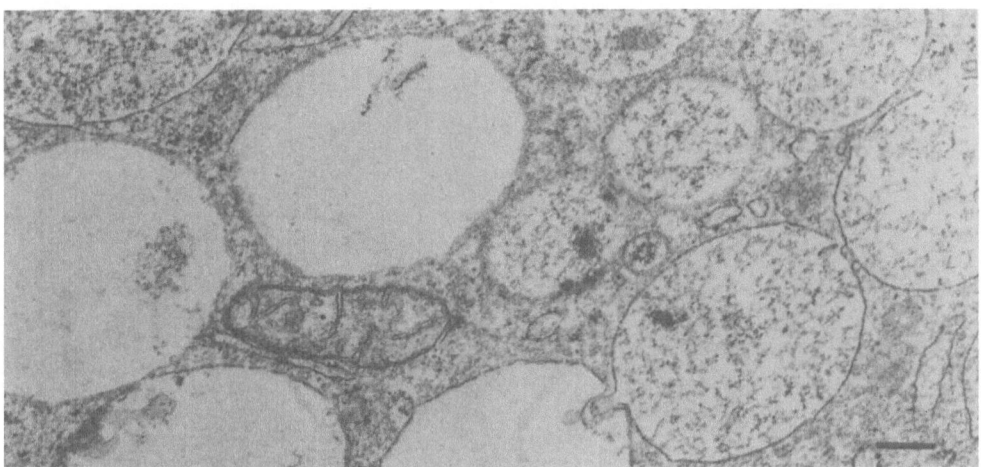

Fig. 4. Vacuoles of type A in a hepatocyte of a patient with mucosulfatidosis. The line indicates the scale of 0.2 micron.

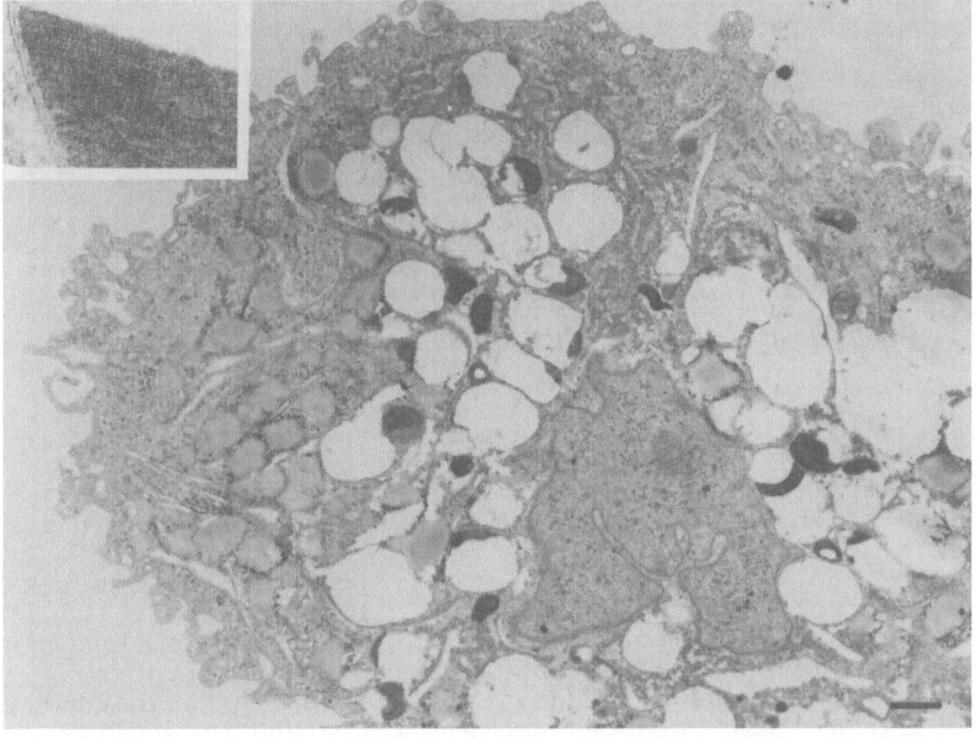

Fig. 5. Vacuoles of type C in a fibroblast cultured from the skin of a patient with fucosidosis. The inset shows a lamellar structure, at higher magnification. The line indicates the scale of 1 micron.

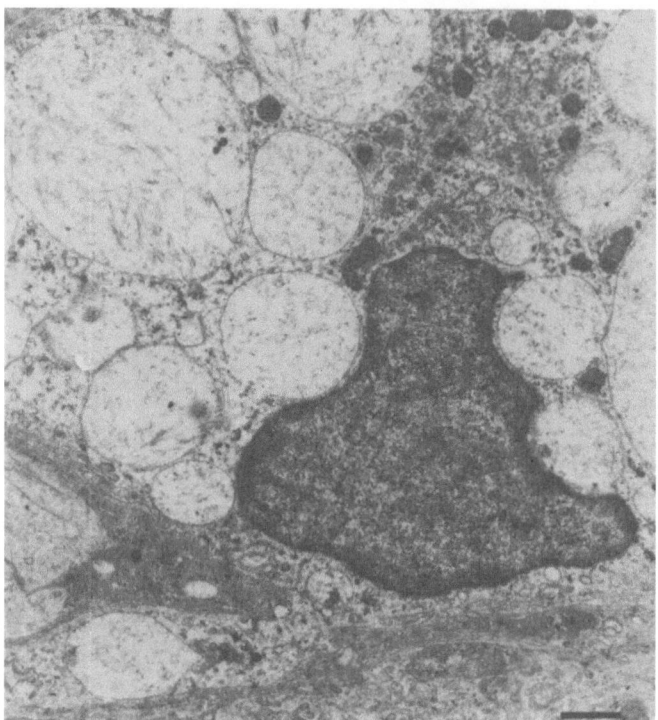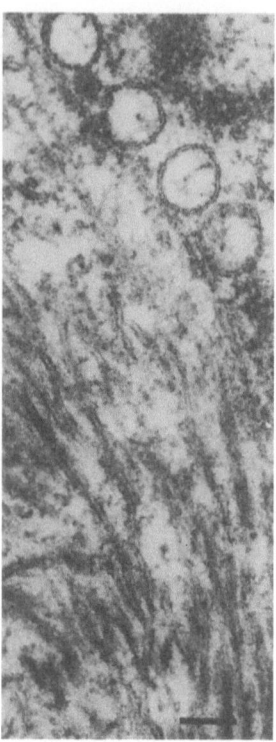

Figs 6 and 7. Part of a Kupffer cell in G_{M1}-ganglio-
sidosis. Clear vacuoles contain various amounts of fine
tubular elements, which are shown at a higher magnification in Fig. 7. The line indicates the scale of respectively 1 and 0.1 micron.

ry striking. In Morquio's syndrome and in type VI mucopolysaccharidosis (see Fig. 3), the vacuoles are mostly
concentrated in Kupffer cells and in macrophages. Only
in fucosidosis were vacuoles of type A observed in the
brain.

Vacuoles of type B are mostly found in nervous tissue. Vacuoles of type C are abundant in the liver and fibroblasts (Fig. 5) of patients with fucosidosis. One may
also mention that in macrophages (24) and in Kupffer
cells (Figs 6 and 7) of patients with G_{M1}-gangliosidosis
the large clear vacuoles contain fine tubules similar to
those observed in Gaucher's disease (8) and in Krabbe's
disease (31) in which cerebrosides are known to accumulate.

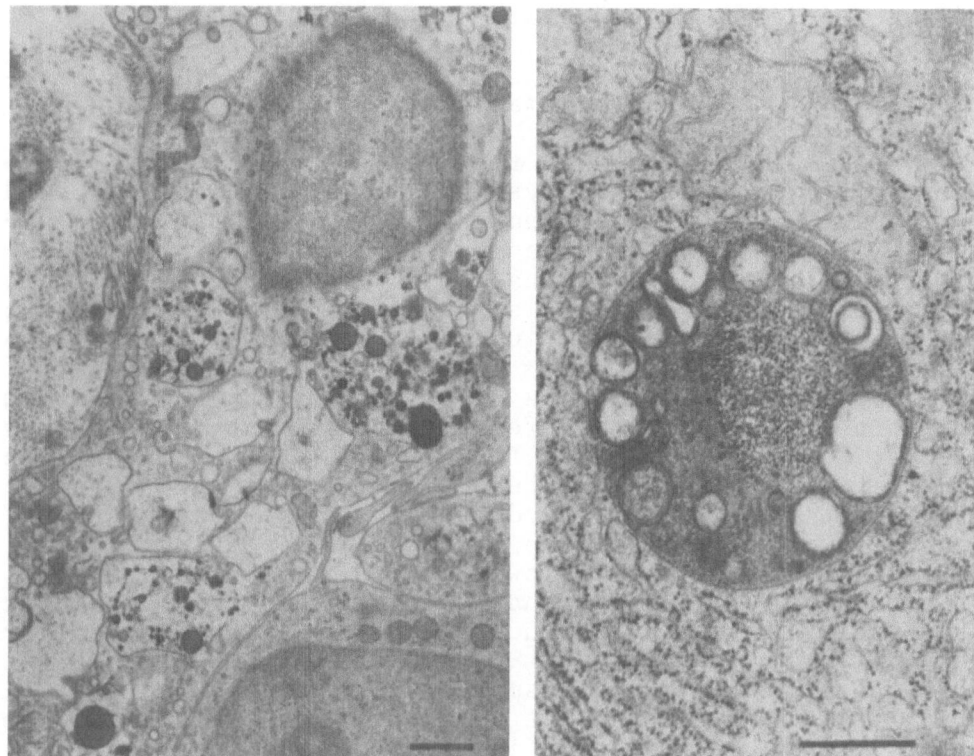

Fig. 8. Fibroblasts in the liver of a patient with lipomucopolysaccharidosis. Most vacuoles of type A contain osmiophilic droplets. The line indicates the scale of 1 micron.

Fig. 9. Lysosome in a hepatocyte of a patient with I-Cell disease. The line indicates the scale of 0.5 miron.

The existence of vacuoles of type C and the presence in the same patients of vacuoles of types A and B are a morphological evidence for the chemical heterogeneity of the depot in lysosomes. This heterogeneity precludes that the storage results from an excess of synthesis since the synthetic pathways for glycolipids and mucopolysaccharides are different and specific. On the contrary, this heterogeneity is easily explained by the lysosomal theory and was predicted by it.

In the liver of patients with I-cell disease, lysosomes are only slightly enlarged and have a polymorphic content (Fig. 9).

The enzymatic evidence

The definitive proof that each form of mucopolysaccharidosis is an inborn lysosomal disease rests on the demonstration of the deficiency of one lysosomal hydrolase
in the tissues of the affected children. Up to now this
conclusive demonstration has only been obtained in the case of fucosidosis, which is due to the complete deficiency
of α-fucosidase (30) and in the case of G_{M1}-gangliosidosis
where a β-galactosidase is lacking (3,18,28).When a complete enzymatic deficiency is demonstrated, there is no doubt
that it is the primary defect that explains the pathological condition. It appears thus that the clinical features
of Hurler's syndrome can result from the complete deficiency of one lysosomal hydrolase. It is expected that
further work, based on the assay of a larger number of
acid hydrolases, will allow to elucidate the cause of other forms of mucopolysaccharidosis. There are good indication that defects of β-glucuronidase (measured on culture
fibroblasts) (16) and of L-iduronidase (12) exist in some patients with gargoylism. In other cases, there is also a partial deficiency of β-galactosidase. This deficiency is restricted to some tissues only and its significance remains obscure (15, 30).
In most cases of mucopolysaccharidosis and also other
diseases where lysosomes are hypertrophied, there is a
large increase in the activity of several, but not all,
acid hydrolases; the pattern of enzyme hyperactivity is
somewhat specific of each disorder. The large increase
in the activity of β-galactosidase in the condition known
as lipomucopolysaccharidosis is particularly striking since it is in contrast with the low activity of the same
enzyme in several other forms of mucopolysaccharidoses.
For this reason, the cases with a high activity of that
enzyme have been referred to as "Gal +" (30).
The hypertrophy of the lysosomal system cannot be
the only cause of the hyperactivity of the acid hydrolases, since this increase varies greatly from enzyme to
enzyme. An alternative explanation would be a greater stability of some hydrolases due to the presence in lysosomes
of a high concentration of substances that might have a
structural similitude to their substrate. In agreement
with this hypothesis, we have found that, in a normal liver homogenate, the termal stability of N-acetyl-β-glucosa-

minidase is increased by the presence of chondroitin sulfate B or of heparan sulfate.

The work on cultured fibroblasts

The observation made by E. Neufeld and her coworkers
(17) that the abnormal mucopolysaccharide metabolism in
fibroblasts cultured from the skin of patients with mucopolysaccharidoses can be corrected by a specific protein
has attracted great interest. The corrective protein is
considered to be the one of which the deficiency in the
patient is responsible for the disease. Each time that
the nature of this correction protein has been identified,
it appeared to be a lysosomal hydrolase. These observations
are in direct agreement with the lysosomal theory.

Conclusion

The hypothesis that mucopolysaccharidoses are due to
the deficit of one acid hydrolase normally present in lysosomes is supported by a growing morphological and enzymological evidence as well as by the recent studies on cultured fibroblasts. This interpretative theory adequately
explains the striking heterogeneity of the storage material in the patients.

References

1. Aleu, F.P., Terry, R.D. and Zellweger, H. Electron
   microscopy of two cerebral biopsies in gargoylism.
   J. Neuropath. Expt. Neurol. 24, 304, 1965.
2. Austin, J.H. Mental Retardation. Metachromatic Leucodystrophy (Sulfatide Lipidosis, Metachromatic, Leucoencephalopathy). In "Medical Aspects of Mental Retardation" (Ch. H. Carter, Ed.). C.C. Thomas, Springfield U.S.A., 768, 1965.
3. Dacremont, G. and Kint, J.A. G_{M1}-ganglioside accumulation and β-galactosidase deficiency in a case of G_{M1}-
   gangliosidosis (Landing disease). Clin. Chim. Acta 21,
   421, 1968.
4. Hers, H.G. Inborn lysosomal diseases. Gastroenterology
   48, 625, 1965.
5. Lagunoff, D., Ross R. and Benditt, E.P. Histochemical
   and electron microscopic study in a case of Hurler's
   disease. Am. J. Path. 41, 273, 1962.
6. Landing, B.H., Silverman, F.N., Craig, J.M., Jacoby,
   M.D., Lahey, M.E. and Chadwick, D.L. Familial neurovisceral lipidosis. Am. J. Dis. Child 108, 503, 1964.

7. Ledeen, R., Salsman, K., Gonatas, J. and Taghavy, A. Structure comparison of the major monosialogangliosides from brains of normal human, gargoylism, and late infantile systemic lipidosis. Part I. J. Neuropathol. Exptl Neurol. 24, 341, 1965.

8. Lee, R.E. The fine structure of the cerebroside occurring in Gaucher's disease. Proc. Nat. Acad. Sci. 61, 484, 1968.

9. Leroy, J.G. and DeMars, R.I. Mutant enzymatic and cytological phenotypes in cultured human fibroblasts. Science 157, 804, 1967.

10. Loeb, H., Tondeur, M., Jonniaux, G., Mockel-Pohl, S. and Vamos-Hurwitz, E. Biochemical and ultrastructural studies in a case of mucopolysaccharidosis "F" (fucosidosis). Helv. Paediat. Acta 24, 519, 1969.

11. Loeb, H., Tondeur, M., Toppet, M. and Cremer, N. Clinical, biochemical and ultrastructural studies of an atypical form of mucopolysaccharidosis. Acta Paediat. Scand. 58, 220, 1969.

12. Matalon, R., Cifonelli, J.A. and Dorfman, A. L-iduronidase in cultured human fibroblasts and liver. Biochem. Biophys. Res. Comm. 42, 340, 1971.

13. McKusick, V.A., Kaplan, D., Wise, D., Hanley, W.B., Suddarth, S.B., Sevick, M.E. and Maumanee, A.E. The Genetic Mucopolysaccharidoses. Medicine 44, 445, 1965.

14. Meyer, K., Bhavanandan, V.P., Yung, D., Lee, L.T. and Howe, C. The keratosulfate-like mucopolysaccharide of chick allantoic fluid. Proc. Nat. Acad. Sci. U.S. 58, 1655, 1967.

15. Murphy, J.V., Wolfe, H.J., Balazs, E.A. and Moser, H.W. A patient with deficiency of arylsulfatases A, B, C and steroid sulfatase, associated with storage of sulfatide, cholesterol sulfate and glycosaminoglycans. In "Lipid Storage Diseases. Enzymatic defects and clinical implications "(J. Bernsohn and H.J. Grossman, Eds). Academic Press, New York, 67, 1971.

16. Neufeld, E.F. Personal communication; see also this symposium.

17. Neufeld, E.F., Barton, R.W., Cantz, M., Derge, J.G., Hall, C.W. and Kresse, H. Deficiency of specific proteins in the mucopolysaccharidoses. This book, 1972.

18. Okada, S. and O'Brien, J.S. Generalized gangliosidosis : β-galactosidase deficiency. Science 160, 1002, 1968.

19. Panizon, F., Sartorelli, C. and Perona, G. La malattia di Morquio e la disostosi spondilo-metafisaria. Acta Paediat. Latina 21, 552, 1968.

20. Sacrez, R., Juif, J.G., Gigonnet, J.M. and Gruner, J. E. La maladie de Landing ou idiotie amaurotique infantile précoce avec gangliosidose généralisée de type G_{M1}. Pédiatrie 22, 143, 1967.
21. Spranger, J., Wiedemann, H.R., Tolksdorf, M., Graucob, E. and Caesar, R. Lipomucopolysaccharidose. Eine neue Speicherkrankheit. Z. Kinderheilk. 103, 285, 1968.
22. Suzuki, K. Ganglioside patterns of normal and pathological brains. In "Inborn disorders of sphingolipid metabolism" (S.M. Aronson and B.W. Volk, Eds). Pergamon Press, New York, 215, 1967.
23. Suzuki, K. Cerebral G_{M1}-gangliosidosis : chemical pathology of visceral organs. Science 159, 1471, 1968.
24. Suzuki, K, Suzuki, K.and Chen,G.C. G_{M1}-gangliosidosis (generalized gangliosidosis). Morphology and chemical pathology. Path. Europ. 3, 389, 1968.
25. Taketomi, T. and Yamakawa, T. Glycolipids of the brain in gargoylism. Japan J. Expt. Med. 37, 11, 1967.
26. Tondeur, M. and Loeb, H. Etude ultrastructurelle du foie dans la maladie de Morquio. Pediat. Res. 3, 19, 1969.
27. Van Hoof, F. and Hers, H.G. L'ultrastructure des cellules hépatiques dans la maladie de Hurler (Gargoylisme). C.R. Acad. Sci. Paris 259, 1281, 1964.
28. Van Hoof, F. and Hers, H.G. Quoted in Ref. 20,1967.
29. Van Hoof, F. and Hers, H.G. L'ultrastructure du foie dans certaines thésaurismoses. Rev. Intern. Hépatol. 17, 815, 1967.
30. Van Hoof, F. and Hers, H.G. The abnormalities of Lysosomal enzymes in mucopolysaccharidoses. European J. Biochem. 7, 34, 1968.
31. Yunis, E.J. and Lee, R.E. Tubules of globoid leukodystrophy : a right-handed helix. Science, 169, 64, 1970.

RECENT OBSERVATIONS ON GAUCHER'S DISEASE

Julian N. Kanfer, Marcia Stein and Christine Spielvogel

Eunice K. Shriver Center at the Walter E. Fernald State

School, Waltham, Massachusetts

INTRODUCTION

Gaucher's disease is a typical "inborn error of metabolism" classified as a sphingolipidosis and is generally characterized by autosomal recessive inheritance. Two distinct clinical types exist. The adult form is the type found most prevelant in the U.S. and is characterized by splenomegaly, the presence of typical "foam cells" in bone marrow aspirates and elevated serum phosphatase. This type is reasonably benign and affected patients usually have elective surgical removal of the spleen when its size becomes excessive. The infantile form is rarely seen in this country and is usually associated with mental retardation and is fatal in infancy (1,2).

Chemical analysis of patients tissue indicated the accumulation of a carbohydrate-containing lipid which was originally believed to be galactocerebroside, the characteristic cerebroside of the central nervous system. Subsequent studies indicated that the material was glucosylceramide (3). This compound is increased some 10-30 fold in spleen tissue and represents an elevation from approximately 0.2 mg/gr in normals to 2-6 mg/gr in Gaucher's disease. The mass of the spleen may increase from a few hundred grams to 1-2 kilos.

The simplest biochemical explanation for the accumulation of a naturally occurring biological material is either an overproduction or, alternatively, a decreased catabolism. Experiments designed to examine these possibilities originally involved incubation of slices of both normal and Gaucher's tissues with either radioactive glucose or galactose (4). The results of these studies indicated that there were no detectable differences between the samples in the ability to incorporate these sugars into glucosyl-

225

ceramide. It was concluded that an overproduction was not responsible for the accumulation of glucosylceramide and therefore, spec-
ulated that a decreased catabolism was the cause.

In 1965, at the Laboratory of Neurochemistry at N.I.N.D.B.,
studies were undertaken in collaboration with Dr. David Shapiro
of the Weizmann Institute to examine this possibility. It was
considered imperative that the metabolism of this sphingolipid be
characterized in normal tissues. In order to accomplish this,
glucosyl-^{14}C ceramide was synthesized by established chemical procedures (5). The hydrolysis of this radioactive compound was studied in normal human and rat spleen to establish the presence and
characterize certain properties of a "glucocerebrosidase" (6).
Once these initial studies were completed, the level of the hydrolase was compared in both normal and Gaucher's tissues (7). The
results indicated that there was a marked decrease of this enzyme
in the pathological tissues. This was the first of the sphingolipidoses for which a specific enzymatic defect was assigned.

At approximately the same time that this work was published,
a brief report (8) appeared describing the decreased hydrolysis of
p-nitrophenyl-β-D-glucoside by Gaucher's tissues. This was largely ignored until it was discovered that such "synthetic" or "artificial" substrates are reasonably accurate tools for the diagnosis
of several specific enzymatic defects. Papers have recently appeared employing 4-methylumbelliferyl-β-D-glucoside for diagnosis of
Gaucher's disease, using white blood cells (9), skin fibroblasts
(10) as well as liver and spleen (11).

G_{M1} gangliosidosis (Pseudo-Hurlers Landings Syndrome) is a
sphingolipidosis in which the accumulation of G_{M1} ganglioside in
tissues was reported (12). This was subsequently explained by a
decreased hydrolysis of p-nitrophenyl-β-galactoside, G_{M1} (13) as
well as mucopolysaccharides and glycoprotein (14). These results
suggested a generalized β-galactosidase deficiency. More recent
publications have reported the accumulation of a heteropolysaccharide, as well as the ganglioside, in such tissues (15,16,17).

These two observations, (a) that Gaucher's disease is diagnosable with a non-specific artificial substrate and (b) that in
a similar disease, G_{M1} gangliosidosis, characterized by a general
β-galactosidase deficiency with an accumulation of both a sphingolipid and a heteropolysaccharide, prompted a search for the accumulation of other carbohydrate-containing materials, in addition to
glucosylceramide in Gaucher's disease.

MATERIALS AND METHODS

Spleen samples were collected and kindly donated by Dr. Hugo
Moser and kept frozen in dry ice from the time obtained. The
tissues were dried either by lyophilization of an aqueous homogenate or by preparation of acetone powders. The scheme for treatment of the sample is given in Figure 1. The dried samples were

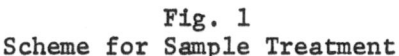

Fig. 1
Scheme for Sample Treatment

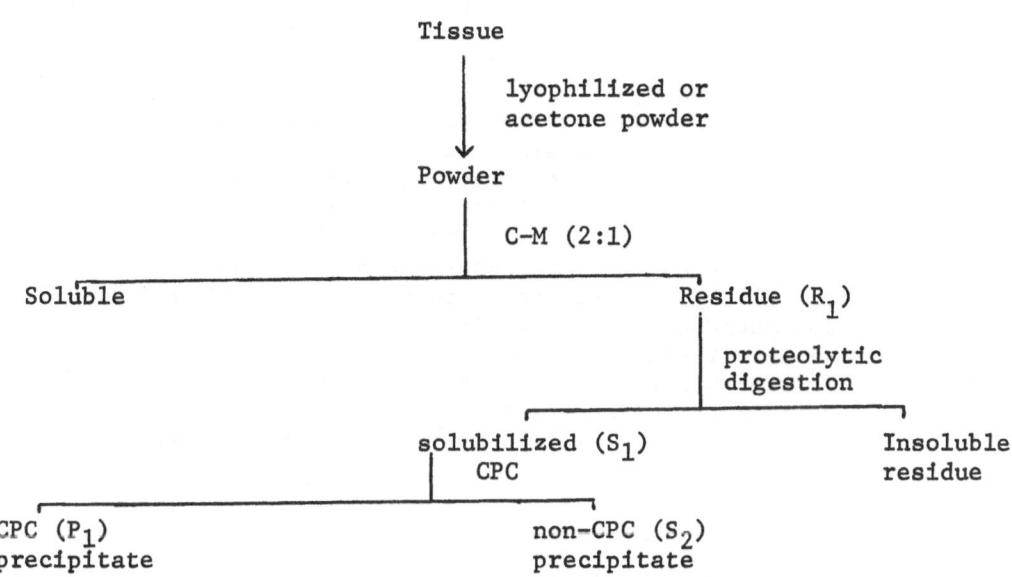

suspended in water, extracted with 20 volumes of C-M (2:1) and partitioned according to the procedure of Folch et al. (18). The lipid
extract was used for the determination of cerebroside content. The
chloroform-methanol insoluble residue (R_1) was homogenized with a
Polytron homogenizer and incubated for 24 hrs. with Papain. The
mixture was centrifuged, the supernatant saved and the insoluble
material incubated with Pronase for 24 hrs. After centrifugation,
the soluble fraction was pooled with the previous extract from the
Papain treatment. The pooled supernates were dialyzed for 48 hrs.
and then lyophilized. The lyophilized residues were dissolved in
water, excess 1% cetyl pyridinium chloride (CPC) solution added
and the tubes stored at $4^{\circ}C$ for 24 hrs. The insoluble precipitate
was harvested by centrifugation and the supernate (non-CPC precipitable) solution was exhaustively dialyzed against water. The CPC
precipitate was dissolved in 1.2 M NaCl and precipitated with 4
volumes of ethanol. This was repeated 3 times. The final precipitate obtained with ethanol was stored as a dry powder.

Sialic acid was determined by the procedure of Aminoff (19)
after hydrolysis at $80^{\circ}C$ for 1 hr. in 0.5 N H_2SO_4. Hexose was
determined by the phenol-H_2SO_4 procedure (20), uronic acid by the
carbozole procedure (21), hexosamine by the Elson-Morgan procedure,
after samples were hydrolyzed for 5 hrs. in 4 N HCl at $100^{\circ}C$ in a
sealed tube under nitrogen (22).

Glucosyl-1-C^{14} ceramide was synthesized as previously described
(5). White blood cells were prepared and the activity of glucocerebrosidase and the hydrolysis of 4-MU-β D glucoside assayed by published procedures (6,7,23).

RESULTS

The analytical values for the individual spleen samples for lipid hexose is presented in Table 1. Thin-layer chromatographic examination of the lipid extract indicated a gross accumulation of material chromatographing with cerebroside standards.

The lipid-free residue was analyzed for several carbohydrate components and these data are also recorded in Table 1.

Since these appeared to be an accumulation of non-lipid carbohydrate containing materials, this was further pursued. Only a single Gaucher's spleen, clinically diagnosed by the presence of "Gaucher's cells" in bone marrow aspirates and splenamegaly, and a single "control" spleen were selected for these studies due to their relative abundance available in the laboratory. The lipid-free residues were treated with aqueous salt solutions in an attempt to extract water soluble carbohydrate materials. Little material was obtained and only slight differences could be observed in hexose, uronic acid and protein between the normals and Gaucher's

TABLE 1
Analysis of Normal and Gaucher's Spleen Tissues

	Lipid hexose*	Hexose**	Hexosamine**	NANA**
Gaucher's				
#1	23.05	.208	.057	.015
#2	28.77	.103	.047	.010
#3	25.29	.135	.037	.013
#4	8.7	.140	--	.006
#5(I)	35	.133	.044	--
#6(I)	25	.119	.038	.006
average:	24.3	.139	.052	.012
Normals				
1	3.97	.115	.05	.006
2	4.0	.136	.026	.008
3	2.03	.081	.019	.0016
4	3.5	.105	.036	0
average:	3.37	.109	.033	.005

*   umoles/gr wet weight tissue

** umoles/mg dry weight lipid-free residue

tissues. This would tend to indicate that most of the excess material was protein-bound. Therefore, the lipid-free residues (R_1)
were treated with two proteolytic enzymes, Papain and Pronase, in
an attempt to liberate the accumulating heteropolysaccharides.
This is essentially the technique used for isolation of glycosaminoglycans (GAG). The supernatant (S_1) from the digestion mixture was fractionated into those compounds precipitating with CPC
(P_1) and those which are non-CPC precipitable (S_2). It should be
noted that a large excess of CPC was used and the mixture was stored overnight at 4°C in order to ensure complete precipitation with
this reagent.

The analytical data on the CPC precipitable materials from
both control and Gaucher's tissues is presented in Table 2. It
is obvious from this data that there is no excessive accumulation
of sulfated mucopolysaccharides in the Gaucher's individuals. The
yields are essentially identical and the gross compositional analyses are similar as judged by cellulose acetate electrophoresis,
the principal compenent being keratin sulfate.

This would tend to indicate that the materials accumulating
should be present in the non-CPC precipitable fraction and this
data is presented in Table 3. It is readily apparent that there
is an approximately 20-fold accumulation of hexose, NANA, hexosamine and fucose in this fraction. The small percentage of uronic
acid containing material would tend to eliminate the usual GAG except for an undersulfated keratin sulfate seen in G_{M1} gangliosidosis
(15,16). The final decision concerning this material will await
further purification, which is currently being undertaken. Paper
chromatographic separation of the hydrolysis products indicated
that galactose (Fig. 2) was the principal aldohexose with traces of
glucose and mannose and glucosamine as the major amino sugar.

TABLE 2

CPC Precipitable

| | yield | Uronic acid | Hexosamine | umoles/gr lipid-free residue | | |
				Fucose	Hexose	NANA
Gaucher's	259	3.5	3.78	0	0.052	0
Normals	240	3.1	1.56	0	0.040	0

TABLE 3

Non-CPC Precipitable

umoles/gr lipid-free residue

	Uronic acid	Hexosamine	Fucose	Hexose	NANA
Gaucher's	2.1	31.8	2.81	46.3	14.2
Normal	0.18	1.13	0.16	2.25	0.54

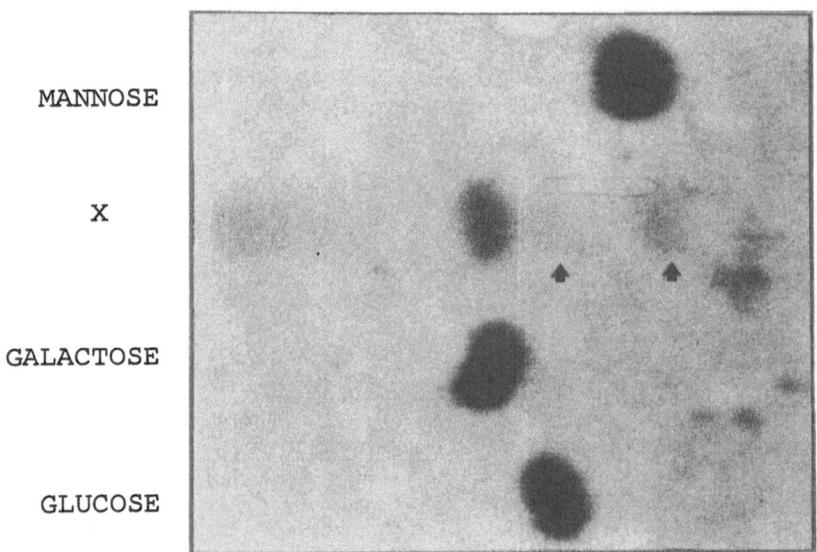

Fig. 2
Paper chromatographic separation of aldohexoses

COMPARISON OF 4-MU-β D GLUCOPYRANOSIDE AND GLUCOSE-^{14}C CEREBROSIDE
CLEAVAGE IN GAUCHER'S DISEASE

During the course of these studies, attempts were made to obtain additional Gaucher's spleen tissue locally. A spleen sample
became available which had, upon analysis, 8.6 umole lipid hexose/
gram tissue. This caused some problems since it could have been
classified either as a high normal or a low Gaucher's. White blood
cells were prepared from this individual and a suitable control.
The hydrolysis of 4-methylumbelliferyl-β D glucoside was examined
and no differences were found, as indicated in Table 4, which would
indicate that the individual was not a Gaucher's. The referring
clinicians were disturbed by these results and continued to feel
that the individual was a Gaucher's due to the presence of foam
cells and splenic hypertrophy. In order to reconcile these differences, the white blood cells were incubated with glucosyl-^{14}C ceramide, and these results are also presented in Table 4. It is apparent that the level of "glucocerebrosidase" activity was diminished
in the suspected Gaucher's as compared to the control sample.

In addition, the opportunity arose to test white blood cells
from an individual previously diagnosed as Gaucher's as judged by
a decreased hydrolysis of 4-MU-β-D glucoside. When incubated with
glucosyl-^{14}C ceramide, no differences were found between the patient
and its control.

Studies on the inhibition of several "lysosomal" hydrolases
of skin fibroblasts by p-chlorophenylmercuriosulfonate has been
undertaken (23). The inhibition of both 4-MU-β-D glucoside and

TABLE 4

Comparison of Hydrolysis of 4-MU-β D-glucoside and
glucosyl-[14]C Ceramide by White Blood Cells

	umoles cleaved/mg protein	
	4-MU-β D-glucoside	Glucosyl-^{14}C ceramide
Suspected Gaucher	1.33	1.6
Mr. C Control	1.715	9.4

glucosyl-^{14}C ceramide by this sulfhydryl-binding in skin fibroblasts from normals and Gaucher's was undertaken. It is apparent
from the results from Fig. 3 that the inhibition of hydrolysis of
the "artificial" substrate by both cell lines is almost identical.
Differences are apparent both between the susceptibility with the
"natural" and "artificial" substrates as well as between Gaucher's
and normal cells.

DISCUSSION

Gaucher's disease is an autosomal recessive disease classically
characterized by the accumulation of glucosyl ceramide. The massive
increase in spleen weight, however, can not be accounted for by the
increase in sphingolipid content alone. The results of the studies
on non-CPC precipitable material would suggest that other heteropolysaccharides also accumulate. The principal carbohydrates appear
to be galactose and glucosamine and sialic acid. The galactose and
glucosamine residues could represent an undersulfated keratin sulfate. An equimolar concentration of these two is probably present

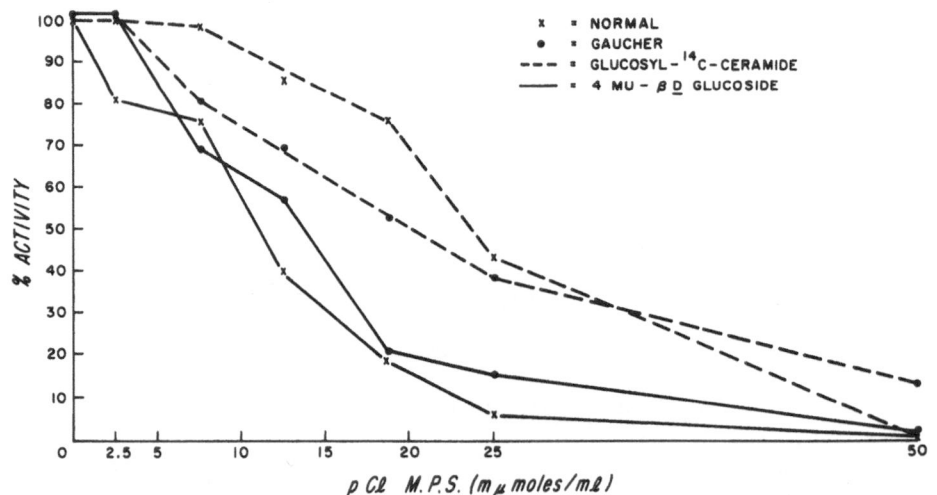

Fig. 3
Inhibition by pCl M-P-S of hydrolysis of 4-MU-β-D-
glucoside and glucosyl-^{14}C cerebroside by normal and
Gaucher's fibroblasts

in such a compound. Therefore, the excess hexose becomes equivalent to the NANA which would suggest the presence of a sialomucopolysaccharide. Studies are currently underway to separate these
two components. The structure of this material is currently unknown. It will be of interest to determine if this is identical
to that which accumulates in tissues of G_{M1} gangliosidosis (15,16,
17). In addition, a similar examination seems warranted of Niemann-
Picks spleen, in which hepatosplenomegaly and the accumulation of a
different sphingolipid occurs, as well as in several diseases of
splenic hypertropy not associated with lipid accumulation. It is
possible that the heteropolysaccharide which accumulates in addition
to cerebroside in Gaucher's may not be related to the β-glucosidase
deficiency. This may merely reflect the accumulation of cellular
structural material in concert with and in response to the storage
of lipid. The role of such compounds in the characteristic pathology of the individual diseases will have to be assessed independently of the lipids.

The levels of several lysosomal acid hydrolases are routinely
assayed in this laboratory. Most are quite reliable and readily
determined. However, the assay of β-$\underline{D}$ glucosidase either as the
4-MU or PNP derivative usually presents difficulties. All determinations are routinely carried out in triplicate in this laboratory. The problem has been that in 5 consecutive attempts to assay
a sample, 300% variation can occur in the triplicates. The sixth
attempt may then turn out to be perfectly satisfactory. This,
coupled with the relatively low absolute activity of β-glucosidase,
approximately 1/1000 that of β $\underline{D}$ N-acetyl glucosaminidase, makes
this a particularly trying assay procedure. The experience cited
in Table 4 also indicates that misdiagnosis may occur when employing an "artificial" substrate as compared to use of the sphingolipid itself as substrate. It should be mentioned that an accurate
unanticipated diagnosis of Gaucher's has been obtained with 4-MU-β
$\underline{D}$ glucoside employing skin fibroblasts.

The conventional dogma has been that of one gene-one enzyme.
However, in the light of multiple enzyme defects found in certain
of the sphingolipidosis, this may have to be modified. Several
lines of evidence point to this need for reappraisal.
1. In generalized gangliosidosis, there is a dimunition of β-
galactosidase activity as assayed with the 4-MU derivatives. This
is also reflected by the inability of tissues from affected patients
to remove the terminal galactose residue of G_{M1} (13,14). However,
the hydrolysis of the β-galactosidic bonds of ceramidegalactoside
and ceramide-lactoside is not affected (24).
2. In Krabbes disease, where ceramide-galactoside accumulates, the
enzymatic problem is a deficiency of ceramide galactoside:βgalac-
tosidase. This is not reflected as a decrease in β-galactosidase
when assayed with an "artificial" substrate (25).
3. In metachromatic leukodystrophy, (MLD) there is sulfatidase
deficiency (26,27). This enzyme is conveniently monitored with an
"artificial" substrate which has been operationally called arylsul-

fatase "A". Although purified "aryl A" is active towards an "artificial" substrate, the presence of a "complimentary" protein is necessary for hydrolysis of sulfatide (28). Recent evidence has been provided for the presence of immunologically detectable but enzymatically inactive aryl "A" in MLD tissues (29,30). A variant form of MLD has been described in which a variety of sulfate containing compounds including steroid sulfates and mucopolysaccharides accumulate (31). There is a deficiency of arylsulfatase A, B and C as well as steroid sulfatase in these tissues.

4. Fabry's disease is characterized by the accumulation of ceramide trihexoside (32) and an α galactosidase deficiency (33). Recent studies have reported the results of the infusion of normal plasma into Fabry's individuals (34). These authors observed a 20-35 fold greater amount of enzyme activity in the recipient than would be predicted from the amount infused, while the levels attained were approximately 150% that of controls.

The deficiency of β-galactosidase in G_{M1} gangliosidosis and ceramide galactoside β galactosidase in Krabbes could be explained by a single gene deficiency affecting a single specific enzyme. However, it would be difficult to reach a similar conclusion concerning the classical MLD and the variant. This dilemma is further compounded by the requirement for a "complementary" fraction sulfatidase activity and the presence of immunologically detectable enzyme protein.

An alternative hypothesis could be that there is a general protein for the hydrolysis of specific bonds, i.e., a β galactosidase, a sulfatase, etc. The specificity for the hydrolysis of a given bond in an specific substrate may be invoked by a specific non-catalytic protein. A classical example of this is the role of α-lactalbumin on tissue UDP-galactose:galactosyl transferase. In nearly all tissues examined including brain, glucosamine is the preferred acceptor for this transferase. However, in the presence of α lactalbumin, glucose is not the preferred acceptor. Thus, brain can be made to synthesize lactose, the milk sugar (35). Such "specific proteins" may also operate with hydrolytic enzymes.

A 1000 fold purification of β-galactosidase from human liver has been reported (36). p-Nitrophenyl-β D galactoside was used as the substrate to monitor this purification. This highly purified enzyme preparation was found inactive toward G_{M1}. It is conceivable that this may be due to removal of a "specific protein" during the extensive purification. For the β-galactosidase deficiencies, the situation with G_{M1} gangliosidosis could be a leaky mutation since there are no zero deficiency. In Krabbes and classical MLD, a specific protein could be absent, while in the MLD variant, a general sulfatase may be absent. The greater amount of galactosidase in Fabry's individuals after plasma infusion could be due to the presence of a "specifier protein" in normal serum which activates the abnormal enzyme.

REFERENCES

1. Fredrickson, D.S., in The Metabolic Basis of Inherited Diseases, by J.B. Stanburg, J.B. Wyngaarden and D.S. Fredrickson, McGraw-Hill, N.Y. 1966, pg. 565.
2. Schettler, G. and Kahlke, W., in Lipids and Lipidosis, G. Schettler ed., Springer-Verlag, N.Y. 1967, pg. 260.
3. Suomi, W.D. and Agranoff, B.W., J. Lipid Res. 6, 211 (1965).
4. Trams, E.G. and Brady, R.O., J. Clin. Invest. 39, 1546 (1960).
5. Kanfer, J., J. Biol. Chem. 240, 609 (1965).
6. Brady, R.O., Kanfer, J. and Shapiro, D., J. Biol. Chem. 240, 39 (1965).
7. Brady, R.O., Kanfer, J.N., Bradley, R.M. and Shapiro, D., J. Clin. Invest. 45, 1112 (1966).
8. Patrick, A.D., Biochem. J. 97, 17c (1965).
9. Beutler, E., Kuhl, W., J. Lab. and Clin. Med. 76, 747 (1970).
10. Beutler, E., Kuhl, W., Trinidad, F., Teplitz, R. and Nadler, H., Amer. J. Human Gen. 23, 62 (1971).
11. Hultberg, B. and Ockerman, P.A., Clin. Chim. Acta 28, 169 (1970).
12. O'Brien, J.S., Stern, M.B., Landing, B.H., O'Brien, J.E. and Donnell, G.N., Amer. J. Dis. of Child. 109, 338 (1965).
13. Okada, S. and O'Brien, J.S., Science 160, 1002 (1968).
14. MacBrinn, M.C., Okada, S., Ho, M.W., Hu, C.C. and O'Brien, J.S., Science 163, 946 (1969).
15. Suzuki, K., Science 159, 1471 (1968).
16. Suzuki, K., Suzuki, K. and Kamoshita, S., J. Neuropath. and Expt'l. Neurol. 28, 25 (1969).
17. Callahan, J.W. and Wolfe, L.S., Biochim. Biophys. Acta 215, 527 (1970).
18. Folch, J., Lees, M. and Sloane-Stanley, G.H., J. Biol. Chem. 226, 497 (1957).
19. Aminoff, D., Biochem. J. 81, 384 (1961).
20. Dubois, M., Gilles, K.A., Hamilton, J.K., Rebers, P.A. and Smith, F., Anal. Chem. 28, 350 (1956).
21. Gregory, J.D., Arch. Biochem. 89, 157 (1960).
22. Davidson, E., in Methods in Enzymology, S.P. Colowick and N.O. Kaplan, ed., Vol. 8, Academic Press, N.Y., 1967, p. 57.
23. Kanfer, J.N., Speilvogel, C. and Milunsky, A., submitted for publication.
24. Brady, R.O., O'Brien, J.S., Bradley, R.M. and Gal, A.E., Biochim. Biophys. Acta 210, 193 (1970).
25. Suzuki, Y. and Suzuki, K., Science 171, 73 (1971).
26. Austin, J.H., Balasubramanian, A.S., Pattabiraman, T.N., Saraswathi, S., Basu, D.K. and Bachhawat, B.K. J. Neurochem. 10, 805 (1963).
27. Jatzkewitz, H. and Mehl, E., J. Neurochem. 16, 19 (1969)
28. Mehl, E. and Jatzkewitz, H., Biochim. Biophys. Acta 151, 619 (1968).
29. Neuwelt, E., Stumpf, D., Austin, J.H. and Kohler, P., Biochim.

Biophys. Acta 236, 333 (1971).

30. Stumpf, D., Neuwelt, E., Austin, J. and Kohler, P., Trans Am. Neurol. Assoc. 96, 1971.

31. Murphy, J.V., Wolfe, H., Balazs, A. and Moser, H.W., in Lipid Storage Diseases, J. Bernsohn and H.J. Grossman, ed., Academic Press, N.Y., 1971, pg. 67.

32. Swelley, C.C. and Klionsky, B., in The Metabolic Basis of Inherited Diseases, J.B. Stanburg, J.B. Wyngaarden and D.S. Fredrickson, ed., McGraw-Hill, N.Y. 1966, pg. 618.

33. Kint, J.A., Science 167, 1268 (1970).

34. Mapes, C.A., Anderson, R.L., Sweeley, C.C., Desnick, R.J. and Krivit, W., Science 169, 987 (1970).

35. Hill, R.L., Brew, K., Vonaman, T.C., Trayer, L.P. and Mattlock, P., Brookhavan Symp. Biol. 21, 139 (1968).

36. Meisler, M.H., Fry, J.B. and Paigen, Fed. Proc. 30, 1118 Abs. (1971).

ACKNOWLEDGEMENTS:

This work was supported by Grants NS 08994, HD 05515 from the U.S.P.H.S. and Grant 724 from the National Multiple Sclerosis Society.

INTERACTION OF ENZYMES WITH LIPID SUBSTRATES

Shimon Gatt, Yechezkel Barenholz, Ilana Borkovski-Kubiler
and Zelina Leibovitz-Ben Gershon

Department of Biochemistry, The Hebrew University-
Hadassah Medical School, Jerusalem, Israel

The recent five to eight years have been characterized by major advances in the enzymology of the complex lipids. This might be exemplified by the characterization of the enzymes which synthesize and degrade the sphingolipids; the identification of separate phospholipases A_1 and A_2; the identification of a new pathway for phosphoglyceride biosynthesis via acyl dihydroxyacetone phosphate and further recognition of the enzymes which synthesize and degrade the glycerophosphatides. A further major advance, pertinent to this symposium, is the recognition that the sphingolipid storage diseases are caused by defects in degradative enzymes. In contrast to this rapid development, identification of the mechanisms of action of these enzymes has been extremely slow. Only scanty information is available to date on the mode of interaction of the enzymes with their respective lipid substrates, either in vivo or in vitro.

The main research effort of our laboratory in the last three years has been directed to investigations on the mechanisms of action and mode of interaction of enzymes acting on complex lipids. Two simultaneous directions were undertaken. In the first, attempts were made to purify the subcellular components which contain the sphingolipid hydrolases and interact these with pure lipid substrates. In the second, the interaction of isolated enzymes with pure substrates was investigated. Only the latter subject will be covered in this presentation and will be exemplified by four enzymes, which represent three types of interaction. A classification of the various types of interactions is presented; this can serve as a general model for enzymes which act on those surface-active lipids classified as "soluble amphipatic molecules" (1).

One of the basic parameters which define an enzyme-substrate interaction is the dependence of the reaction rate on substrate concentration (V/S curve). With most enzymes, the kinetics of this interaction follows the Michaelis-Menten theory; the V/S curve is a rectangular hyperbola and the double reciprocal presentation of the same data (V^{-1}/S^{-1} curve), is a straight line. The latter curve will deviate from linearity and the V/S curve from the hyperbolic shape, in those cases where the kinetic determinants that control the enzyme-substrate interaction are not constant throughout the range of substrate concentrations used in the experiment. This might occur when a substrate or a product is also an inhibitor or when the affinity alters because of a change in the structure or conformation of the enzymatic protein, such as with allosteric enzymes. It might however also occur if the substrate undergoes a change which depends on its own concentration. Enzymes acting on "soluble amphipatic lipids" are examples of this phenomenon.

Numerous examples are available of hyperbolic V/S curves, obtained with enzymes acting on lipid substrates. However, a theoretical consideration will compel us to conclude that with "soluble amphipats", hyperbolic V/S curves should be an exception rather than the rule. At low concentrations, compounds of this type are present in true molecular solution in aqueous media ("monomers"). Above a certain concentration, which is characteristic for each compound (the "critical micellar concentration" - CMC), but which might be influenced by the composition of the medium used for dissolution, a phase transition occurs. The concentration of the monomers is maximal at the CMC. Above this concentration the monomer level is constant and all excess substance aggregates into micelles. It is unlikely that the parameters of interaction of the enzyme with the micelles will be exactly the same as with the monomers; a change in the shape of the V/S curve is therefore expected at a substrate concentration equalling the critical micellar concentration.

Emphasis must be put on an important point which has frequently been overlooked and which is responsible for erroneous V/S curves. Below the CMC, the values on the abcissa are correctly presented, since the concentration of the substrate available for interaction with the enzyme equals the number of monomeric molecules in the solution. Above the CMC, where part or even most of the lipid is present as micelles rather than as monomers, the values on the X-axis, while equalling the total concentration, do not any longer represent the "true" concentration of the substrate as related to its interaction with the enzyme. This scale is correct only in the extreme case, where, for the purpose of interaction with the enzyme, each monomeric molecule in the micelle is statistically equal to a monomeric molecule in solution; such a case must, logically be an exception. This argument might be illustrated with lysolecithin as substrate. Egg lysolecithin has an aggregation number of 180 (2), i.e. above the CMC,180 molecules aggregate to form one micelle. It is improbable that these 180 molecules of the compact micelle have an equal chance of colliding with enzyme molecules as have 180 monomers of lysolecithin. Conversely, an opposite extreme case might be argued, where one enzyme molecule interacts with only one micelle of lysolecithin. Then, to double the substrate "units" above the CMC (i.e., to get a number of micelles which equals the number of monomers), the concentration of the substrate will have to be increased by 180 times that of the CMC. A correct presentation of the V/S curve for the latter case will therefore require that the concentration scale of the abcissa above the CMC be shortened 180 fold. The "activity" of the micelle (i.e., the number of enzyme molecules which can interact with and bind to one micelle) is most likely somewhere in between the above two extreme cases; the "true" concentration scale above the CMC is therefore not known.

Fig. 1 presents a classification of the four basic forms of V/S curves, obtained with lipid amphipatic substrates; they will be hitherto referred to as types I, II, III and IV. Examples for each of these are scattered throughout the literature. For the purpose of this concise presentation, they will be exemplified only by data of enzymes investigated in our laboratory.

Type I is the classical Michaelis-Menten type V/S curve. It is obtained in cases of enzymes acting on lipid substrates where, under the experimental conditions used, there is no monomer-micelle transition. This type occurs with many enzymes which act on "swelling amphipats" (1) or on lipid substrates dispersed by detergents. The latter cases are best exemplified with the sphingolipid hydrolases where the V/S curves were hyperbolic (for references on these enzymes, see ref. 3). As will be shown below, it might also be erroneously obtained when the CMC is very low, and the assay procedure is not sensitive enough to detect deviations from the hyperbolic shape below the CMC.

Type II. The V/S curve is hyperbolic to a certain substrate concentration, then "breaks" and the curve becomes parallel to the abcissa. Similarly, the straight line in the V^{-1}/S^{-1} presentation breaks and is followed by a second line, parallel to the abcissa. This is the case where the enzyme utilizes monomers but probably not micelles of the substrate. The curve becomes parallel since the concentration of the monomers above the CMC is constant. This concentration will remain constant and equals the CMC even when substrate molecules are removed by the action of the enzyme, due to a rapid disaggregation of micelles.

This case usually cannot be differentiated from that discussed above, where the enzyme utilizes also the micelles but the "activity" of one micelle equals that of a monomer, and where the values on the X-axis have not been corrected for the aggregation number. If the aggregation number is high, the curve beyond the "break" will, in this case, not be parallel but will have a very shallow upward slope.

Type III. The V/S curve is hyperbolic to a certain concentration, then "breaks" and rates decrease. In the V^{-1}/S^{-1} presentation, the straight line "breaks" and is succeeded by a second straight line with an upward slope. This is the case where the enzyme utilizes monomers but probably not micelles, and where the micelles either inhibit the enzyme or interfere with the action of the enzyme on substrate monomers.

Type IV. The V/S curve is sigmoidal, though the sigmoid is usually not symmetrical. This is the case where the enzyme utilizes micelles but not monomers (or utilizes the latter at much lower rates).

The patterns belonging to types II - IV will now be exemplified by the following four enzymes: Soluble and particulate lysolecithinase of rat brain (4,5), and soluble (6,7) or microsomal (8-10) base-acetyl coenzyme A acetyl transferases of the yeast Hansenula ciferri. Each enzyme was analyzed for the following four parameters: 1. Dependence of the reaction rates on enzyme concentration (V/E). 2. Dependence of the reaction rates on substrate concentration (V/S). 3. Dependence of the V/S curves on enzyme concentration. 4. Effect of albumin on either V/E or V/S.

1. Soluble lysolecithinase of rat brain (Type II). Lysolecithinase of brain tissue is mostly particulate or microsomal; a small part of the total activity of brain homogenate is present in the 100,000 xg supernatant as a soluble protein. The soluble enzyme (as well as

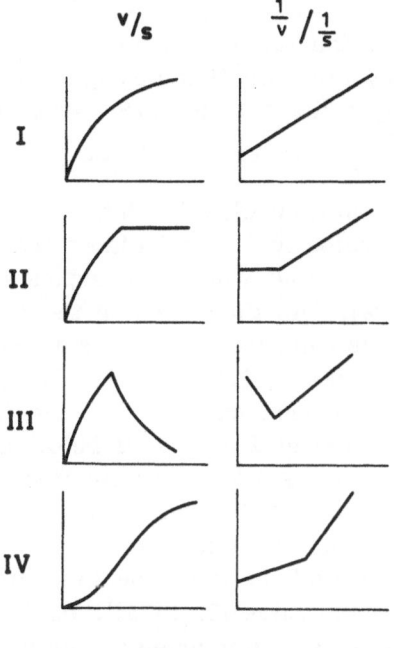

Fig. 1

Classification of the V/S and V^{-1}/S^{-1} curves as related to the four types of interactions of enzymes with "soluble amphipatic molecules".

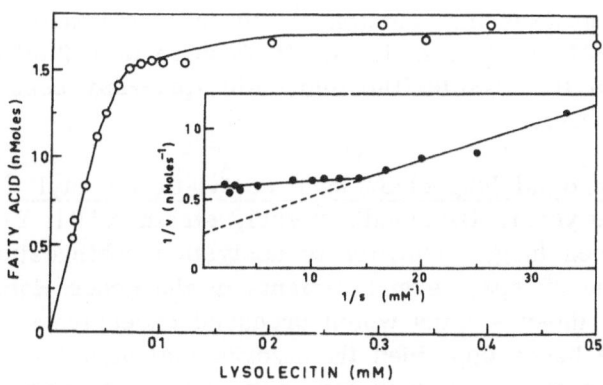

Fig. 2

V/S and V^{-1}/S^{-1} curves of the soluble lysolecithinase.

a small portion of the particulate enzymes which could be solubilized) were further purified by treatment with protamine sulfate and ammonium sulfate, followed by gel filtration through Sephadex G-50. The V/E curves were straight lines. The V/S curve (Fig. 2) was of type II.

The V^{-1}/S^{-1} presentation clearly shows that the curve does not reach the maximal velocity, as calculated from the descending portion of the curve (i.e., that which corresponds to the hyperbolic portion of the V/S curve). As discussed in the introduction, this is the case where the enzyme utilizes substrate monomers, but probably not micelles. Using tritium-labeled lysolecithin of high specific activity, we could show that the enzyme indeed utilized the substrate at a concentration of $1 \mu M$, well below any reported value of CMC for this compound. A close examination of Fig. 2 shows that beyond the "break", the V/S curve is not completely parallel, but has a very shallow upward slope. As discussed in the introduction, it is impossible to distinguish between the two alternatives - a. the enzyme does not utilize the micelles at all, or b. the enzyme utilizes micelles, but one micelle of 180 monomeric units is equivalent to one substrate "unit". The concentration at which the "break" in the V/S curve occurred was independent of protein concentration; this suggested that, contrary to the particulate or microsomal lysolecithinase (see below), the substrate was not adsorbed onto non-specific sites of the soluble enzyme. Albumin had little effect at low concentrations; at albumin to substrate ratios of 0.2 or more, inhibition ensued. As will be shown later, lysolecithin binds to albumin and the enzyme most probably utilizes that portion of the substrate monomers which remain free. At an albumin to substrate ratio of 0.2 or more, the concentration of free lysolecithin molecules probably becomes limiting and rates decrease.

2. Microsomal long-chain base acetyl-CoA acetyl transferase (type IV). The yeast, Hansenula ciferri, strain NRRL Y-1031, F60-10, produces large quantities of acetylated sphingosine bases (11). We tested 25 species and variants of the genus Hansenula and found that only those strains which produced excessive quantities of the sphingosine bases contained the microsomal acetyl transferase (12). This enzyme transferred the acetyl group of acetyl CoA to free or N-acetylated sphingosine base as well as to primary amines of 6-18 carbon atoms. Using these amines, maximal rates were obtained with hexadecyl or octadecylamines. The V/E curves were straight lines. The V/S curves, when determined at a fixed con-

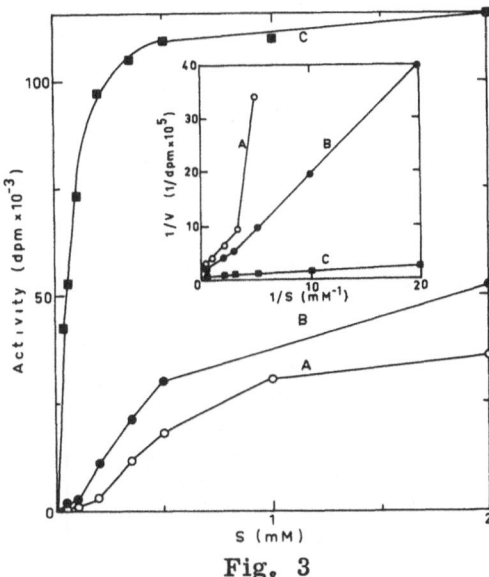

Fig. 3

V/S and V^{-1}/S^{-1} curves of the microsomal acetyltransferase.

centration of the base and varying concentrations of acetyl CoA, were hyperbolic. This agrees with the theoretical consideration, since the acetyl CoA is present in a true, molecular solution. However, when the acetyl CoA concentration was fixed and that of the base varied, two types of curves were obtained (Fig. 3).

Using dihydrosphingosine (● — ●) or hexadecylamine (o — o) the curves were sigmoidal (type IV); with N-acetyl phytosphingosine as substrate (■ — ■), the curve was hyperbolic (type I). The V^{-1}/S^{-1} presentation corroborated these conclusions. In accord with the assumption that type IV represents those cases where the enzyme utilizes micelles but not monomers, back extrapolation of the ascending portions of the two sigmoidal V/S curves intersected the abcissa at values very close to the critical micellar concentrations of the two bases (the measured CMCs of dihydrosphingosine and hexadecylamine were 0.08 and 0.2 mM, respectively). These points of intersection were independent of protein concentration. Concerning the hyperbolic shape of the curve using N-acetyl phytosphingosine, this probably represents an example of a type I curve, obtained with a type IV enzyme-substrate interaction, because of insufficient experimental sensitivity. This compound showed no CMC even at concentrations as low as 1 μM. The sensitivity of the assay procedure was not sufficient to determine the reaction rates at such low concentrations; the portion of the V/S curve below the CMC is therefore absent from the V/S curve and the curve is hyperbolic.

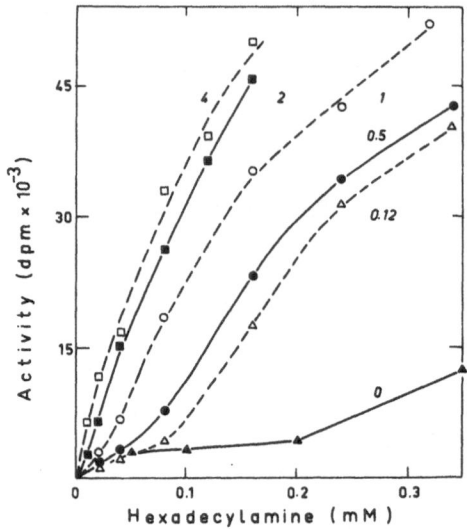

Fig. 4

V/S curves of the microsomal acetyltransferase at several albumin to amine ratios.

The sigmoidal V/S curves could be changed into hyperbolas by albumin (Fig. 4). This experiment was performed using several fixed albumin to substrate ratios. These molar ratios are represented by the number on each curve. The sigmoidity of the curves decreased at ratios up to 1.0. At ratios of 2 or more, the curves were hyperbolic.. Fig. 5 shows the same data in the double reciprocal presentation; at molar ratios of 2 or more, the V^{-1}/S^{-1} curves were straight lines. In separate experiments we found that albumin did not inhibit even when in a 24 fold molar excess over the base. Fig. 5 also shows that the maximal velocities were the same, in the absence or presence of albumin. The stimulatory effect of albumin at low substrate concentrations suggests that while the enzyme does not utilize free monomers of the bases, it transfers the acetyl group to albumin-bound monomers. Albumin thus substitutes for the micellar aggregate which is probably required for binding to the enzyme. At the optimal albumin to amine ratio, all substrate molecules are equally "recognized" by the enzyme and the V/S curve is hyperbolic.

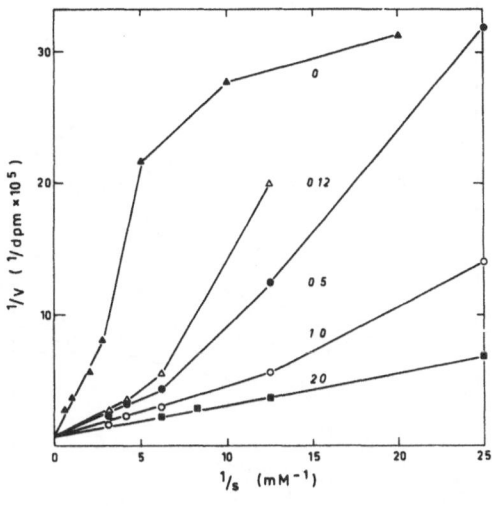

Fig. 5

Double reciprocal presentation of the data of Fig. 4.

3. Type III enzymes. Two enzymes which yielded V/S curves
of type III were investigated, a particulate or microsomal lysolecithinase and a soluble amine-acetyl CoA acetyl transferase. There are
numerous differences between these two enzymes and they will therefore be discussed separately.

a. Microsomal or particulate lysolecithinase of rat brain. No
clear cut separation could be obtained between the "particulate" enzyme
which sedimented at 25,000 xg and the "microsomal" enzyme which
sedimented at 100,000 xg. The ratio of the two depended on the method
employed for subcellular fractionation. No differences with regard to
the properties discussed below could be detected between these two
fractions. For the purpose of this discussion, they will therefore be
treated as one enzyme, and for simplicity will be designated as the
"microsomal lysolecithinase".

The V/E curves obtained with this enzyme were irregular. Two
types of curves were obtained when reaction rates were plotted against
enzyme concentration; these depended on the concentration of the
substrate (Fig. 6; the numbers represent the respective substrate
concentrations). At lysolecithin concentrations up to about 0.05 mM,
the V/E curves were straight lines and reaction rates increased with

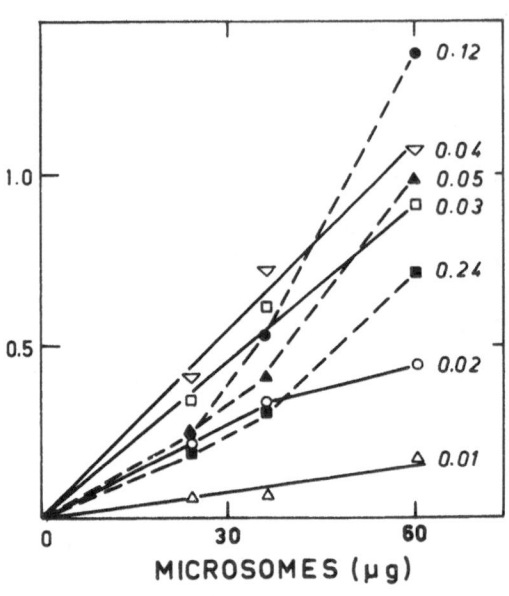

Fig. 6

V/**E** curves of the microsomal lysolecithinase at several substrate concentrations.

increasing substrate concentrations. At concentrations of about 0.1 mM substrate or more, the curves deviated from linearity and were of parabolic shape. Furthermore, at these concentrations, reaction rates decreased with increasing substrate concentration; this is a consequence of the type III shape of the V/S curve (Fig. 7), where substrate concentrations above 0.05-0.1 mM inhibited the reaction. The parabolic shape of the V/**E** curves, i.e., increasing specific activities with increasing protein concentrations, suggests that the degree of inhibition by the substrate depends on the substrate to protein ratio.

The V/S curves obtained with the microsomal lysolecithinase (Fig. 7) were typically of type III, suggesting that the enzyme utilized lysolecithin monomers, and that micelles of the substrate were inhibitory. The inversion points (i.e., the substrate concentration resulting in the maximal rate and above which the V/S curve descended), depended on the enzyme concentration (Fig. 8). It is evident that increasing the concentration of the enzymatic protein (the following concentrations were used; 22 μg - open circles, 66 μg - full circles and 154 μg - squares) shifted the inversion points to higher substrate concentrations.

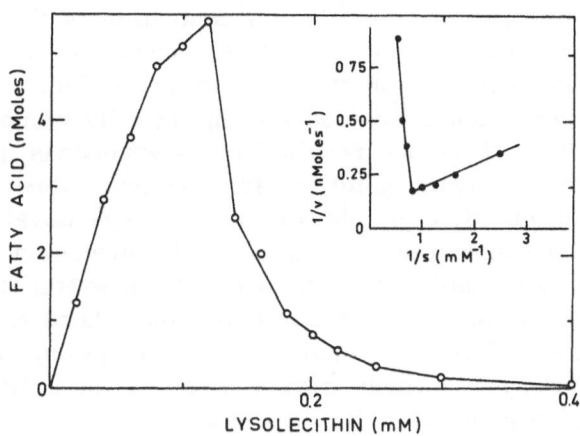

Fig. 7

V/E and V^{-1}/S^{-1} curves of the microsomal lysolecithinase.

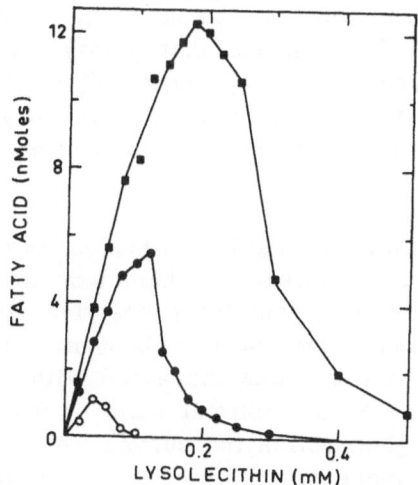

Fig. 8

V/S curves of the microsomal lysolecithinase at three enzyme concentrations.

Since we assumed that the inversion point is related to the CMC of the substrate, the latter being a thermodynamic property, the results of Fig. 8 suggest that the effective concentration of the substrate in solution is decreased through non-specific adsorption onto, or binding to the particulate protein. In the V/S curves of Fig. 8, the values on the abcissa were not corrected for the quantity removed by such an adsorption. This therefore resulted in an erroneous designation of the values of the inversion points of the abcissa. Since increasing the enzyme concentration will result in greater removal of substrate by adsorption, the experimental values of the inversion points will move to higher substrate concentrations. Back extrapolation of the inversion points to zero enzyme concentration (where none of the substrate is removed from the solution by adsorption) yielded a value of about 0.02-0.04 mM, which is very close to the critical micellar concentration of egg or liver lysolecithin.

Fig. 9 shows the existence of the above mentioned adsorption onto the enzymatic protein. Tritium-labelled lysolecithin was mixed, at 0° with the particulate enzyme and the protein was then sedimented, in the cold, by centrifugation. The results (Fig. 9, curve A) show that only about 10% of the substrate was recovered in the supernatant, demonstrating that about 90% was bound to the protein and sedimented with it. Curve B of Fig. 8 shows that if this experiment was repeated in the presence of serum albumin, about 50% of the radioactive compound was recovered in the supernatant. This suggests that the albumin competes with the particulate protein for non-specific binding of lysolecithin.

Addition of albumin to reaction mixtures increased the reaction rates. Fig. 10 shows the effect of albumin on the V/E curves (the numbers on the curves represent the respective albumin to lysolecithin ratios). Without albumin (R=0) or at suboptimal ratios, the curves were parabolic and reaction rates increased with increasing albumin to lysolecithin ratios. At the optimal ratio of 0.5, the curve was a straight line; at higher ratios the curves were straight but the rates decreased with increasing ratios. Fig. 11 shows the effect of albumin (at the optimal ratio of 0.5) on the V/S curve. Addition of albumin converted the type III curve (Fig. 11, curve A) to type I, i.e., the curve became hyperbolic (Fig. 11, curve B).

The albumin effects may be explained as follows: Because of nonspecific adsorption of lysolecithin onto the particulate protein, the enzyme is partly inhibited even below the inversion point. This inhi-

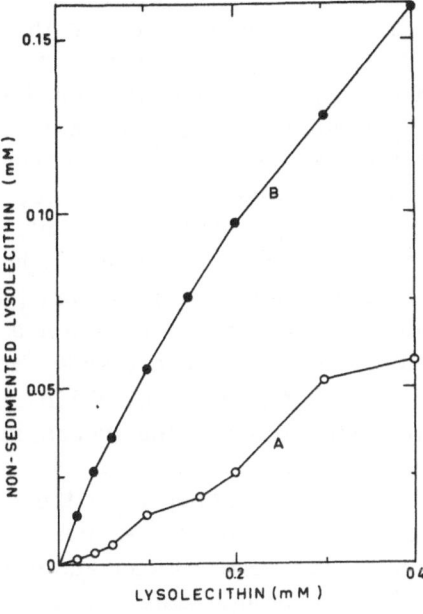

Fig. 9

Adsorption of lysolecithin onto rat brain microsomes in the absence and presence of albumin.

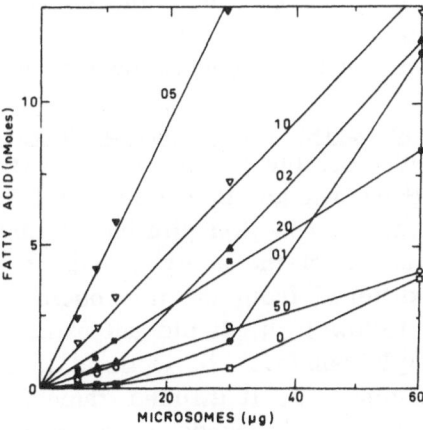

Fig. 10

V/E curves of the microsomal lysolecithinase at several albumin lysolecithin ratios.

bition becomes more pronounced above the inversion point, when there are probably monomers as well as micelles in the medium. Albumin, by binding the substrate (see Fig. 9), removes the inhibitory lyso-lecithin from the enzymatic particle and thereby increases the reaction rates. In the presence of microsomes and albumin, the substrate will be present in four phases: Monomers (whose concentration will be constant as long as there are micelles), micelles, albumin-bound lyso-lecithin and microsome-bound lysolecithin. Mainly the free monomers are available for interaction with the enzyme. When albumin concen-trations are increased, more substrate gets bound to this protein, thereby causing micelles to break up to maintain a constant level of monomers. A more detailed analysis, not shown in the Figures, showed that at suboptimal albumin to lysolecithin ratios, the V/S curves were still of type III, although the inversion points were moved to higher substrate concentrations. At the optimal ratio, where probably all micelles have disappeared from the medium, the curve was of type I, (i.e., hyperbolic). At ratios above the optimum, albumin inhibited the reaction. The excess albumin most likely reduced the concentration of the monomers available to the enzyme and thereby lowered the reaction rates.

Stimulation of the reaction rates by protein other than albumin, is shown in Fig. 12. Increasing quantities of heat-denatured micro-somes were added to reaction mixtures of lysolecithin and native microsomes. The denatured microsomes, because of their consider-able adsorptive capacity, competed with the enzymatic protein for the non-specific bound substrate and, similarly to albumin, relieved the inhibition of the enzyme by the adsorbed substrate.

b. <u>Soluble amine acetyl-CoA acetyl transferase.</u> This enzyme, which is localized in the soluble portion of the extract of H. ciferri could be purified by Sephadex gel filtration and DEAE-cellulose chro-matography. It catalyzed a reaction similar to that of the microsomal enzyme, i.e., the transfer of the acetyl group of acetyl CoA to primary amines. It however differed from the microsomal enzyme in its sub-strate specificity, as follows: a. It did not utilize sphingosine bases as substrates for acetyl transfer. b. Optimal transfer rates were obtained with dodecylamine. c. It utilized glucosamine, arylamines and catecholamines ; these compounds were not acted upon by the microsomal preparation.

Furthermore, Fig. 13 shows that this enzyme is of type III with amines of 12-16 carbon atoms, which form micelles in the experimental

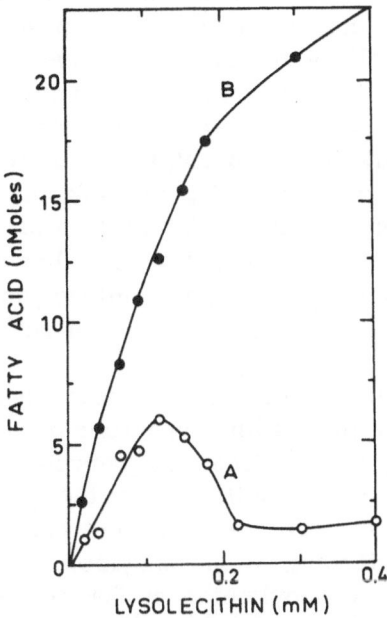

Fig. 11

V/S curves of the microsomal lysolecithinase in the absence and presence of albumin.

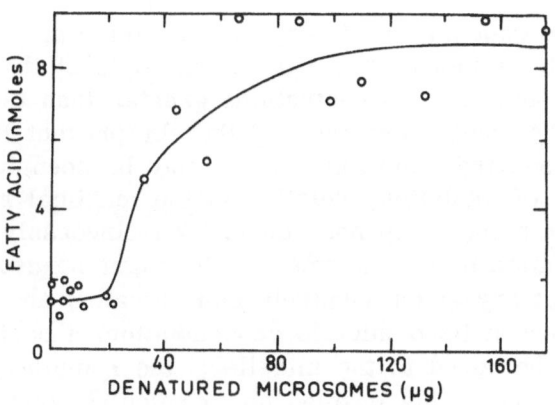

Fig. 12

Effect of heat-denatured microsomes on the rates catalyzed by the microsomal lysolecithinase.

concentration range. It is of interest and in accord with the theoretical consideration that those amines which did not have a monomer-micelle transition (C_6-C_{10} as well as the aryl- and catecholamines) yielded hyperbolic (i.e., type I) V/S curves. The inversion points obtained using the dodecyl, tetradecyl and hexadecylamines were in good agreement with the critical micellar concentrations of these compounds. According to the definition of type III, this enzyme utilized monomers, but not micelles. The mechanism of interaction of this soluble enzyme with its substrate thus contrasts sharply with that of the microsomal acetyltransferase, which using the same amines yielded sigmoidal curves of type IV, (i.e., utilizing micelles and not monomers).

There were several interesting differences between the soluble acetyltransferase and the preceeding type III-enzyme, the microsomal lysolecithinase, as follows: a. The V/E curves were straight. b. The inversion points were unaffected by the quantity of enzymatic proteins suggesting that the substrate was not removed from the medium by non-specific binding to the enzyme. Fig. 14 shows three V/S curves obtained with dodecylamine at 1.8 (o — o), 5.4 (● — ●) and 10.8 (□ — □) μg of the enzyme; all three had identical inversion points. c. Albumin increased the reaction rates, using the long-chain amines (while having no similar effect with the water-soluble amines), but did not eliminate the inversion points. This is exemplified by the experiment shown in Fig. 15, where V/S curves of tetradecylamine are presented at several ratios of albumin to amine (the numbers on the curve represent the respective molar ratios).

The above data may be interpreted as follows. Being of type III, the enzyme utilizes monomers, but not micelles of the amines. Once micelles form (at amine concentrations greater than the CMC) they combine with the soluble enzyme and thereby prevent its catalytic activity of the substrate monomers. It may be seen from Fig. 14 that the degree of inhibition, relative to the maximal rates attained at the inversion points, depended on and was inversely proportional to the concentration of the enzyme. This might be explained by assuming that at any given substrate concentration above the CMC (which determines a fixed micelle concentration) a certain fixed quantity of enzyme will be bound to the micelles; the remaining enzyme is free for catalytic action. This enabled us to calculate the quantity bound to the micelles by using the following two equations: At an enzyme concentration E_1 the rate will be $V_1 = k_3$ ($E_{1\ total} - E_{bound}$); at E_2, the corresponding rate will be $V_2 = k_3$ ($E_{2\ total} - E_{bound}$). Since V_1, V_2,

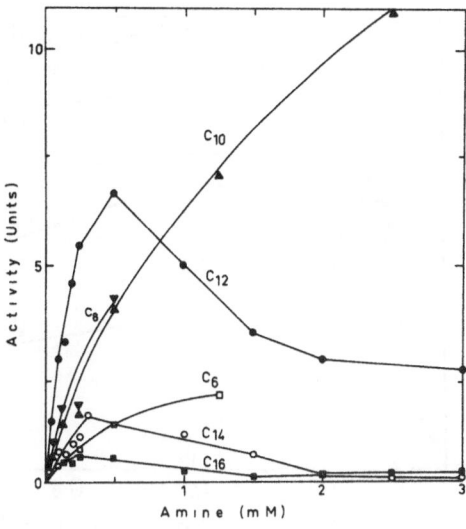

Fig. 13

V/S curves of the soluble acetyltransferase with amines of 6-16 carbon atoms.

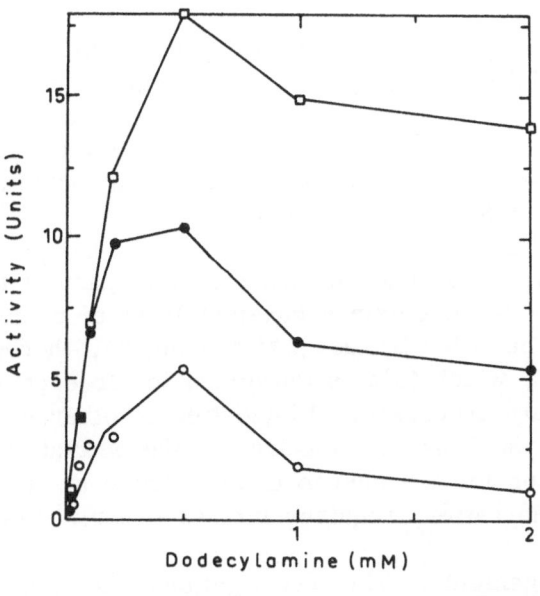

Fig. 14

V/S curves of the soluble acetyltransferase at three enzyme concentrations.

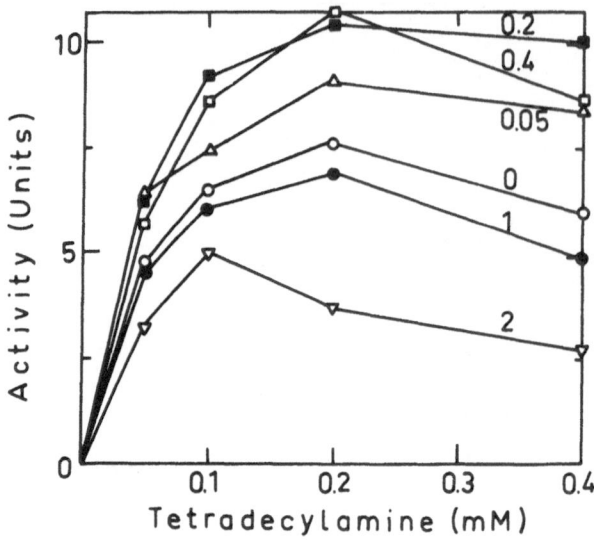

Fig. 15

V/S curves of the soluble acetyltransferase at several albumin to tetradecylamine ratios.

$E_{1\ total}$ and $E_{2\ total}$ are experimental values, E_{bound} could be calculated. Using the data of Fig. 14, the calculated average value was 1.4 µg of enzymatic protein bound to the micelles at 2 mM dodecylamine. The above assumptions stipulate that beyond the "inversion point", the rates should be proportional not to the total enzyme concentration, but to $E_{free} = E_{total} - E_{bound}$.

When albumin is added to the medium, part of the amine binds to this protein. To maintain a constant level of monomers in the solution, some micelles break up to monomers, thereby releasing "bound enzyme", which is thus converted to "free enzyme" and the reaction rates are increased. Elucidation of other effects of albumin on this system, such as the reasons for the activation below the inversion point or for the shapes of the curves at or above an optimal albumin to amine ratios, requires further experimentation.

Acknowledgements. The investigations discussed in this presentation were supported in part by a U.S. Public Health Service Grant (NS-02967). The technical assistance of Miss I. Edelman and Mrs. A. Geresh in parts of these investigations is acknowledged.

SUMMARY

The various interactions of enzymes with lipid substrates which belong to the "soluble amphipats" (1), were classified into four types, as follows.

Type I, consists of those cases in which a monomer-micelle transition is absent in the experimental conditions.

Type II, consists of those cases in which the enzyme utilizes monomers of the substrate but probably not .micelles.

Type III, consists of those cases in which the enzyme utilizes monomers of the substrate and micelles inhibit the reaction.

Type IV, consists of those cases in which the enzyme utilizes micelles of the substrate but probably not monomers.

The interactions of types II, III and IV were exemplified by experiments done in our laboratory on four enzymes: a. Soluble lysolecithinase (type II); b. microsomal lysolecithinase (type III); c. soluble amine acetyl CoA acetyltransferase (type III) and d. microsomal base acetyl CoA acetyltransferase (type IV). Each enzyme was analyzed for the following four parameters: 1. Dependence of reaction rates on enzyme concnetration (V/E curves). 2. Dependence of reaction rates on substrate concentration (V/S curves). 3. Dependence of the V/S curves on enzyme concentration. 4. Effect of albumin on the V/E and V/S curves. The conclusions drawn from these experiments were related to the theoretical aspects of the enzyme-substrate interactions, pertaining to each of the above types.

REFERENCES

1. D. Chapman, Introduction to Lipids, McGraw Hill, 1969.
2. N. Robinson and L. Saunders, J. Pharm. Pharmacol., 11 (1959) 115T.
3. S. Gatt, in Lipids, Methods in Enzymology, vol. XIV, J.M. Lowenstein, ed., Academic Press, 1969, p. 134.
4. Z. Leibovitz and S. Gatt, Biochim. Biophys. Acta, 164 (1968) 439.
5. Z. Leibovitz-Ben Gershon, I. Borkovski-Kubiler and S. Gatt, submitted for publication.

6. Y. Barenholz, I. Edelman and S. Gatt, Israel J. Chem.,
        (1971) in press.
7. Y. Barenholz, I. Edelman and S. Gatt, submitted for publication.
8. Y. Barenholz and S. Gatt, Biochem. Biophys. Res. Comm.,
        35 (1969) 676.
9. Y. Barenholz and S. Gatt, Israel J. Chem., 8 (1970) 149p.
10. Y. Barenholz and S. Gatt, submitted for publication.
11. F. H. Stodola, L. J. Wickerham, C. R. Scholfield and H. J. Dutton,
        Arch. Biochem. Biophys. 98 (1962) 176.
12. Y. Barenholz, I. Edelman and S. Gatt, Biochim. Biophys. Acta,
        in press.

PROBLEMS IN PRENATAL DIAGNOSIS USING SPHINGOLIPID HYDROLASE ASSAYS

J. Alexander Lowden and Marie-Anne LaRamee

Research Institute, The Hospital for Sick Children,

Toronto, Ontario, Canada

When Dr. Volk asked for my title last spring I thought that a rather mundane study of changes in sphingolipid hydrolase activity during growth and development would demonstrate some points about sphingolipid turnover. We wanted to know why certain organs store particular sphingolipids although they apparently have adequate levels of enzyme activity. During the interim several unrelated bits of information have stimulated a change in this plan. I am becoming concerned about our rapid advance into the service approach to prenatal diagnosis using assays of enzyme activity in amniotic fluid as well as in cultured amniocytes. It is certainly true that the feasibility of monitoring pregnancies in high-risk families is the most hopeful and important development in the history of sphingolipid biology. I want to discuss, today, some of the dangers inherent in our as yet early knowledge. I am worried that we may think we know more than we really do and in our ignorance we may make wrong decisions which can feasibly destroy the credibility of the entire programme. I shall talk today only about sphingomyelinase, β-galactosidase and hexosaminidase but the problems mentioned probably apply equally to many other hydrolases.

SPHINGOMYELINASE

The Niemann-Pick diseases were classified ten years ago by Crocker (1) on phenotypic grounds into 4 relatively distinct types (Table I). Subsequently Brady et al (2) and Schneider and Kennedy (3) showed that in Types A and B, there was an absolute defect in sphingomyelinase activity. In Type C disease (3, 4) however, enzyme activity is normal and Spence (5) has recently found that in Type D, the Nova Scotian variety, the enzyme activity is

257

greater than normal.

TABLE I

CLASSIFICATION OF NIEMANN-PICK DISEASES

Type		Life Span	Sphingomyelinase Activity
A	classical infantile usually Jewish visceral and neurological	0- 2 years	absent (2, 3)
B	non-neurological visceral and pulmonary	?	absent (2, 3)
C	juvenile visceral and neurological	3- 5 years	normal - low normal (3, 4)
D	Nova Scotia neurological and visceral	15-20 years	elevated (5)

Using presently available methods it should be possible, in families in which there is an index case, to make a prenatal diagnosis of Type A or B disease. Schneider et al (6) have recently examined a 19 week foetus from a mother who had previously had a child that died with classical Type A disease. Sphingomyelinase activity was negligible in acetone powders of cultured amniocytes obtained at 13 weeks gestation although glucocerebrosidase activity in the same cells was normal. The foetus had increased levels of sphingomyelin in liver, minimal enzyme activity in liver and brain and evidence of lipid storage by both light and electronmicroscopy. Thus at 19 weeks of gestation the foetus had advanced Niemann-Pick disease. The authors, quite properly, note that postnatal attempts at treating the disease are meaningless. Treatment must be prevention and presently prevention requires an index case. Type A and B Niemann-Pick heterozygotes can be detected by assaying sphingomyelinase activity in leucocytes and the enzyme is also present in serum. Furthermore, most cases of classical Type A disease are in Jewish infants (7) that is within a defined population group. Thus like Tay-Sachs disease, Type A Niemann-Pick disease fits all criteria for a mass carrier screening programme and theoretically the disease is preventable without waiting for an index case.

Two problems trouble me. In Toronto, in the past 7 years with a Jewish population of over 100,000 I have seen only one case of Type A disease — and that in a French-Canadian Catholic infant. The disease is rare and carrier screening therefore is of

questionable economic reality. Secondly, at present, it is not
possible to distinguish Type A and Type B heterozygotes nor
probably is it possible to subclassify affected foetuses except on
the basis of previously affected children. Both will have absent
sphingomyelinase activity, but the prognosis for children with Type
B disease however is quite different. In the Toronto area there
are two Type B patients, one was originally presented as case 18
by Crocker and Farber (8). She is now 25 years old. She has
recently graduated from teachers college. She has had a splenectomy, has a large liver and pulmonary involvement, and although
she is well below the third percentile for height and weight, she
has been a remarkably active girl and can now make a valid contribution to society. Schneider and Kennedy (3) found almost no
sphingomyelinase activity in her spleen. The second child is now
six years old. She is only at the third percentile for height and
has pronounced hepatosplenomegaly. Pulmonary infiltration is
sufficient to cause some distress with prolonged exertion but she
also is surprisingly active. Her I.Q. is 126. Assays of sphingomyelinase in her leucocytes revealed a complete absence of activity.
Both her parents and her sibling are presumed heterozygotes (Table
II). While these patients undoubtedly have a disease which will
shorten their life it does not compare with the problems of the
Type A child and the validity of arguments in favour of abortion
of foetuses with Type B disease must be questioned. The older of
these girls comes from a Jewish family — like most cases of Type
A disease. I believe therefore that, until we can distinguish
biochemical genotypes, mass carrier screening for sphingomyelinase-
deficient heterozygotes amongst Ashkenazi Jews should not be done.

TABLE II

SPHINGOMYELINASE ACTIVITY IN LEUCOCYTES IN
TYPE B NIEMANN-PICK DISEASE

	Sphingomyelinase activity $\mu\mu$moles/mg prot./hr.
Patient	0.00
Mother	5.7
Father	14.4
Brother	14.2
Normal Controls mean $\pm$ S.D. (16)	38.3 $\pm$ 19.3

β-GALACTOSIDASE

Defects in β-galactosidase activity have been described in two phenotypically different disorders (9). Type 1 G_{M1} gangliosidosis occurs in young infants, is characterized by visceral, skeletal and dermal changes as well as by profound psychomotor deterioration and leads to death in early infancy (10). Type 2 disease occurs later in childhood and has a more protracted course. The affected children often survive till 7-10 years of age. They have no visceromegaly and no skeletal abnormalities (11).

O'Brien (12) described two distinct enzyme-active bands visualized on starch gel electrophoresis and claimed that in Type 1 disease both were absent while in Type 2 disease only the faster-migrating band was lost. Recently Pinsky and Powell (13) noted that fibroblasts grown in culture from these two types of gangliosidoses do retain β-galactosidase activity. The Type 1 tissue has an enzyme which is heat stable and has a pH optimum at 3.75 while the Type 2 cells retain an enzyme that is unstable when heated at 42° and has a pH optimum of 4.25. In testing amniocytes for β-galactosidase activity in high risk pregnancies for G_{M1} gangliosidosis the findings described by Pinsky and Powell should be borne in mind. The enzyme activity of cultured fibroblasts can alter during sub cultures. We do not know much about the β-galactosidases of the two different types of cells in amniotic fluid and because amniocytes are more difficult to grow it is possible that a four-week culture may have low levels of enzyme. How can we be sure that this enzyme activity indicates a heterozygote foetus? It may be residual activity of only one of the enzymes as described by Pinsky and Powell (13). The other enzyme may be absent.

HEXOSAMINIDASE

Perhaps the most exciting developments in this field have been made in the enzymology of the G_{M2} gangliosides — particularly Tay-Sachs disease. In 1969 O'Brien and Okada (14) clearly demonstrated that patients with Tay-Sachs disease have little or no hexosaminidase A activity and that carriers have a decreased activity. Our results (Table III) are in agreement with their findings. They also mentioned (15) that pregnancy affected hexosaminidase activity. Because mass carrier screening programmes are certain to be plagued with pregnant women who want to know if they will have a child with Tay-Sachs disease we decided to examine this point. We used the heat denaturation enzyme assay system (14) to study hexosaminidases in the serum of 82 pregnant women (Fig. 1). We found that total activity rose to 10 times non-pregnant levels during gestation and that most of this increase was due to a rise in the heat stable or B enzyme. Hexosaminidase A also rose but at a slower rate. Thus by 3 months gestation all pregnant women

TABLE III

HEXOSAMINIDASE ACTIVITY IN SERUM

	Total mμ moles/ml	%A	Number of Sera assayed
Normal	531 ± 119	70.6 ± 11.9	70
Obligate heterozygote	495 ± 95	40.5 ± 6.8	20
Homozygote	445 ± 70	<1%	6

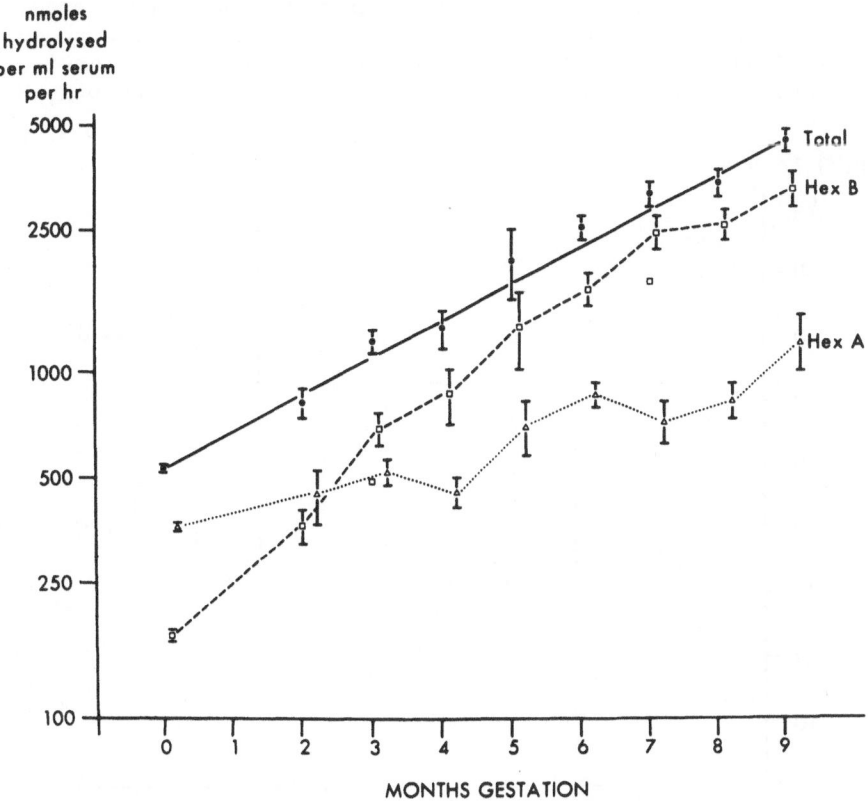

Fig. 1. Change in serum hexosaminidase activity during pregnancy.
Points shown are means ± S.E. The calculated regression line is
plotted only for the total activity figures ($\log_e$ of regression
coef. = 0.94). The crossover point when B becomes greater than
A is at 2 months gestation.

tested as heterozygotes. When we examined leucocyte activity
(Fig. 2) however we found that although the total activity rose
the percentage in the B fraction was unchanged and carriers could
be clearly distinguished from non-carriers. In the post partum
period hexosaminidases fell rapidly in serum and the usual A > B
distribution was seen by 48 hours after delivery (Fig. 3). We
hypothesized that the increased B enzyme came from placenta and
supported this claim with preliminary data from Walker et al (16).
The carrier state can be detected in women during pregnancy but it
is essential in screening programmes to know which women are
pregnant.

     Subsequently we have examined these enzymes on cellulose
acetate electrophoresis. Electrophoresis was performed in a
Gelman Sepratek apparatus in phosphate-citrate buffer (0.2M,pH 7.0)
at 6 mA for 20 minutes. The enzymes migrated towards the anode.
After migration was complete the strip was closely applied to a
second strip soaked with a 1 mM solution of methylumbelliferyl-
β-D-N-acetylglucosaminide in phosphate-citrate buffer, (0.04M,pH 4.1).

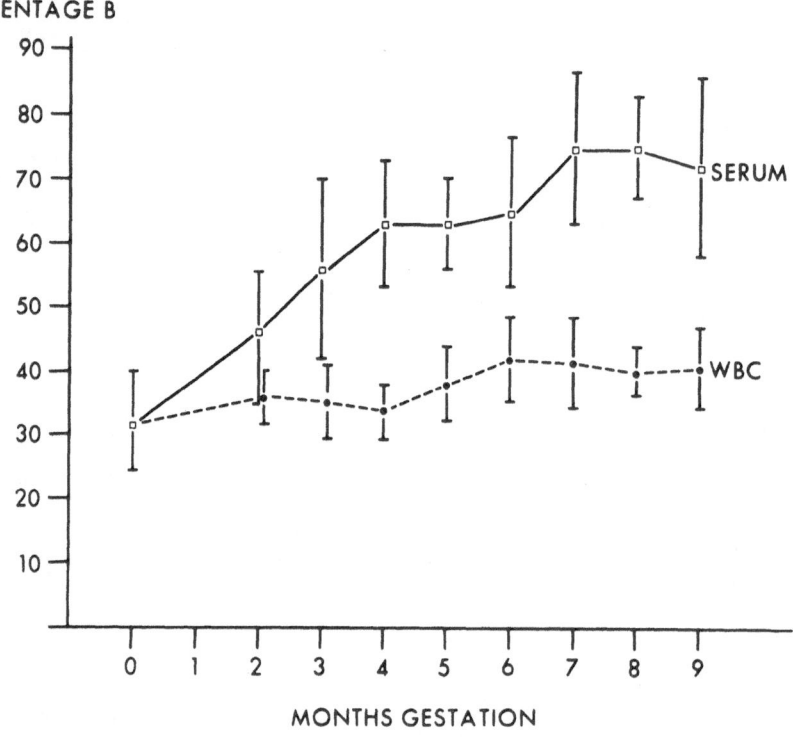

Fig. 2. Percentage of total hexosaminidase in the heat-stable
("B") fraction in serum and leucocytes during pregnancy.

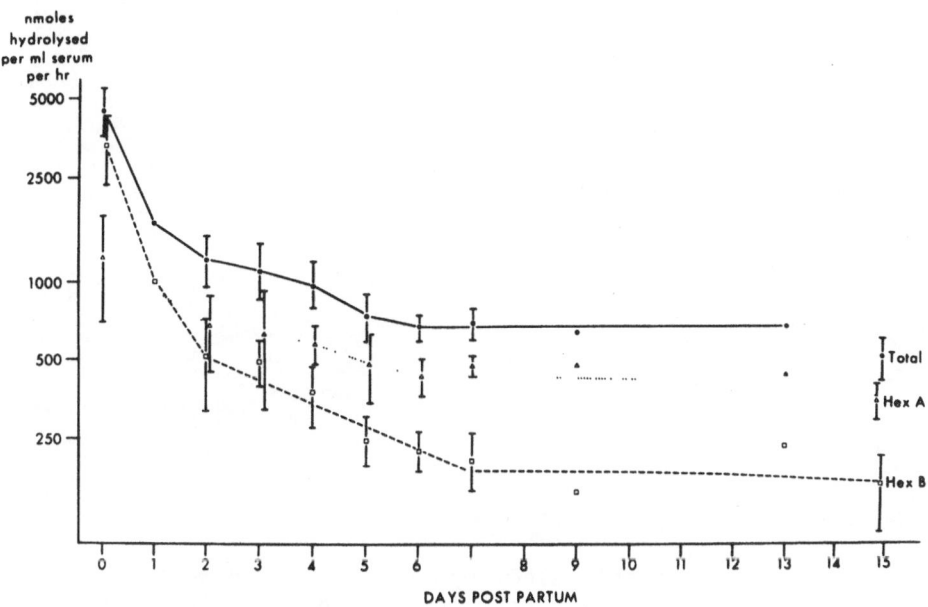

Fig. 3. Change in serum hexosaminidase activity in post-partum women. Points shown are means ± S.D. Note the normal A > B distribution of activities has returned in all patients studied by 3 days.

The two strips were placed in a closed container in a 37° incubator for 30 minutes. The strip was then exposed to ammonia vapours and the fluorescent spots visualized under ultraviolet light. The following slides are indeed not good and can only attempt to convey my points. Anyone who has tried to photograph fluorescing methylumbelliferone on acetate strips will appreciate the technical problems. In the first slide (Fig. 4) we see a standard separation of sera from a normal person, a heterozygote, a child with Tay-Sachs disease and a pregnant woman. All display three bands. The slowest band I have called C. It is faint in all sera, but prominent in serum from a patient with Tay-Sachs disease. Heating at 50° for four hours at pH 4.0 destroys all the activity in the fast or A band but does not affect the B band.

    When we examined placenta, amniotic fluid and foetal liver we found little enzyme that corresponds to the heat-stable or so-called B band in serum. Instead (Fig. 5) we found a large C band with an obvious A band. In liver from older children the B band gradually

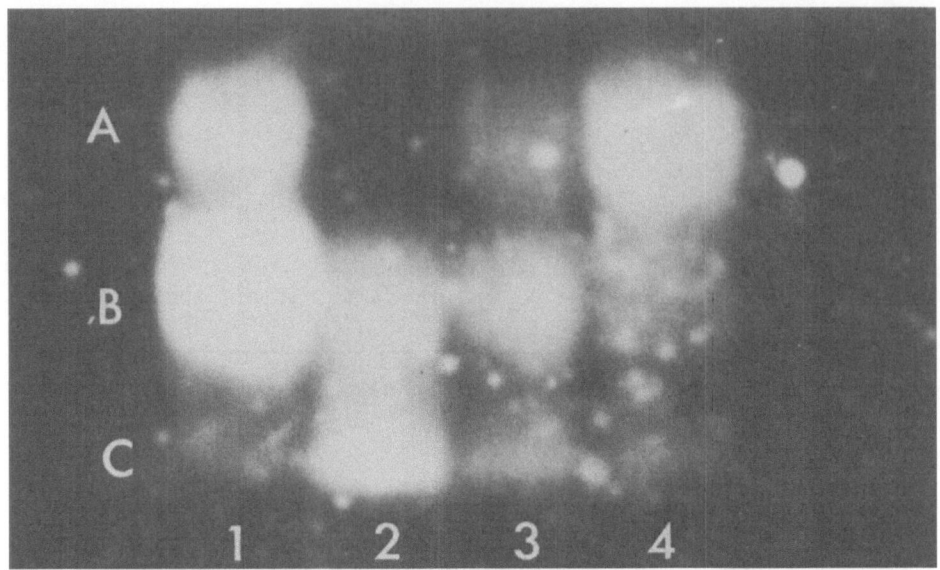

Fig. 4. Cellulose acetate electrophoretogram of hexosaminidases from sera, 1. pregnant women near term, 2. child with Tay-Sachs disease, 3. heterozygote and 4. normal. Conditions of electrophoresis and enzyme location described in text.

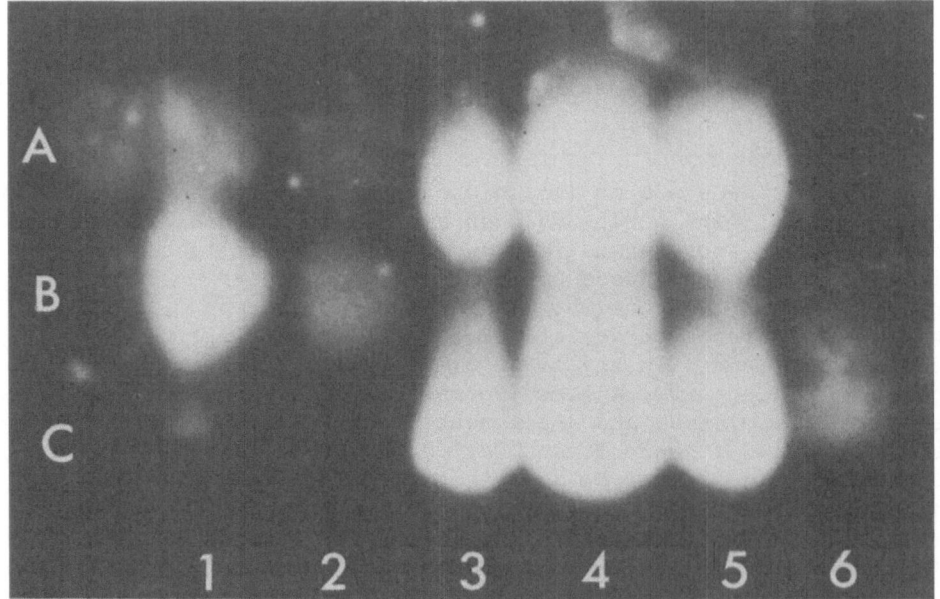

Fig. 5. Cellulose acetate electrophoretogram of hexosaminidases. 1, pregnant serum, 2. carrier serum, 3. foetal liver, 4. adult liver, 5, placenta, 6. amniotic fluid. Conditions of electrophoresis and enzyme location described in text.

becomes obvious. Assays of heat stable enzymes in amniotic fluid
or amniocytes are thus not really comparable with serum assays.
The residual enzyme is quite different in each case.

To emphasize this point we assayed hexosaminidases in serum
and leucocytes from a child with Tay-Sachs disease (Table IV).
Although we found no heat-labile serum enzyme, the leucocyte
activity fell 12.5% on heating for four hours. Examination of the
leucocytes from this patient shows a large C and a smaller B, but
no A band. If the B band enzyme is heat-stable, then the heat-
labile enzyme must be in the C band.

Although Schneck et al (17) and O'Brien et al (18) have
reported the successful prenatal diagnosis of high-risk pregnancies
for Tay-Sachs disease I believe the problem is not a simple one.

Our findings indicated not two but three distinct hexosaminidase bands. One is the heat-labile A band, one is the heat-stable
B enzyme of serum and the third is a tissue enzyme, C, which is
partly heat-denaturable. With low hexosaminidase A activity,
simple heat denaturation may not be adequate to differentiate
between an affected foetus and some carrier foetuses with low
hexosaminidase A activity.

The solution to these problems is not far away. Methods are
available for the separation and purification of the individual
enzyme species (19, 20). If antibodies can be prepared for each
type of enzyme, and if they do not cross-react, it will be
possible to assay the enzyme both immunochemically and by the
chemical substrates. This double testing for amniotic cells

TABLE IV

HEXOSAMINIDASES IN TAY-SACHS DISEASE

	Total acitivity	Heat-stable activity
	n moles/hr.	
Serum*	460	460
Leucocytes[o]	1600	1400

*calculated per ml serum

[o]calculated per mg leucocyte protein

and fluid would provide a safer set of criteria on which to make a
prenatal diagnosis of Tay-Sachs disease. Perhaps immunochemical
methods can be applied to other sphingolipid hydrolases and can be
used to solve some of the problems of prenatal diagnosis of the
G_{M1} gangliosidoses or the Niemann-Pick diseases.

REFERENCES

1. Crocker, A.C. The cerebral defect in Tay-Sachs disease and
    Niemann-Pick disease. J. Neurochem. 7: 69, (1961).

2. Brady, R.O., Kanfer, J.N., Mock, M.B. and Fredrickson, D.S.
    The metabolism of sphingomyelin, II. Evidence of an
    enzymatic deficiency in Niemann-Pick disease. Proc. Nat.
    Acad. Sci. U.S.A. 55: 366, (1966).

3. Schneider, R.B. and Kennedy, E.P. Sphingomyelinase in normal
    human spleens from subjects with Niemann-Pick disease.
    J. Lip. Res. 8: 202, (1967).

4. Lowden, J.A. and LaRamee, M.A. Sphingomyelinase in Type C
    Niemann-Pick disease. Arch. Neurol. Submitted, October 1971.

5. Spence, M.W. personal communication.

6. Schneider, E.L., Ellis, W.G., Brady, R.O., McCulloch, J.R. and
    Epstein, C.J. Prenatal Niemann-Pick disease: Biochemical and
    histological examination of a 19 gestational week fetus.
    Submitted for publication, September 1971.

7. Fredrickson, D.S. in The Metabolic Basis of Inherited Disease.
    Stanbury, J.B., Wyngaarden, J.B. and Fredrickson, D.S. eds.
    New York, McGraw-Hill, 1966, p. 586.

8. Crocker, A.C. and Farber, S. Niemann-Pick Disease: A review
    of eighteen patients. Medicine 37: 1, (1958).

9. Derry, D.M., Fawcett, J.S., Andermann, F. and Wolfe, L.S.
    Late infantile systemic lipidosis. Major monosialoganglio-
    sidosis, delineation of two types. Neurology 18: 340, (1968).

10. Lowden, J.A., Olivares, R., and Reilly, B.J. Infantile G_{M1}
    gangliosidosis. Arch. Neurol. Submitted, October 1971.

11. Wolfe, L.S., Callahan, J., Fawcett, J.S., Andermann, F. and
    Scriver, C.R. G_{M1}-gangliosidosis without chondrodystrophy
    or visceromegaly: Beta-galactosidase deficiency with
    gangliosidosis and the excessive excretion of a keratan
    sulfate. Neurology 20: 23, (1970).

12. O'Brien, J.S., Okada, S., Ho, M.W., Fillerup, D.L., Veath, M.L. and Adams, K. in Lipid Storage Diseases. Enzymatic and clinical implications. Bernsohn, J. and Grossman, H.J. eds. New York, Acad. Press, 1971, p. 225.

13. Pinsky, L. and Powell, E. G_{M1}-gangliosidosis Types 1 and 2: Enzymatic differences in cultured fibroblasts. Nature 228: 1093, (1970).

14. Okada, S. and O'Brien, J.S. Tay-Sachs Disease: Generalized absence of a Beta-D-N-Acetylhexosaminidase component. Science 165: 698, (1969).

15. O'Brien, J.S., Okada, S., Chen, A. and Fillerup, D.L. Tay-Sachs disease. Detection by serum hexosaminidase assay. New Eng. J. Med. 283: 15, (1970).

16. Walker, P.G., Woollen, M.E. and Pugh, D. N-acetyl-β-glucosaminidase activity in serum during pregnancy. J. Clin. Path. 13: 353, (1960).

17. Schneck, L., Valenti, C., Amsterdam, D., Freidland, J., Adachi, M., and Volk, B.W. Prenatal diagnosis of Tay-Sachs disease. Lancet I: 582, (1970).

18. O'Brien, J.S., Okada, S., Fillerup, D.L., Veath, M.L. Adornato, B., Brenner, P.H. and Leroy, J.G. Tay-Sachs disease: Prenatal diagnosis. Science 172: 61, (1971).

19. Frohwein, Y.Z. and Gatt, S. Isolation of β-N-Acetyl-hexosaminidase, β-N-Acetylglucosaminidase, and β-N-Acetyl-galactosaminidase from calf brain. Biochem. 6: 2775, (1967).

20. Robinson, D. and Stirling, J.L. N-Acetyl-β-glucosaminidases in human spleen. Biochem. J. 107: 321, (1968).

RADIOACTIVE PRECURSOR INCORPORATION INTO LIPIDS OF HUMANS WITH CEREBRAL LIPIDOSES:1-^{14}C-GLUCOSAMINE, U^{3}H-SERINE, AND ^{3}H-ACETATE*

Robert M. Burton, S. Handa**, R. E. Howard*** and T. Vietti

Departments of Pharmacology, Pediatrics, and Pathology and The Beaumont-May Institute of Neurology, Washington University Medical School, St. Louis, Missouri 63110

Our laboratory as part of the Beaumont-May Institute of Neurology has long been interested in hereditary neurological diseases in humans and in the study of the normal development of the nervous system. These latter studies have been employing small animals primarily the rat and, in a few instances, the rhesus monkey and minipig. Recently, some of our results on the metabolism of glycolipids have been summarized in a review entitled "Factors affecting Incorporation of Precursors into body constituents - A review of common sense considerations with glycolipids or examples" (2). In an effort to translate the information gained from laboratory animal experiments to the human and to gain further insight into human cerebral lipidosis, we have entered a long term collaborative study with a number of departments at Washington University Medical School and St. Louis Children's Hospital. Our objectives are to make and correlate studies of the clinical, pathological, electron microscopic and biochemical aspects of hereditary neurological diseases.

The following report contains some of our results from administering D-(1-^{14}C)-glucosamine to a patient with gangliosidoses and two patients with suspected Niemann-Pick's disease. One of the latter patients also received ^{3}H-acetate and the other DL-(^{3}H)-serine.

Lipidoses study protocol: Patients were selected following clinical diagnoses and judged to be in the terminal phase of the disease. Written permission of the parents and autopsy permit

*Supported by USPHS grants N501575-14 and FR37
**Address: Biochemistry Dept., Tokyo University, Japan
***Address: Pathology Dept., Texas University, San Antonio, Texas

were obtained and the study cleared by the clinical research committee and the radiation hazard committee. The sterile solution
of the radioactive precursor was administered intraveneously.
Initial blood specimens were drawn in EDTA coated syringes at one
minute, 5, 30 and 60 minutes. Thereafter blood specimens (5 ml)
were collected daily. Urine was collected by an indwelling catheter and feces in plastic diapers. Mucous secretions were obtained by aspiration. At death, the autopsy was performed as quickly
as possible - generally within 4 hours. Tissue specimens were
processed immediately and the remaining tissue frozen for future
use.

    <u>Radioactive precursors:</u> D-(1-^{14}C)- glucosamine$_3$HC$_1$ (0.5mCi;
49 mg), DL-(^{3}H)-serine (3.0mCi;2.15 mg), and sodium ^{3}H-acetate
(3.0mCi;2.06 mg) were obtained from the New England Nuclear Corpor-
ation, Boston. The precursors were dissolved in 1.ml each of 70%
ethanol in sterile tubes and the solvent removed. They were then
dissolved in 3 ml sterile normal saline and sterilized by millipore filtration. The 3 ml were injected and the needle flushed
with 2 ml of sterile saline.

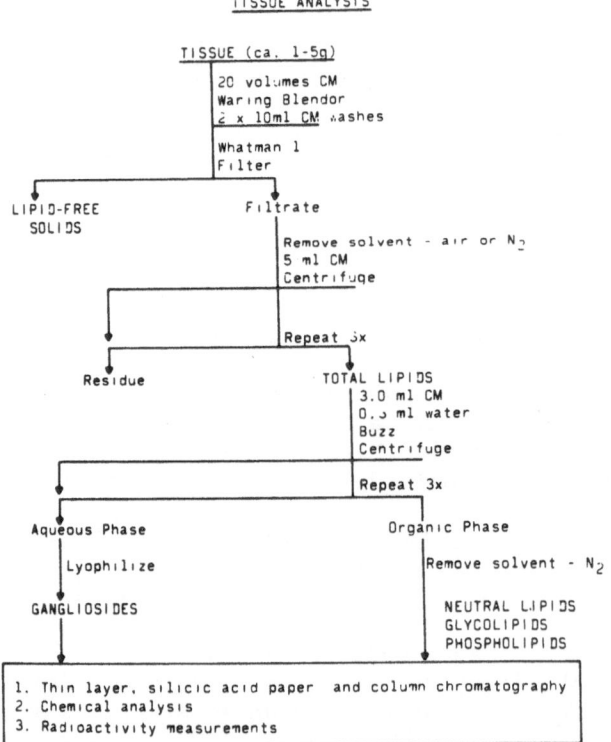

Fig. 1. Tissue analysis flow chart.

<u>Chemical procedures</u>: Immediately following autopsy, part of all organs removed were weighted, extracted by chloroform-methanol (2-1) and filtered through Whatman No. 1 paper and processed essentially by the Folch-Pi partition procedure (6,7) as illustrated in the flow chart (Fig. 1).

Gangliosides were separated into individual species by thin layer chromatography. Each plate contained three aliquots for quanitation and a reference aliquot and/or ganglioside mixture to locate the specific band for each species. (Fig. 2).

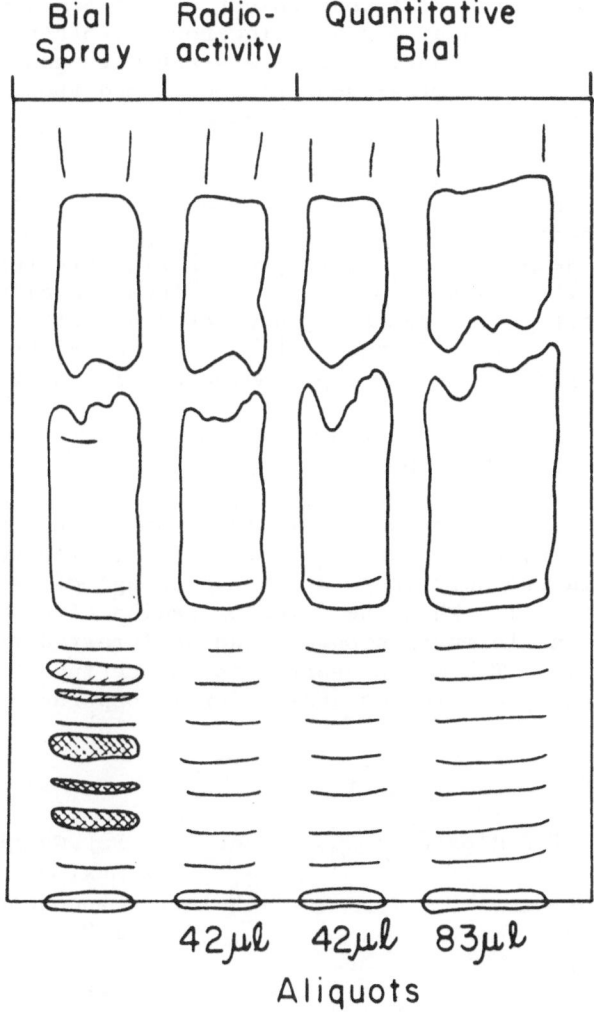

Fig. 2. Diagram of thin layer plate for determining the specific radioactivity of each ganglioside type.

Details of the chromatographic procedure and the identification of
each ganglioside are described by Handa and Burton (8). Other
lipids were separated on Whatman No. SG-81 employing several solvent systems. Radioactive measurements were made using the Packard Tri-Carb liquid scintillation spectrometer 3375. The silica
gel was removed from the TLC plates and counted directly in tolu-
ene-Omnifluor and aqueous solutions were measured in dioxane-
Omnifluor-naphthalene. Corrections for quenching was determined
by either external or internal standards technique.

Case history summaries: The patient with gangliosidoses was
a female Negro who apparently developed normally from birth for
about 2 years when her normal development ceased and she began to
regress. At age 4 brain biopsy and electron microscopy coupled
with a red spot in the macula were consistant with ganglioside
storage disease. The chemical analysis confirmed the ganglioside
storage and identified the glycolipid as Gm2 (5).

The two patients with apparent Niemann-Pick's disease were
siblings of Protestant German decent. The older, a male, died at
age 4 and the younger, a female, expired at age 5. Both followed
essentially the same clinical course, exhibiting progressive
jaundice from birth and slow physical and mental development followed by spasticity of extremities, decreased alertness, and coma
in the last year of life. A red spot in the macula, bone marrow
aspiration, and electron microscopy indicated Niemann-Picks disease.

RESULTS AND DISCUSSION

The general pattern of sphingolipid accumulation in brains of
several species, including man, is similar - only the temporal
factor is altered probably in relationship to age of maturity and/
or length of life (1). Thus the choice of radioactive precursors
for studying human lipidosis probably can be inferred from small
animal experiments. Table I presents data indicating that ^{14}C-
glucosamine is the precursor of choice for incorporation into
gangliosides.

TABLE I

Incorporation of Radioactive Substances into Rat Gangliosides

Precursor	% Maximum Relative Incorporation
1-^{14}C-Glucosamine	100
1-^{14}C-Galactose	58
1-^{14}C-Glucose	28
3-^{14}C Serine	9
4-^{14}C Aspartic Acid	1

It was found that $1-^{14}C$ glucosamine resulted in the gangliosides being labelled in the aminosugar moieties (2,3):

neuNAc	-	gal	-	galNAc	-	gal	-	glc	-	sph
36%		0%		28%		0%		0%		0%

	neuNAc		ste
	36%		0%

Glucose and galactose labelled all of the sugar and aminosugar moieties, while serine introduced the radioactive label primarily into sphingosine. ^{14}C from aspartic acid was randomly distributed perhaps showing a preference for the fatty acid. Other experiments have shown that ^3H-acetate results in labelling of the fatty acids and, with time, the hydrocarbon portion of the sphingosine.

The administration of $D-(1-^{14}C)$-glucosamine to the three patients resulted in initial high blood levels of soluble radioactivity in the blood plasma. After 60-90 minutes little soluble radioactivity could be detected, however, the blood glycoproteins were highly labelled with carbon-14 reaching a maximum at 6-12 hours. The radioactivity was present as N-acetyl glucosamine and N-acyl neuraminic acid. The half-time for loss of blood glycoprotein radioactivity is about four days (9). The rate of urinary excretion of radioactivity was initially high and decreased with time. After one month, about 50% of the administered radioactivity had been excreted in the urine. Mucous secretions accounted for approximately 4%. No detectable radioactivity was found in the feces. Respiratory loss as carbon dioxide was not measured.

Incorporation of $D-(1-^{14}C)$-glucosamine radioactivity into red blood cell lipids was observed (9). Radioactivity increased from initial low levels to a maximum at 13 to 15 days post-administration. Thereafter a slow decrease was observed. While part of the radioactivity appeared in cholesterol by non-specific labelling, i.e., metabolism of the ^{14}C-glucosamine to ^{14}C-acetate, the largest part of the radioactivity was found in the globoside, galNAc-gal-gal-glc-ceramide, and specifically in the N-acetyl galactosamine.

The radioactivity incorporated into various tissues of the gangliosidosis patient is presented in Table II and compared with that of the Niemann-Pick female. It is apparent that the radioactivity resides in the brain tissue for both patients; the gangliosidosis patient has more radioactivity than the NP.

TABLE II

Radioactivity Incorporated into Tissues

Tissue	D-(1-^{14}C)-Glucosamine		^{3}H-Serine	^{3}H-Acetate
	AFI*	NP**	NP**	NP***
	cpm/g.WW		cpm/g.WW	cpm/g.WW
Cerebellum	2080	456	3364	4675
Liver	28	53	1708	4975
Kidney	12	27	1212	3539
Spleen	10	5	450	7594
Lymph Nodes	27	23	1642	9467
Fat		15	583	

* Gangliosidoses
** Niemann-Picks - female sibling
***Niemann-Picks - male sibling

Table III presents the radioactivity for each ganglioside type expressed as cpm per gram of wet weight tissue. Most of the radioactivity in the gangiosidoses patient is present as the stored ganglioside Gm2 (4.8 umoles neuNAc/g.WW) and can be compared to the NP patient where the radioactivity is only 15 cpm/g.WW for Gm2 (0.065 umoles neuNAc/g.WW). The NP patient contained most of her radioactivity in ^{G}D16 (0.2 umoles neuNAc/g.WW). The amino sugar moieties of the gangliosides contained all of the radioactivity.

TABLE III

D-1-^{14}C)-Glucosamine Radioactivity Incorporated
into Cerebellum Gangliosides

Ganglioside		AFI*	NP**
		cpm/g.WW Tissue	
Gm2	gal NAc-gal-glc-Cer		
	NeuNAc	1670	15
Gml	gal-galNAc-gal-glc-Cer		
	NeuNAc	--	27
Gdla	gal-galNAc-gal-glc-Cer		
	NeuNAc NeuNAc	64	51
Gdlb	gal-galNAc-gal-glc-Cer		
	NeuNAc		
	NeuNAc	146	308
Gtl	gal-galNAc-gal-glc-Cer		
	NeuNAc NeuNAc		
	NeuNAc	64	12

* Gangliosidoses
** Niemann-Pick - female

The results from the administration of ^{3}H-serine and ^{3}H-acetate are less specific. The data shown in Table II indicates that lipids in all the tissues contained radioactivity. No definative pattern emerges for the tritium distribution as for the ^{14}C-glucosamine. It is suggestive that the brain tissue contained more serine tritium than other tissues. Brain does contain large amounts of sphingo lipids and serine labels the sphingosine moiety. On the other hand the acetate tritium is higher in spleen and lymph nodes. Acetate tritium labels fatty acids. However, the incorporation of serine and acetate is accompanied by considerable non-specific labelling.

It is difficult to draw conclusions from these studies except to note that the patterns of _in vivo_ incorporation of selected precursors appear to be consistant with the laboratory animal studies.. The appearance of most of the ^{14}C radioactivity in ganglioside Gm2 is expected since this is the stored ganglioside. It was observed earlier that ganglioside metabolism, hence more total radioactivity in Gm2, seems to occur more rapidly in cerebellum than in frontal cortex (5). With the advent of coupled gas liquid chromatography-mass spectrometry, it is now possible to carry out studies of this type with normal humans but avoiding the dangers of radiation damage since stable isotopes serve as the label (11).

REFERENCE

1. Burton, R. M. in "Lipids and Lipidoses" Schettler, G.(Editor) Berlin, Heidelberg, New York, Springer-Verlag (1967) p 122.

2. Burton, R. M. Lipids 5 475 (1970).

3. Burton, R. M., Garcia-Bunuel, L., Golden, M., and Balfour, Y. Biochem. 2 580 (1963).

4. Burton, R. M. and Gibbons, J. M., Biochim. Biophys. Acta 84 220 (1964)

5. Burton, R. M., Handa, S., Howard, R. E. and Vietti, T. Path. europ. 3 424 (1968)

6. Folch-Pi, J., Ascoli, I., Lees, M., Meath, J. A., and LeBaron, F. N., J. Biol. Chem. 191 833 (1951)

7. Folch-Pi, J., Lees, M. and Sloane-Stanley, G.H., J. Biol. Chem. 226 497 (1957)

8. Handa, S. and Burton, R.M., Lipids 4 205 (1969)

9. Handa, S., Burton, R. M., Howard, R. E. and Vietti, T., Lipids (submitted)

10. Luse, S. in "Inborn Disorders of Sphingolipid Metabolism",
     Aronson, S. M. and Volk, B. W. (Editors), Oxford, New York,
     Pergamon Press (1966) p93.

11. Rynhagen, R., W ikstron, S., and Woller, G. R., Anal. Chem.
     <u>37</u> 435 (1965).

AN INVESTIGATION OF THE METABOLISM OF TAY-SACHS GANGLIOSIDE

SPECIFICALLY LABELED IN CRITICAL PORTIONS OF THE MOLECULE

R. O. Brady, J. F. Tallman, W. G. Johnson and J. M. Quirk

Lab. of Neurochemistry, NINDS, NIH, Bethesda, Md. 20014

& Dept. of Biochem., Georgetown Univ., Washington, D. C.

Investigations which provided for a demonstration of an enzymatic deficiency in Tay-Sachs disease varied considerably in design from the basic pattern of experimentation which proved so useful for unravelling the metabolic abnormalities in related disorders of lipid metabolism. For example, in order to elucidate the etiology of Gaucher's disease, Niemann-Pick disease, and Fabry's disease, the principal sphingolipid which accumulates in the tissues of patients with these disorders was labeled with radiocarbon-^{14}C or radiohydrogen-^{3}H in a critical portion of the molecule. The metabolism of these labeled compounds was then examined in the following fashion. Enzymes which catalyzed the initial step in the catabolism of the accumulating substances were identified and partially purified from appropriate mammalian tissues. The conditions which influenced the activity of these enzymes were ascertained. The optimal pH for the reactions was determined, the Michaelis constant for each enzyme was defined, and the products of the reactions were identified. When these parameters were clearly established in control human tissue preparations, the activity of the enzyme suspected of being involved in the pathogenesis of the disease was determined in similar specimens obtained from patients with these disorders of lipid metabolism. This technique was used with success for identifying the deficiency of glucocerebrosidase in Gaucher's disease, sphingomyelinase in Niemann-Pick disease, and ceramidetrihexosidase in Fabry's disease[1].

Not so for Tay-Sachs disease. The discovery of the nature of the enzymopathy in this condition was hampered by two serious obstacles. The first was the extreme difficulty encountered in the preparation of labeled Tay-Sachs ganglioside (G_{M2}) for metabolic studies. The second was the false lead obtained through experiments with artificial chromogenic substrates. By analogy with the demonstrations of deficiencies of catabolic enzymes in the previously mentioned sphingolipidoses, it was assumed that a similar type of metabolic defect probably occurred in Tay-Sachs disease. The most likely site of such a lesion was a missing hexosaminidase[2]. However, in 1968, Sandhoff, Andreae, and Jatzkewitz reported that total hexosaminidase activity was usually higher than normal in brain tissue obtained from patients with the classic form of Tay-Sachs disease[3]. This observation was confirmed by Dr. Edwin H. Kolodny in this laboratory, and because of this finding, we undertook the preparation of G_{M2} specifically labeled in the N-acetyl-neuraminic acid portion of the molecule in order to investigate whether the catabolism of this ganglioside could be initiated by the hydrolytic cleavage of sialic acid from this molecule. The requisite sialic acid-labeled G_{M2} was prepared through a combination of biosynthetic and selective enzymatic degradative procedures[4]. When the metabolism of this labeled compound was investigated, a novel enzymatic reaction was discovered in a number of tissues in which N-acetylneuraminic acid was cleaved from G_{M2}. The other product of the reaction was shown to be asialo-G_{M2} in enzyme preparations obtained from rat small intestinal tissue[5]. Muscle tissue also contained a significant amount of G_{M2} sialidase activity, and therefore the functioning of this enzyme was investigated in muscle biopsy specimens from control human sources and in muscle tissue obtained from patients with Tay-Sachs disease. The activity of this sialidase was identical in the control and Tay-Sachs muscle tissue preparations.

TABLE I

G_{M2}SIALIDASE ACTIVITY IN HUMAN MUSCLE TISSUE PREPARATIONS

Source	Sialic acid cleaved
	pmoles/mg protein/hr
Controls (4)	389.
Tay-Sachs disease (4)	351.

These observations were reported in April 1969[6].

At this point it was apparent that a deficiency of G_{M2} sialidase was not responsible for the accumulation of ganglioside in the brains of patients with Tay-Sachs disease. We therefore sought to determine whether the metabolic lesion was a diminution of activity of a particular hexosaminidase isozyme which catalyzed the cleavage of N-acetylgalactosamine from G_{M2}. In order to carry out this investigation, we modified the procedure for preparing sialic acid-labeled G_{M2} and used N-acetylgalactosamine-$[^{14}C]$ as the precursor in vivo. With this radioactive aminosugar, both the N-acetylgalactosaminyl and N-acetylneuraminyl moieties of G_{M2} become labeled. The potential radioactive products of enzymatic hydrolysis of this labeled ganglioside are easily separable by ion exchange chromatography since the sialic acid is strongly charged and the hexosamine is neutral at alkaline pH. With this doubly labeled substrate, it was shown that the cleavage of N-acetylgalactosamine was catalyzed by an enzyme in normal human muscle tissue and that this enzyme was totally inactive in muscle tissue preparations obtained from patients with Tay-Sachs disease[7].

TABLE II

G_{M2} HEXOSAMINIDASE ACTIVITY IN HUMAN MUSCLE TISSUE

Source	Hexosamine cleaved pmoles/mg protein/hr
Controls (4)	304
Tay-Sachs disease (3)	0

While these experiments convincingly demonstrated an abnormality of ganglioside metabolism in tissue of patients with Tay-Sachs disease, they did not provide evidence whether the molecule of N-acetylgalactosamine was cleaved prior or subsequent to the hydrolysis of the molecule of N-acetylneuraminic acid. Furthermore, we were especially interested in investigating the metabolism of G_{M2} in brain tissue of patients with Tay-Sachs disease since significant quantities of G_{M2} accumulate only in this organ. We therefore undertook metabolic studies with labeled gangliosides in mammalian brain preparations. Lysosomes obtained from fresh rat and human brain tissue contain an enzyme which catalyzes the cleavage of N-acetylgalactosamine from G_{M2}. The other product of the reaction was shown to be hematoside (G_{M3}) [8]. In order to facilitate the investigation of the activity of this enzyme in human brain tissue preparations, we prepared G_{M2} specifically labeled in the N-acetylgalactosaminyl portion of the molecule. A solubilized enzyme preparation was obtained from young rat brain tissue which catalyzed the transfer of N-acetylgalactosamine from uridine diphosphate N-acetylgalactosamine to hematoside (Reaction 1) [9].

$$\text{NeuNAc-Gal-Glc-Cer} + \text{UDP-GalNAc}[^{14}C] \xrightarrow{\text{transferase}}$$

$$\text{GalNAc}[^{14}C]\text{-(NeuNAc)-Gal-Glc-Cer} + \text{UDP}$$

Using this hexosamine-labeled G_{M2}, we compared the activity of G_{M2} hexosaminidase in control fresh human brain lysosome preparations with that in biopsy specimens obtained from patients with Tay-Sachs disease. This hexosaminidase was virtually absent in the brain lysosome preparations obtained from patients with Tay-Sachs disease[8].

TABLE III

G_{M2} HEXOSAMINIDASE ACTIVITY IN HUMAN BRAIN LYSOSOMES

Source	Hexosamine cleaved pmoles/mg protein/hr
Controls (7)	154
Tay-Sachs disease (3)	2

G_{M2} sialidase was essentially the same in the lysosomes obtained from the controls and the patients with Tay-Sachs disease. These findings provide support for the concept that the hexosaminidase isozyme which has been shown with artificial substrates to be deficient in Tay-Sachs disease[10] does indeed play a role in the catabolism of G_{M2}.

These observations require that one inescapable fact be constantly born in mind; viz., G_{M2} accumulates in the nervous system of patients with Tay-Sachs disease in spite of the apparent functioning of G_{M2} sialidase. This reaction is clearly demonstrable in enzyme preparations of brain tissue from patients with the classic and variant forms of Tay-Sachs disease. Furthermore, hexosaminidase B may be increased many fold in the brains of patients with the classic form of Tay-Sachs disease. This enzyme can catalyze the hydrolysis of asialo-G_{M2} (at least in vitro) which is formed by the G_{M2} sialidase. The pathogenesis of Tay-Sachs disease may rest in part on a limitation of the availability of the sialidase route for G_{M2} catabolism. Our kinetic data seem to indicate that the sialidase pathway is slightly more active than the hexosaminidase in most tissues. In brain both pathways may be required to dispose of G_{M2} during the neonatal period of very rapid ganglioside turnover in this organ. The important observation was made in the course of these experiments that the activity of the sialidase does not increase in brain tissue of patients with Tay-Sachs disease. This situation is in direct contrast with the usual finding in lipid storage diseases in that there is generally a marked enhancement of the activity of sphingolipid hydrolases other than the one directly involved in the hereditary disease process[11] This lack of increased G_{M2} sialidase is also in sharp contrast with the augmentation of hexosaminidase B activity in brain tissue of patients with the classic form of Tay-Sachs disease. We are therefore tempted to conclude that the activity of the sialidase under consideration is not coordinated with requirements for G_{M2} catabolism. If the sialidase were inducible in brain in a manner which has been shown in peripheral tissues for other sphingolipid hydrolases[12], there might be a much lesser accumulation of ganglioside in the brains of patients with Tay-Sachs disease.

There are a number of other factors which also could contribute to the accumulation of G_{M2} in Tay-Sachs disease, and we shall mention only 4 at this time. 1. It is possible that there is an unfavorable spatial relationship regarding the accessibility of asialo-G_{M2} to hexosaminidase B. This argument seems partially refuted by the observation that the quantity of asialo-G_{M2} which accumulates in brain tissue of patients with total hexosaminidase deficiency is between 4 and 5 times greater than that in patients with the classic form of Tay-Sachs disease[13]. This finding suggests that some catabolism of asialo-G_{M2} does occur via hexosaminidase B in Tay-Sachs patients with a deficiency of hexosaminidase A only. 2. The accumulating G_{M2}, which is itself an inhibitor of hexosaminidase activity[14], could impede the catabolism of asialo-G_{M2} via hexosaminidase B. 3. There is a difference in the optimal pH for the sialidase and hexosaminidase enzymes in brain lysosomes. The optimum pH for hexosaminidase is 5.1, whereas for sialidase it is pH 4.4. It is not yet possible to determine the conditions of acidity which prevail naturally within the lysosomes. However, it is certainly possible that the hydrogen ion concentration in the microenvironment of these enzymes may play an important regulatory function and have a directing influence on the catabolism of G_{M2} via these alternative routes in brain. 4. A heretofore entirely unsuspected mechanism may contribute to the accumulation of G_{M2} in Tay-Sachs disease. It has been conceived by one of us (WGJ) that catalytically inactive hexosaminidase A (cross reacting material) may be synthesized and such a protein may even be present in augmented quantity in the brain of patients with Tay-Sachs disease. The question then arises whether this metabolically unreactive protein (or fragment thereof) would bind G_{M2} and impair its catabolism via the existing sialidase pathway. In this regard, the particularly significant observation has been made of a marked accumulation of G_{M2} in purified lysosomes obtained from brain tissue of a patient with Tay-Sachs disease in which the activity of lysosomal hexosaminidase B was increased 4-fold over that in control human lysosome preparations. Although the stoichiometry and mechanism of such a putative inhibitor are certainly not

established at this time, we feel the concept is of sufficient
potential significance that it should be offered as a speculation
at this time.

In a comprehensive examination of the pathogenesis Tay-Sachs
disease, one is required to attempt to provide an explanation for
the lack of accumulation of significant quantities of G_{M2} and
asialo-G_{M2} in peripheral organs of patients with the conventional
form of this disorder. One of the principal factors involved may
be the fact that the concentration of gangliosides in most visceral
organs is about 1 percent of that in brain. One wonders if the
presumed lesser quantity of G_{M2} turned over in these organs can be
catabolized via the sialidase and hexosaminidase B to a sufficient
extent to prevent extensive accumulation of G_{M2} in these tissues.
Furthermore, in some extra-neural tissues, the specific activity of
G_{M2} sialidase is considerably greater than that in brain. For
example, in heart muscle preparations, it is 6 times greater than
that in brain homogenates[5]. However, we need further investigation
of the rate and quantity of ganglioside turnover in extra-neural
tissues before attempting a critical assessment of this possibility.
Moreover, it probably will ultimately be necessary to isolate and
characterize the enzymes involved in G_{M2} catabolism to determine
if they are indeed similar in various organs and can therefore be
presumed to participate in ganglioside metabolism in an analogous
manner.

We have begun some experimentation in this direction. Hexosaminidase A has been purified to homogeneity from human urine
through a combination of ammonium sulfate precipitation, gel
filtration, and anion and cation exchange column chromatography[15].
The purified enzyme is 6000-fold enriched over the original specific
activity of hexosaminidase A in unfractionated urine. The pure
enzyme catalyzes the hydrolysis of 6 mmoles of N-acetylglucosamine
from 4-methylumbelliferyl-β-$\underline{D}$-N-acetylglucosaminide per mg of
protein per hour. However, the amount of N-acetylgalactosamine
cleaved from aminosugar-labeled G_{M2} was 6 orders of magnitude less
than that which occurred with the fluorogenic substrate. The
paucity of catalytic activity with the natural glycolipid may be
due to a deleterious alteration of the structure or configuration
of the excreted enzyme. Another aspect which had to be considered
was the possibility that this low activity was due to unphysiological
conditions of assay in the completely aqueous assay system in vitro.
In order to try to obtain some insight regarding this potential
limitation, we examined the effect of adding purified hexosaminidase
A to fresh brain lysosomes obtained from a patient with total
hexosaminidase deficiency. The addition of urinary hexosaminidase
A did not increase the cleavage of hexosamine-labeled G_{M2} in this
experiment.

TABLE IV

CATABOLISM OF TAY-SACHS GANGLIOSIDE IN BRAIN LYSOSOMES FROM A
CONTROL AND A PATIENT WITH TOTAL HEXOSAMINIDASE DEFICIENCY

Source of Lysosomes	Moiety cleaved	
	GalNAc	NeuNAc
	picomoles/mg protein/hr	
Control	186	216
Patient	0	225
Patient + purified urinary Hex. A	0	*

* Not determined

Again, G_{M2} sialidase is within the normal range in the lysosomes
obtained from the patient with total hexosaminidase deficiency.
Although these experiments do not exclude the possibility of a
missing cofactor in the lysosomal preparation from the patient with
total hexosaminidase deficiency, we consider this an unlikely
explanation for the failure of urinary hexosaminidase A to cleave
G_{M2}. We tentatively conclude that even though the hexosaminidase
is active with the artificial fluorogenic substrate, it is altered
in some fashion so that it has lost the ability to catalyze the
cleavage of G_{M2}. We also conclude from these experiments that
urine is an unsatisfactory source of hexosaminidase A for attempting
to treat patients with Tay-Sachs disease by enzyme replacement
therapy. We are currently exploring the activity of hexosaminidases
towards G_{M2} which have been obtained from other human tissues such
as placenta.

Regardless of the source from which hexosaminidase is obtained,
an overriding limitation of replacement therapy for patients with
Tay-Sachs disease is the serious doubt whether parenterally administered enzymes will cross the blood-brain barrier in its natural
state. In the event that they do not, other modes of delivery will
have to be explored. Among the alternative possibilities is the
administration of hexosaminidase via an indwelling ventricular
catheter. Still other procedures may be imagined. One is the
possibility of chemically modifying the enzyme so that it can
cross the blood-brain barrier. Alternatively, the barrier itself
may be temporarily opened[16]. There is the even more remote
possibility that techniques will become available through which
deficient cells can be transduced and eventually produce sufficient
quantities of the requisite enzyme[17].

It is quite apparent that we still have much to unravel before the pathogenesis of Tay-Sachs disease is completely understood. It is also evident that considerable progress in this regard should be forthcoming in the relatively near future because of several recent developments in this area of research. The preparation of G_{M2} specifically labeled in various portions of the molecule provides us with the ability to assess precisely the extent of G_{M2} metabolism via the hexosaminidase and sialidase pathways. The development of procedures for the purification of hexosaminidase A from different human sources coupled with our ability to examine its catalytic activity with the hexosamine-labeled G_{M2} will be immensely helpful for exploring the possible therapeutic usefulness of these preparations for enzyme replacement trials. We expect that immunochemical studies with purified hexosaminidase preparations will show whether cross-reacting protein is produced in the classic and variant forms of Tay-Sachs disease. We anticipate that we will be able to determine whether such material contributes to the accumulation of G_{M2} and the attendant pathologic reactions in patients with Tay-Sachs disease.

REFERENCES

1. Brady, R. O. Cerebral lipidoses. Ann. Rev. Med. 21, 317 (1970).

2. Brady, R. O. The sphingolipidoses. New Eng. J. Med., 275, 312 (1966).

3. Sandhoff, K., Andreae, U., and Jatzkewitz, H. Deficient hexosaminidase activity in an exceptional case of Tay-Sachs disease with additional storage of kidney globoside in visceral organs. Life Sci., 7, 283 (1968).

4. Kolodny, E. H., Brady, R. O., Quirk, J. M., and Kanfer, J. N. Preparation of radioactive Tay-Sachs ganglioside labeled in the sialic acid moiety. J. Lipid Res., 11, 144 (1970).

5. Kolodny, E. H., Kanfer, J. N., Quirk, J. M., and Brady, R. O. Properties of a particle-bound enzyme from rat intestine that cleaves sialic acid from Tay-Sachs ganglioside. J. Biol. Chem., 246, 1426 (1971).

6. Kolodny, E. H., Brady, R. O., Quirk, J. M., and Kanfer, J. N. Studies on the metabolism of Tay-Sachs ganglioside. Federation Proc., 28, 596 (1969).

7. Kolodny, E. H., Brady, R. O., and Volk, B. W. Demonstration of an alteration of ganglioside metabolism in Tay-Sachs disease. Biochem. Biophys. Res. Commun., 37, 526 (1969).

8. Tallman, J. F., Brady, R. O., and Johnson, W. G. Manuscript
    in preparation.

9. Quirk, J. M., Tallman, J. F., and Brady, R. O. The preparation
    of trihexosyl- and tetrahexosylgangliosides specifically labeled
    in the N-acetylgalactosaminyl moiety. J. Labeled Compounds,
    in press.

10. Okada, S., and O'Brien, J. S. Tay-Sachs disease: generalized
    absence of a beta-D-N-acetylhexosaminidase component. Science,
    165, 698 (1969).

11. Brady, R. O., O'Brien, J. S., Bradley, R. M., and Gal, A. E.
    Sphingolipid hydrolases in brain tissue of patients with
    generalized gangliosidoses. Biochim. Biophys. Acta, 210,
    193 (1970).

12. Kampine, J. P., Kanfer, J. N., Gal, A. E., Bradley, R. M., and
    Brady, R. O. Response of sphingolipid hydrolases in spleen and
    liver to increased erythrocytorrhexis. Biochim. Biophys. Acta,
    137, 135 (1967).

13. Suzuki, Y., Jacob, J. C., Suzuki, K., Kutty, K. M., and Suzuki,
    K. G_{M2} gangliosidosis with total hexosaminidase deficiency.
    Neurology, 21, 313 (1971).

14. Frohwein, Y. Z., and Gatt, S. Enzymatic hydrolysis of sphingo-
    lipids. VI. Hydrolysis of ceramide glycosides by calf brain
    β-N-acetylhexosaminidase. Biochemistry, 6, 2783 (1967).

15. Johnson, W. G., and Brady, R. O. Purification of hexosaminidase
    A. in S. P. Colowick and N. O. Kaplan (Eds.) Methods in
    Enzymology, Academic Press, N. Y., in press, 1972.

16. Rapoport, S. I., Hori, M., and Klatzo, I. Reversible osmotic
    opening of the blood brain barrier. Science, 173, 1026 (1971).

17. Merril, C. R., Geier, M., and Petricciani, J. C. Bacterial
    virus gene expression in human cells. Nature, 233, 398 (1971).

ACKNOWLEDGMENT

We thank the National Tay-Sachs & Allied Diseases
Association, Inc. and the Tay-Sachs Association of Maryland,
Inc. for their generous aid to J.F.T. during the course of
this work.

CHEMISTRY AND METABOLISM OF GLYCOSPHINGOLIPIDS IN FABRY'S DISEASE

Charles C. Sweeley,[1] Carol A. Mapes,[1] William Krivit[2] and
Robert J. Desnick[2,3]

[1] Department of Biochemistry, Michigan State University,
East Lansing, Michigan 48823; [2]Department of Pediatrics,
University of Minnesota Medical School, Minneapolis,
Minnesota; [3]Dight Institute of Genetics and Department
of Pediatrics, University of Minnesota Medical School,
Minneapolis, Minnesota

INTRODUCTION

Fabry's disease is a systemic metabolic disorder of glycosphingolipid metabolism (Sweeley and Klionsky, 1963). It can be
recognized clinically in childhood or early adolescence by cutaneous vascular lesions (angiokeratoma) and periodic episodes of fever
and pains in the extremities (Sweeley and Klionsky, 1966). With
increasing age, these symptoms are usually accompanied by proteinuria and gradual development of renal dysfunction. A significant
mortality occurs in the fourth and fifth decades from renal failure
or cardiovascular complications. Pedigree studies (Opitz et al.,
1965) and linkage data (Johnston, Warland, and Weller, 1966;
Johnston et al.,1969) indicate that the metabolic defect in Fabry's
disease is transmitted by an X-linked gene. The most severely
affected individuals are, therefore, hemizygous males, although
some heterozygous females also have significant clinical manifestations.

Histochemical studies of abnormal blood vessels, kidney and
other tissues reveal the widespread occurrence of vacuoles in which
deposits of a birefringent crystalline lipid can be found

(Pompen, Ruiter, and Nyers, 1947; Scriba, 1950). The accumulated lipid from the kidneys of two patients with Fabry's disease was identified as a mixture of two neutral glycosphingolipids, galactosylgalactosylglucosylceramide (CTH) and galactosylgalactosylceramide (CDH) (Sweeley and Klionsky, 1963; Sweeley and Klionsky, 1964). The general chemical nature of the stored glycosphingolipids was confirmed in subsequent analyses of kidneys and other tissues from patients (Miyatake, 1969; Schibanoff, Kamoshita and O'Brien, 1969) and levels of these lipids were established in their plasma and urine (Christensen-Lou, 1966; Vance, Krivit and Sweeley, 1969; Desnick, Sweeley, and Krivit, 1970; Philippart, Sarlieve, and Manacorda, 1969; Kremer and Denk, 1968).

The first evidence of a deficiency of a catabolic enzyme was reported in 1967 when very low enzymatic activity of ceramide trihexosidase was found in particulate fractions from small intestinal mucosa of a patient with Fabry's disease, whereas comparable fractions from normal tissue catalyzed the hydrolysis of the terminal galactose residue of CTH (Brady et al., 1967). More recently, it was shown that normal plasma contains measurable levels of ceramide trihexosidase, but this enzymatic activity is absent from the plasma of hemizygous patients with Fabry's disease (Mapes, Anderson, and Sweeley, 1970). The general absence of this galactosidase activity was therefore presumed to be responsible for the accumulation of CTH in this glycosphingolipidosis.

Efforts directed toward the eventual control of Fabry's disease have been initiated. It has been shown, for example, that affected males can be diagnosed by amniocentesis and measurement of the galactosidase activity in cultured fetal fibroblasts (Brady, Uhlendorf, and Jacobson, 1971) and the possibility of diagnosis by determination of CTH levels in the cultured fetal cells has been discussed (Desnick and Sweeley, 1971). A pilot study on enzyme replacement by plasma infusion has been reported (Mapes et al., 1970), in which it was found that enhanced galactosidase activity could be measured in plasma from hemizygous patients following infusion of normal plasma. The possibility of therapeutic control as an alternative to amniocentesis and abortion of the affected fetus is especially attractive in this glycosphingolipidosis. The clinical course of the disease is prolonged and adults can expect to live a reasonably full and normal life if the periodic crises of pain can be controlled and if the gradual deposition of sphingolipids can be prevented.

This review summarizes recent studies of the chemical structures of CDH and CTH from normal and Fabry tissues, some properties of the plasma ceramide trihexosidase, and replacement of this enzymatic activity in patients by plasma infusions and kidney transplantations.

THE ACCUMULATED GLYCOSPHINGOLIPIDS

The mixture of accumulated neutral glycosphingolipids from fresh or formalin-fixed Fabry kidney can be separated readily into two components by silicic acid chromatography. The major component (CTH) was shown to be galactosyl-(1→4)-galactosyl-(1→4)-glucosyl-(1→1')-ceramide by gas chromatographic studies of methanolysis products before and after permethylation, periodate oxidations of CTH, and mild acid hydrolysis products (Sweeley, Snyder, and Griffin, 1970). This structure was subsequently verified by independent chemical studies (Miyatake, 1969).

Studies of the stereochemical configurations of the glycosidic linkages in this lipid have resulted in a controversy. Early findings by nuclear magnetic resonance spectroscopy indicated that the anomeric configurations of the internal galactose and the glucose residues were β, but the terminal galactose of Fabry kidney CTH was assigned the β configuration (Sweeley, Snyder, and Griffin, 1970) while an α configuration was assigned to the terminal galactose of CTH from mouse Nakahara–Fukuoka sarcoma (Kawanami, 1967). At about the same time Kint (1970) reported that leukocytes from patients with Fabry's disease were deficient in an α-galactosidase activity measured with the artificial substrates, p-nitrophenyl-α-D-galactopyranoside and 4-methylumbelliferyl-α-D-galactopyranoside. This finding was soon confirmed (Clarke et al., 1970; Romeo and Migeon, 1970) and it was also found that the α-galactosidase activity of cultured fibroblasts was extremely low for patients. Of more significance is the fact that enzymatic studies of CTH hydrolysis with galactosidases of known anomeric specificity also support the view that the terminal galactose residue has an α configuration. Evidence of this kind, reported almost simultaneously by several groups (Hakomori et al., 1971; Li and Li, 1971; and Bensaude, Callahan and Philippart, 1971), was based on the conversion of CTH to lactosylceramide and free galactose by an α-galactosidase from ficin and small intestine. Similar results were obtained more recently for CTH isolated from normal and Fabry kidney, using an α-galactosidase from coffee beans (Clarke, Wolfe, and Perlin, 1971). Finally, evidence for an α configuration has been found in several studies of nuclear magnetic resonance spectra of intact CTH and its trimethylsilyl derivative (Hakomori et al., 1971; Clarke, Wolfe, and Perlin, 1971; Handa et al., 1971). The 220 MHz spectra of free CTH in pyridine-d_5 containing a trace of D_2O were particularly useful (Clarke, Wolfe, and Perlin, 1971), and should be a standard method for studies of glycolipid configurations.

We have compared 100 MHz spectra of trimethylsilyl derivatives of reference oligosaccharide alditols with that of the galactosyl-(1→4)-galactosyl-(1→4)-sorbitol derived from Fabry CTH and have concluded that our previous assignment of a β configuration to the

terminal galactose of this lipid was in error (Laine, Griffin, and
Sweeley, unpublished studies). Our results are, therefore, in
agreement with other nuclear magnetic resonance spectroscopic
studies and support the enzymatic studies with artificial substrates and specific galactosidases. Convincing evidence has thus
been obtained in support of the complete structure shown below for
CTH, galactopyranosyl-α(1→4)-galactopyranosyl-β(1→4)-glucopyranosyl-
β(1→1')-ceramide, from kidney of Fabry patients and from normal
kidney.

The second component (CDH) from Fabry kidney was shown to be
galactosyl-(1→4)-galactosyl-(1→1')-ceramide (Sweeley, Snyder, and
Griffin, 1970). Impure fractions of this lipid contained substantial proportions of a sulfur-containing component (Sweeley and
Klionsky, 1966) and it is possible that abnormal amounts of a
sulfatide of unknown composition may accompany the two neutral
glycosphingolipids in kidneys from these patients (Gregoire,
Jonniaux, and Voet, 1971). Abnormal amounts of digalactosylceramide have been found only in kidney, urinary sediment and
pancreas (Sweeley and Klionsky, 1963; Miyatake, 1969; Schibanoff,
Kamoshita and O'Brien, 1969; Christensen-Lou, 1966) in contrast to
the widespread occurrence of CTH deposits in Fabry's disease.
Nuclear magnetic resonance spectroscopy of the borohydride reduction product from the galactosyl-(1→4)-galactose moiety has
indicated that the terminal galactose residue has an α glycosidic
linkage. The two neutral glycosphingolipids are, therefore,
exactly analogous structurally in the galactosyl-α(1→4)-galactose
portions, and it is reasonable to assume that their accumulation
can be accounted for by the same enzymatic deficiency.

METABOLIC ORIGIN OF ACCUMULATED GLYCOSPHINGOLIPIDS IN FABRY'S DISEASE

Normal kidney contains CTH and CDH (Mårtensson, 1966) and it is likely that a substantial proportion of the accumulated lipid in endothelial and epithelial cells of the glomerulus and of Bowman's space can be accounted for by interruption of the normal cellular turnover of these constituents. The same mechanism might be responsible for the slow formation of lipid deposits in the epithelial cells of the distal tubule, which can be detected readily in urinary sediment of patients with Fabry's disease (Desnick, Sweeley, and Krivit, 1970; Philippart, Sarlieve and Manacorda, 1969).

A second source of material might be the catabolic formation of CTH from globoside, which has recently been shown to have an internal galactose with an α-glycosidic linkage, 2-acetamido-2-deoxygalactopyranosyl-β(1→3)-galactopyranosyl-α(1→4)-galacto-pyranosyl-β(1→4)-glucopyranosyl-β(1→1')-ceramide(Hakomori et al., 1971; Yamakawa, Nishimura and Kamimura, 1965). The enzymatic conversion of globoside to CTH with a β-N-acetylhexosaminidase from jack bean is known (Li and Li, 1971). The incomplete turnover of kidney globoside, a major constituent of the kidney pool of glyco-sphingolipids (Mårtensson, 1966), is therefore another potential source of large amounts of the accumulated CTH in kidney cells. A similar mechanism might account for CTH deposits in other visceral organs where globoside is a known constituent of membranes.

A third source of cellular deposits of CTH is the circulating neutral glycosphingolipids in plasma and erythrocytes, the latter probably being the richest source of globoside in man (Yamakawa, Nishimura and Kamimura, 1965; Sweeley and Dawson, 1969). The site where red cell globoside is metabolized has not yet been settled, although turnover studies of labeled red cell glycosphingolipids in the pig suggest that globoside and CTH might be released from senescent red cell membranes directly into the plasma (Dawson and Sweeley, 1970). Sequential hydrolysis of the sugar units in the plasma itself or in cells which are rich in the lysosomal glycosyl hydrolases would lead to increased levels of plasma and tissue CTH, respectively, in the absence of ceramide trihexosidase activity. This mechanism is also consistent with the accumulation of CTH in endothelial, perithelial, and smooth-muscle cells of blood vessels throughout the body of Fabry patient.

THE ENZYMATIC DEFICIENCY OF α-GALACTOSIDASE ACTIVITY

An enzymatic defect in biopsied small intestine from two patients with Fabry's disease was reported by Brady et al. (1967). After cholate pre-treatment of a crude homogenate of mucosal cells, aliquots of 20,000xg supernate were incubated with a preparation of uniformly ^{3}H-labeled CTH. The level of ceramide trihexosidase

activity in the tissue was determined from the radioactivity in
upper phase containing liberated galactose. Under these conditions
the normal enzymatic activity was about 6.3 nmoles of substrate
hydrolyzed per mg protein per hour. The enzymatic activity in
preparations from the two patients was less than 0.5% of normal
levels, and about 30% of normal activity was observed with a
heterozygote. Similar findings were later obtained with assays of
ceramide trihexosidase activity in acetone powders from control and
Fabry kidney (Dubach, Enderlin and Mannhart, 1969).

Early attempts by us to determine whether added lysosomal
ceramide trihexosidase from porcine liver and kidney would be
active in plasma at pH 7 led to the discovery of enzymatic activity
in normal human plasma (Mapes, Anderson and Sweeley, 1970).
Aliquots (0.5 ml) of plasma were incubated for 4 hours with 100
nmoles of unlabeled CTH, and liberated galactose was determined by
an end-point assay with galactose dehydrogenase. A bimodal curve
of enzymatic activity versus pH indicated that there might be two
forms of ceramide trihexosidase in plasma, with pH optima at 5.4
and 7.2. Normal levels of enzymatic activity were about 8 ± 2
nmoles of galactose liberated per ml of plasma per hour at pH 5.4
and 17 ± 2 nmoles per ml per hour at pH 7.2. There was no ceramide
trihexosidase at either pH in plasma from hemizygous Fabry patients,
while heterozygotes had 20-30% of normal total ceramide trihexosidase activity, all of which was present as the pH 5.4 form (Mapes
et al., 1970).

The two forms of plasma ceramide trihexosidase activity have
been separated by Cohn fractionation (Mapes and Sweeley, in
preparation). The form designated component A had optimal
enzymatic activity at pH 5.4 and the second form (component B) had
optimal activity at pH 7.2. Most of the activity of component A
occurred in fraction IV-1 when Cohn Method 6 (Cohn et al., 1946)
was used to separate the plasma proteins, and most of component B
activity was recovered in fraction I, as shown in Table I. Variable
amounts of both forms of ceramide trihexosidase were bound to the
serum albumin fraction (V in Table I), accounting for 15-20% of the
total enzymatic activity of each component. Since similar binding
of enzymatic activity of components A and B was demonstrated with
added bovine serum albumin, it is unlikely that the activity in
Cohn fraction V represents separate forms of enzymatic activity.

Neuraminidase treatment of component A converted it into
another enzymatically active form with optimal ceramide trihexosidase activity at pH 7.2 (Mapes and Sweeley, in preparation). An
extract of Cohn fraction IV-1 was made in 0.5 M citrate-phosphate
buffer at pH 5.4 and then solid neuraminidase from *Clostridium
perfringens* was added. After incubation for 3 hours at 37° aliquots
were assayed for ceramide trihexosidase activity over a pH range

Table 1

Ceramide Trihexosidase Activity of Cohn Fractions from Human Plasma

Fraction	% of Total Plasma Protein	Specific Activity[*]		Units/Liter Plasma	
		pH 5.4	pH 7.2	pH 5.4	pH 7.2
I	5.1	0.01	0.80	----	2320
II + III	26.7	0.01	0.01	----	----
IV-1	5.8	1.10	0.01	3520	----
IV-4	6.6	0.01	0.01	----	----
V	53.8	0.023	0.016	699	486
Super. V	2.0	0.01	0.01	----	----

[*]Spec. Act. = nanomoles galactose liberated per 4 hrs per mg protein.

4.6 to 8.0. Controls in which neuraminidase was omitted were treated under identical conditions. The effect of neuraminidase on the enzymatic activity of the component A form of ceramide trihexosidase is shown in Fig. 1. After the incubation there was substantial activity at pH 7.2 but at pH 5.4 the activity had disappeared completely, within the limits of the assay we used. The control had no measureable activity at pH 7.2 although about 30% of the ceramide trihexosidase activity at pH 5.4 was lost during the incubation. This is explained by the instability of component A, which had a half-life of about 5 hours under the conditions of the experiment.

These studies suggest that component A of plasma ceramide trihexosidase is a sialoglycoprotein and that component B is a structurally related glycoprotein which is devoid of sialic acid residues that are susceptible to the *Cl. perfringens* neuraminidase. It has not been proved by these experiments that the A and B components only differ in their sialic acid content, but such a conclusion is certainly a possibility. It is consistent with the observed effect of neuraminidase on other serum enzymes (Parker and Bearn, 1962), and is analogous to the observation that aryl-sulfatase A can be converted to the B form by neuraminidase treatment, and that many lysosomal enzymes can be converted from acidic to basic forms by this method (Goldstone, Konecny, and Koenig, 1971).

Kint utilized the artificial substrates, p-nitrophenyl-α-D-galactopyranoside and 4-methylumbelliferyl-α-D-galactopyranoside, to demonstrate an α-galactosidase deficiency in the leukocytes of hemizygotes and heterozygotes with Fabry's disease (Kint, 1970). This technique was subsequently used to confirm the deficiency of

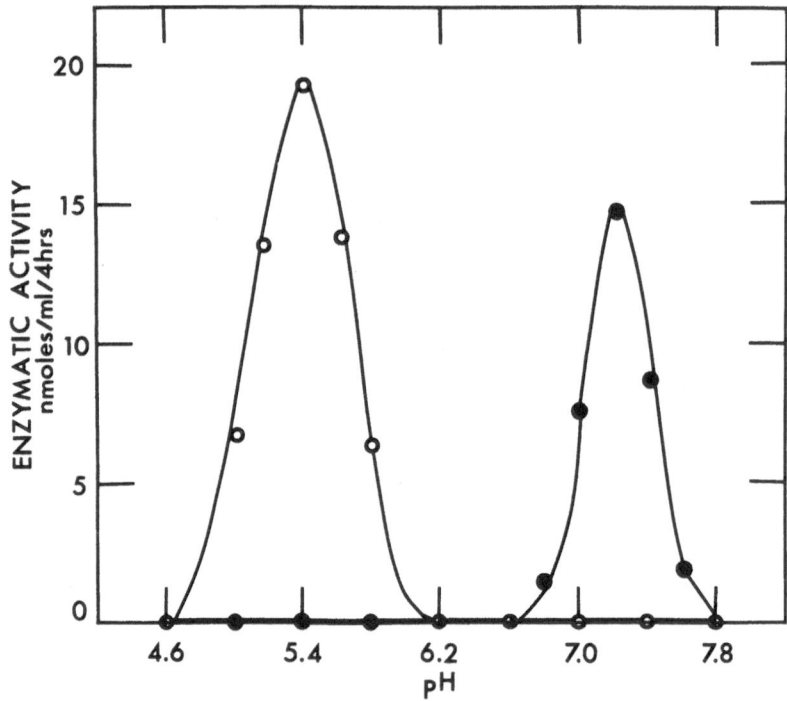

<u>Figure 1</u>. Effect of neuraminidase treatment on the pH optimum
of ceramide trihexosidase component A, derived from Cohn
fraction IV-1. The comparison is between neuraminidase-
treated (-•-) and control (-o-) incubations, carried out as
described in the text.

α-galactosidase activity in cloned and uncloned cultured normal and
Fabry fibroblasts (Romeo and Migeon, 1970) and cultured amniotic
cells from a hemizygous fetus with this disorder (Brady, Uhlendorf,
and Jacobson, 1971). It has been assumed that the artificial substrates can be used to measure ceramide trihexosidase activity,
although it has been difficult to prove that the same enzymatic
activity is measured with CTH and artificial substrates. In another
glycosphingolipid disorder, Krabbe's globoid cell leukodystrophy,
there is evidence that different enzymes are responsible for
galactosylceramide β-galactosyl hydrolase activity and 4-methyl-
umbelliferyl-β-<u>D</u>-galactoside β-galactosyl hydrolase activity
(Suzuki and Suzuki, 1971). Studies of serum enzymatic activity
were made with both substrates, but a deficiency of galactocerebrosidase activity was not accompanied by deficiency of activity
for the artificial substrate in homozygous Krabbe patients (Suzuki
and Suzuki, 1971).

In view of the ease of analysis for α-galactosidase activity with the fluorogenic substrate, as compared with the ceramide trihexosidase assay with CTH, we developed a method for determination of α-galactosidase activity in human plasma with 4-methylumbelliferyl-α-D-galactopyranoside (Desnick et al., in review). The standard reaction mixture contained 15 μmoles of citrate-phosphate buffer (pH 4.6), 50 μl of serum or fresh heparinized plasma, and 1500 nmoles of 4-methylumbelliferyl-α-galactoside or 500 nmoles of 4-methylumbelliferyl-β-galactoside in a final volume of 350 μl. After incubation at 37° for two hours (α) or 0.5 hours (β), the reaction was terminated by addition of 4.65 ml of 0.1 M ethylenediamine buffer (pH 11.2). A fluorescence assay of the liberated methylumbelliferone was carried out with a Turner fluorimeter (Model 110) with 365 nm (excitation) and 450 nm (fluorescence) filters. Under the conditions of this assay, the reaction rate was linear and proportional to enzyme concentration (volume of plasma used). Normal levels of α-galactosidase and β-galactosidase activities in plasma are shown in Table II along with the very low levels that were observed for α-galactosidase activity in plasma from hemizygotes with Fabry's disease. Intermediate levels of α-galactosidase activity were observed in plasma from heterozygotes, as expected.

Table II

Galactosidase Activity in Normal and Fabry Plasma[*]

Subject	α-Galactosidase	β-Galactosidase
	(nmoles substrate cleaved/hr/ml)	
Hemizygotes (9)	0.33 - 0.68	1.3 - 4.3
Heterozygotes (5)	2.8 - 6.2	1.7 - 3.8
Controls (15)	7.8 - 13.1	1.1 - 5.7

[*]These assays were carried out with the artificial substrate, 4-methylumbelliferyl-α-D-galactopyranoside, as described in the text.

ENZYME REPLACEMENT IN FABRY'S DISEASE

The replacement of active enzymes in patients with genetically determined enzymatic deficiences now appears to be a potential therapeutic approach to the treatment of these disorders. Several studies carried out with cultured cells have provided evidence that antibodies (Tulkens, Trouet, and van Hoof, 1970) and enzymes (Porter, Fluharty, and Kihara, 1971) in the medium can penetrate the cell membrane and are transported through the cytoplasm to lysosomes. It is expected, therefore, that circulating lysosomal enzymes added by infusions or injection of pure enzymes will be enzymatically active in cells where storage of lipids has occurred. Furthermore, factors which are now assumed to be lysosomal enzymes can "leak" from normal cultured cells into the medium, and correct the metabolic defect in various mucopolysaccharidoses in culture (Fratantoni, Hall, and Neufeld, 1969). It may be that lysosomal enzymes of a transplanted normal organ such as kidney will provide enzymatic activity to other organs by this same mechanism through secretion from normal cells and plasma transport to target organs. Studies of the feasibility and therapeutic potential of plasma infusions (Mapes et al., 1970) and kidney transplantation (Desnick et al, in review; Philippart et al., 1972) have been reported.

A pilot study of plasma infusion was initially carried out with two hemizygous patients with Fabry's disease (Mapes et al., 1970). Both patients had characteristic clinical symptoms and the levels of CTH in their plasma and of CDH and CTH in their urinary sediment were consistently elevated. Ceramide trihexosidase activity measured with the CTH assay was absent in both patients' plasma samples.

Normal plasma was obtained by plasmapharesis of heparinized blood from cross-matched donors with normal ceramide trihexosidase activity. The patients were infused with 550 and 600 ml of normal plasma, respectively. Plasma was assayed by the CTH method for enzymatic activity (component B) and for CTH levels for a period of two weeks. Measureable enzymatic activity was found in the plasma of these patients after infusion and in six hours the activity had risen to maximum levels, which were approximately 150% of the average normal activity in plasma. Afterwards a complex turnover curve was obtained, suggesting that enzymatic activity was lost rapidly during the first day, but at a slower rate for the following six days. After a week, activity could no longer be detected. Unexpectedly, there was a marked enhancement of ceramide trihexosidase activity in these patients, since the levels increased to peaks which were well beyond those anticipated by dilution of the infused activity in the recipient blood volume.

We are unaware of any published mechanisms which would uniquely account for the enhancement. However, attention might be directed to an analogous phenomenon in patients with von Wille-brand's disease, a syndrome in which there is an inherited deficiency of Factor VIII or antihemophilic factor. In the von Willebrand's patient, plasma Factor VIII activity reaches levels about 8-fold greater than predicted from the amount of plasma infused. The peak of activity is reached several hours after infusion, which is similar to our findings in the Fabry study. In both cases, the enhancement obtained *in vivo* could not be reproduced *in vitro* by incubation of donor and abnormal plasma together.

Attempts were made more recently to obtain additional information about the enhancement effect following plasma infusions to

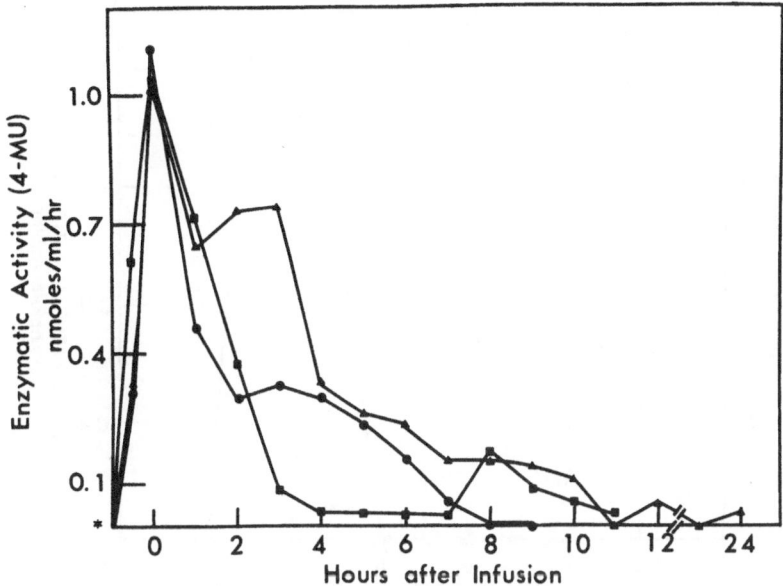

Figure 2.   Plasma α-galactosidase activity in three hemizygous
patients with Fabry's disease after infusion of normal plasma.
Enzymatic activity was determined with 4-methylumbelliferyl-α-
D-galactopyranoside, as described in the text.

Fabry patients.   In these experiments, 4-methylumbelliferyl-α-D-
galactopyranoside was used instead of CTH for the assays of plasma
enzymatic activity.   As summarized in Figure 2, measurable activity
was present in the plasma for several hours post-infusion.   Rapid
turnover occurred in all three of the hemizygous patients, and the
half-life of enzymatic activity ranged from 1 to 4 hours.   However,
there was no enhancement of the α-galactosidase activity in these
patients, in contrast to the results obtained with CTH in the
previous studies.

It is apparent that different enzymes are monitored by the
natural glycosphingolipid substrate and the artificial substrate,
although both of these assays represent a determination of α-gal-
actosyl hydrolase activity.   We have carried out an additional
plasma infusion to prove this point.   A male hemizygous patient was
administered the usual amount of normal plasma by infusion, and
post-infusion enzymatic activity was then monitored by three different methods, two of which utilized the CTH substrate while the
third was carried out with the 4-methylumbelliferyl-α-galactoside
substrate.   Galactose liberated from CTH was determined enzymatically
with galactose dehydrogenase, as previously described (Mapes,
Anderson, and Sweeley, 1970), and separate aliquots were used to

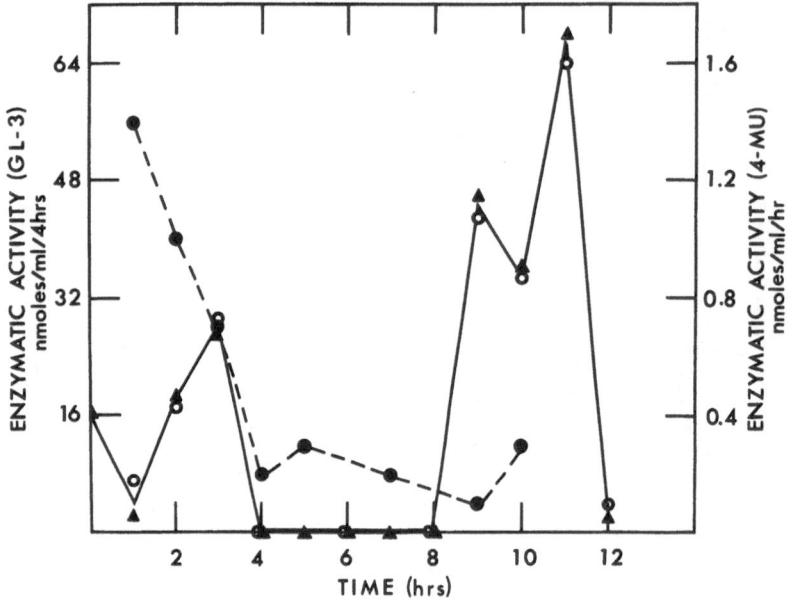

<u>Figure 3</u>. Plasma α-galactosidase activity in a patient with
Fabry's disease after infusion of normal plasma. After
incubation of aliquots of plasma with CTH (GL-3), assays of
liberated galactose were made with galactose dehydrogenase
(-▲-) and by gas-liquid chromatography (-○-); assays were
also made on separate aliquots with 4-methylumbelliferyl-α-<u>D</u>-
galactopyranoside (-●-).

determine galactose by gas chromatography.

Free sugars were eluted with 5 ml of water from a mixed-bed
resin composed of equal quantities of Amberlite CG-120 (H⁺) and
CG-400 (OH⁻) used to desalt the aliquot of upper phase after CTH
incubation with plasma. The eluates were evaporated to dryness and
the residues dissolved in a small volume of methanol-water (9:1).
The solution was pipeted onto Whatman No. 1 filter paper and galactose was separated from glucose in isopropanol-acetic acid-water
(3:1:1). Recovery of reference galactose was about 95%. Samples
eluted from the paper were evaporated to dryness and trimethylsilyl
derivatives were prepared with bistrimethylsilyltrifluoracetamide
in dimethylformamide. Analyses by gas chromatography were carried
out on 3% SE-30 at 170°. As shown in Figure 3, both methods gave
the same result (within experimental error), indicating marked
enhancement of ceramide trihexosidase activity which was maximum
10-12 hours after the infusion. In contrast to these results, there
was only one initial peak of α-galactosidase activity, shortly after
completion of the infusion, and the same rapid turnover previously

observed with the artificial substrate was obtained.

There are presently no clinical indications suggesting that plasma infusions will have a therapeutic value in the treatment of Fabry's disease. On the contrary, this procedure has probably aggravated the condition of several patients with severe renal dysfunction. Furthermore, the failure to obtain prolonged lowering of plasma levels of CTH by this approach raise questions about the effectiveness small amounts of plasma ceramide trihexosidase will have when administered by infusion. Nevertheless, these studies should provide some insight into those factors involving metabolic transformations of lysosomal hydrolases that will have to be controlled for effective delivery of enzymatic activity to a particular target organ.

Ceramide trihexosidase replacement by transplantation of enzymatically active tissue is an alternative therapeutic approach that is presently being evaluated. Renal transplantation is logical since patients with Fabry's disease develop azotemia and ultimately suffer from total renal failure. To date seven renal transplantations have been carried out on Fabry patients (J. Ackerman, Michigan State University; M. Philippart, University of California at Los Angeles; L. Wolfe, McGill University, private communications). Two of them were transplanted within the past several months in Minnesota with kidneys obtained from cadaver donors. A third kidney was transplanted into one recipient, wherease the other was nephrectomized and splenectomized prior to transplantation. The levels of α-galactosidase activity (4-methylumbelliferyl-α-galactoside assay) and CTH levels in plasma and urine are being determined periodically in both recipients. Preliminary findings indicate clinical improvement in both patients and biochemical alterations in the levels of active enzyme and CTH concentration in plasma. Long-term evaluation will be necessary to determine the success of enzyme-producing tissue transplantation in the metabolic control of Fabry's disease and possibly other inborn errors of metabolism. As advances in transplantation immunobiology occur, it is possible that transplantation of patients with Fabry's disease, even before manifest renal insufficiency, may provide a practical treatment of the biochemical and clinical abnormalities of this disorder.

Acknowledgment

This investigation has been supported in part by research grants from the USPHS (AM 12434, AM 14470, CA 08101, CA 08832, GM 01156, and RR-400).

References

1. Bensaude, I., J. Callahan, and M. Philippart, "Fabry's Disease as an α–Galactosidosis: Evidence for an α–Configuration in Trihexosyl Ceramide," Biochem. Biophys. Res. Commun., 43, 913 (1971).

2. Brady, R. O., A. E. Gal, R. M. Bradley, E. Mårtensson, A. L. Warshaw, and L. Laster, "Enzymatic Defect in Fabry's Disease: Ceramide Trihexosidase Deficiency," New. Engl. J. Med., 276, 1163 (1967).

3. Brady, R. O., B. W. Uhlendorf, and C. B. Jacobson, "Fabry's Disease: Antenatal Detection," Science, 172, 174 (1971).

4. Christensen-Lou, H. O., "A Biochemical Investigation of Angio-keratoma Corporis Diffusum," Acta Path. Microbiol. Scand.,68, 332 (1966).

5. Clarke, J. T. R., J. Knaack, J. C. Crawhill, and L. S. Wolfe, "Ceramide Trihexosidosis (Fabry's Disease) Without Skin Lesions," New Engl. J. Med., 284, 233 (1971).

6. Clarke, J. T. R., L. S. Wolfe, and A. S. Perlin, "Evidence for a Terminal α–D–Galactopyranosyl Residue in Galactosyl-galactosylglucosylceramide from Human Kidney," J. Biol. Chem., 246, 5563 (1971).

7. Cohn, E. J., L. E. Strong, W. L. Hughes, Jr., D. J. Mulford, J. N. Ashworth, M. Melin, and H. L. Taylor, "Preparation and Properties of Serum and Plasma Proteins IV. A System for the Separation into Fractions of the Protein and Lipoprotein Components of Biological Tissues and Fluids," J. Am. Chem. Soc., 68, 459 (1946).

8. Dawson, G. and C. C. Sweeley, "In Vivo Studies on Glycosphingo-lipid Metabolism in Porcine Blood," J. Biol. Chem., 245, 410 (1970).

9. Desnick, R. J., K. Y. Allen, S. J. Desnick, and W. Krivit, "α–Galactosidase Activity in Plasma, Serum, Leukocytes, and Urine from Hemizygotes with Fabry's Disease and Normal Individuals," in review.

10. Desnick, R. J., K. Y. Allen, J. Najarian, R. Simmons, and W. Krivit, "Fabry's Disease: Correction of the Enzymatic Defect by Renal Transplantation," J. Lab. Clin. Invest., in review.

11. Desnick, R. J. and C. C. Sweeley, "Prenatal Detection of Fabry's Disease," in "Antenatal Diagnosis," A. Dorfman (editor), Univ. of Chicago Press, Chicago, 1971.

12. Desnick, R. J., C. C. Sweeley, and W. Krivit, "A Method for the Quantitative Determination of the Neutral Glycosphingolipids in Urine Sediment," J. Lipid Res., 11, 31 (1970).

13. Dubach, U. C., F. Enderlin, and M. Mannhart, "Absent Renal Ceramide Trihexosidase Activity in Fabry's Disease," Germ. Med. Mth., 14, 34 (1969).

14. Fratantoni, J. C., C. W. Hall, and E. F. Neufeld, "The Defect in Hurler and Hunter Syndromes. II. Deficiency of Specific Factors Involved in Mucopolysaccharide Degradation," Proc. Nat. Acad. Sci., 64, 360 (1969).

15. Goldstone, A., P. Konecny, and H. Koenig, "Lysosomal Hydrolases: Conversion of Acidic to Basic Forms by Neuraminidase," FEBS Letters, 13, 68 (1971).

16. Gregoire, P. E., G. Jonniaux, and W. Voet, "Etude des Glycolipides Urinaires dans la Maladie de Fabry," Clin. Chim. Acta, 33, 387 (1971).

17. Hakomori, S. I., B. Siddiqui, Y. T. Li, S. C. Li, and C. G. Hellerqvist, "Anomeric Structures of Globoside and Ceramide Trihexoside of Human Erythrocytes and Hamster Fibroblasts," J. Biol. Chem., 246, 2271 (1971).

18. Handa, S., T. Ariga, T. Miyatake, and T. Yamakawa, "Presence of α-Anomeric Glycosidic Configurations in the Glycolipids Accumulated in Kidney with Fabry's Disease," J. Biochem. (Tokyo), 69, 625 (1971).

19. Johnston, A. W., P. Frost, G. L. Spaeth, and J. H. Renwick, "Linkage Relationships of the Angiokeratome (Fabry) Locus," Ann. Hum. Genet., 32, 369 (1969).

20. Johnston, A. W., B. J. Warland, and S. D. V. Weller, "Genetic Aspects of Angiokeratome Corporis Diffusum," Ann. Hum. Genet. 30, 25 (1966).

21. Kawanami, J., "Lipid of Cancer Tissues. II. Neutral Glycolipids of Nakahara-Fukuoka Sarcoma Tissue," J. Biochem. (Tokyo), 62, 105 (1967).

22. Kint, J. A., "Fabry's Disease, α-Galactosidase Deficiency," Science, 167, 1268 (1970).

23. Kremer, G. J., and R. Denk, "Angiokeratoma Corporis Diffusum (Fabry). Lipoidchemische Untersuchungen des Harnsediments," Klin. Wschr., 46, 24 (1968).

24. Laine, R. L., C. A. Griffin, and C. C. Sweeley, unpublished studies.

25. Li, Y. T., and S. C. Li, "Anomeric Configuration of Galactose Residues in Ceramide Trihexosides", J. Biol. Chem., 246, 3769 (1971).

26. Mapes, C. A., R. L. Anderson, and C. C. Sweeley, "Trihexosyl Ceramide:Galactosyl Hydrolase in Normal Human Serum and Plasma and its Absence in Patients with Fabry's Disease," FEBS Letters, 7, 180 (1970).

27. Mapes, C. A., R. L. Anderson, C. C. Sweeley, R. J. Desnick, and W. Krivit, "Enzyme Replacement as a Possible Therapy for Fabry's Disease, an Inborn Error of Metabolism," Science, 169, 987 (1970).

28. Mapes, C. A. and C. C. Sweeley, "Separation of Plasma Ceramide Trihexosidase into Two Forms by Cohn Fractionation," in preparation.

29. Mårtensson, E., "Neutral Glycolipids of Human Kidney. Isolation, Identification and Fatty Acid Composition," Biochim. Biophys. Acta, 116, 296 (1966).

30. Miyatake, T., "A Study on Glycolipids in Fabry's Disease," Jap. J. Exp. Med., 39, 35 (1969).

31. Opitz, J. N., F. C. Stiles, D. Wise, R. R. Race, R. Sanger, G. R. von Gemmingen, E. G. Cross, and W. P. de Groot, "The Genetics of Angiokeratoma Corporis Diffusum (Fabry's Disease), and its Linkage with Xg(a) Locus," Am. J. Hum. Genet., 17, 325 (1965).

32. Parker, W. C., and A. G. Bearn, "Studies on the Transferrins of Adult Serum, Cord Serum, and Cerebrospinal Fluid," J. Exp. Med., 115, 83 (1962).

33. Philippart, M., S. S. Franklin, A. Gordon, D. Leeber, and A. R. Hull, "Studies on the Metabolic Control of Fabry's Disease Through Kidney Transplantation," in "Sphingolipids, Sphingolipidoses and Allied Disorders," B. W. Volk and S. M. Aronson (editors), Plenum Press, New York, 1972.

34. Philippart, M., L. Sarlieve, and A. Manacorda, "Urinary Glyco-
    lipids in Fabry's Disease: Their Examination in the Detec-
    tion of Atypical Variants and the Presymptomatic State,"
    Pediatrics, 43, 201 (1969).

35. Pompen, A. W. M., M. Ruiter, and H. J. G. Wyers, "Angiokeratoma
    Corporis Diffusum (universale) Fabry, as a Sign of an
    Unknown Internal Disease. Two Autopsy Reports," Acta Med.
    Scand., 128, 234 (1947).

36. Porter, M. T., A. L. Fluharty, and H. Kihara, "Correction of
    Abnormal Cerebroside Sulfate Metabolism in Cultured Meta-
    chromatic Leukodystrophy Fibroblasts," Science, 172, 1263
    (1971).

37. Romeo, G., and B. R. Migeon, "Genetic Inactivation of α-Galacto-
    sidase Locus in Carriers of Fabry's Disease," Science, 170,
    180 (1970).

38. Schibanoff, J. M., S. Kamoshita and J. S. O'Brien, "Tissue
    Distribution of Glycosphingolipids in a Case of Fabry's
    Disease," J. Lipid Res., 10, 515 (1969).

39. Scriba, K., "Zur Pathogenese des Angiokeratoma Corporis
    Diffusum Fabry mit Cardio-vasorenalem Symptomenkomplex,"
    Verh. Deutsch. Ges. Path., 34, 221 (1950).

40. Suzuki, Y., and K. Suzuki, "Krabbe's Globoid Cell Leukodystro-
    phy: Deficiency of Galactocerebrosidase in Serum, Leukocytes,
    and Fibroblasts," Science, 171, 73 (1971).

41. Sweeley, C. C. and G. Dawson, "Lipids of the Erythrocyte," in
    "The Red Cell Membrane, Structure and Function," G. Jamieson
    and T. J. Greenwalt (editors), J. B. Lippincott, Philadel-
    phia, 1969.

42. Sweeley, C. C. and B. Klionsky, "Fabry's Disease: Classifica-
    tion as a Sphingolipidosis and Partial Characterization of a
    Novel Glycolipid," J. Biol. Chem., 238, 3148 (1963).

43. Sweeley, C. C. and B. Klionsky, "Fabry's Disease: The Isolation
    and Characterization of a Ceramide Trihexoside from Kidney,"
    Abstracts Sixth Int. Congr. Biochem., New York, 1964.

44. Sweeley, C. C. and B. Klionsky, "Glycolipid Lipidosis: Fabry's
    Disease," in "The Metabolic Basis of Inherited Disease," J.
    B. Stanbury, J. B. Wyngaarden and D. S. Fredrickson (editors),
    2nd ed., p. 618, McGraw-Hill, New York, 1966.

45. Sweeley, C.C., P.D. Snyder, and C.E. Griffin, "Chemistry of
     Glycosphingolipids in Fabry's Disease," Chem. Phys. of
     Lipids, 4, 393 (1970).

46. Tulkens, P., A. Trouet, and F. van Hoof, "Immunological
     Inhibitions of Lysosome Function," Nature, 228, 1282 (1970).

47. Vance, D.E., W. Krivit, and C.C. Sweeley, "Concentrations of
     Glycosyl Ceramides in Plasma and Red Cells in Fabry's
     Disease," J. Lipid Res., 10, 188 (1969).

48. Yamakawa, T., S. Nishimura, and M. Kamimura, "The Chemistry
     of the Lipids of the Posthemolytic Residue or Stroma of
     Erythrocytes. XIII. Further Studies on Human Red Cell
     Glycolipids," Jap. J. Exp. Med., 35, 201 (1965).

THE CHEMICAL PATHOLOGY OF TAY-SACHS DISEASE[x]

Konrad Sandhoff and Horst Jatzkewitz

Max-Planck-Institut für Psychiatrie,

Neurochemische Abteilung, München, Germany

In his review on sphingolipidoses (1) which appeared in the New England Journal of Medicine in 1966, R.O. Brady predicted that a sphingolipodystrophy remains to be discovered where abnormal quantities of the entire globoside molecule might accumulate because of attenuation of a hexosaminidase that catalyses the hydrolysis of the terminal N-acetylgalactosamine.

In 1967, this missing link in Brady's enumeration was detected (12). But strange to say it was a biochemically exceptional form of Tay-Sachs disease with all the typical clinical symptoms and additionally visceral involvement. Accordingly, Tay-Sachs ganglioside and its neuraminic acid-free residue were accumulated in the brain of this non-Jewish boy, aged two and a half years at death, the kidney globoside being deposited in the visceral organs (Fig.1). Since all the accumulated substances contained ß-linked N-acetylgalactosamine in the terminal position of the oligosaccharide chain it seemed reasonable to assume a deficient ß-N-acetylhexosaminidase. Indeed, a generalized ß-N-acetylhexosaminidase deficiency could

---

[x]This paper includes the presentations of H. Jatzkewitz and K. Sandhoff: "The Chemical Pathology of Tay-Sachs Disease", and of K. Sandhoff and H. Jatzkewitz: "Characterization of Two Human Hexosaminidases Involved in Tay-Sachs Disease".

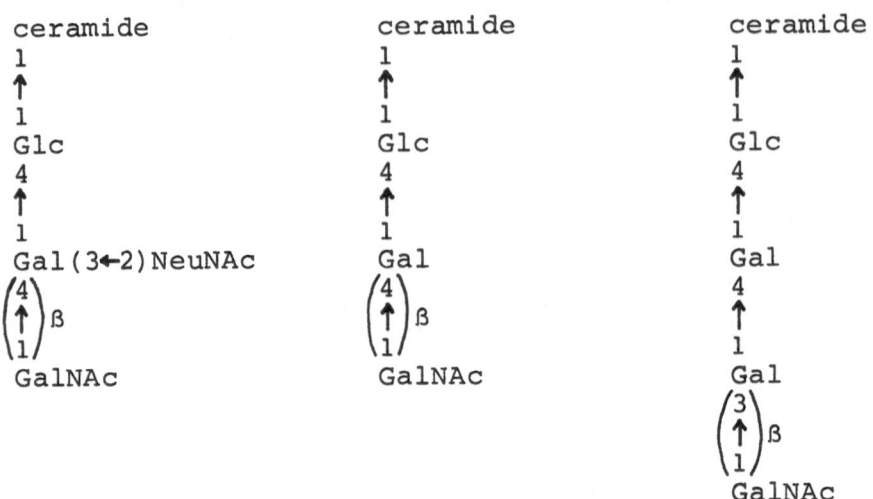

TAY-SACHS   TRIHEXOSYLCERAMIDE   KIDNEY GLOBOSIDE
GANGLIOSIDE
  (TSG)   (THC)

FIG. 1.-Lipids accumulated in Tay-Sachs disease with
visceral storage of kidney globoside. Ceramide = N-acyl-
sphingosine; Glc = D-glucose; Gal = D-galactose;
GalNAc = N-acetyl-D-galactosamine; NeuNAc = N-acetylneuraminic acid.

be established using p-nitrophenyl-ß-D-glucosaminide or
-galactosaminide as substrates (12). Thus the reason
for the excessive accumulation of the Tay-Sachs
ganglioside, its neuraminic acid-free residue in brain
and kidney globoside in the visceral tissues of a
gangliosidosis could be assumed for the first time.

    In conventional cases of Tay-Sachs disease,
however, with the accumulation of Tay-Sachs ganglioside
and its neuraminic acid-free residue in the brain only,
ß-N-acetylhexosaminidase activity was present and even
somewhat higher than in normal tissues of comparable
age (Fig. 2).

    Another possibility, although less probable, of a
deficient N-acetylneuraminidase, preventing the
degradation of Tay-Sachs ganglioside could also be
excluded: The neuraminidase activity in normal controls,
in the exceptional case of Tay-Sachs disease and in the
conventional cases was the same towards labelled Tay-
Sachs ganglioside (TSG) (= ganglioside G_{M2}) and

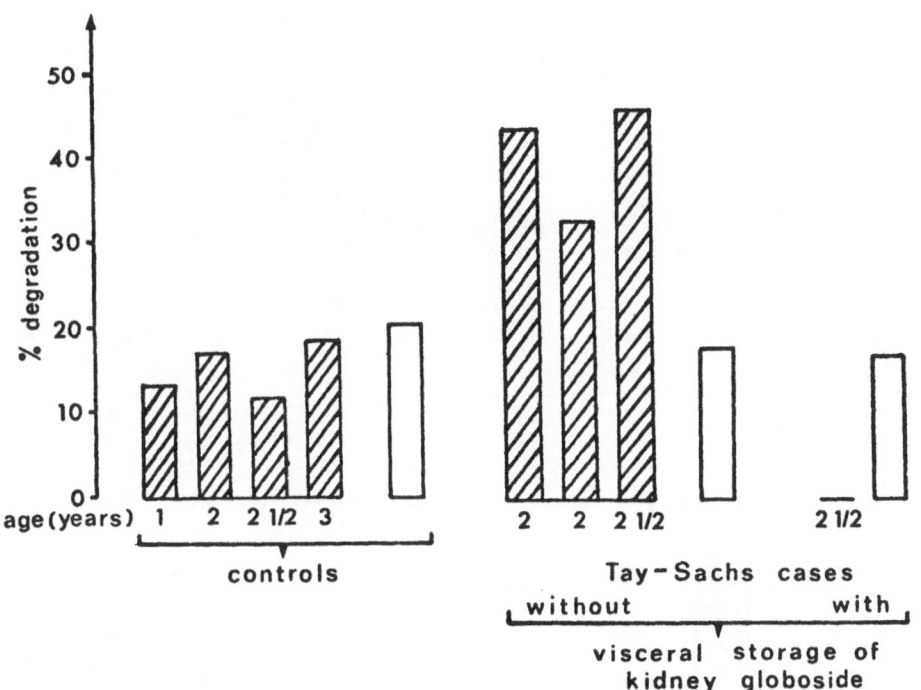

FIG. 2.-Hexosaminidase ⬚ and neuraminidase ☐ activity
in normal and Tay-Sachs brain tissues (12). Substrate
for the assay of hexosaminidase activity: p-nitrophenyl-
ß-D-N-acetylglucosaminide, for the assay of neuraminidase activity: tritium labelled hematoside. The ordinate
shows the product formed, expressed as a percentage of
the substrate used.

hematoside (= ganglioside G_{M3}) (Fig. 2) (12).

The elimination of the apparent contradiction
concerning the N-acetylhexosaminidase activity in the
different cases was initiated by the work of Robinson
and Stirling (7). They could show that human N-acetylhexosaminidase exists in two multiple forms with
different electrophoretic mobilities. The acidic form
was termed "hexosaminidase A", the basic form "hexosaminidase B". While these authors demonstrated the
resolution of these two compounds by starch gel
electrophoresis using 4-methylumbelliferyl N-acetyl-ß-
D-glucosaminide as substrate, we achieved the separation
by isoelectric focussing identifying enzymic activity
again with the corresponding p-nitrophenyl derivative
as substrate (9).

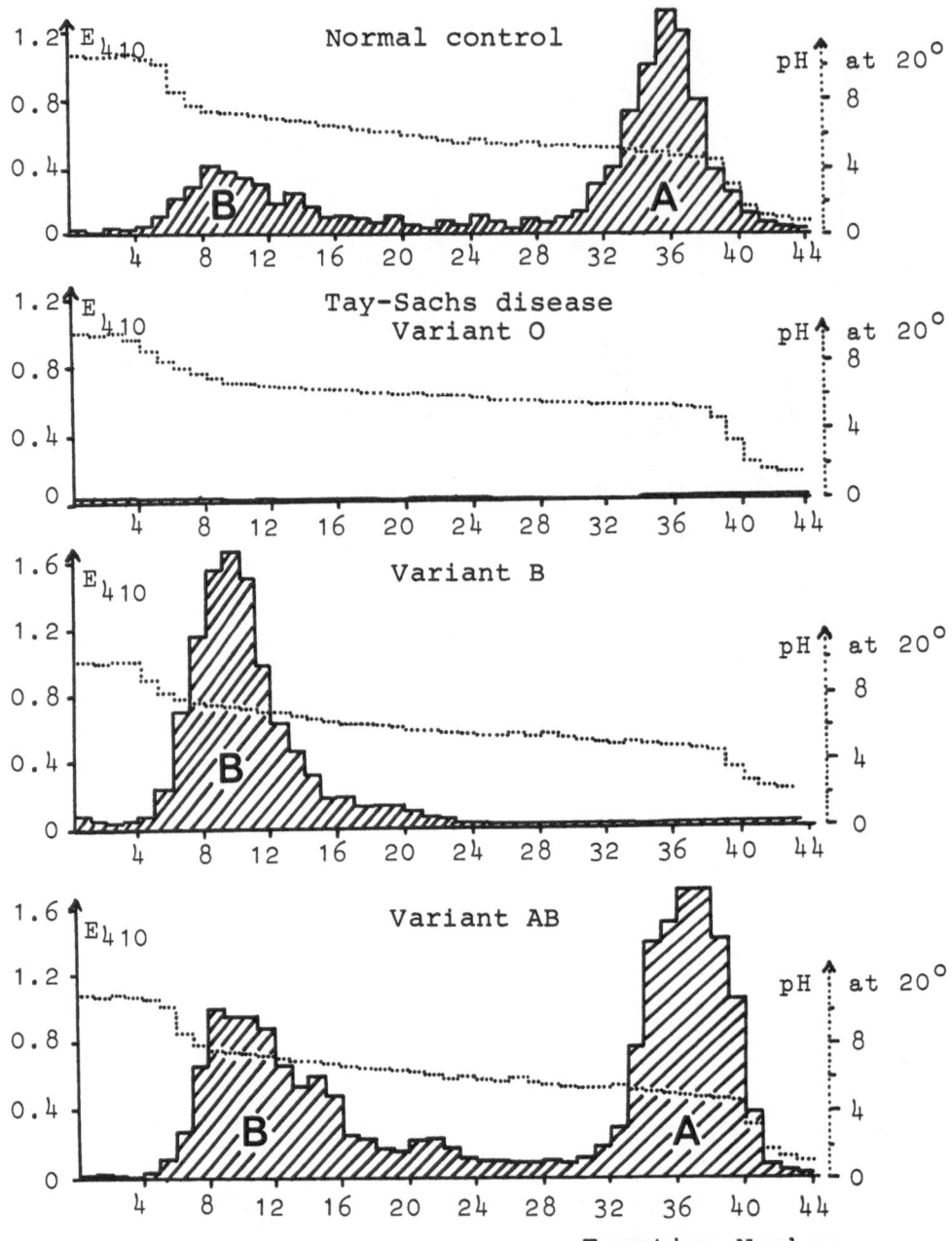

FIG. 3.-Variation of ß-N-acetylhexosaminidase pattern
in the brain tissue of three variants of Tay-Sachs
disease (10, 13). Method: Isoelectric focussing (·····pH).
Assay of activity: Extinction at 410 nm with p-nitro-
phenyl-ß-N-acetylglucosaminide as substrate.

As expected, both hexosaminidases were absent in the case of Tay-Sachs disease with the additional storage of kidney globoside (Fig.3). Two further cases of conventional Tay-Sachs disease were investigated. In one of them hexosaminidase A activity was lacking, while the B-form activity was increased. In the other case, both activities (A and B) were present, and increased in the brain tissue. Thus, at the first glance, there seemed to be a more detailed information about the increased hexosaminidase activity seen in cases of conventional Tay-Sachs disease but again no correlation between the hexosaminidase activities and the accumulated glycolipids was recognizable. However, when investigating two more brain tissues of the conventional type of Jewish origin, the A activity again was missing, thus independently and simultaneously (10) confirming the results obtained in 1969 by Okada and O'Brien (6) with tissues from the conventional type when using starch gel electrophoresis for the resolution of the multiple forms as described by Robinson and Stirling.

Obviously, there exist three enzymatically different variants of Tay-Sachs disease: one character-

TABLE 1.-Acid hydrolase activities (μmoles of substrate cleaved/g of wet tissue/min) in the brain tissue of three variants of Tay-Sachs disease in comparison to other pathological and to normal controls (13)

Subjects	Acid-phos-phatase	ß-Galac-tosi-dase	ß-Glu-cosi-dase	ß-N-Acetyl-glucosamini-dase A	B
Normal controls	0.75	0.08	0.025	0.32	0.21
Tay-Sachs tissues — Variant 0	1.38	0.18	0.37	0.04	0.004
Tay-Sachs tissues — Variant B	1.16	0.12	0.23	<0.02	1.71
Tay-Sachs tissues — Variant AB	1.30	0.13	0.18	0.88	0.86
Other pathol. tissues — G_{M1}-Gangliosidosis	0.89	0.012	0.09	1.46	0.54
Other pathol. tissues — Gaucher (inf.)	0.92	0.06	0.007	0.38	0.34
Other pathol. tissues — Gargoylism	1.18	0.04	0.05	1.12	0.48
Other pathol. tissues — Juv.amaur.idiocy	0.71	0.07	0.05	0.30	0.18
Other pathol. tissues — Niemann-Pick	0.84	0.09	0.08	0.76	0.79

ized by the absence of both hexosaminidases A and B,
therefore termed "variant O", one with an absence of the
hexosaminidase A and an active hexosaminidase B, therefore called "variant B", and one with both hexosaminidase A and B activities enhanced in brain, named
"variant AB" (10). Intermediate stages are conceivable
and have already been detected in juvenile cases (15).

Since the hexosaminidase A and B are lysosomal
enzymes, some other lysosomal acid hydrolase activities
in the brain tissue of these three variants of Tay-
Sachs disease were determined and compared to other
pathological and normal controls (Table 1). It seems
that the diminuation of one glycosidase (e.g. hexosaminidase) activity induces an increase of other glycosidase
(e.g. glucosidase) activities (13).

Now the next question arises: Is there any correlation between the enzymic alterations in the three
variants of Tay-Sachs disease and the different lipid
patterns? In order to determine this lipids quantitatively, a thin-layer densitometric micromethod was developed
with a standard deviation of 2-5 per cent (5).

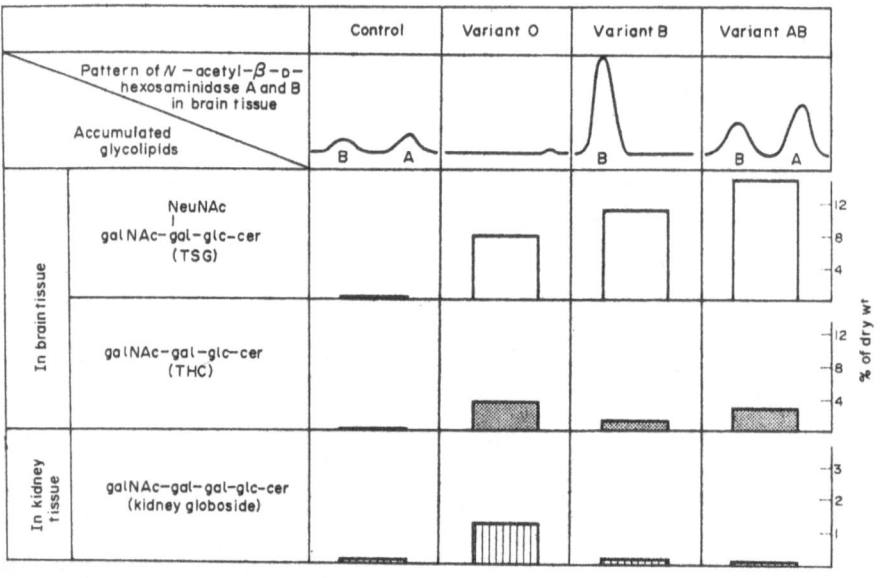

FIG. 4.-Correlation between the alteration of the hexosaminidase pattern and the glycolipid accumulation in
three variants of Tay-Sachs disease (13).

Let us first consider the amount of lipids involved in
Tay-Sachs disease (Fig.4). The storage patterns of these
lipids in the nervous tissue exhibited characteristic
differences for the three variants (13). In all cases
the accumulation of the Tay-Sachs ganglioside (TSG) was
most pronounced. It was accompanied by a minor storage
of the corresponding sialic acid-free trihexosylceramide (THC) of this ganglioside. The variant O
(3 cases) shows the relatively lowest amount of TSG and
the relatively highest amount of the THC in the nervous
tissue. Furthermore, this variant shows an extensive
storage of kidney globoside in the visceral organs. The
level of this lipid is approximately normal in the
organs of the other variants. The two variants AB
(1 case) and B (3 cases) apparently differ from each
other in the extent to which the TSG and THC were
accumulated. This extent was higher in the variant AB.

   The content of lipids typical for the white matter
(Fig.5), was reduced to very low values (13). The amount

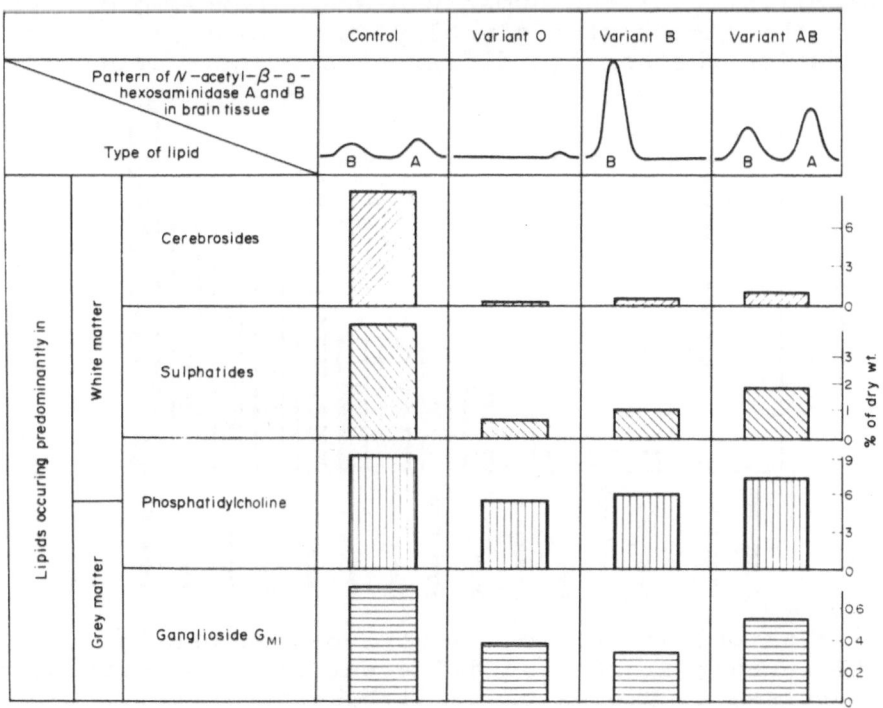

FIG. 5.-Content of some brain lipids (grey and white
matter) in three variants of Tay-Sachs disease in
comparison to normal control. Lipid content is expressed
as percentage of dry weight.

of cerebrosides, for instance, was 2.5 per cent of the
normal in the variant O. The levels of the cerebroside
sulphates and of the C_{24}-sphingomyelin were also
distinctly reduced; all these changes being the
expression of pronounced secondarily initiated demyelination. The greatest decrease of these lipids was
observed in the variant O, the lowest in the variant AB.

Now, for conclusion, let us go back to Fig. 4: It
can be assumed that the lipid storage patterns result
from the corresponding enzyme alterations in the three
variants. More evidence, however, has been obtained
after the hexosaminidases were purified and their
action investigated not only on artificial chromogenic
but on their physiological substrates.

Frohwein and Gatt (2) demonstrated in 1967 that a
particulate ß-N-acetylhexosaminidase preparation from
calf brain degraded the glycosphingolipids accumulated
in Tay-Sachs disease. This fact encouraged us to study
the specificity of the human ß-N-acetylhexosaminidases
against the accumulated glycolipids in order to answer
the question whether the different storage effects in

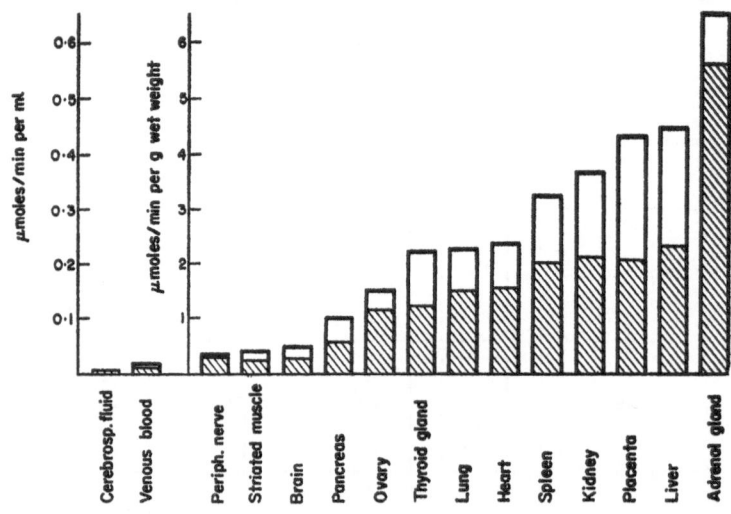

FIG. 6.-Variations in the N-acetyl-ß-D-hexosaminidases
A and B in body fluids and different organs. Activities
are expressed as µmoles of p-nitrophenyl-N-acetyl-ß-D-
glucosaminide split per min and per ml fluid or g wet
weight (3). Lower (hatched) sections: N-acetyl-ß-D-
hexosaminidase A. Upper (clear) sections: N-acetyl-ß-D-
hexosaminidase B. Each column corresponds to the average
of three determinations.

the three variants of Tay-Sachs disease are caused by
the respective ß-N-acetylhexosaminidase alterations.

The distribution of the two ß-N-acetylhexosaminidases, A and B, in various human organs is demonstrated
in Fig. 6 (3). Both enzymes A and B are widely distributed, but show quite different levels in the tissues
studied. Since liver tissue showed high activities of
both enzymes and was available, we used it as starting
material for the enzyme purification. Using conventional
techniques like gelfiltration, ion exchange chromatography and isoelectric focussing, the enzymes A and B
were purified 4 and 2 thousandfold respectively (14).

The purified hexosaminidases exhibited ß-N-acetyl-
glucosaminidase- and -galactosaminidase activity,
cleaving the p-nitrophenyl derivative of N-acetylglucosamine 8 to 10 times more rapidly than that of
N-acetylgalactosamine (7,14). This ratio changed with
ageing of the enzymes to about 15:1 after several months
in favour of the ß-N-acetylglucosaminidase activity.
Both enzymes were optimal active at acidic pH values

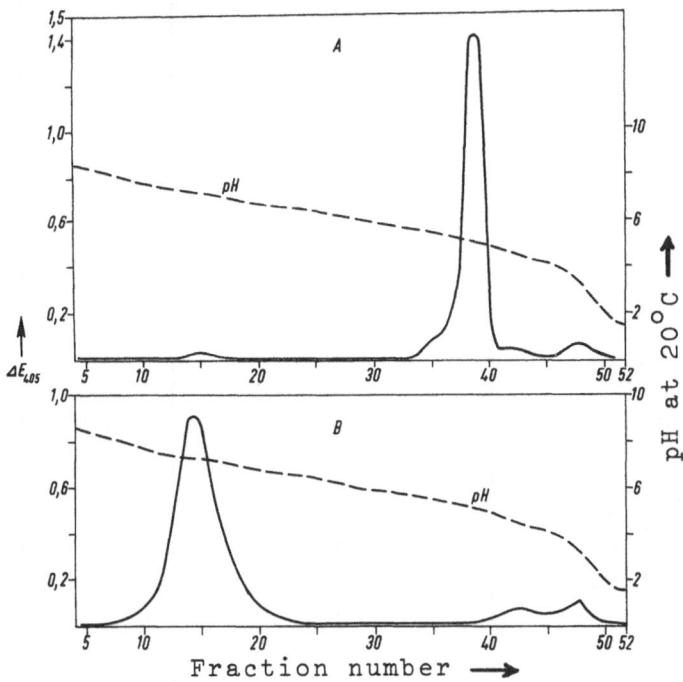

FIG. 7.-Isoelectric focussing of the purified ß-N-acetylhexosaminidases A and B (14). ——: ß-N-acetylhexosaminidase activity; ---: pH at 20°C.

around pH 4.4. They exhibited the same apparent molecular
weight of about 130.000, estimated by gelfiltration.
They were relatively stable when stored at 0°C, pH 5.
Pure enzyme B preparations showed later by isoelectric
focussing a second, rather inhomogeneous enzyme peak
between pH 3.3 and 4.3 (Fig.7). Additionally we found

TABLE 2.-Inhibition constants K_i (mM) for some competitive (c) and noncompetitive (nc) inhibitors of the
ß-N-acetylhexosaminidases A and B, using chromogenic
substrates (14). S_1 = p-Nitrophenyl-N-acetyl-ß-D-glucosaminide; S_2 = p-Nitrophenyl-N-acetyl-ß-D-galactosaminide.

Substrates / Inhibitors	ß-N-Acetylhexosaminidase A		ß-N-Acetylhexosaminidase B	
	S_1	S_2	S_1	S_2
Acetate(c)	7	9	20	13
Jodacetate(c)	56	40	57	42
Acetamide(c)	3	3	9	7
Glucosamine-HCl(c)	18	22	24	27
Galactosamine-HCl(c)	38	34	44	61
N-Acetylglucos-amine(c)	8	10	5	4
N-Acetylgalactos-amine(c)	0.4	0.6	0.7	0.6
N-Acetylglucos-aminolactone(c)	3×10^{-4}	1×10^{-4}	1×10^{-4}	1×10^{-4}
Tay-Sachs ganglioside(c)	0.3	0.4	0.2	0.4
Trihexosyl-ceramide(c)	0.03	0.03	0.03	0.03
Trihexosylceramide in 0.15% crude sodium tauro-cholate solution(c)	0.02	–	0.01	–
N-Ethylmaleimide(nc)	24	no inhi-bition	27	no inhi-bition
Silver nitrate(nc)	0.02	0.02	0.02	0.01
Aluminium chloride(nc)	121	114	83	138

some evidence that the A-enzyme was later partly transformed to a ß-N-acetylhexosaminidase having the same
isoelectric point as the B-enzyme.

A close relationship between enzymes A and B was
revealed by kinetic studies (7,14). For both enzymes
similar pH-profiles, Michaelis- and inhibition constants
were found. The ß-N-acetylglucosaminidase- and ß-N-acetyl-
galactosaminidase activities of both enzymes were inhibited to the same degree by the same inhibitor as it can
be seen in Table 2, where the inhibition constants for
a number of inhibitors are presented.

It should be noted that the Tay-Sachs ganglioside
and its asialo residue, trihexosylceramide, are strong
competitive inhibitors for both enzymes. Furthermore
mixed substrate analysis revealed that one and the same
active site of ß-N-acetylhexosaminidase A catalyzes the
degradation of ß-N-acetylgalactosaminides and ß-N-acetyl-
glucosaminides (14). The same was found for the B enzyme.
Further evidence for the close relationship between
enzymes A and B was found in vivo: The lack of both
enzyme activities in variant O (10,12) indicates to a
common genetic control, which is furthermore supported
by the fact that both enzyme activities in the heterozygotes of this variant are reduced to about 50% of
normal control (4).

For the investigation of the specificity of these
closely related ß-N-acetylhexosaminidases A and B

TABLE 3.-Michaelis constants K_m [mM] and maximum velocities V_{max} [µmoles/(min x mg protein)] of ß-N-acetylhexosaminidases A and B (14).

Substrate	ß-N-Acetyl-hexosaminidase A		ß-N-Acetyl-hexosaminidase B	
	K_m	V_{max}	K_m	V_{max}
p-Nitrophenyl-N-acetyl-ß-D-glucosaminide	0.67	117	0.67	73
p-Nitrophenyl-N-acetyl-ß-D-galactosaminide	0.16	9.5	0.15	4.8
Trihexosylceramide	0.2	1.1	0.2	1.1
Kidney globoside	0.15	0.2	0.2	0.2

towards the glycosphingolipids accumulated in Tay-Sachs
disease we found it very convenient to radioactively
label the sphingosine moiety of the substrates by
catalytic hydration of the double bond, using tritium
gas (13,14). So we could get specific activities in the
range of 150 µCi/µmole.

Both enzymes A and B readily degraded the neutral
glycosphingolipids trihexosylceramide and kidney
globoside (Table 3)(14). On the other hand the main
storage compound, Tay-Sachs ganglioside, was cleaved
only by the prolonged action of a concentrated ß-N-acetylhexosaminidase A preparation (11). One mg of the purified
ß-N-acetylhexosaminidase A cleaved about 50 µmoles trihexosylceramide per hour, but only 0.2 µmoles Tay-Sachs
ganglioside in 24 hours. Using ß-N-acetylhexosaminidase
B, no significant degradation of the ganglioside was
found.

It should be mentioned that trihexosylceramide was
degraded by the enzymes A and B only in the presence of
a crude taurocholate preparation (Fig.8)(14). Other
detergents,like pure sodium taurocholate, desoxycholate,
cholate, Triton X-100 and Cutscum had only little or no
effect.

According to these in vitro results it can be
assumed, that the storage of Tay-Sachs ganglioside in
variants O and B is caused by the deficiency of ß-N-
acetylhexosaminidase A (Fig.4). The storage of tri-

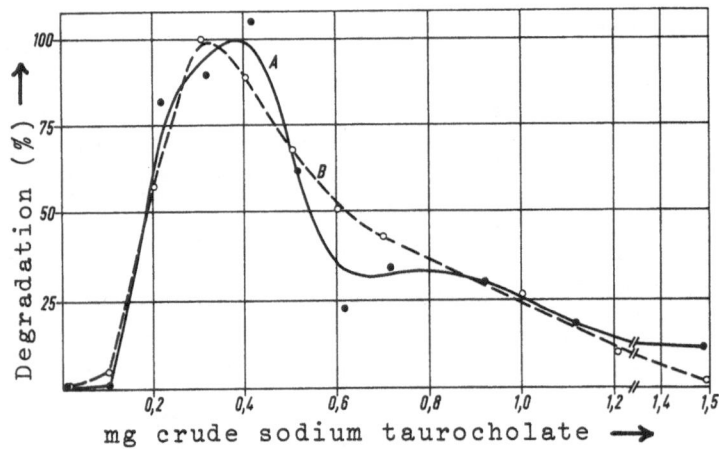

FIG. 8.-Degradation of trihexosylceramide in the
presence of crude sodium taurocholate. Enzyme: purified
ß-N-acetylhexosaminidases A and B (14).

TABLE 4.-Degradation of Tay-Sachs ganglioside (TSG) by a crude mixture of both N-acetyl-ß-D-hexosaminidases A and B in relation to the degradation of p-nitrophenyl-N-acetyl-ß-D-glucosaminide (13).

	µmoles TSG split/mol p-nitrophenyl-N-acetyl-ß-D-glucosaminide split[x]	
Control	0.7	(0.6-0.8)
Variant O	0	
Variant B	0	
Variant AB	0.1	(0.0-0.2)
Control + variant AB (1:1)	0.5	(0.2-0.8)

[x]Mean values of two or three experiments. Maximum deviations in brackets. The values are calculated from 24 h incubations with TSG and from 30 min incubations with the chromogenic substrate.

hexosylceramide can easily be explained in variant O, where both ß-N-acetylhexosaminidases A and B are missing. The same holds true for the accumulation of kidney globoside in the visceral tissues. The storage of trihexosylceramide in the variants B and AB, however, is more difficult to explain, since the B enzyme or the A and B enzymes are still able to hydrolyze trihexosylceramide (13). The accumulation in these variants may be due to the embedding of the trihexosylceramide in the lamellae of the membranous cytoplasmic bodies (MCB's)(8,16), whereby this substrate may partly be withdrawn from the action of the enzymes.

It is difficult to explain the storage of glycolipids in the nerve tissue of the patient afflicted with the variant AB. Both ß-N-acetylhexosaminidases A and B from this case exhibited normal properties in cleaving chromogenic substrates and trihexosylceramide and had normal heat stability (13). But preliminary experiments demonstrated that the ß-N-acetylhexosaminidase A in the variant AB is essentially reduced in its ability to split Tay-Sachs ganglioside (Table 4)(13). This enzyme alteration may be the cause for the ganglioside storage in this variant. In conclusion the different storage patterns can be attributed to the corresponding ß-N-acetylhexosaminidase alterations in the three variants.

REFERENCES

(1) Brady, R.O. The sphingolipidoses, New Engl. J. Med. 275, 312 (1966).

(2) Frohwein, Y.Z., and Gatt, S. Enzymatic hydrolysis of sphingolipids. VI. Hydrolysis of ceramide glycosides by calf brain ß-N-acetylhexosamini- dase, Biochemistry 6, 2783 (1967).

(3) Harzer, K., and Sandhoff, K. Age-dependent variations of the human N-acetyl-ß-D-hexosaminidases, J. Neurochem. 18, in press (1971).

(4) Harzer, K., and Sandhoff, K. Enzymatische Unter- suchungen im Blut von Überträgern einer Variante der Tay-Sachsschen Erkrankung (Variante O), Klin. Wschr., in press (1971).

(5) Harzer, K., Wässle, W., Sandhoff, K., and Jatzkewitz, H. Densitometrische Mikrobestimmung von Lipiden nach Dünnschichtchromatographie des Gesamtlipidextrakts, Z. analyt. Chem. 243, 527 (1968).

(6) Okada, S., and O'Brien, J.S. Tay-Sachs disease: Generalized absence of a beta-D-N-acetyl- hexosaminidase component, Science, N.Y., 165, 698 (1969).

(7) Robinson, D., and Stirling, J.L. N-Acetyl-ß- glucosaminidases in human spleen, Biochem. J. 107, 321 (1968).

(8) Samuels, S., Korey, S.R., Gonatas, J., Terry, R.D., and Weiss, M. Studies in Tay-Sachs disease. IV. Membranous Cytoplasmic Bodies, J. Neuropath. exp. Neurol. 22, 81 (1963).

(9) Sandhoff, K. Auftrennung der Säuger-N-Acetyl-ß-D- hexosaminidase in multiple Formen durch Elektro- fokussierung, Hoppe-Seyler's Z. physiol. Chem. 349, 1095 (1968).

(10) Sandhoff, K. Variation of ß-N-acetylhexosaminidase- pattern in Tay-Sachs disease, FEBS Letters 4, 351 (1969).

(11) Sandhoff, K. The hydrolysis of Tay-Sachs ganglioside (TSG) by human N-acetyl-ß-D-hexosaminidase A, FEBS Letters 11, 342 (1970).

(12) Sandhoff, K., Andreae, U., and Jatzkewitz, H. Deficient hexosaminidase activity in an exceptional case of Tay-Sachs disease with additional storage of kidney globoside in visceral organs, Path. europ. 3, 278 (1968).

(13) Sandhoff, K., Harzer, K., Wässle, W., and
      Jatzkewitz, H. Enzyme alterations and lipid
      storage in three variants of Tay-Sachs disease,
      J. Neurochem. 18, in press (1971).
(14) Sandhoff, K., and Wässle, W. Anreicherung und
      Charakterisierung zweier Formen der mensch-
      lichen N-Acetyl-ß-D-hexosaminidase, Hoppe-
      Seyler's Z. physiol. Chem. 352, 1119 (1971).
(15) Suzuki, Y., and Suzuki, K. Partial deficiency of
      hexosaminidase component A in juvenile G_{M2}-
      gangliosidosis, Neurology 20, 848 (1970).
(16) Suzuki, K., Suzuki, K., Rapin, I., Suzuki, Y., and
      Ishii, N. Juvenile G_{M2}-gangliosidosis, Clinical
      variant of Tay-Sachs disease or a new disease,
      Neurology, Minneap. 20, 190 (1970).

SANDHOFF'S DISEASE: STUDIES ON THE ENZYME DEFECT IN HOMOZYGOTES AND DETECTION OF HETEROZYGOTES

Edwin H. Kolodny, M.D.

Eunice Kennedy Shriver Center for Mental Retardation, Inc., at the Walter E. Fernald State School, Waltham, Mass.; and J.P. Kennedy Memorial Laboratories, Massachusetts General Hospital, Boston, Mass.

Three varieties of G_{M2}-gangliosidosis have been described. These can be distinguished by: their clinical presentation; the nature of lipid storage; and the nature of the enzyme deficiency. In Tay-Sachs disease, the most common form of G_{M2}-gangliosidosis, G_{M2} ganglioside accumulates within the nervous system and there is a deficiency of hexosaminidase A [1,2]. In the United States, most of the children afflicted with this disease have been of Jewish parentage. A much rarer type of G_{M2}-gangliosidosis known as Juvenile G_{M2}-gangliosidosis [3,4,5] has in common with Tay-Sachs disease the central nervous system accumulation of G_{M2} ganglioside and deficiency of hexosaminidase A. However, these biochemical abnormalities are less severe than in Tay-Sachs disease.

Another type of G_{M2}-gangliosidosis, first described in 1968 by Sandhoff, et al [6] and Pilz, et al [7] is associated with: central nervous system storage of G_{M2} ganglioside and its corresponding asialo derivative; accumulation of globoside within visceral organs; and deficiency in the activities of both the A and B forms of hexosaminidase. Suzuki, et al [8] have recently reported detailed morphological and biochemical studies in another patient with this disease. They confirmed the essential findings of Sandhoff and his coworkers and described in addition a marked increase in the water-extractable hexosamine in cerebral gray matter. A patient with this disease studied by Strecker,

et al (9) showed a marked increase in the daily urinary excretion
of N-acetylneuraminic acid and of oligosaccharides containing in
variable amounts mannose and N-acetylglucosamine. Brief mention
of additional patients with this disease have been made by O'Brien
(10), Raine (11), Okada, et al (12), Desnick, et al (13), and
Tateson and Bain (14).

   We have had the opportunity to study two patients with this
rare disease and to investigate their families. This report
compares the chemical findings of the liver of one of these
patients with those of the liver of a patient with Tay-Sachs
disease. Some of the properties of the hexosaminidase activity
present in the liver of the patient with Sandhoff's disease are
also described. The activity of hexosaminidase in the serum from
both patients with Sandhoff's disease and from various members of
their families was also studied. Criteria have been developed for
the detection of heterozygous carriers of this disorder and these
are also presented.

CASE REPORTS

Case 1

   This boy (K.G.) was born on Feb. 8, 1969, to unrelated parents
of French-English extraction. He was the third boy and fifth child
in the family. His early development was normal. However, at the
fifth month he could not roll over and his spontaneous activity was
reduced. Thereafter, his development was slow. In the seventh
month, cherry-red spots were visualized in both maculae. At age 10
months, during a hospitalization because of pneumonia, a bone
marrow aspirate revealed the presence of foam cells. On examination
at age 14 months, the child did not reach for objects and visual
following could not be demonstrated. The optic discs were pale, the
gag reflex was decreased, and muscle tone was increased. Generalized
seizures occurred and the head size began to increase. The EEG
showed generalized slowing with frequent spike activity in the left
anterior cerebral hemisphere. He was readmitted at age 19 months
because of an upper respiratory tract infection. At the time of
his final hospital admission at age 22 months, he could no longer
swallow. He died after a two-week hospitalization.

   Pathological Findings. The autopsy was performed by Dr. H.
Frame at the A. Barton Hepburn Hospital, Ogdensburg, New York.
Permission to open the head was not granted. The head circumference
was 51 cm. and there was emaciation. Otherwise, the gross examination was unremarkable. The microscopic examination
(Dr. V. Hymen) revealed central clusters of large foamy macrophages within the lymphoid aggregates of the spleen. Foamy
macrophages were also seen in the liver, pancreas, and bone
marrow. There was fine vacuolization in the epithelium of renal

convoluted tubules. Stains for fat were positive in these regions.

Sections of the lower thoracic spinal cord demonstrated
nerve cells with pale-staining cytoplasm swollen to one and one-
half times their normal size. In frozen sections, these cells
stained with the PAS and cresyl-violet stains. Stains for
myelin demonstrated demyelinization of the lateral columns.

Electron microscopic studies of sections from the spinal cord
and several of the visceral organs will be presented in a
separate report.

Case 2

This male child (J.C.) was born on March 10, 1968, the second
child of nonconsanguineous, white, non-Jewish parents. Birth
weight was 7 pounds, 3 ounces. His development was slow. He was
described as a nervous and irritable child who was sensitive to
sound. During a hospitalization at 14 months for a respiratory
tract infection and otitis media, cherry-red spots were visualized
in both maculae. The EEG showed considerable paroxysmal activity
with suggestive spikes preceding some high voltage waves. The EMG
and sensory and motor nerve conduction studies were normal. On
examination at age 2 he was apathetic but made some following
movements to light with either eye. The optic discs were pale.
On a recent examination at age $3\frac{1}{2}$ years, he was blind but his
hearing seemed normal. His startle reaction was mild and his
extremities were limp.

METHODS OF STUDY

Tissue Specimens

Specimens of liver tissue were obtained at autopsy from a
$3\frac{1}{2}$ year old girl who died of head injuries in an automobile
accident, from a $3\frac{1}{2}$ year old boy with the typical features of
Tay-Sachs disease and a deficiency of serum hexosaminidase A and
from case 1. Each autopsy was performed less than eight hours
after death and all fresh unfixed tissues were kept frozen at
-20 °C until analysis.

Fractionation of Major Constituents

A dry powder was prepared from 5 grams of liver with ice-
cold acetone. To one gram of this powder, 20 ml of chloroform:
methanol (2:1) were added and the mixture refluxed for one hour.
The extract was filtered while hot and then the residue was
returned to the flask, another 20 ml of chloroform:methanol(1:1)was

added and again refluxed for one-half hour. The mixture was
filtered and the filtrates combined. After adding 10 ml of chloroform to the filtrate, the mixture was partitioned according to the
procedure of Folch, et al (15). Water was used to form two phases.
The lower phases were washed twice with theoretical upper phase
water (chloroform:methanol:water, 3:48:47). The combined upper
phases were exhaustively dialyzed against water, lyophilized, and
weighed. The weight of the chloroform:methanol insoluble residue
was determined after drying in a vacuum desiccator. To determine
proteolipid protein, the procedure of Lees was employed (16).
Aliquots of the lower phases were brought to dryness, dissolved in
0.5N NaOH containing 5% sodium dodecyl sulfate and heated at 75°C
for 12 hours. This hydrolysate was then assayed by the method of
Lowry, et al (17), using Versatol (Warner-Chilcott) as a protein
standard.

Lipid Analysis

One-half of each lower phase was brought to dryness and dissolved in a few mls of chloroform. The mixture was separated on a
1 X 20 cm column of silicic acid according to the method of
Vance and Sweeley (18) employing successively 100 ml of chloroform, 10 ml of ethyl acetate, 400 ml of acetone:methanol (9:1) and
100 ml of methanol. Total cholesterol in the chloroform fraction
was determined by the method of Franey and Amador (19). Total
phosphorous in the methanol fraction was determined by the procedure
of Bartlett (20).

Chromatographic Standards

Authentic glycolipids were prepared or purchased for the
analysis of neutral glycolipids and gangliosides by preparative
thin-layer chromatography. Cerebrosides were purified from a
Folch lowerphase extract of bovine brain. Ceramide dihexoside,
ceramide trihexoside (galactosylgalactosylglucosylceramide) and
globoside were prepared from human red blood cell stroma by the
method of Hakomori and Strycharz (21). Sulfatide was purchased
from Supelco. The asialo derivatives of Tay-Sachs ganglioside
(G_{A2}) and G_{M1} ganglioside (G_{A1}) (22) were prepared by hydrolysis
of the respective parent gangliosides as previously described (23).
The gangliosides used as standard compounds were prepared from
bovine brain according to the procedure of Kanfer (24) and
fractionated into individual species using the column chromatographic method of Penick, et al (25).

Analysis of Neutral Glycolipids

The acetone:methanol fraction from the column was brought to dryness, dissolved in 4 ml of chloroform, and 4 ml of 0.6N methanolic sodium hydroxide was added. After one hour at room temperature, 4.8 ml of 0.5N methanolic hydrochloric acid, 6.8 ml of water and 13.6 ml of chloroform were added, the solution mixed and centrifuged. The upper phase was discarded and the lower phase was washed twice with 20 ml methanol:water (1:1) and then brought to dryness. This procedure was employed to remove contamination by phospholipids.

The neutral glyolipids were separated on thin layer plates of silica gel G in chloroform:methanol:water (100:42:6). With this system cerebroside, ceramide dihexoside, and G_{A1} were clearly separated from other compounds. Sulfatide and ceramide trihexoside migrated together but were free of other glycolipids. G_{A2} and globoside were also obtained together as a distinct band. These five major bands were identified with iodine vapor, individually scraped from the plates and eluted in columns with chloroform: methanol: water (10:5:1). In order to separate sulfatide and ceramide trihexoside, they were subjected to thin layer chromatography on silica gel G using n-propanol: water:15 N ammonium hydroxide (6:2:1) as solvent. Similarly, globoside and G_{A2} were separated by double development of a silica gel G plate in chloroform:methanol:water (65:25:4). The sugar content of the individual glycolipid fractions eluted from the silica gel was determined with the micro-orcinol procedure of Folch and Greaney (26).

Ganglioside Analysis

The gangliosides present in the upper phases from the liver tissues were separated by thin-layer chromatography on silica gel G in chloroform:methanol:2.5N ammonium hydroxide (60:35:8) followed by development in n-propanol:water (8:2). The reference compounds were identified with iodine vapor. Corresponding bands from liver samples were scraped off the plate, hydrolyzed in 0.05N sulfuric acid for one hour at 80°C and then subjected to the procedure of Aminoff (27) for the quantitative estimation of N-acetylneuraminic acid.

Preparation of Liver Hexosaminidase

A soluble preparation of liver hexosaminidase was obtained by triturating 50 mg of the acetone powder with 15 ml of 0.01M

potassium phosphate buffer containing 3.8 mg/ml sodium taurocholate. After one hour, the mixture was centrifuged at 30,000 x g.
The supernatant which resulted was termed "crude liver hexosaminidase".
Fractionation of the crude enzyme was performed on columns of DEAE-
cellulose according to a modification of the technique of Young,
et al (28). Identical closed columns 1.6 X 23 cm were utilized in
conjunction with a peristaltic pump so that all of the columns were
eluted simultaneously. A linear gradient of sodium chloride in
0.01M potassium phosphate buffer pH 6.0 was used for elution of the
columns. Contiguous fractions of high activity were pooled and
concentrated by ultrafiltration with an Amicon UM-10 membrane to a
protein content of one mg per ml.

Assay of Liver Hexosaminidase

The incubation mixture for the determination of liver
hexosaminidase consisted of: 5-20 μgms of enzyme protein; 8
μmoles of phosphate-citrate buffer pH 4.4; 200 mμmoles of 4-methyl-
umbelliferyl-β-D-N-acetylglucosaminide or -galactosaminide in a
total volume of 0.2 ml. After incubation for one hour at 37°C,
2.5 ml of 0.17M glycine-carbonate buffer pH 9.9 was added and the
amount of fluorescence present measured on an Aminco-Bowman spectrofluorometer with incident wavelength 366 mμ and emission wavelength 446 mμ.

Incubations with G_{A2}-C^{14} (25 mμmoles) or globoside (72 mμmoles)
contained 20-40 μgms of enzyme protein, 5 μmoles of phosphate-citrate
buffer pH 4.4, and 0.19 mg of sodium taurocholate in a total volume of
50 μl. The G_{A2}-C^{14} was prepared by mild acid hydrolysis of Tay-Sachs
ganglioside labeled with radioactivity in both the N-acetylgalactosaminyl
and N-acetylneuraminyl portions of the molecule (23, 29). Incubations
with enzyme from control liver were terminated after two hours while
the Sandhoff disease liver enzyme mixture was maintained at 37°C
with occasional shaking for 17 hours. The amount of N-acetylgalactosamine cleaved from the G_{A2}-C^{14} was determined as described previously
(29) while that released following incubation with globoside was
demonstrated through a modification of the Elson-Morgan procedure (30).

Assay of Serum Hexosaminidase

Serum hexosaminidase determinations were performed according
to a modification of the method of O'Brien et al. (31). Heat
inactivation of 100 μl of a 1:10 dilution of serum was carried
out at 49° C for two hours. The enzyme reaction mixture included

100 μl of 2 mM solution of 4-methylumbelliferyl-β-D-N-acetylglucos-aminide in 0.04M citrate-phosphate buffer pH 4.4. The reaction was stopped and the amount of fluorescence determined as described for the liver hexosaminidase.

Electrophoresis of Hexosaminidase

Electrophoresis of liver hexosaminidase was performed on cellulose acetate strips using 1-5 μl of enzyme according to the method of Suzuki, et al (8). The intensity of the fluorescence present after the incubation step was increased by the addition of a few drops of concentrated ammonium hydroxide to the incubation chamber.

The techniques used for the electrophoresis of white blood cell hexosaminidase was the same as that described for the liver enzyme. White blood cells were prepared from 10 ml of venous blood according to the dextran sedimentation method (32). The white cell pellet was treated twice with 2 ml of ice-cold acetone, centrifuged and finally dried in a vacuum desiccator. Hexosaminidase was extracted from the acetone powder by triturating 1 mg with 0.4 ml of 0.01M phosphate buffer pH 6.0 containing 3.8 mg/ml of sodium taurocholate for one hour. Following centrifugation, aliquots of the supernatant solution were applied to a cellulose acetate strip and electrophoresed as described.

RESULTS

Diagnosis of Sandhoff's Disease

In both patients, the initial diagnosis of the Sandhoff variant of G_{M2}-gangliosidosis was made after low levels of hexosaminidase were found in specimens of their serum (Table 1) following a four-hour incubation. None of the control patients shown in Table 1 had a history of diabetes mellitus or chronic illness.

Chemical Analyses of Liver

The major constituents of the liver acetone powder are shown in Table 2. On a dry weight basis, there was a larger amount of lipid extracted from the liver of case 1 than from the control liver. This is reflected in the higher values for upper phase

solids, gangliosides, cholesterol, phospholipid and neutral glycolipid. Upper phase solids, gangliosides and phospholipids were also
increased in the liver of the patient with Tay-Sachs disease but
the difference was not as large as in the Sandhoff's disease liver.

Table 1

Serum hexosaminidase in patients with
Sandhoff's disease, Tay-Sachs disease and controls

	Total Activity (mμmoles/ml serum/hour)	Hexosaminidase A (%)
Case 1	33.9	60.1
Case 2	11.3	58.3
Controls (48)	413–1364	50–67.2
Tay-Sachs disease (7)	867–1687	2.5–7.5

Table 2

Major constituents of liver

	dry wt. %		
	Control	Tay-Sachs	Sandhoff
C:M insoluble residue	90.26	86.60	83.08
Proteolipid protein	0.35	0.56	0.52
Upper phase solids	0.58	1.03	1.77
Cholesterol	0.02	0.02	0.03
Phospholipid	3.31	4.16	4.32
Neutral glycolipid	0.05	0.04	0.14
Gangliosides	0.06	0.10	0.18

Analysis of the liver glycolipids revealed a marked accumulation
of both G_{A2} and globoside (Table 3). Together these two glycolipids accounted for more than 92% of all neutral glycolipid
whereas in the control liver they comprised only 12% of the total
glycolipid. The Tay-Sachs liver contained only a slight increase
in G_{A2} and no increase in globoside. In the liver of the patient

Table 3

Glycolipid composition of liver

Glycolipid	(mμmoles/gm dry wt)		
	Control	Tay-Sachs	Sandhoff
cerebroside	581	389	443
ceramide dihexoside	161	105	120
ceramide trihexoside	68	40	188
G_{A2}	57	81	2425
globoside	85	62	9790
G_{A1}	69	67	67
sulfatide	145	197	124

with Tay-Sachs disease the amount of G_{M2} ganglioside (Table 4) was five times the level of the control while there was a 32-fold increase in G_{M2} in the liver of case 1. There were several individual bands of ganglioside in each of the liver upper phase extracts which migrated more slowly than G_{M1} but did not exactly co-chromatograph with the authentic bovine brain polysialogangliosides used as reference compounds. These were therefore grouped together and their amountcalculated from an average molecular weight of 1838, the molecular weight of disialoganglioside.

Table 4

Ganglioside composition of liver

Ganglioside	(mμmoles/gm dry wt)		
	Control	Tay-Sachs	Sandhoff
G_{M3}	363	572	316
G_{M2}	29	152	915
G_{M1}	29	30	23
Slower-moving	29	25	91

Table 5

Substrate specificity of liver hexosaminidase

| Substrate | Hexosaminidase activity (mµmoles/mg protein/hr) | |
	Control	Sandhoff
4-MUB-β-D-N-acetylglucosaminide	633.0	7.8
4-MUB-β-D-N-acetylgalactosaminide	250.0	3.2
G_{A2}	19.5	0
globoside	16.2	0

Crude Liver Hexosaminidase

The pH optimum for the crude enzyme from both the control and
Sandhoff disease liver was found to be 4.0 using 4-methylumbelliferyl-
β-D-N-acetylglucosaminide. The substrate specificities of the crude
enzyme are shown in Table 5. With the 4-methylumbelliferyl
glycosides, there is an 80-fold difference in specific activity
between the control liver enzyme and the enzyme from the liver of
case 1. Both the Sandhoff enzyme and the control enzyme show a
2.5-fold difference between the level of N-acetylglucosaminidase
and the level of N-acetylgalactosaminidase. The hydrolysis of
G_{A2} and globoside by the crude enzyme of the control liver occurred
at 3% of the rate shown for the 4-methylumbelliferyl derivatives.
With the crude enzyme from the Sandhoff disease liver no hydrolysis
of either G_{A2} or globoside could be detected even after a prolonged
incubation (17 hours).

Fractionation of Liver Hexosaminidase

The distribution of activity after fractionation of the crude
enzyme preparations on DEAE-cellulose is shown in figure 1. The
control enzyme preparation yielded three peaks of enzyme activity.
Peak I had the same electrophoretic mobility on cellulose acetate
as the hexosaminidase B band in the crude enzyme preparation.
Similarly, peak III migrated on cellulose acetate the same
distance as the hexosaminidase A band of the crude enzyme. The
electrophoretic mobility of peak II was in between that of peaks
I and III. Concentrates from peaks I and III of the Sandhoff
disease enzyme fractionation migrated with cellulose acetate
electrophoresis in a manner identical with peaks I (hexosaminidase B)

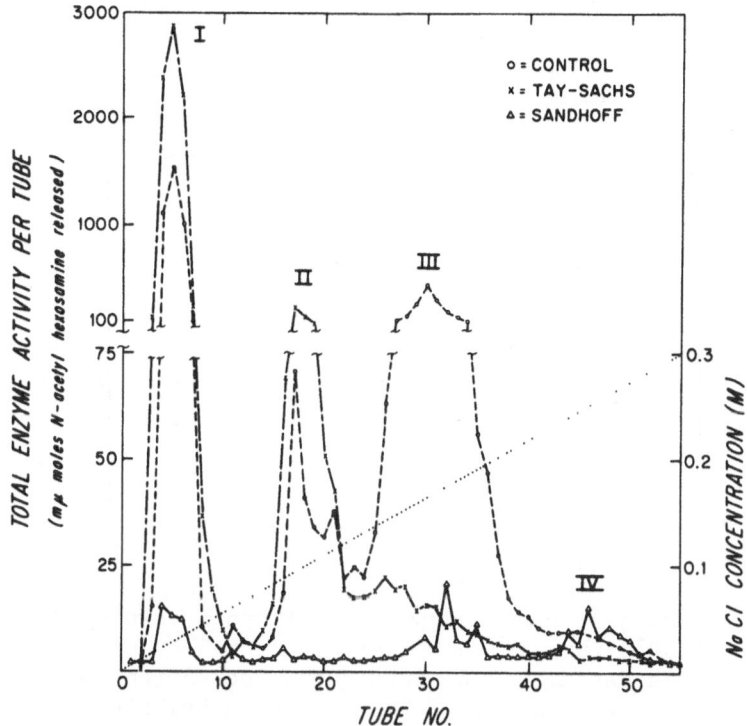

Figure 1. Fractionation of crude liver hexosaminidase on DEAE-cellulose. Crude enzyme (7½ ml.) was placed on a column 1.6 X 23 cm. and eluted with a linear gradient of sodium chloride in 0.01M phosphate buffer pH 6.0. Five ml fractions were collected.

and III (hexosaminidase A) respectively from control liver. There was no enzyme activity in the fractions from the separation of the crude Sandhoff enzyme which corresponded to peak II of the control liver. However, for the Sandhoff enzyme there was a definite increase in activity in an area beyond peak III, designated as peak IV.

The pH optimum for peak I was 4.2-4.9, for peak II, 4.5-4.9 and for peak III, 4.0-4.6. The pH optima of these peaks in the Tay-Sachs and Sandhoff enzymes did not differ from the control enzyme.

Examination of the thermolability of enzyme activity in peak III (hexosaminidase A) suggested certain differences (Figure 2). Heating the enzyme from the Sandhoff peak III for 10 minutes at 50°C resulted in loss of approximately 30% of its activity but with further heat treatment there was very little additional loss of enzyme activity. The initial loss in activity of the control enzyme in peak III was slower so that a 30% loss did not occur until 30 minutes of heating. Also with further heating there was

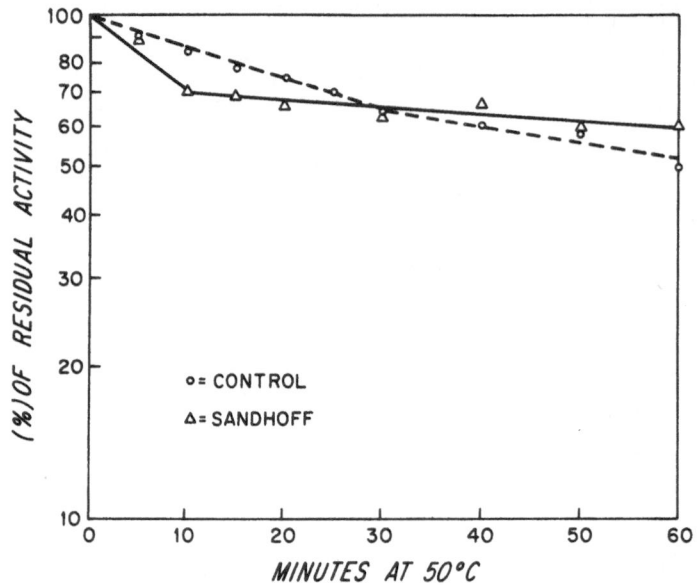

Figure 2. Aliquots of enzyme from peak III in a volume of 100 μl were heated at 50°C for varying intervals from 5-60 minutes. Enzyme activity was determined by subsequent incubation of the heat-treated fractions with 100 μl of 2mM 4-methylumbelliferyl-β-D-N-acetylglucosaminide in 0.08M citrate-phosphate buffer pH 4.4.

continued loss of activity.

        Employing the 4-methylumbelliferyl glycosides as substrates, it was also noted that the relative proportions of N-acetylglucosaminidase and N-acetylgalactosaminidase activity present in the individual peaks (Table 6) differed between the control and Sandhoff enzymes. In the control and Tay-Sachs liver hexosaminidase components there was considerably more N-acetylglucosaminidase activity than N-acetylgalactosaminidase activity.   In the residual activity present in the Sandhoff enzyme fractions, the reverse was found, namely more N-acetylgalactosaminidase activity than N-acetylglucosaminidase activity.

Serum hexosaminidases

        The range of total serum hexosaminidase for the parents of cases 1 and 2 was 333-545 mμmoles/ml serum/hour (Figure 3). In only two of the 48 control patients was the amount of total enzyme activity in this same low range. In contrast, the activity of serum hexosaminidase in six members of the family of case 1 (G. family), and three members of the family of case 2 (C. family) was in this range or below. These findings suggested that hetero-

Table 6

Substrate specificity of hexosaminidase components

DEAE-Cellulose Column Fraction	Control	N-acetylglucosaminidase / N-acetylgalactosaminidase Tay-Sachs	Sandhoff
I ("B" Component)	3.6	4.1	0.5
II	1.7	3.1	-
III ("A" Component)	4.9	-	0.4
IV	-	-	0.75

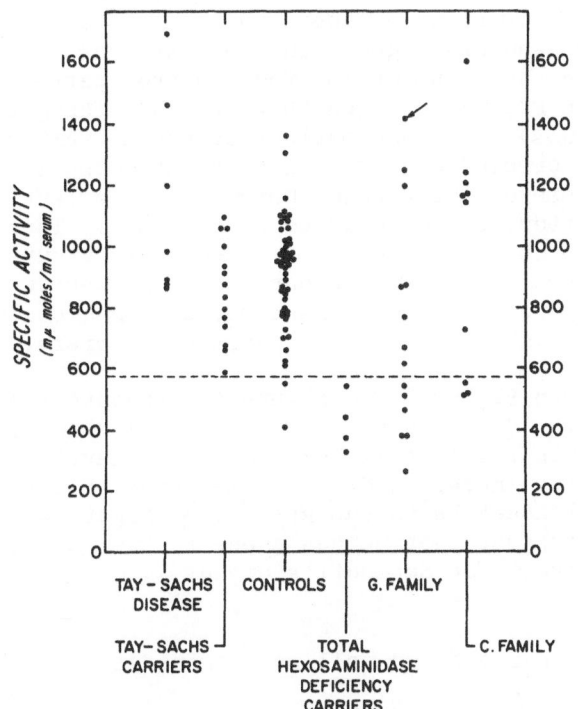

Figure 3.   Total hexosaminidase in the serum of patients with Tay-Sachs disease, obligate heterozygotes for Tay-Sachs disease, control patients, the parents of two patients with Sandhoff's disease, and various members of the families of these two patients.   The individual in the G. family indicated by the arrow is a diabetic.

zygotes for Sandhoff's disease might possibly be distinguished by low levels of total serum hexosaminidase activity.

Recognition of heterozygotes for Sandhoff's disease was also facilitated by determination of the fraction of total serum hexosaminidase which was stable to heating at 49°C for two hours (hexosaminidase B). In the four obligate heterozygotes for Sandhoff's disease this fraction varied between 18.7% and 31.5% (Figure 4). The hexosaminidase B fraction in all of the control sera was above this range, while in four members of the G. family and two members of the C. family the percent hexosaminidase B fell within the heterozygote range.

If the heterozygote range is increased to include a gray zone between 32 and 36%, then two additional members of the G. family and one more member of the C. family, indicated by circles in Figure 4, are included. The total serum hexosaminidase of each of these three (Figure 3) was in the same low range as shown for the obligate heterozygotes. Thus, by the criteria of low total hexosaminidase and low percent B, these individuals are considered carriers of the Sandhoff gene. In contrast, the total hexosaminidase activity in the serum of the four control patients shown in the gray zone in Figure 4 ranged above the heterozygote level (between 798 and 1031). The one patient of the C. family in the gray zone who is not circled had a total hexosaminidase level of 1175. Therefore, because of their total hexosaminidase levels, none of these five individuals are regarded as carriers. The levels of hexosaminidase B in the two control patients in Figure 3 with total serum enzyme levels in the carrier range were well above the gray zone in Figure 4 and thus these patients also could be excluded from the ranks of Sandhoff's disease carriers.

The arrows in Figure 3 and Figure 4 designate the same patient in the G. family. He is an elderly individual with diabetes mellitus. Although his total serum hexosaminidase level is high (Figure 3), a finding often noted in diabetes mellitus, his percentage of serum hexosaminidase B is in the gray zone (Figure 4). Genetic considerations suggest that he has a one in two chance of being a carrier of the trait for Sandhoff's disease.

White blood cell hexosaminidase

The differences in the ratio of hexosaminidases A to B in heterozygotes for the two forms of infantile G_{M2}-gangliosidosis are reflected in white blood cells as well as serum. These differences are illustrated qualitatively in Figure 5. In carriers of Tay-Sachs disease (lane 2), the hexosaminidase B band predominates while in carriers of Sandhoff's disease (lane 3) the A band comprises the major fraction of the total.

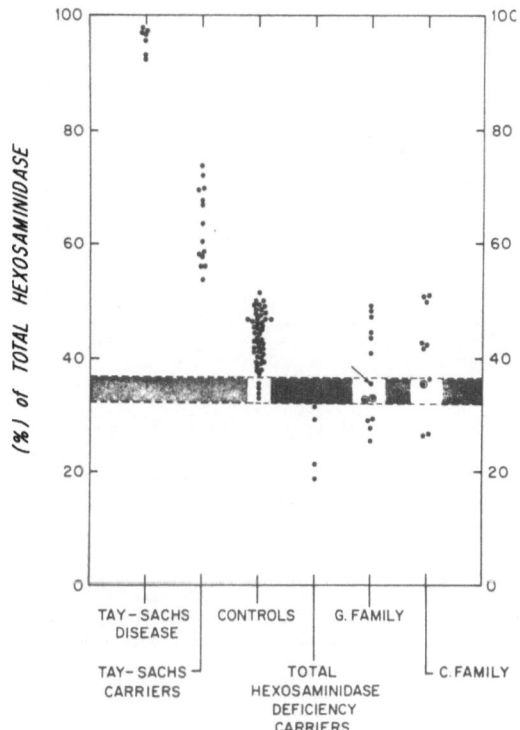

Figure 4. Percent of total hexosaminidase in the B form in the
serum of patients with Tay-Sachs disease, obligate heterozygotes
for Tay-Sachs disease, control patients, the parents of two patients with Sandhoff's disease and various members of the families
of those two patients. The individual in the G. family indicated
by the arrow is the same individual marked by an arrow in Figure 3.
The three dots in the gray zone which are circled represent individuals with low levels of total serum hexosaminidase.

DISCUSSION

    The clinical course of both patients was typical of classical
Tay-Sachs disease. In both, there occurred progressive psychomotor
retardation, primary optic atrophy, cherry-red spots in the maculae,
increased motor response to sound, seizures and enlarging head size.
One notable clinical difference from Tay-Sachs disease was the presence of foam cells in the bone marrow of case 1. This finding was
not reported by either Pilz et al (7) or Suzuki, et al (8) in their

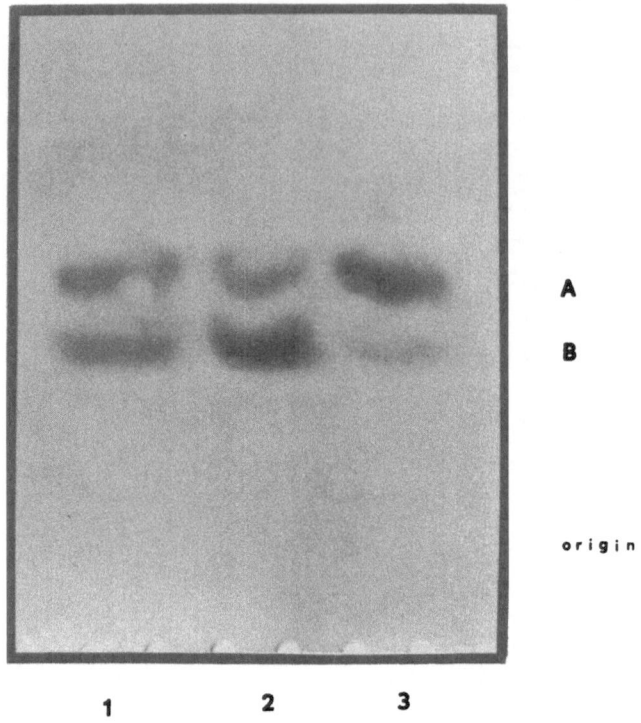

Figure 5. Separation of white blood cell hexosaminidases on a
Beckman cellulose acetate electrophoresis strip. Equal amounts of
enzyme activity were placed at the origin. Lane 1 - control;
lane 2 - obligate heterozygote for Tay-Sachs disease; lane 3 - maternal uncle of case 2.

cases. However, if other cases can be shown to demonstrate this
change, bone marrow biopsy may prove a useful technique in the
clinical differentiation of this disease from Tay-Sachs disease.

The light microscopic findings in the spinal cord of case 1
are indistinguishable from the findings of classical Tay-Sachs
disease. However, unlike Tay-Sachs disease, there was histological
evidence of lipid storage in every visceral organ that was examined.
These findings are similar to those in previously reported cases of
so-called Tay-Sachs disease with visceral involvement (33, 34). In
view of our present knowledge regarding the heterogeneity of infantile amarotic idiocy, it is likely that these earlier cases would
now be regarded as examples of Sandhoff's disease.

The major findings on chemical analysis of the liver of case 1 were a marked increase in G_{M2} ganglioside, its asialo derivative and in globoside. Although G_{M2} ganglioside is also increased in the liver of patients with Tay-Sachs disease, there was a six-fold difference in the amount of accumulation of this substance in the case 1 liver as compared to the Tay-Sachs liver.

Common to the chemical structure of each of the three lipids which were stored in the liver of case 1 is a terminal N-acetylgalactosamine moiety. Enzymatic hydrolysis of G_{M2} has been demonstrated with both crude enzyme preparations from muscle (29) and purified liver hexosaminidase (35). Globoside and G_{A2} have also been degraded using preparations of hexosaminidase (35, 36). Furthermore, kinetic studies have indicated similar rates of hydrolysis of these two glycolipids by hexosaminidase A and B (36). Therefore, the deficiency of total hexosaminidase in Sandhoff's disease probably accounts for the storage of these substances in this disease.

In several of the inborn errors of metabolism, study of the residual enzyme activity has contributed to a better understanding of the relationship between the genetic defect and the enzyme abnormality. Examples of diseases of sphingolipid metabolism studied in this way include metachromatic leukodystrophy (7), G_{M1}-gangliosidosis(38), and Fabry's disease (13). Investigation of the residual hexosaminidase activity in the liver of case 1 disclosed the presence of two components with the same electrical charge as hexosaminidase A and B as judged by their behavior on DEAE-cellulose and cellulose acetate electrophoresis. Further, there was no difference in the pH optimum of the Sandhoff enzyme compared with normal hexosaminidase. This finding is in contrast to the report of Tateson and Bain (14) who found a shift in the pH optimum from pH 4.5 to pH 5.5.

However, a change was observed in the thermolability of the hexosaminidase A component suggesting the possibility that there may be a structural defect in the Sandhoff enzyme. This defect may be close to the catalytic site, thus accounting for the low levels of activity characterizing this enzyme.

The residual enzyme in the Sandhoff liver was also characterized by a change in the ratio of N-acetylglucosaminidase to N-acetylgalactosaminidase activity present as compared to the normal enzyme. In the crude liver enzyme this ratio was approximately 2.5 to 1 but in the components separated by DEAE-cellulose chromatography there was greater N-acetylgalactosaminidase activity than N-acetylglucosaminidase activity. The reason for this difference is not known. It could result from a structural alteration similar in type in both of the major components of the hexosaminidase in Sandhoff's disease.

Heterozygotes for Sandhoff's disease are characterized both

by low levels of total serum hexasaminidase and a low value for
the percentage of hexosaminidase B. These changes are due princi-
pally to a reduction in the absolute amount of hexosaminidase B
present in their serum.

Stirling and Robinson (39) have shown that by treatment with
neuraminidase, hexosaminidase A may be converted to a form indistinguishable from hexosaminidase B on electrophoresis. Also, in
Tay-Sachs disease there is an absence of hexosaminidase A and an
increase in hexosaminidase B (1, 2). These two observations have
raised the question whether the A form of hexosaminidase is derived from the B form through the action of one or more sialyl
transferases. However, the manner in which the gene for Sandhoff's
disease is expressed in the carrier state does not support this
hypothesis. There is a greater reduction in the amount of the B
form than in the amount of the A form in carriers of the disease.
If hexosaminidase B were the precursor of hexosaminidase A, the
reverse might have been expected.

Multienzyme deficiencies have been observed in at least two
other inborn errors of sphingolipid metabolism, G_{M1}-gangliosidosis
(40) and metachromatic leukodystrophy with total sulfatase deficiency (41). The molecular basis for these deficiencies is not yet
known. One explanation, suggested by Murphy, et al (41), is that
a polypeptide subunit common to each of the enzyme components is
missing. Proof of this hypothesis will have to await purification
of these enzymes and analysis of their structure.

Prenatal diagnosis of Sandhoff's disease is possible. We
have successfully monitored a pregnancy at risk for this disease
in the C. family (42). However, the relative rarity of the gene
for Sandhoff's disease makes it unlikely that mass screening for
heterozygotes will disclose very many couples with a risk for bearing a child with Sandhoff's disease. This is in contrast to Tay-
Sachs disease where a discrete high-risk population exists.

SUMMARY

Two non-Jewish male infants are described with the typical
clinical presentation of Tay-Sachs disease. In the serum of both
there was marked deficiency of total hexosaminidase activity. The
anatomical study of one of these patients revealed histologic evidence of lipid storage in spinal cord, bone marrow, liver, spleen,
pancreas and kidney. Chemical analysis of the liver disclosed significant storage of G_{M2} ganglioside, the asialo-derivative of G_{M2}
(G_{A2}) and globoside.

The hexosaminidase activity present in this liver degraded the specific glycosides of 4-methylumbelliferyl at a little more than 1% of the rate observed with the control enzyme. However, no hydrolysis of G_{A2} or globoside could be demonstrated with the residual enzyme. The pH optimum for the enzyme was the same as that found for the control enzyme. Differences between the control enzyme and the hexosaminidase present in Sandhoff's disease were found for thermolability of component A and for the ratio of N-acetylglucosaminidase to N-acetylgalactosaminidase activity.

Total serum hexosaminidase activity in the parents of the two patients was reduced. The fraction which was heat stable was also diminished. These two findings were used to identify the relatives of these patients who were carriers of the gene for Sandhoff's disease.

The molecular defect in Sandhoff's disease was considered. It is probable that both hexosaminidase A and B are formed from a common precursor and that in Sandhoff's disease a structural defect similar in both forms diminishes their catalytic activity.

ACKNOWLEDGEMENTS

Grateful acknowledgement is given to Drs. G. Selby, J. Ryder, C. Jacobson, B. Musselman, A. Wright, and A. Milunsky for referring cases 1 and 2 for helping in the study of these patients. The invaluable assistance of Drs. H. Frame, V. Hymen and E. P. Richardson in the pathological examination of case 1 is noted with appreciation. To Mr. G. Sheng I am indebted for expert and devoted technical assistance. This work was supported by U. S. Public Health Service grant HD 05515.

REFERENCES

1. Okada, S. and O'Brien, J. Science 165, 698 (1969).

2. Sandhoff, K. FEBS Letters 4, 351 (1969).

3. Volk, B. W., Adachi, M., Schneck, L., Saifer, A. and Kleinberg, W. Arch. Path. 87, 393 (1969).

4. Suzuki, K., Suzuki, K., Rapin, I., Suzuki, Y., and Ishii, N.

   Neurology 20, 190 (1970).

5. Menkes, J. H., O'Brien, J. S., Okada, S., Grippo, J., Andrews,
    J. M., and Cancilla, P. A. Arch. Neurol. 25, 14 (1971).

6. Sandhoff, K., Andreae, U., and Jatzkewitz, H. Life Sciences I
    283 (1968).

7. Pilz, H., Muller, D., Sandhoff, K. and ter Meulen, V. Deutsch.
    Med. Wochschr. 39, 1833 (1968).

8. Suzuki, Y., Jacob, J. C., Suzuki, K., Kutty, K. M. and Suzuki,
    K. Neurology 21, 313 (1971).

9. Strecker, G. and Montrevil, J. Clin. Chem. Acta 33, 395
    (1971)

10. O'Brien, J. S. Lancet ii, 805 (1969).

11. Raine, D. N. Lancet ii, 959 (1969).

12. Okada, S., Veath, M. L., Leroy, J. and O'Brien, J. S. Am. J.
    Hum. Genet. 23, 55 (1971).

13. Desnick, R. J., Sharp, H. L. and Krivit, W. Abs. Int'l Cong.
    Human Genetics. p. 57 (1971).

14. Tateson, R. and Bain, A. D. Lancet ii, 612 (1971).

15. Folch, J. Lees, M. and Sloane Stanley, G. H. J. Biol. Chem.
    226, 497 (1957).

16. Lees, M. Unpublished.

17. Lowry, O. H., Rosebrough, N. J., Farr, A. L. and Randall, R. J.
    J. Biol. Chem. 193, 265 (1951).

18. Vance, D. E. and Sweeley, C. C. J. Lipid Res. 8, 621 (1967).

19. Franey, R. and Amador, E. Clin. Chem. Acta 21, 255 (1968).

20. Bartlett, G. R. J. Biol. Chem. 234, 466 (1959).

21. Hakomori, S. and Strycharz, G. D. Biochemistry 7, 1279 (1968).

22. Nomenclature is that of Svennerhilm, L. J. Neurochem. 10,
    613 (1963).

23. Kolodny, E. H., Kanfer, J., Quirk, J. M., and Brady, R. O.
    J. Biol. Chem. 246, 1426 (1971).

24. Kanfer, J. N., in J. Lowenstein (editor), Methods in Enzymology, Vol. 14, Academic Press, New York, p. 660 (1969).

25. Penick, R. J., Meisler, M. H., and McCluer, R. H. Biochim. Biophys. Acta 116, 279 (1966).

26. Folch, J. and Greaney, J. Unpublished.

27. Aminoff, D. Biochem. J. 81, 384 (1961).

28. Young, E., Ellis, E., Lake, B. and Patrick, A. FEBS Letters 9, 1 (1970).

29. Kolodny, E. H., Brady, R. O. and Volk, B. W. Biochem. Biophys. Res. Comm. 37, 526 (1969).

30. Morgan, W. T. J. and Elson, L. A. Biochem. J. 28, 988 (1934).

31. O'Brien, J. S., Okada, S., Chen, A. and Fillerup, D. New Engl. J. Med. 283, 15 (1970).

32. Kampine, J. P., Brady, R. O., Kanfer, J. N., Feld, M., and Shapiro, D. Science 155, 86 (1967).

33. Turban. Thesis. Freiburg (1944).

34. Norman, R. M., Urich, H., Tingey, A. H. and Goodbody, R. A. J. Path. Bac. 78, 409 (1959).

35. Sandhoff, K. FEBS Letters 11, 342 (1970).

36. Kolodny, E. H. Unpublished.

37. Stumpf, D. and Austin, J. Arch. Neurol. 24, 117 (1971).

38. Pinsky, L., Powell, E. and Callahan, J. Nature 228, 1093 (1970).

39. Robinson, D. and Stirling, J. L. Biochem. J. 107, 321 (1965).

40. Ho, M. W., and O'Brien, J. S. Science 165, 611 (1969).

41. Murphy, J. V., Wolfe, H. J., Balazs, E. A., and Moser, H. W., in J. Bernsohn and H. Grossman (Editors), Lipid Storage Diseases, Academic Press, New York, p. 67 (1971).

42. Kolodny, E. H., Jacobson, C. and Uhlendorf, W. Unpublished.

AN UNUSUAL CASE OF G_{M2}-GANGLIOSIDOSIS WITH DEFICIENCY OF HEXOSAMINIDASE A AND B[*]

F. Van Hoof, Ph. Evrard and H.G. Hers

Laboratoire de Chimie Physiologique and Département de Neurologie Infantile, Université de Louvain, Louvain, Belgium.

In this report, we briefly describe a patient with G_{M2}-gangliosidosis having a deficiency in both isoenzymes of N-acetyl-β-hexosaminidase and displaying several clinical, ultrastructural and enzymatic particularities.

Case report

C.P., a non-Jewish girl, is now 5 years old. Since the age of 18 months, she developed a slowly progressive psychomotor regression accompanied by frequent episodes of inappropriate laughter, palpebral and peribuccal myoclonic movements and akinetic attacks. She was first admitted to the unit of Neuropediatrics when she was 3 years old. At that time, she was still able to walk a few steps. The neurological examination revealed a bilateral pyramidal syndrome with more prominent spasticity of the lower extremities and a marked axial hypotony. There was an intense acousticomotor response ("startle reaction") and episodic troubles of deglutition. The speed of conduction in peripheral nerves was diminished. Spleen and liver were normal in size. Funduscopy and electroretinography, bone X-Ray, circulating lymphocytes, bone marrow and urinary mucopolysaccharides were normal.

---

[*]Supported by the Belgian FRSM and by NIH Grant AM-9235. We are grateful to Dr. G. Jonniaux for the analysis of brain gangliosides.

At the time of the first admission to the hospital the child had received for many months large amounts of diphenylhydantoin and of barbiturates and displayed symptoms of drug intoxication including hypertrophy of the gums, elevated level of serum SGPT transaminase and ultrastructural alteration of the liver (Fig. 4). These symptoms progressively disappeared after cessation of diphenylhydantoin treatment and transitory intellectual improvement was noted.

These clinical features are reminiscent of the late infantile G_{M2}-gangliosidosis (1, 3, 5, 11). The child has been under regular clinical control for the last two years. The psychomotor state is slowly regressing, with spastic quadriparesis, but the visual function remains normal.

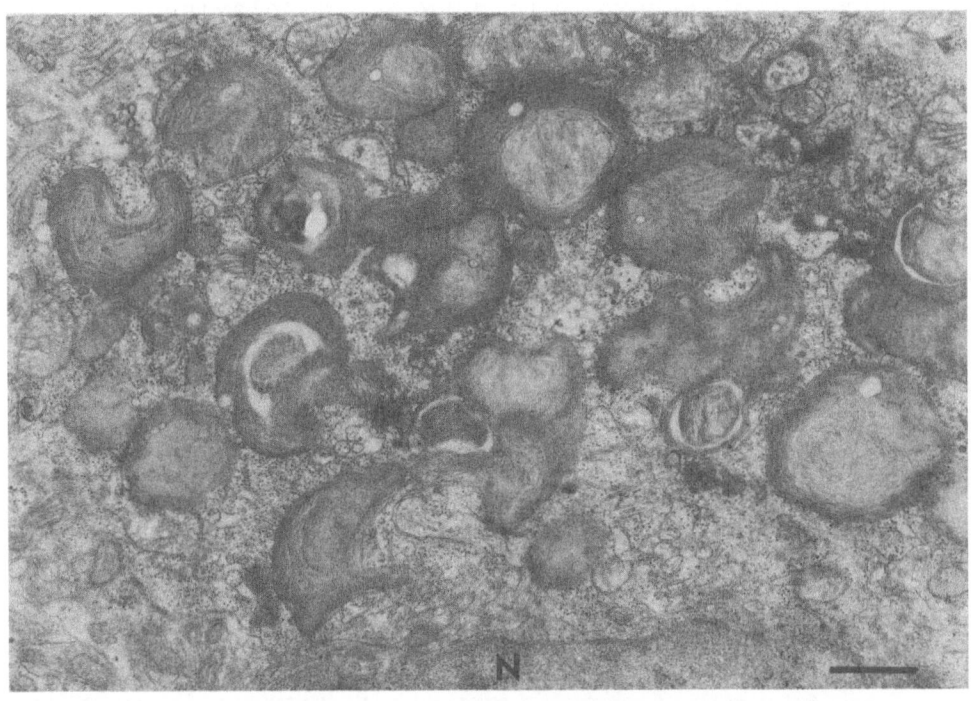

Fig. 1. Perikaryon of a brain neurone. Polymorphic cytoplasmic inclusions. The periodicity of the lamellar material is approximately 6.5 to 7 nm. N : nucleus. The line indicates the scale of one micron.

Morphology

<u>Brain</u> : A biopsy was obtained from the second occipital circonvolution, 3 months after cessation of the drug treatment. On semi-thin sections, the cytoplasm of the neurons was ballooned and small refringent inclusions were seen in the glial cells.

Electron microscopy revealed numerous polymorphic inclusions, ranging from 1 to 5 microns in diameter, in the neurones, mainly in the perikaryon. They were limited by a unit membrane and their periphery was made of concentric lamellae whereas the central core contained irregularly oriented membranes, granular material and small round osmiophilic bodies (Fig. 1). Other inclusions were similar to the "membranous cytoplasmic bodies" of Tay-Sachs disease or to the zebra bodies of Hurler's syndrome. This aspect of the neurones was reminiscent of that seen by Suzuki et al. in juvenile G$_{M2}$-gangliosidosis (5).

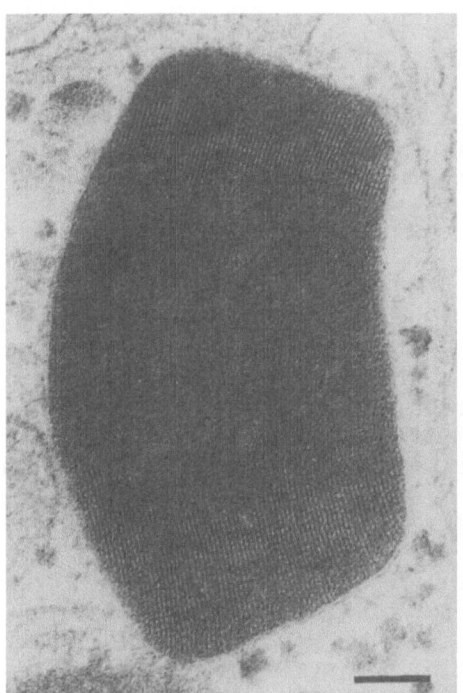 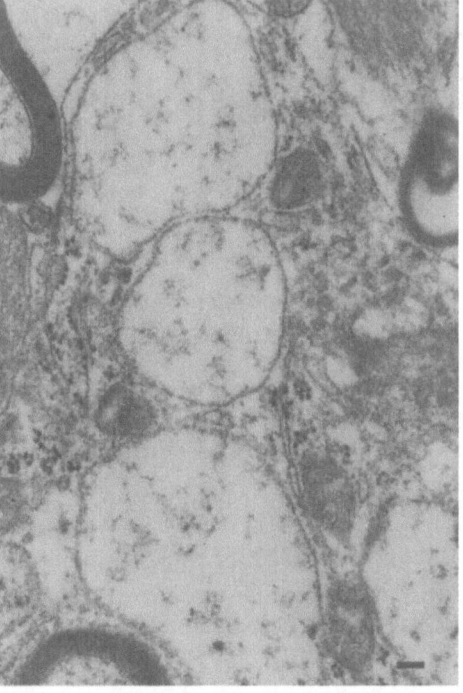

Fig. 2 . Brain, grey matter. Lamellar inclusion in a glial cell. The line indicates the scale of 0.1 micron.

Fig. 3. Brain, white matter. Clear vacuoles delimited by a single membrane, in the cytoplasm of a glial cell. The line indicates the scale of 0.1 micron.

The glial cells in the grey matter contained numerous smaller osmiophilic inclusions, ranging from 0.2
to 1 micron. These inclusions were surrounded by a unit
membrane and contained homogeneously lamellar material
with a periodicity of 6.0-6.5 nm (Fig. 2). The oligodendroglial cells of the white matter contained similar
storage granules and, less often, clear vacuoles (Fig.3).
Osmiophilic lamellar inclusions were also observed in
the endothelial cells of brain capillaries.

Liver : The ultrastructure of the liver was examined at
two occasions; a first biopsy was taken at the time of
diphenylhydantoin intoxication and a second one 3 months
later. In both biopsies no normal dense bodies were seen,
but instead there were many vacuoles, ranging from 1 to
3 microns in diameter. These vacuoles were delimited by
a single membrane and contained polymorphic material and
pseudomyelinic figures (Fig. 4). In some of them cytoplasmic constituents were present, indicating that they
were lysosomal autophagic vacuoles.
    In the first biopsy, there was a marked dilatation
of the endoplasmic reticulum (Fig. 4). This abnormality
had completely disappeared in the second biopsy. The
other constituents of the hepatocytes were normal.
    The Kupffer cells contained numerous rounded clear
vacuoles, similar to those seen in mucopolysaccharidosis (8).

Chemistry

The chemical analysis of the brain was performed
by Dr. G. Jonniaux, Laboratoire de Biologie Médicale,
Université de Bruxelles. In both the white and the grey
matter, G_{M2}-ganglioside was present in a large excess,
its sialic acid content reaching approximately 50 % of
that of the total gangliosides (normal value 0.5 to 2 %).

Enzymology

A series of lysosomal enzymes were assayed in liver,
leucocytes and urine at the time of drug intoxication
and again three months later; at this second occasion,
the brain was also analysed. The results of these analyses are shown in Table 1. In most samples there was a
remarkable diminution in the total hexosaminidase activity that is compatible with the diagnosis of Sandhoff's
disease. However, a very intriguing finding was that the
hexosaminidase activity was only slightly subnormal in
liver at the time of the first biopsy, but dropped to
very low values after cessation of diphenylhydantoin administration.

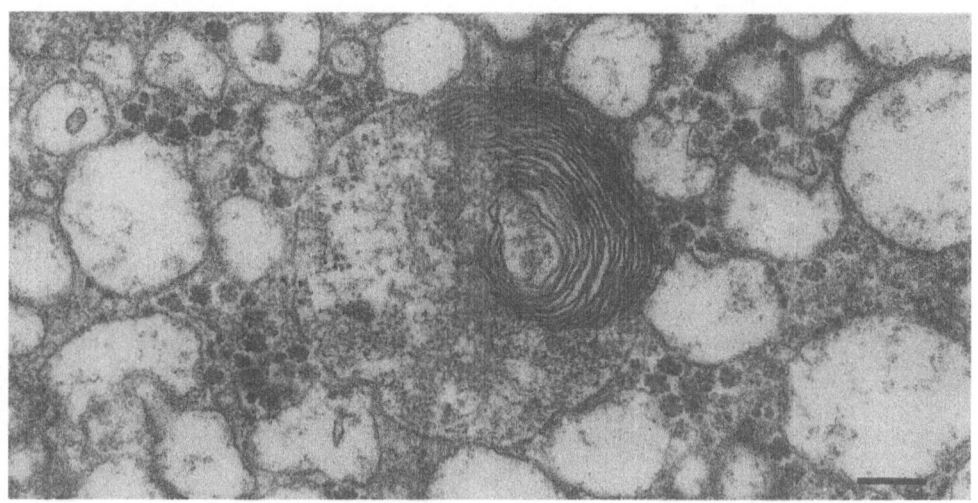

Fig. 4. Fragment of the cytoplasm of a hepatocyte
at the time of diphenylhydantoin intoxication. In the
center of the figure, a vacuole containing lamellar deposits and fine granular material. The surrounding cytoplasm contains enlarged cysternae of mostly agranular
endoplasmic reticulum, and some glycogen α-particles.
The line indicates the scale of 0.2 micron.

    In contrast to this enzymatic deficiency, there
was a large increase in the activity of many other acid
hydrolases in liver, brain and leucocytes similar to
what has been previously described in several pathological conditions in which the lysosomes are hypertrophied
(9, 10).
    Serum hexosaminidase was assayed at four occasions,
by a method (7) derived from that of O'Brien et al. (2)
and of Young et al. (12). Like in Sandhoff's disease,
the activity was only 2 to 5 % of the controls. 80 to
90 % of the residual activity disappeared after 2 hours
incubation at 50° and pH 4.4. This thermolability is
characteristic of hexosaminidase A. Other lysosomal enzymes were present in serum at levels higher than normal.
    Hexosaminidase activity in the serum of the parents
of the propositus was 40 to 50 percent of the normal value : similar results were obtained in two obligate heterozygotes of Sandhoff's disease.

TABLE I - ACTIVITY OF LYSOSOMAL ENZYMES (percent of the mean normal value)[1]

ACID HYDROLASES	LIVER		BRAIN		LEUCOCYTES		URINE	
	I	II	Gray matter	White matter	I	II	I	II
N-acetyl-β-galactosaminidase	84	1	18	17	18	5	3	2
N-acetyl-β-glucosaminidase	24	0.5	6	4	4	11	3	4
α-L-arabinosidase	395	-	*173*	297	93	82	58	42
α-L-fucosidase	224	-	290	232	*104*	-	67	32
α-D-galactosidase	555	-	*342*	464	*282*	161	90	51
β-D-galactosidase	461	-	*146*	395	181	151	66	98
α-D-glucosidase	463	-	275	333	-	-	*114*	-
β-D-glucosidase	-	-	625	1000	-	-	-	-
β-D-glucuronidase	306	-	*138*	278	49	99	75	55
α-D-mannosidase	306	-	*180*	*233*	244	230	91	61
β-D-xylosidase	*155*	-	775	1000	74	-	57	155
Cathepsin D	-	-	*150*	133	675	-	-	-
β-glycerophosphatase	-	-	428	555	-	-	91	-
nitrophenylphosphatase	*145*	-	*200*	485	-	-	97	-
nitrocatecholsulfatase	-	-	-	-	-	233	156	32
Palmitate esterase	-	-	-	-	-	780	-	-

[1]Values in italics are not significantly different from normal.

Experiments in animals

Diphenylhydantoin was administered to mice at a dose of 300 mg/kg per day, which killed seven out of ten animals in four weeks. This treatment failed to induce any significant increase in the activity of N-acetyl-β-glucosaminidase or N-acetyl-β-galactosaminidase. Ultrastructural examination of the liver of these animals showed only a moderate increase in the amount of small elements of the smooth endoplasmic reticulum.

Discussion

If one assumes that the nearly normal activity of hexosaminidases A and B in the first liver biopsy is the result of diphenylhydantoin intoxication, our patient has the enzymatic hallmark of Sandhoff's disease (4,6). However, the clinical picture differs largely from that of Sandhoff's and Tay-Sachs diseases (3,4,6) which are characterized by a more rapid development and an early appearance of ophthalmological disturbances.

Many drugs are known to stimulate the synthesis of enzymes in the liver, particularly of those bound to the endoplasmic reticulum. In our case, we do not know the intracellular localisation of the hexosaminidase in the first biopsy. It is clear however that this activity in the liver did not prevent the lysosomal overloading and did not improve the clinical condition.

Experiments in animals failed to provide any information about the effect of diphenylhydantoin on the activity of N-acetyl-β-hexosaminidase.

References

1. Bernheimer, H. and Seitelberger, F. Über das Verhalten der Ganglioside im Gehirn bei 2 Fällen von spätinfantiler amaurotischer Idiotie. Wien.Klin. Wochschr. 80, 163, 1968.
2. O'Brien, J.S., Okada, S., Chen, A. and Fillerup, D.L. Tay-Sachs Disease. Detection of Heterozygotes and Homozygotes by Serum Hexosaminidase Assay. New Engl. J. Med. 283, 15, 1970.
3. O'Brien, J.S., Okada, S., Ho, M.W., Fillerup, D.L., Veath, M.L. and Adams K. Ganglioside storage diseases. Federation Proc. 30,956, 1971.
4. Sandhoff, K., Andreae, U. and Jatzkewitz, H. Deficient hexosaminidase activity in an exceptional case of Tay-Sachs disease with additional storage of kidney globoside in visceral organs. Life Sciences 7, 283, 1968.

5. Suzuki, K., Suzuki, K., Rapin, I., Suzuki, Y. and Ishii, N. Juvenile G_{M2}-gangliosidosis. Clinical variant of Tay-Sachs disease or a new disease. Neurology 20, 190, 1970.

6. Suzuki, Y., Jacob, J.C., Suzuki, K., Kutty, K.M. and Suzuki, K. G_{M2}-gangliosidosis with total hexosaminidase deficiency. Neurology 21,313, 1971.

7. Van Hoof, F. In preparation.

8. Van Hoof, F. and Hers, H.G. L'ultrastructure des cellules hépatiques dans la maladie de Hurler (Gargoylisme). C.R. Acad. Sci. Paris 259, 1281, 1964.

9. Van Hoof, F. and Hers, H.G. The abnormalities of lysosomal enzymes in mucopolysaccharidoses. European J. Biochem. 7, 34, 1968 .

10. Van Hoof, F. and Hers, H.G. The mucopolysaccharidoses as "lysosomal diseases". This book, 1972.

11. Volk, B.W., Adachi, M., Schneck, L., Saifer, A. and Kleinberg, W. G_S-Ganglioside Variant of Systemic Late Infantile Lipidosis. Arch. Pathol. 87, 393, 1969.

12. Young, E.P., Ellis, R.B., Lake, B.D.and Patrick, A.D. Tay-Sachs disease and related disorders : fractionation of brain N-acetyl-β-hexosaminidase on DEAE-cellulose. FEBS Letters 9, 1, 1970.

SANDHOFF'S DISEASE: ULTRASTRUCTURAL AND BIOCHEMICAL STUDIES

R. J. Desnick,* P. D. Snyder, S. J. Desnick,*
W. Krivit, and H. L. Sharp

Department of Pediatrics and *Dight Institute for
Human Genetics, University of Minnesota Medical School,
Minneapolis, Minnesota 55455

INTRODUCTION

Sandhoff's disease results from the deficient activity of both
N-Acetyl-β-hexosaminidase A and B (14,17,19-22) and is characterized
by the neural and visceral deposition of G_{m2} ganglioside, its asialo
derivative (NAcgal-gal-glc-cer) and globoside (NAcgal-gal-gal-glc-
cer) in affected individuals (Figure 1) (3,6,9,10,14,19-22,24,25).

The clinical features and course of this disorder are similar
to those of Tay-Sachs disease, a metabolically related sphingolipidosis which results from deficient activity of hexosaminidase A only
(11,17,22). Specific clinical and pathologic findings (Table 1) as
well as the biochemical documentation of the specific enzymatic deficiencies provide the distinction between these two disease entities.
To date, no patients with Sandhoff's disease have had Jewish ancestry,
whereas a well-documented Jewish predilection occurs among patients
with Tay-Sachs disease; presumably, many cases of Sandhoff's disease
have previously been misdiagnosed as Tay-Sachs disease.

In both disorders, clinical onset occurs during the first few
months of life, when the subtle signs of delayed motor development
may be noted. During the next six months, little, if any, progress
is made in motor or mental development. Signs of primary optic
atrophy and the classic bilateral "cherry red" macular degeneration
can be observed early in both diseases. In contrast to patients
with Tay-Sachs disease, the physical sign of hyperacusis may not be
discerned in Sandhoff's disease. Cardiovascular symptoms have been
reported as the presenting symptom in Sandhoff's disease (6); these
patients may have cardiomegaly and a pansystolic murmur of mitral
insufficiency when associated with significant left-sided heart

failure.   Electrocardiographic findings range from mild left ventricular hypertrophy to severe changes compatible with endocardial
fibroelastosis; minor electrocardiographic changes have been previously reported in patients with Tay-Sachs disease (16).   Minimal
hepatosplenomegaly may be present and subtle roentgen skeletal
changes similar to those seen in patients with mucopolysaccharidoses
may be detected in patients with Sandhoff's disease (6).

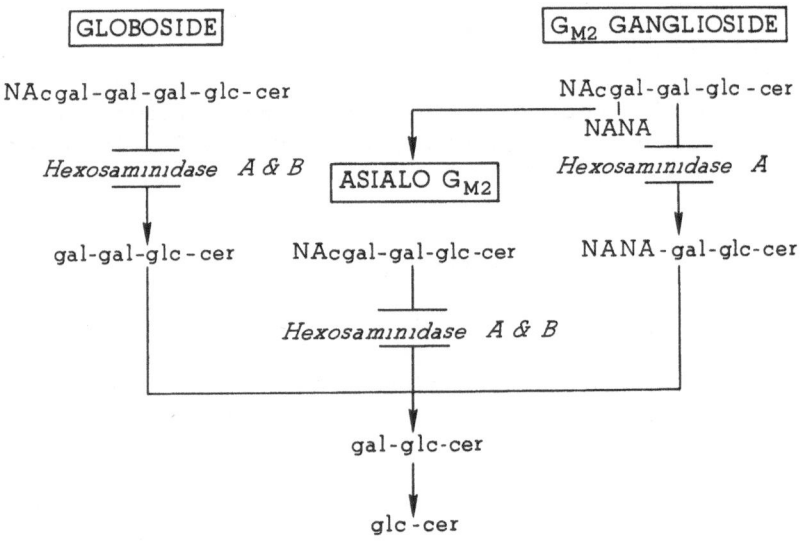

Figure 1.   Three glycosphingolipids with terminal NAcgal moieties
accumulate in neural and visceral tissue resulting from deficient
hexosaminidase A and B activities in Sandhoff's disease.   Cer=
ceramide, gal=galactose, glc=glucose, NAcgal=N-acetyl-galactosamine.

     By twelve months, these patients have bilateral pyramidal tract
abnormalities, including increased tendon reflexes, spasticity and
positive Hoffmann's and Babinski's signs.   Their ability to sit,
push backwards, transfer objects from hand to hand, in addition to
smiling and laughing appropriately, have usually been lost by one
year.   EEG changes indicate diffuse and multifocal CNS dysfunction,
with excessive delta wave activity and multifocal spikes.   After
twelve months, psychomotor degeneration is progressive with myoclonic jerks involving the face, trunk and limbs, symmetrically
increased muscle tone, spastic quadriplegia and constantly abducted
lower limbs, which are flexed at the knees and plantar flexed at
the the ankles.   The course is progressively downhill and death
usually occurs due to pneumonia between 22 and 36 months of life.

Table 1. CLINICAL AND PATHOLOGIC COMPARISON OF SANDHOFF'S AND
TAY-SACHS DISEASES

Clinical Manifestations	Sandhoff's Disease (Deficient Hex A & B)	Tay-Sachs Disease (Deficient Hex A)
CNS Deterioration	+ +	+ +
"Cherry-Red" Macular Degeneration	+ +	+ +
Hyperacusis	+/-	+ +
Cardiomegaly	+	-
Hepatosplenomegaly	+/-	-
Roentgen Skeletal Abnormalities	+	-
Bone Marrow Histiocytosis	-	-
Jewish Predilection	-	+
Pathological Manifestations		
Lysosomal Lipid Accumulation		
Brain	+ +	+ +
Visceral	+ +	+

MORPHOLOGIC STUDIES

Materials and Methods

Brain biopsies were obtained at craniotomy. Percutaneous liver
biopsies were obtained with a 1.2 mm Menghini needle by previously
described procedures (23). Specimens were fixed in neutralized
formalin for light microscopy and stained with hematoxylin and eosin
and PAS. A portion of the specimen was fixed for electron microscopy in Millonig's buffer containing 1.25% glutaraldehyde and 1.25%
osmic acid. After 1 to 1 1/2 hours, the tissue was dehydrated in
alcohol and propylene oxide and embedded in Epon. Thin sections,
stained with uranyl acetate and lead hydroxide, were examined in a
Phillips 200 electron microscope. One micron sections, fixed as
above and stained with methylene blue-Azure II, were examined under
the light microscope.

Results

Pathologically, the accumulation of glycosphingolipid results
in morphologic alterations in the brain similar to that in Tay-Sachs
disease, but the visceral accumulation of glycosphingolipid in
Sandhoff's disease morphologically differentiates the two disease
processes (Table 1). Figure 2 is a photomicrograph of a one micron
section of grey matter demonstrating the compact cytoplasmic accumulation of lipid within swollen neurons, a more dispersed accumulation

within the astrocytes and the deposition of lipid within the endothelial cells of a cerebral vessel. The cytoplasm of the neuronal
cells is pale, vacuolated and contains fine granules which are
positive for PAS, Oil Red O and Luxol fast blue; the nucleus is
often eccentrically displaced. Macrophages are abundant in the
neuropil which stain positively with the above lipid stains. Figure
3 is an electron photomicrograph showing that the neuronal lipid
accumulation is predominantly arranged as parallel or concentrically
lamellar membranes within the cytoplasmic lysosomes. In contrast,
smaller multivesicular bodies are predominantly seen within the
astrocytes (Figure 4) and similar multivesicular bodies are observed
in the capillary endothelium of the brain (Figure 5).

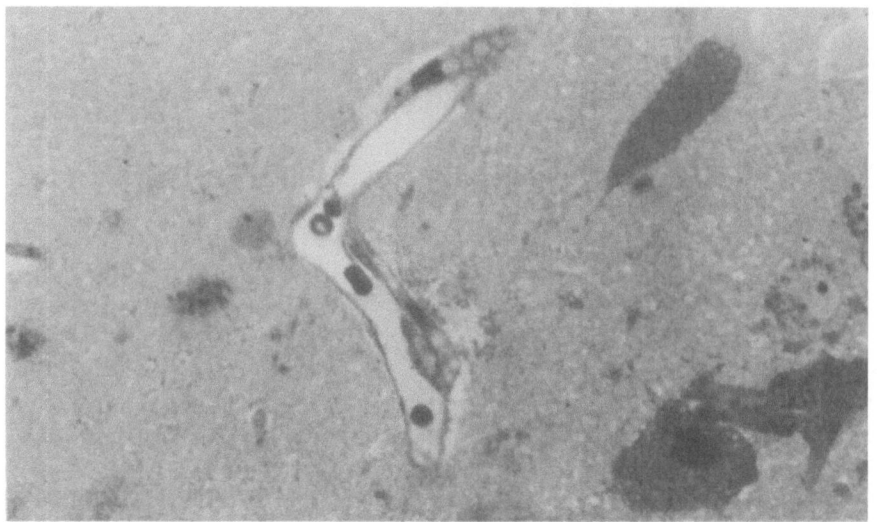

Figure 2. Photomicrograph exhibiting ballooned neurons in a one
micron section of cerebral grey matter from a one year old patient
with Sandhoff's disease, taken at the time of craniotomy. Closely
packed lipid spheres eccentrically displace the nucleus while a
more dispersed lipid accumulation is seen within the cytoplasm of
astrocytes. Lipid can also be visualized within blood vessel endothelium. X 500, Stained methylene blue-Azure II.

In the hepatocytes (Figure 6), lysosomes containing lamellar
structures, which eventually become as large as nuclei, are easily
demonstrated in one micron sections fixed in osmic acid and glutaraldehyde and subsequently stained with methylene blue-Azure II.
Unfortunately, the visceral lipid deposition is obscured during
formalin fixation, which presumably accounts for the previous
failure to recognize this disorder, even at autopsy. Figure 7 shows
the ultrastructure of a portion of the hepatocyte cytoplasm which

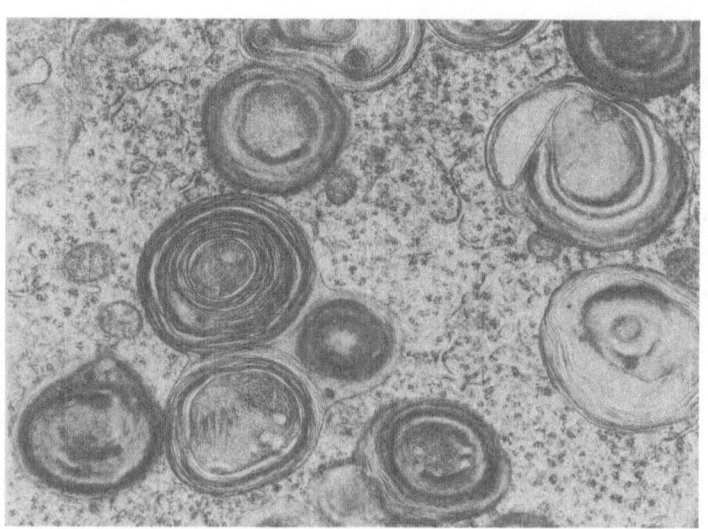

Figure 3. Electron micrograph of the cytoplasm of a neuron with its dispersed ribosomes. The abnormal lipid accumulation is arranged predominantly in a concentric lamellar configuration (membranous cytoplasmic bodies). X 31,700.

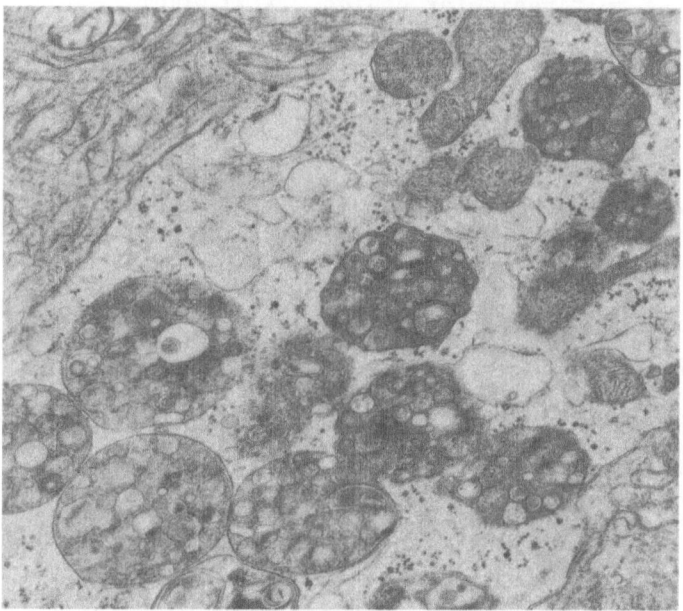

Figure 4. Electron micrograph of the cytoplasm of an astrocyte. The lipid accumulates predominantly in the form of multivesicular bodies. X 31,700.

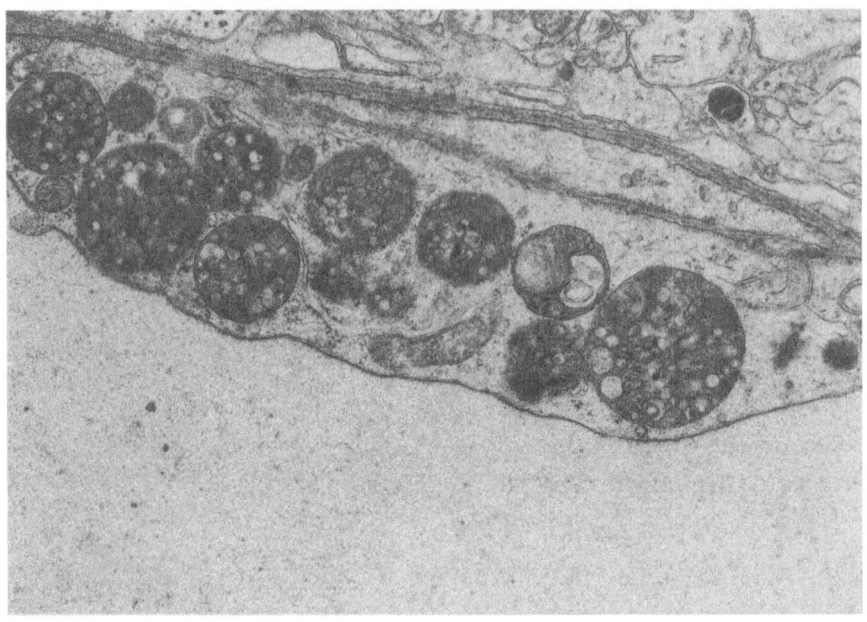

Figure 5. Electron micrograph of the vascular endothelium of a
blood vessel in cerebral grey matter. Lipid accumulation is visualized again as multivesicular bodies. X 31,700.

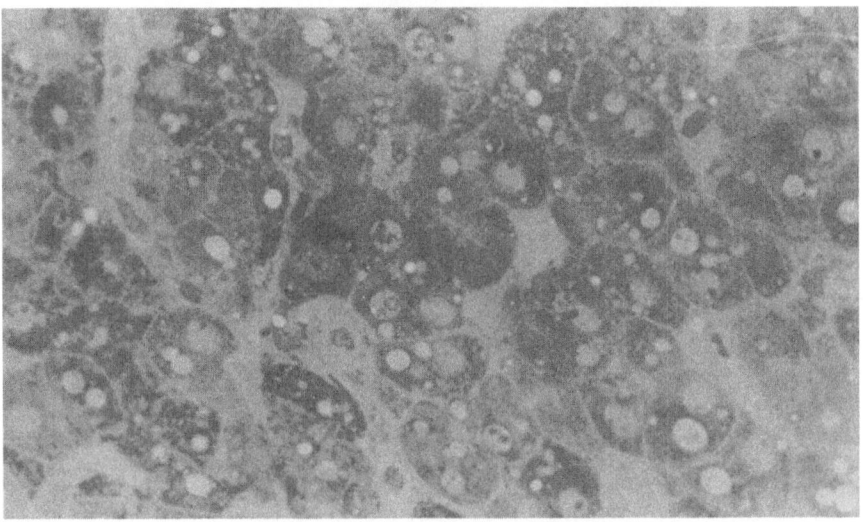

Figure 6. Photomicrograph of a one micron section of the hepatic
parenchyma. The cytoplasm contains variable-sized vacuoles, many
of which contain myelin figures. Only an occasional neutral lipid
droplet is seen. X 500, Stained methylene blue-Azure II.

reveals multiple lysosomes containing tightly laminated dense osmo-
philic structures against a background of finely particulate matter;
the glycogen rosettes, mitochondria, and endoplasmic reticulum appear
normal.   Figure 8 is an electron photomicrograph of tissue obtained
by rectal biopsy.   Although normal on light microscopy, ultrastructural examination of rectal tissue demonstrates both membranous
cytoplasmic and multivesicular bodies within the vascular endothelium
as well as in the neurons.   Essentially every tissue examined under
the electron microscope contains similar lipid accumulation.

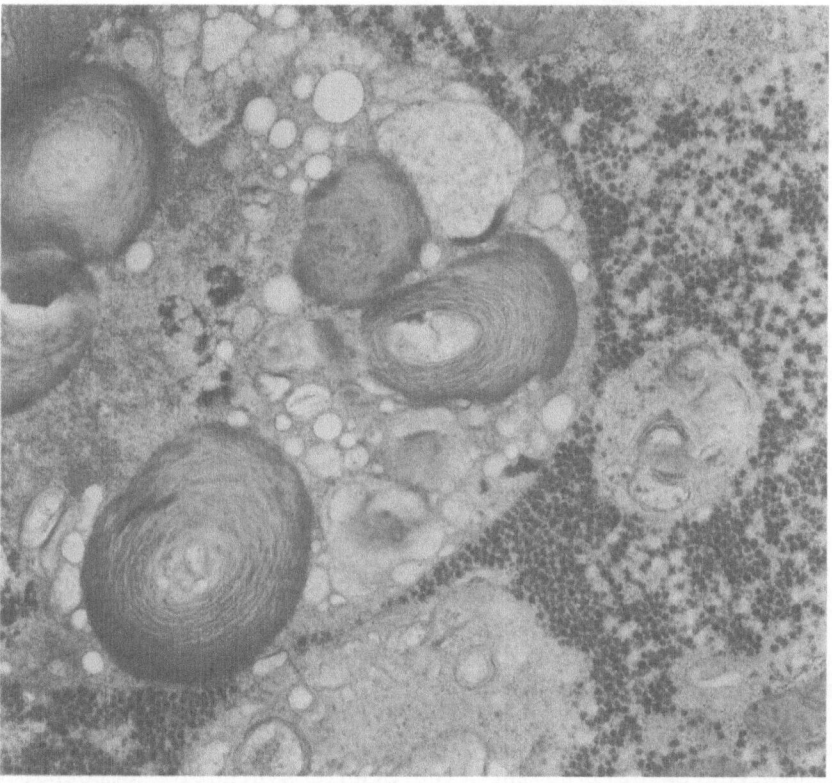

Figure 7.   Electron micrograph of a small portion of the hepatic
cell cytoplasm.   Very large lysosomes are present by one year of
age which contain tightly laminated concentric lipid configurations.
The lysosome also contains fine particulate matter; otherwise the
glycogen rosettes, mitochondria and rough and smooth endoplasmic
reticulum are normal in appearance.   X 22,600.

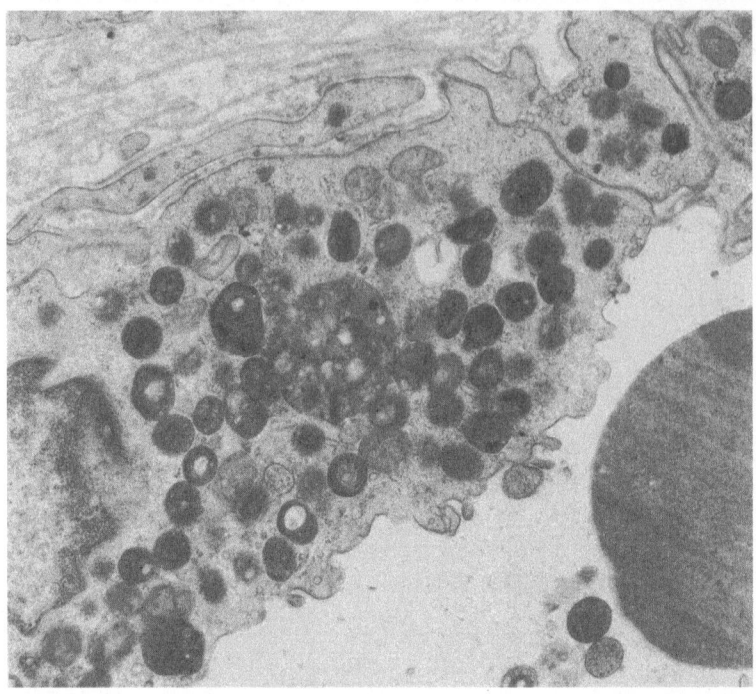

Figure 8.   Electron micrograph of a rectal blood vessel.   Lipid
accumulated in the endothelial wall as membranous cytoplasmic
bodies and multivesicular bodies.   A red blood cell is observable
in the lower right hand border.   X 22,600.

BIOCHEMICAL STUDIES

Materials and Methods

Previously reported methods were used for the collection and
determination of the glycosphingolipid concentrations in urinary
sediment (1,2) and plasma (27,28).   Hexosaminidase A and B activities
were determined in plasma and cultured skin fibroblasts by the
methods of O'Brien et al.(8) and Okada et al.(12), respectively;
these procedures utilize the fluorogenic synthetic compound, 4-
methylumbelliferyl-N-acetyl-β-D-glucosaminide, as enzyme substrate.

Hepatic tissue (4-17 mg wet weight) obtained by percutaneous
biopsy (23) was homogenized in 1.0 ml of 0.04 M citrate-phosphate
buffer, pH 4.4; 0.1 ml aliquots were diluted to 1.0 ml in the same
buffer and assayed by the plasma method.   Hepatic hexosaminidase

activity is expressed as nanomoles substrate cleaved per mg wet weight per hour. Platelets were isolated from fresh, citrated whole blood, twice washed with buffered saline (pH 7.4), and homogenized in 0.04 M citrate-phosphate buffer (pH 4.4). The reaction mixture totaled 150 microliters:50 μl of 1:10 diluted whole platelet homogenate and 100 μl of 1.0 mM fluorogenic substrate; the plasma methodology was used to assay the platelet reaction mixture. Protein was determined by the method of Lowry et al.(7) and the platelet hexosaminidase activity expressed as nanomoles substrate cleaved per mg protein per hour. Cerebrospinal fluid and the media from cultured fibroblasts were assayed by the plasma methodology and hexosaminidase activity expressed as nanomoles substrate cleaved per ml per hour.

Hexosaminidase A and B were concentrated from fresh normal plasma for subsequent infusion by the following procedure utilizing sterile technique. Fresh, heparinized plasma (500-750 ml) was fractionated with solid $(NH_4)_2SO_4$ to 33% saturation at 4°C. After 3 hours, the precipitated protein was removed by centrifugation (35,000 X g for 20 min.). The supernatant fraction was saved and solid $(NH_4)_2SO_4$ was added to 60% saturation. After centrifugation as above, the precipitate was dissolved in a minimal volume of sterile distilled water and exhaustively dialyzed for 48 hours at 4°C. against multiple changes of sterile distilled water. The dialysate was concentrated under N_2 with a Diaflo ultrafiltration apparatus to a final volume of 70-75 ml. Following millipore filtration, an aliquot of the concentrate was pyrogen tested (5). The final concentrate, which contained 60-65% of the original plasma hexosaminidase A and B activities in 10% of the original volume, had less than 1 μg/ml $(NH_4)_2SO_4$, 140-150 meq/L of sodium, 8-16 gm % protein, and was pyrogen free.

Fresh whole plasma (100 ml) or the fractionated plasma concentrate (75 ml) was infused into the patient over a 2-hour period. Blood samples (200 μl) for plasma enzymatic assay were obtained by hourly heel puncture before, during and for 6 hours after infusion, then every 2 hours for 18 hours, and subsequently, every 24 hours for seven days. Plasma hexosaminidase activity was assayed immediately and aliquots were frozen for subsequent analyses. Blood was obtained for plasma glycosphingolipid determinations before and either 8 or 24 hours post-infusion. Daily 24-hour urinary sediment collections were obtained during the infusion studies for glycosphingolipid analyses.

Results

The diagnosis of Sandhoff's disease and its differentiation from Tay-Sachs disease requires biochemical documentation. Thus, the biochemical diagnosis of this disorder can be easily accomplished by the demonstration of (1) the accumulation of the glycosphingolipid substrate, globoside (NAcgal-gal-gal-glc-ceramide), in urinary sediment (1,6) or plasma (6) and/or (2) the deficient activities of the enzymes, hexosaminidase A and B (6,8,10,12,22-24) in various tissues and fluids.

Urinary sediment glycosphingolipid analysis provides a simple screening procedure for the biochemical diagnosis of various glycosphingolipidoses (1,2), including Sandhoff's disease. Figure 9 is a thin layer chromatogram of the urinary sediment glycosphingolipids from a patient with Sandhoff's disease and her twin brother; the significant visceral accumulation of globoside (GL-4) is diagnostic of Sandhoff's disease (2) and therefore, differentiates this disorder from Tay-Sachs disease. Subsequent quantitation of the urinary sediment globoside demonstrates levels 10-50 fold greater than normal control levels (2).

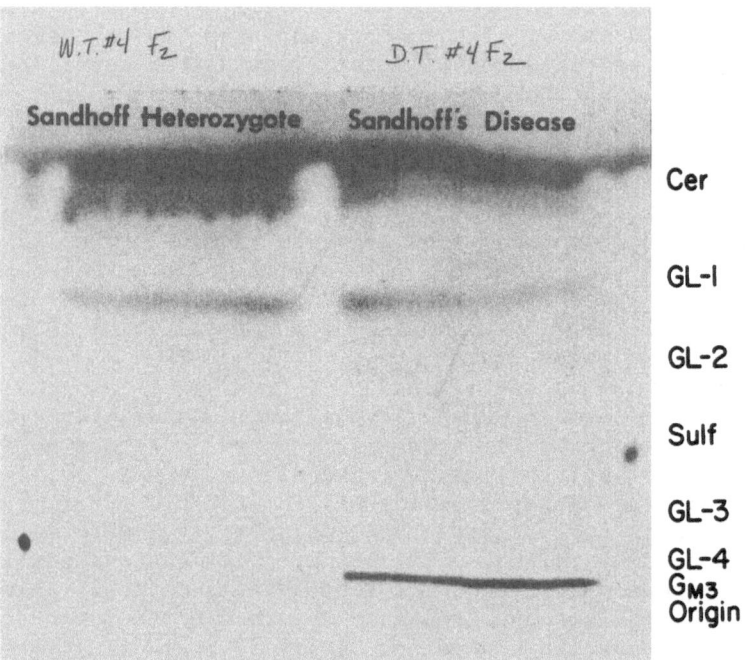

Figure 9. Thin-layer chromatogram of 24-hour urinary sediment glycosphingolipids from a homozygote and heterozygote for Sandhoff's disease at age 4 months, demonstrating the diagnostic accumulation of globoside (GL-4) in the sediment of the homozygote.

Table 2 indicates the total hexosaminidase activity in the plasma, platelets, cerebrospinal fluid, liver and cultured skin fibroblasts from a homozygote and heterozygotes for Sandhoff's disease and appropriate age-matched controls. Consistently, in each

Table 2. TOTAL HEXOSAMINIDASE ACTIVITY IN VARIOUS TISSUES FROM HOMOZYGOTES AND HETEROZYGOTES WITH SANDHOFF'S DISEASE AND NORMAL CONTROLS

	Plasma (nm/ml/hr)	Platelets (nm/mg protein/hr)	CSF (nm/ml/hr)	Liver (nm/mg wet tissue/hr)	Cultured Skin Fibroblasts (nm/mg/wet cells/hr)
Homozygote, D.T.	32	5.7	11	0.9	13.4
Heterozygote, W.T.	886			118	166
Normal Infant Control Mean and Range	1,731 1,040-2,720 (n=12)	280 197-377 (n=6)	152 113-194 (n=6)	236 164-295 (n=6)	274 212-376 (n=6)
Adult Heterozygotes					
T.T., Father	296			48	
J.T., Mother	600			81	
Normal Adult Control Mean and Range	661 430-1,160 (n=19)			99 93-106 (n=6)	

of these sources, the deficient hexosaminidase A and B activities could be demonstrated in the homozygote.

Figure 10 shows the pedigree of an informative family in which two children had Sandhoff's disease, their respective levels of total plasma hexosaminidase activity, and the percent of hexosaminidase B activity. When compared to age-matched controls, the father and the male twin could be easily identified as heterozygotes. However, the plasma enzymatic activities of the mother, an obligate heterozygote, were within the adult normal range, suggesting that the plasma assay is not totally reliable for heterozygote identification.

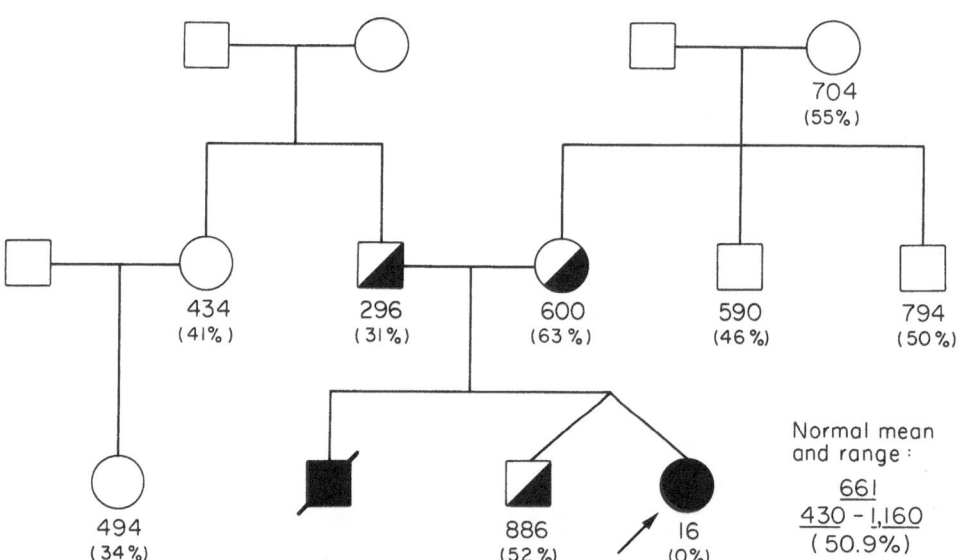

Figure 10. Pedigree of a family with Sandhoff's disease indicating the plasma total hexosaminidase activities and percent hexosaminidase B for various members.

Therefore, the hexosaminidase activities were determined in hepatic tissue obtained by percutaneous biopsy from the family members. Table 3 demonstrates the intermediate levels of hexosaminidase activity in both the mother and father and a significant decrease in the percent of hexosaminidase B activity, respectively; these values are compatible with the parents'obligate heterozygosity. The intermediate level of total hepatic hexosaminidase activity confirmed the plasma heterozygote identification of the male twin (W.T.) when compared to the levels of normal infantile hexosaminidase activity.

Table 3. LIVER HEXOSAMINIDASE A AND B ACTIVITY IN HOMOZYGOTES AND
HETEROZYGOTES WITH SANDHOFF'S DISEASE AND NORMAL CONTROLS

Patients	Total A and B Activity (nmoles A & B/mg wet tissue/hr)	% B Activity
Homozygote, D.T.	0.9	0
Heterozygote, W.T.	118	34.5
Normal Infant Control Mean and Range (n=6)	236 (164-295)	35.4 (33.0-37.7)
Adult Heterozygotes		
T.T., Father	48	19.2
J.T., Mother	81	21.8
Normal Adult Control Mean and Range (n=6)	99 (99-106)	34.0 (32.4-36.6)

The patient with Sandhoff's disease was placed on a galactose-
free dietary regimen in order to test the hypothesis (13) that the
rate of accumulation of galactose-containing glycosphingolipid substrates might be decreased. Plasma levels of glycosphingolipids
were determined with the patient on a regular infantile diet for
five months, and subsequently on a galactose-free diet for three
months. Figure 11 shows the concentration of plasma globoside and
the percent globoside of total plasma galactosphingolipids (lactosyl
+ trihexosyl + tetrahexosyl ceramides + G_{m3} ganglioside) during
regular and galactose-free dietary regimens. Although a sharp decrease in the plasma globoside level occurred three days after initiation of the galactose-free diet, the levels of globoside did not
remain decreased and, in fact, progressively increased during this
period. The percent globoside of total galactosphingolipid was not
significantly different during either dietary regimen.

Sandhoff's disease provides the unique opportunity to attempt
enzyme replacement in a disorder in which two enzymatic activities
are deficient. Enzyme replacement studies were carried out by infusion of fresh, whole plasma and fractionated plasma concentrates
containing the active hexosaminidases. The results of analyses for
total hexosaminidase activity in the plasma of the recipient after
four separate enzyme infusions are shown in Figure 12. Maximal
enzymatic activity for each infusion occurred immediately following
infusion (0 hour), and attained levels expected from dilution of the
enzymatic activity infused in the recipient's blood volume. The
enzymatic activity decreased rapidly with a $T_{1/2}$ of approximately
2-4 hours. Infusion of the fractionated plasma concentrates resulted
in maximal enzymatic activity 60 to 195 percent greater than that
attained with fresh, whole plasma in similar volumes. Detectable
enzymatic activity above pre-infusion levels was not observed after

30 hours post-infusion. The hexosaminidase B activity was approximately 50% of the total hexosaminidase activity, reflecting the percentage in the infused plasma.

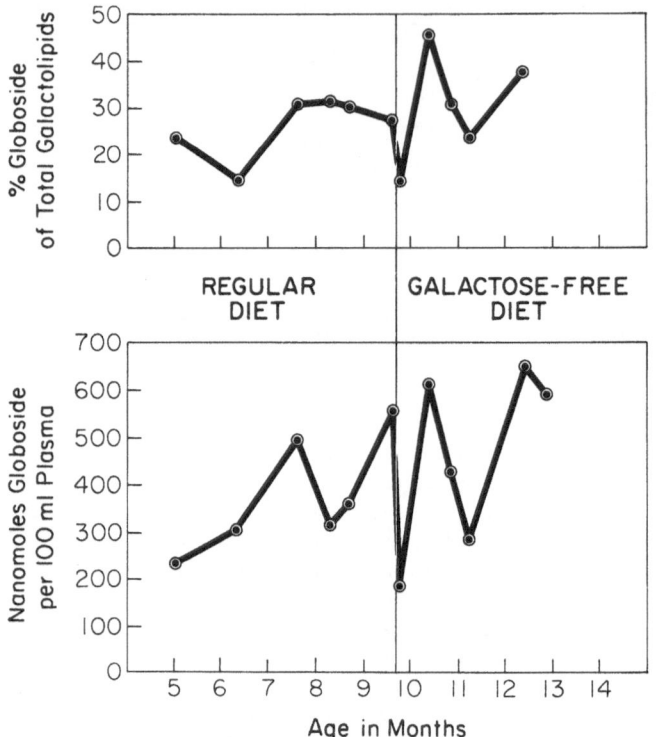

Figure 11. Changes in the concentration of plasma globoside (NAcgal-gal-gal-glc-ceramide) and percent globoside of the total plasma galactosphingolipids in a homozygote with Sandhoff's disease during regular and galactose-free dietary regimens.

Table 4 indicates the changes in the plasma glycosphingolipid concentrations 24 hours post-infusion of the whole plasma (Infusion 1, Figure 12) and 8 hours post-infusion of the fractionated plasma concentrate (Infusion 3, Figure 12). A significant increase in the levels of the glycosphingolipids distal to the enzymatic blocks was demonstrated after both infusions (Table 4). The levels of hematoside (G_{m3} ganglioside), which is a product of hexosaminidase A activity (18) were increased over pre-infusion levels by 44 and 39% at 8 and 24 hours post-infusion, respectively. The levels of trihexosyl ceramide, the product of hexosaminidase A and B activity (22), were increased over pre-infusion levels by greater than 100% after both infusions. Furthermore, the levels of plasma glucosyl ceramide, the common catabolic product of both enzymes, were increased 71 and 442% at 8 and 24 hours post-infusion, respectively.

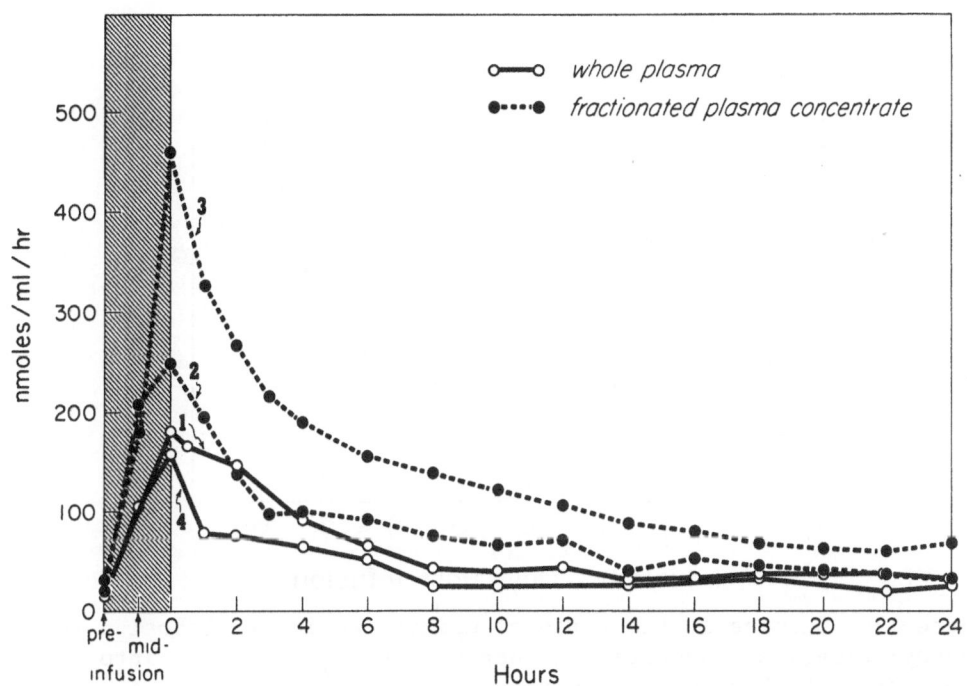

Figure 12. Enzyme replacement studies in Sandhoff's disease: plasma total hexosaminidase activities in a homozygote with Sandhoff's disease after infusions of normal whole plasma (Infusions 1 and 4) and fractionated plasma concentrates (Infusions 2 and 3). Enzymatic activity is expressed as nanomoles of substrate hydrolyzed per milliliter of plasma per hour.

Table 4. CHANGES IN PLASMA GLYCOSPHINGOLIPID CONCENTRATIONS PRE- AND POST-INFUSION IN A HOMOZYGOTE WITH SANDHOFF'S DISEASE

	Whole Plasma Infusion 24 hrs Post-Infusion % Change	Plasma Concentrate Infusion 8 hrs Post-Infusion % Change
Glucosyl Ceramide	+ 442	+ 71
Lactosyl Ceramide	− 7	+ 102
Trihexosyl Ceramide	+ 139	+ 110
Tetrahexosyl Ceramide	+ 27	− 32
Hematoside	+ 390	+ 44

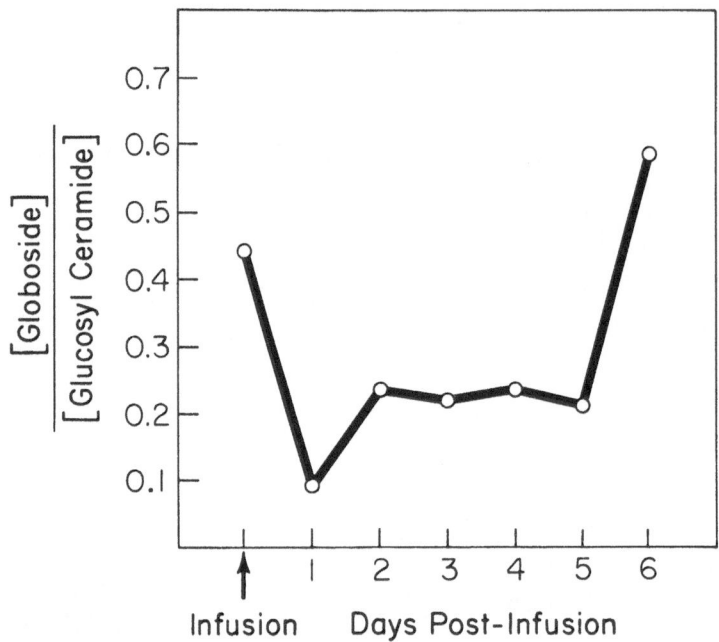

Figure 13.   Changes in the ratio of urinary sediment globoside to
glucosyl ceramide concentrations during a plasma infusion into a
homozygote with Sandhoff's disease.

      The glycosphingolipid levels were determined in urinary sedi-
ment collected daily during an infusion study. Figure 13 indicates
the changes in the ratio of globoside to glucosyl ceramide concentrations for six days following a plasma infusion. The ratio significantly decreases on days one through five following infusion and
returns to pre-infusion levels on the sixth day. These data indicate
a decrease in the urinary sediment globoside concentration and a
concomitant increase in the level of glucosyl ceramide; these results
are compatible with active hexosaminidases catabolizing accumulated
renal globoside.

                              DISCUSSION

      Sandhoff's disease is an autosomal recessive inborn error of
glycosphingolipid metabolism resulting from the deficient activities
of N-acetyl-β-hexosaminidase A and B. Clinical manifestations of
this disorder are very similar to those in Tay-Sachs disease, a
related glycosphingolipidosis, and their distinction requires biochemical and/or morphologic confirmation. In both diseases, hexosaminidase A activity is deficient, resulting in the predominantly
neural deposition of G_{m2} ganglioside and its asialo derivative; the

deposition of these glycosphingolipids in cerebral tissue is manifested by similar neurological symptoms in both disorders. The
visceral manifestations in Sandhoff's disease result from the concomitant deficiency of hexosaminidase B activity and the subsequent
visceral accumulation of its glycosphingolipid substrates, asialo-
G_{m2} and globoside.

Ultrastructural examination of all tissues obtained from
patients with Sandhoff's disease reveals significant lysosomal lipid
deposition (6,25). In cerebral grey matter, the neurons contain
predominantly membranous cytoplasmic bodies, whereas multivesicular
bodies are more abundant in astrocytes. The cerebral blood vessel
endothelium contains both multivesicular and membranous cytoplasmic
bodies. This ultrastructural observation may be related to the
cardiovascular pathology which occurs in Sandhoff's, but not in
Tay-Sachs disease; the significant lipid deposition in vascular
endothelium may result from endothelial cell glycosphingolipid synthesis and/or pinocytosis of the accumulated globoside from the
plasma of these patients.

In the hepatocyte lysosomes, lipid accumulation progresses with
age; the hepatic lysosomes were twice normal size at three months of
age and by one year of age, many of these lysosomes were distended
by membranous lipid deposits to a diameter equal to that of the
hepatic cell nucleus (6). Although no specific ultrastructural
change was observed, the extensiveness, size and variation of the
membranous lipid deposits within the lysosomes, particularly in the
hepatocytes, were different than that occurring in other storage
diseases described in the literature. It is important to note that
routine formalin fixation obscures the visceral lipid accumulation;
however, one micron sections fixed for electron microscopy and
stained with methylene blue-Azure II reveal the visceral lysosomal
lipid deposition by light microscopy.

The biochemical diagnosis of homozygous individuals with Sandhoff's disease can easily be made in patients presenting with the
clinical symptomatology of Tay-Sachs disease, especially in non-
Jewish patients. Markedly increased levels of globoside in urinary
sediment and plasma will diagnose affected individuals; no increase
in the levels of globoside was found in the urinary sediment of
patients with Tay-Sachs disease. Determination of hexosaminidase A
and B activities, using synthetic substrates, in biopsied tissue,
peripheral leukocytes, platelets, cerebrospinal fluid, cultured
skin fibroblasts or plasma of suspected individuals will confirm the
diagnosis. Heterozygosity for the Sandhoff gene can be more reliably detected by the hexosaminidase activities in tissue than in
plasma (23). Appropriate age-matched controls must be assayed for
accurate heterozygote identification. Heterozygous individuals can
be detected by the above enzymatic techniques or by the demonstration

of morphologic changes in biopsied hepatic or rectal tissue.

Based on tissue culture galactose incorporation studies, it has been postulated (13) that a galactose-free diet might decrease the rate of synthesis and subsequent accumulation of galactosphingo- lipids in disorders in which these lipids cannot be catabolized. Therefore, a galactose-free dietary regimen was initiated in a patient with Sandhoff's disease. The results indicated a progres- sive increase in the levels of plasma globoside with age. Presum- ably, the other metabolic sources of galactose, i.e. epimerase conversion of glucose to galactose, provided sufficient endogenous galactose for galactosphingolipid synthesis.

Enzyme replacement studies were carried out in the patient with Sandhoff's disease; these studies were not considered therapeutic but an extension of the biochemical and physiologic studies of this disorder. The levels of maximal enzymatic activity attained were consistent with those expected from dilution of the enzymatic acti- vity infused in the recipient's blood volume. Enzymatic activity decreased rapidly suggesting possible compartmentalization of the active enzyme. The changes in the plasma glycosphingolipid concen- trations indicated active substrate catabolism by the infused enzymes. Urinary sediment was obtained before and following an enzyme replace- ment study to determine possible changes in the glycosphingolipids of desquamated kidney cells. A decrease in the ratio of globoside to glucosyl ceramide, the substrate and distal catabolic product of hexosaminidase A and B activities, was demonstrated one to five days post-infusion, returning to pre-infusion levels on the sixth day. These data suggest that the active enzyme might enter renal cells and catabolize the accumulated kidney globoside. Subsequently, these cells would be desquamated into the urine and their globoside concentration quantified by urinary sediment lipid analysis. These findings are supported by previous studies demonstrating the ability of enzymes to enter cells in vivo (4) and in culture (15).

The nature of the genetic defects in Sandhoff's and Tay-Sachs diseases has been the subject of recent speculation (24,26). We would propose another model for the explanation of these enzymatic deficiencies on the molecular level. This model requires the basic assumption that the enzymes, hexosaminidase A and B, are multimers, and have at least one common glycopolypeptide or polypeptide subunit, denoted O. Each enzyme has at least one other different subunit; thus, hexosaminidase A has polypeptide subunits O and A and hexo- saminidase B has subunits O and B.

It has been recently demonstrated using natural substrates (22) that both hexosaminidase A and B are catabolically active on asialo- G_{m2} and globoside and that only hexosaminidase A hydrolyzes the terminal hexosamine from G_{m2} ganglioside. Thus, in Tay-Sachs disease, the deficient hexosaminidase A activity and increased hexosaminidase B activity accounts for the marked accumulation of G_{m2} ganglioside and the lesser accumulation of its asialo derivative. On the molecular level, it is suggested that Tay-Sachs disease results from an autosomal structural mutation in the A subunit rendering hexosaminidase A catabolically inactive on natural and synthetic substrates.

It is proposed that in Sandhoff's disease, the genetic defect is a single autosomal structural mutation in the common 0 subunit, which alters the active sites of both hexosaminidase A and B and renders these enzymes non-catalytic on both natural and synthetic substrates. These deficiencies are consistent with the systemic deposition of G_{m2} ganglioside, its asialo derivative and globoside, the glycosphingolipid substrates which accumulate in Sandhoff's disease.

Recently, Sandhoff (17,22) has reported another variant of Tay-Sachs disease also characterized by the accumulation of G_{m2} ganglioside, asialo-G_{m2} and globoside. Hexosaminidase A and B were only partially active on natural substrates, but when artificial substrates were utilized, the activities of both hexosaminidase A and B were significantly increased over normal levels. It is suggested that the structural defect in the new variant results from an amino acid substitution in the common 0 subunit. However, this mutation is located at a site which alters the catalytic activity of both enzymes toward natural substrates, leading to decreased reaction velocities. This results in the accumulation of the respective glycosphingolipid substrates. The cells respond to this lipid accumulation by increasing the number and area of lysosomal membranes with a concomitant increase in the activity of lysosomal enzymes per gram of tissue. Presumably, these partially catalytic hexosaminidases also are increased in quantity. Thus, if the mutant conformation of the 0 subunit can result in normal catalytic activity towards synthetic substrates, an apparent increase of hexosaminidase activities would result. This is consistent with the observed biochemical findings in this new variant and a single structural mutation.

REFERENCES

1. Desnick, R.J., Dawson, G., Desnick, S.J., Sweeley, C.C. and Krivit, W. New Eng. J. Med., 284:739, 1971.

2. Desnick, R.J., Sweeley, C.C., and Krivit, W. J.Lipid Res., 11:31, 1970.

3. Grégoire, P.E., Jonniaux, G., Loeb, H., Voet, W., and Capelle,R.
    Rev. Franc. Etud. Clin. Biol., 14:568, 1969.

4. Hug, G. and Schubert, W.K., J. Cell Biol., 35:1, 1967.

5. Kim, Y.B. and Watson, D.N. J. Exp. Med., 131:161, 1970.

6. Krivit, W., Desnick, R.J., Lee, J., Wright, F., Sweeley, C.C.,
    Snyder, P.D., and Sharp, H.L. Amer. J. Med., in press.

7. Lowry, O.H., Rosebrough, N.J. Farr, R.L. and Randall, R.J.,
    J. Biol. Chem., 193:265, 1951.

8. O'Brien, J.S., Okada, S., Chen, A. and Fillerup, D.L. New Eng.
    J. Med., 283:15, 1970.

9. O'Brien, J.S., Okada, S., Ho, M.W., Fillerup, D.L., Veath, M.L.
    and Adams, K. in Lipid Storage Diseases, Bernsohn, J. and
    Grossman, H.J., editors, New York: Academic Press, Inc., 1971,
    p. 225-273.

10. O'Brien, J.S., Okada, S., Ho, M.W., Fillerup, D.L., Veath, M.L.
    and Adams, K. Fed. Proc., 30:956, 1971.

11. Okada, S., and O'Brien, J.S. Science, 165:698, 1969.

12. Okada, S., Veath, M.L., Leroy, J. and O'Brien, J.S. Amer. J.
    Human Genet., 23:55, 1971.

13. Philippart, M. Proceedings of the Soc. for Ped. Res., 1971,
    p. 61. Presented at the Soc. for Ped. Res., April, 1971,
    Atlantic City, New Jersey.

14. Pilz, H., Müller, D., Sandhoff, K. and Ter Meulen, V. Deut.
    Med. Wochschr., 93:1833, 1968.

15. Porter, M.T., Fluharty, A.L. and Kihara, H. Science, 172:1263,
    1971.

16. Rodriquez-Torres, R., Schneck, L. and Kleinberg, W. Bull. N.Y.
    Acad. Med., 47:717, 1971.

17. Sandhoff, K. FEBS Lett., 4:351, 1969.

18. Sandhoff, K. FEBS Lett., 11:342, 1970.

19. Sandhoff, K., Andreae, U. and Jatzkewitz, H. Path. Europ.,
    3:278, 1968.

20. Sandhoff, K., Andreae, U. and Jatzkewitz, H. Life Sciences, 1:283, 1968.

21. Sandhoff, K. Jatzkewitz, H. and Peters, G. Naturwissenschäften, 56:356, 1969.

22. Sandhoff, K., Harzer, K., Wässle, W. and Jatzkewitz, H. J. Neurochem., in press.

23. Sharp, H.L. and Desnick, R.J. Gastroenterology, 60:752, 1971.

24. Snyder, P.D., Krivit, W. and Sweeley, C.C. J. Lipid Res., in press.

25. Suzuki, Y., Jacob, J.C., Suzuki, K., Kutty, K.M. and Suzuki, K. Neurol., 21:313, 1971.

26. Tateson, R. and Bain, A.D. Lancet, ii:612, 1971.

27. Vance, D.E. and Sweeley, C.C. J. Lipid Res., 8:621, 1967.

28. Vance, D.E., Krivit, W. and Sweeley, C.C. J. Lipid Res., 10:188, 1969.

ACKNOWLEDGMENTS

We are indebted to Miss Linda Kern and Mr. Mohanreddy Raman for their excellent technical assistance.

This investigation was supported in part by research grants (CA 11996, CA 07306, CA 08101, CA 08832 and AM 14470) from the National Institutes of Health, a grant (RR-400) from the General Clinical Research Centers Program of the Division of Research Resources, National Institutes of Health, a grant (CRES-259) from the National Foundation, a grant (71-778) from the American Heart Association, a grant from the National Cystic Fibrosis Research Foundation, a grant from the Thomey Lipid Diseases Research Fund, University of Minnesota and graduate school grants from the University of Minnesota.

BIOCHEMICAL STUDIES ON G$_{M1}$-GANGLIOSIDOSIS AND CERAMIDE TRIHEXOSIDOSIS

L. S. Wolfe, J. T. R. Clarke and R. G. Senior

The Donner Laboratory of Experimental Neurochemistry,
Montreal Neurological Institute, McGill University,
Montreal, Canada.

G$_{M1}$-GANGLIOSIDOSIS

Two clinical forms of G$_{M1}$-gangliosidosis are now recognized (9,15,25). In Type I (generalized gangliosidosis) the disease is apparent at birth or soon after and mental and motor retardation progress rapidly to cause death before two years of age. This is associated with an abnormal facial appearance, prominent hepatosplenomegaly and marked skeletal abnormalities. In Type II (late infantile or juvenile G$_{M1}$-gangliosidosis), the disease onsets after 6 months and although the psychomotor deterioration is similar to Type I it progresses more slowly, and death can occur anytime between 3 and 10 years. There is little characteristic about the child's appearance, the liver and spleen are not enlarged unduly and the skeletal abnormalities are minor, although in recent reports they are possibly of diagnostic value. O'Brien has recently reviewed the clinical and biochemical abnormalities in this disease (15). In both types, G$_{M1}$-ganglioside and its asialo-derivative accumulate in greatly increased amounts in brain and peripheral neurones in intracellular organelles with very similar properties and appearance to the membranous cytoplasmic bodies seen in Tay Sachs disease (19,20). G$_{M1}$-ganglioside is also present in increased quantities in non-neural tissues (liver, spleen, cultured fibroblasts) in both types but the visceral accumulation is much more marked in the Type I form (3,15,20,25). β-Galactosyl hydrolase activity (pH 4-5) to artificial substrates and to G$_{M1}$-ganglioside is greatly diminished (1-5% of normal) in the brain of both types. However, in the liver, in leukocytes and in cultured fibroblasts the deficiency of this enzyme activity is greater in the Type I than in the Type II form. The two clinical types appear to be determined by different mutant genes affecting the activity of β-galactosyl hydrolases (16). Different tissues have different complements of this group of lysosomal hydrolases to specific lipid or non-lipid substrates. The precise differences in β-galactosyl hydrolase activity in the two types of diseases towards a variety of natural substrates is at present unknown. Present evidence suggests that β-galactosyl hydrolase activity specifically to terminal galactose molecules β-linked glycosidically to N-acetyl hexosamine whether in glycolipids or in glycoproteins is the basic enzyme deficiency in both forms of the disease.

Glycopeptide Accumulation in G_{M1}-gangliosidosis

A characteristic histopathological feature of routine preparations of the liver and kidney in G_{M1}-gangliosidosis is the presence of a marked vacuolization of the liver parenchymal cells and the renal tubular epithelium (9). Further, the ultrastructure of material accumulating in histiocytes in the liver is markedly different to that seen in neurones. This led Suzuki in 1968 to investigate further the chemical pathology of the liver and spleen. Non-lipid hexosamine and galactose was increased greatly over normal although there was considerable variability from case to case (18). A highly water soluble mucopolysaccharide fraction was isolated from delipidized liver which contained predominantly glucosamine and galactose in approximately equal amounts and small amounts of mannose, galactosamine and fucose (18,20). On the basis of the carbohydrate composition and electrophoretic mobility, Suzuki suggested this material was like skeletal keratan sulfate, but markedly undersulfated. In addition a sialomucopolysaccharide was found in the ganglioside fraction which also contained mainly glucosamine and galactose (20). These compounds were not found in brain. Our studies at this time showed that in Type II G_{M1}-gangliosidosis the urine contained abnormal quantities of glycopeptides, not precipitable by cetyl pyridinium chloride which contained predominantly glucosamine and galactose with negligible uronic acid, sialic acid (9.5% by wt.) and very little sulfate (25). At that time we regarded this material as undersulfated keratan sulfate-like glycopeptides. The excessive excretion of the keratan sulfate-like glycopeptides has also been confirmed in the Type I form (17). We then obtained frozen liver samples of a Type I case and found that it also contained greatly increased amounts (25-30 mg/gm wet wt.) of glucosamine and galactose-containing glycopeptides (2). A convenient method was found for separating and isolating a major proportion of these compounds without resorting to multiple enzyme digestions. If the liver was simply homogenized in 10 rather than 20 volumes of chloroform-methanol (2:1 by vol.) because of their high water solubility, the bulk of these glycopeptides partitioned into the upper aqueous phase along with the gangliosides. The gangliosides could be completely removed by repeated extractions of the dried material with dry chloroform-methanol (2:1) in which the glycopeptides were insoluble. Subsequent fractionations on DEAE-Sephadex and Biogel P-10, P-4, and P-2 columns showed that we were dealing with glucosamine and galactose-containing glycopeptides of molecular weights from 2000 - 10,000. Approximately 50% of the fraction had molecular weights estimated by molecular sieve chromatography of 2000-4000. The compositions of these fractions were all very similar; glucosamine and hexose (mainly galactose) in almost equimolar proportions, no fucose, approximately 5% N-acetyl-neuraminic acid, negligible sulfate and 2-9% protein. We hypothesized that these glycopeptides were derived from the partial degradation of skeletal keratan sulfate which had been desulfated enzymatically but the carbohydrate chain could not be metabolized further due to the absence of β-galactosyl hydrolases which normally removed galactose units at chain termini or branch points. We suggested that this defect may account for the skeletal abnormalities seen particularly in the Type I form of the disease (3,25).

We now realize that the situation is much more complex and these conclusions were premature. Our evidence published last year was not adequate to implicate the keratan sulfates as the sole source of the glycopeptide accumulations in G_{MI}-gangliosidosis liver. Several other glycoproteins contain multiple N-acetyl-glucosamine-galactose units. Therefore, we decided to re-examine in more detail the structure of the various glycopeptide fractions. We needed considerably more material than was available in our previous studies, and were fortunate to get further pieces of frozen liver post-mortem from G_{MI}-gangliosidosis Type I cases from Dr. J. A. Lowden, Hospital for Sick Children, Toronto, Dr. Irwin Schafer, Dept. of Pediatrics, University Hospitals of Cleveland, and from a new case diagnosed at the Montreal Children's Hospital. We report here our preliminary findings on a glycopeptide fraction isolated from the aqueous Folch upper phases in these cases.

The yield of the unfractionated glycopeptide fractions freed of gangliosides was 6-10 mg/gm wet weight. After chromatography on Biogel P-10 the glycopeptide fractions from each of the three cases showed similar profiles. A small anthrone positive peak was observed at the void volume followed by an incompletely resolved peak at Ve/Vo (elution vol./void vol.) 2.37 and a major peak at 3.25 representing 60 percent of the material applied to the column. This major fraction (150 mg) from the liver of one case (K-2B) was used for the analyses reported here. The retention properties on Biogel P-4 columns indicated that the apparent M.W. was 2000. The glycopeptides were non-reducing. They showed no MN or AB blood group activity. The specific optical rotation was $[\alpha]_D^{24}$ = +1.5 (c=2.4, H_2O) compatible with all β-linked sugars. The composition of the fraction which accounts for 86% of the dry weight is shown in Table I.

Table I. Analysis of glycopeptide fraction K-2B

	μmoles/gm
Gal	1253
Man	1000
GlcNAc	1812
GalNAc	trace
NeuNAc	76
fuc	0
glc	0
xyl	0
uronic acid (carbazole)	0
sulfate (benzidine)	trace
Lowry protein (% by wt)	(9.0)

We decided to carry out periodate oxidation (Smith degradation) steps on this glycopeptide fraction. Our reasoning was that
if the glycopeptide fraction contained essentially straight chain
repeating GlcNAc - Gal units linked as in desulfated keratan sulfates then it should not be markedly degraded by periodate oxidation except for one terminal sugar on each chain (11). If significantly more periodate was consumed than expected for keratan sulfates, then either the glycopeptide is more branched with more
terminal sugars or the linkages are other than through the 3
position of galactose or the 3 or 4 positions of N-acetylglucosamine. The sequential periodate (Smith) degradation procedure we
used was based on that of Jamieson, Jett and DeBernardo (13).
Glycopeptide fraction K-2B was oxidized by 15 mM sodium meta-
periodate for 12 hours at 37°. The excess periodate was determined spectrophotometrically before being consumed by 50% aqueous
ethylene glycol and the oxidized sample reduced with a 10-fold
excess of sodium borohydride at 4° buffered to pH 8.0 with borate
buffer. The excess borohydride was destroyed by the addition of
acetic acid and the sample desalted on a Biogel P-4 column. The
appropriate carbohydrate-containing eluate was hydrolysed in 0.1 N
H_2SO_4 at 37° for 5 hours, neutralized and separated on another
Biogel P-4 column. The changes in the carbohydrate composition of
glycopeptide fraction K-2B after two steps of periodate oxidation
expressed in terms of molar ratios of constituent based on mannose
as 2.0 are shown in Table II. These results are consistent with
an empirical formulation of the carbohydrate chain as $Man_2GlcNAc_4Gal_3$
before periodate oxidation becoming $Man_2GlcNAc_4$ after the first Smith
degradation and $Man_2GlcNAc$ after the second associated with appropriate molecular weight changes as seen by the elution volumes on
Biogel P-4. The first Smith degradation consumed 3.4 μmoles of
periodate/mg material and gave rise to 1.85 μmoles of formate.
The amount of formate formed was sufficient to account for the
periodate consumed. Thus, the first step destroyed terminal neutral
hexoses exclusively and this hexose was galactose. If the apparent

Table II. Molar ratio of components of glycopeptide K-2B
after sequential periodate oxidations

	Before Periodate	1st Step	2nd Step
Man	2.0	2.0	2.0
Gal	2.6	0.2	0.2
GlcNAc	3.7	3.8	0.6
Biogel P-4, Ve/Vo	1.4	1.6	1.7

molecular weight estimated from elution volumes from Biogel columns
is around 2000, then three moles of galactose were destroyed. In
the second Smith degradation 2.0 μmoles/mg of periodate were consumed. Since terminal N-acetylated hexosamines consume 1 mole of
periodate/mole then the consumption can account for a loss of three
moles of hexosamine leaving 1 mole unattacked. No mannose was
oxidized.

We conclude from these results that a quantitatively important proportion of the glycopeptide accumulation in G_{M1}-gangliosidosis
liver is due to a class of compounds which are highly branched. The
periodate oxidation experiments do not suggest structures like undersulfated skeletal or corneal keratan sulfates. The polysaccharide
structure contains terminal galactose (possibly 3) subterminal
N-acetylglucosamine (possibly 3) and a core of two mannose units
and one N-acetylglucosamine. These structural features resemble
an MN-active glycopeptide isolated from human erythrocytes which
contain three non-reducing branches attached to a mannose core (23).
We wish to emphasize that these are preliminary results obtained on
only one fraction of a complex mixture of glycoprotein materials
accumulating in the viscera in G_{M1}-gangliosidosis. We cannot exclude completely the presence of partially degraded keratan sulfate
species since recent enzymatic degradation studies of Hirano and
Meyer indicate the great complexity and heterogeneity in the oligosaccharide sequences of corneal and cartilaginous keratan sulfates
(12). We suggest that the enzyme deficiency in G_{M1}-gangliosidosis
Types I or II is in β-galactosyl hydrolase(s) specific to terminal
galactose units β-linked glycosidically to an N-acetylated hexosamine which leads to the accumulation of both glycolipids and
glycoproteins containing these terminal sequences.

CERAMIDE TRIHEXOSIDOSIS

In the last 8-10 years much interest has developed in the
neutral glycosphingolipid storage disease variously called Fabry's
disease, angiokeratoma corporis diffusum, hereditary dystopic
lipidosis, α-galactosidosis, and now, ceramide trihexosidosis. The
terms Fabry's disease and angiokeratoma corporis diffusum evoke

images of the pathognomonic skin rash which has brought the vast
majority of patients with the disease to light. The terms hereditary dystopic lipidosis and α-galactosidosis are imprecise in light
of all we know about the disease today. Since heterozygous female
carriers of the disease rarely have the characteristic skin lesions,
but may develop significant renal impairment (6,24); and since at
least two male patients have been described who lacked the lesions
but who had all the biochemical features of the disease (5), we
favor the term ceramide trihexosidosis. It is biochemically precise
without implying any fixed clinical presentation.

The demonstration by Sweeley and Klionsky (21) of a massive
accumulation of trihexosylceramide in the kidney of a patient who
had died of Fabry's disease opened the way to a definitive understanding of the pathogenesis of the disease. Brady and his group
(1), using the labelled natural substrate, demonstrated a defect in
the catabolism of trihexosylceramide in patients with Fabry's
disease. Subsequently, Kint (14) showed, using artificial substrates, a deficiency of nonspecific α-galactosidase activity in
peripheral leukocytes from similar patients. This was difficult
to reconcile with the generally held view that the linkages in the
oligosaccharide portion of trihexosylceramide were all of the
β stereoconfiguration (22).

Structure of Galactosylgalactosylglucosylceramide

In a re-examination of the relationship between the accumulation of trihexosylceramide and the nonspecific α-galactosidase
deficiency observed in ceramide trihexosidosis, we have been able
to show that normal and Fabry's trihexosylceramide both contain
terminal α-D-galactopyranosyl residues (4). This conclusion was
based on the results of physicochemical, chemical and enzymic
studies which are summarized in Table III. The first clue to the
presence of a terminal α-galactosidic linkage in trihexosylceramide
was the optical rotation of the pure compound. With the use of
the molecular rotations of lactosylceramide, prepared by the partial hydrolysis of brain ganglioside, and the appropriate methyl-
D-galactosides, and applying Hudson's rules, the calculated rotation of a trihexosylceramide containing a single α-D-galactopyranosyl residue is almost identical to the observed rotations (Table
III). The nmr spectra of the intact glycosphingolipids recorded in
pyridine-d5 at 100 and 220 Megahertz contained three doublets in
the region of the anomeric protons. The chemical shifts and
coupling constants of these doublets confirmed the presence of two
β-D-glycopyranosides and a single α-D-glycopyranoside. Although
these data were considered conclusive evidence for the presence
of an α-D-galactopyranosyl residue, whether it was terminal or
internal was unknown.

Table III. Evidence for a Terminal α-D-galactopyranosyl
Residue in Trihexosylceramide

	Lactosylceramide	CTH
Optical rotation $[\alpha]_D^{23}$ (in pyridine)	-12 (C=2.1)	+23 (C=7.5)
NMR spectra of anomeric protons	δ=4.70 ppm, J=7.5Hz δ=4.90 ppm, J=7.5Hz	δ=4.74 ppm, J=7.6Hz δ=4.94 ppm, J=7.5Hz δ=5.45 ppm, J=4.1Hz
Chemical hydrolysis (% hydrolysis in 0.3N HCl at 60° for 2 hrs)	46%	70%
Enzymic hydrolysis α-galactosidase (coffee bean)	0	+
β-galactosidase (E. coli)	+	0

The proof that the α-D-galactopyranosyl residue is terminal
rests on the results of the chemical and enzymic hydrolysis of the
terminal galactosidic linkage. For these studies, we employed trihexosylceramide and lactosylceramide labelled in the terminal galactose moiety by oxidation with D-galactose oxidase and reduction of
the resulting hexodialdose with tritiated sodium borohydride. We
found that the terminal galactosidic linkage of trihexosylceramide
was more acid labile than the terminal β-galactosidic linkage of
lactosylceramide. We also found that the terminal galactosidic
linkage of trihexosylceramide was susceptible to hydrolysis by an
α-galactosidase purified from green coffee beans (7), but was
completely resistant to hydrolysis by E. coli β-galactosidase. The
only products of the reaction were unreacted trihexosylceramide and
lactosylceramide. These results not only add further evidence for
the α-stereoconfiguration of one of the galactosyl residues in
trihexosylceramide, but they also show that it is the terminal
galactosyl residue. Furthermore, they indicate that the
α-galactosidase deficiency observed in Fabry's disease is a direct
reflection of the deficiency of trihexosylceramide:galactosyl
galactohydrolase.

We also undertook some nmr studies of globoside purified from
normal human kidney. The absorption of the anomeric protons is not
well resolved at 100 Megahertz but at 220 Megahertz four well-
defined doublets were observed. Three of these have the spectral

characteristics of β-anomeric protons (δ_1=4.69 ppm, J=8.0Hz; δ_2=4.88 ppm, J=7.5Hz; δ_3=4.99 ppm, J=8.1Hz), and one has the features of an α-anomeric proton (δ_4=5.36 ppm, J=3.9Hz). This is strong evidence that human kidney globoside has the same configuration as globoside from erythrocytes and fibroblasts as shown by Hakomori and his group (10). On the basis of these studies and the fatty acid compositions, a precursor-product relationship between globoside and trihexosylceramide probably obtains in human kidney as Dawson and Sweeley (8) suggested from studies of the metabolism of globoside in pigs.

Renal Transplantation in a Case of Ceramide Trihexosidosis

We would like to report now some studies we have undertaken on a patient with ceramide trihexosidosis who underwent bilateral nephrectomies followed by renal homotransplantation because of his progressive renal failure. We had demonstrated histological and biochemical features typical of Fabry's disease in this patient although he had no angiokeratomas (5). The analysis of kidney tissue taken at nephrectomy demonstrated a 20-fold excess of glycolipid hexose (Table IV). Enzyme assays were done on fresh tissue within 15 minutes of its excision. Using trihexosylceramide tritiated in the terminal galactose and p-nitrophenyl-α-D-galactopyranoside, we were able to demonstrate marked concomitant deficiencies of trihexosylceramide-galactosyl galactohydrolase and nonspecific α-D-galactosidase in the kidney tissue. It is interesting, however, that the pH optima of the hydrolysis of the two substrates was different. Studies in normal human kidney showed that the optimum pH for the hydrolysis of trihexosylceramide was about 3.6. On the other hand, the pH optimum using p-nitrophenyl-α-D-galactopyranoside was 5.4 to 5.6. Similar differences in pH optima were observed in the hydrolysis of various α-galactosides (such as trihexosylceramide, melibiose and p-nitrophenyl-α-D-galactopyranoside) by coffee bean α-galactosidase.

Table IV. Lipid composition of human kidney

Specimen	Water Content %	Total Lipids	Glycolipid Hexose	Lipid P	Ganglioside NANA
			mg/g wet wt.		μg/g wet wt.
Controls					
1	81.4	34.5	0.27	0.48	16.4
2	80.9	36.1	0.25	0.52	12.4
Fabry's					
A.H.	70.5	77.2	5.80	0.49	29.8

Table V.   Effect of Renal Homotransplantation
on Urinary and Plasma CTH Levels

	Urine	Plasma
	(μmoles/24 hr)	(μmoles/100 ml)
Preoperative	0.749	0.45-0.75
Postoperative (assays during 1st 4 mo.)	0.100-0.175	0.45-1.11
Normal	0.014-0.033 (4)	0.20-0.40 (6)

Prior to renal transplantation, the patient was excreting over 700 nmoles of trihexosylceramide per day in his urine (Table V). Postoperatively, this fell markedly to 100 to 150 nmoles per day, which is still, however, 4-8 times normal. The excretion of digalactosylceramide fell from 300-400 nmoles per day to zero. The elevated levels of trihexosylceramide in the patient's plasma were essentially unchanged by peritoneal dialysis, hemodialysis, bilateral nephrectomies or renal transplantation.

The transplanted kidney appeared therefore to be contributing little, if anything, to the metabolism of circulating trihexosylceramide. The elevated excretion of trihexosylceramide in the urine after transplantation could be explained in at least three ways. First, the catabolic potential of the donor kidney might be inadequate to handle the trihexosylceramide delivered to it by the circulation. Secondly, the catabolism of endogenous trihexosylceramide by the donor kidney might be impaired by immunosuppressive therapy. Thirdly, and most likely, the trihexosylceramide in the patient's urine might be derived from desquamated epithelial cells from the mucosa of his own bladder and urethra. The second alternative is easiest to rule out, and is currently under investigation. The first possibility will be resolved when the analysis of the glycosphingolipid content of the donor kidney is done.

On the basis of these findings, it appears that renal transplantation has little place in the treatment of the nonuremic patient with ceramide trihexosidosis.

Acknowledgements

This research was supported by a grant MT-1345 to L.S.W. from the Medical Research Council of Canada and Medical Research Council of Canada Fellowships to Dr. Clarke and Dr. Senior.

REFERENCES

1. Brady, R. O., Gal, A. E., Bradley, R. M., Martensson, E.,
    Warshaw, A. L. and Laster, L. Enzymatic defect in Fabry's
    disease: ceramide trihexosidosis deficiency. New Engl. J.
    Med. 276, 1163. 1967.

2. Callahan, J. W. and L. S. Wolfe. Isolation and characteriza-
    tion of keratan sulfates from the liver of a patient with
    G_{M1}-gangliosidosis Type I. Biochim.Biophys.Acta 215, 527,
    1970.

3. Callahan, J. W., Pinsky, L. and Wolfe, L. S. G_{M1}-gangliosidosis
    (Type II): Studies on a Fibroblast Cell Strain. Biochem. Med.
    4, 295, 1970.

4. Clarke, J. T. R., Wolfe, L. S. and Perlin, A. S. Evidence for
    a Terminal α-D-Galactopyranosyl Residue in Galactosylgalacto-
    sylglucosylceramide from Human Kidney. J. Biol. Chem. 246,
    5563, 1971.

5. Clarke, J. T. R., Knaack, J., Crawhall, J. C. and Wolfe, L. S.
    Ceramide trihexosidosis (Fabry's Disease) without skin lesions.
    New Engl. J. Med. 284, 233, 1971.

6. Colley, J. R., Miller, D. L., Hutt, M. S. R., Wallace, H. J.
    and deWardener, H. E. The renal lesion in angiokeratoma
    corporis diffusum. Brit. Med. J. 1, 1266, 1958.

7. Courtois, J. E. and Petek, F., in E. F. Neufeld and V. Ginsburg
    (Editors), Methods in Enzymology, Vol. VIII, Academic Press,
    New York, p. 565, 1966.

8. Dawson, G. and Sweeley, C. C. In vivo Studies on Glycosphingo-
    lipid Metabolism in Porcine Blood. J. Biol. Chem. 245, 410,
    1970.

9. Derry, D. M., Fawcett, J. S., Andermann, F. and Wolfe, L. S.
    Late Infantile Systemic Lipidosis. Neurology 18, 340, 1968.

10. Hakomori, S-I, Siddiqui, B., Li, Y-T, Li, S-C and Hellerqvist,
    C. G. Anomeric Structures of Globoside and Ceramide Tri-
    hexoside of Human Erythrocytes and Hamster Fibroblasts.
    J. Biol. Chem. 246, 2271, 1971.

11. Hirano, S., Hoffman, P. and Meyer, K. The Structure of Kerato-
    sulfate of Bovine Cornea. J. Org. Chem. 26, 5064, 1961.

12. Hirano, S. and Meyer, K. Enzymatic Degradation of Corneal
     and Cartilaginous Keratosulfates. Biochem. Biophys. Res.
     Comm. 44, 1371, 1971.

13. Jamieson, G. A., Jett, M. and DeBernardo, S. L. The Carbo-
     hydrate Sequence of the Glycopeptide Chains of Human Trans-
     ferrin. J. Biol. Chem. 246, 3686, 1971.

14. Kint, J. A. Fabry's disease: alpha galactosidase deficiency.
     Science 167, 1268, 1970.

15. O'Brien, J. S., Okada, S., Ho, Mae Wan, Fillerup, D. L.,
     Veath, M. Lois and Adams, K. Ganglioside storage diseases.
     Fed. Proc. 30, 956, 1971.

16. Pinsky, L., Powell, E. and Callahan, J. G$_{M1}$-gangliosidosis
     Types 1 and 2; enzymatic differences in cultured fibroblasts.
     Nature 228, 1093, 1970.

17. Severi, F., Magrini, U., Tettamanti, G., Bianchi, E. and
     Lanzi, G. Infantile G$_{M1}$-gangliosidosis. Helv. Paed. Acta 26,
     192, 1971.

18. Suzuki, K. Cerebral G$_{M1}$-gangliosidosis: Chemical Pathology of
     Visceral Organs. Science 159, 1471, 1968.

19. Suzuki, K., Suzuki, K. and Chen, G. C. Morphological, Histo-
     chemical and Biochemical Studies on a Case of Systemic Late
     Infantile Lipidosis. J. Neuropath. Exptl. Neurol. 27, 15,
     1968.

20. Suzuki, K., Suzuki, K. and Kamoshita, S. Chemical pathology
     of G$_{M1}$-gangliosidosis. J. Neuropath. Exptl. Neurol. 28,
     25, 1969.

21. Sweeley, C. C. and Klionsky, B. Fabry's disease: Classifica-
     tion as a sphingolipidosis and partial characterization of a
     novel glycolipid. J. Biol. Chem. 238, PC3148, 1963.

22. Sweeley, C. C., Snyder, P. D., Jr., and Griffin, C. E.
     Chemistry of Glycosphingolipids in Fabry's Disease. Chem.
     Phys. Lipids 4, 393, 1970.

23. Thomas, D. B. and Winzler, R. J. Structure of Glycoproteins of
     Human Erythrocytes. Biochem J. 124, 55, 1971.

24. Wallace, H. J. Angiokeratoma corporis diffusum. Brit. J.
     Dermat. 70, 354, 1958.

25. Wolfe, L. S., Callahan, J., Fawcett, J. S., Andermann, F. and Scriver, C. R. G_{M1}-gangliosidosis without chondrodystrophy or visceromegaly. Neurology 20, 23, 1970.

CHEMICAL PATHOLOGY OF

TAY-SACHS DISEASE IN THE FETUS[*]

Larry Schneck, Masazumi Adachi and Bruno W. Volk

Isaac Albert Research Institute of the Kingsbrook
Jewish Medical Center and the Department of Neurology,
Kingsbrook Jewish Medical Center, and Veterans Admini-
stration Hospital, Brooklyn, New York.

Prenatal diagnosis of Tay-Sachs disease not only offers a
means for effective pregnancy management, but it also provides a
unique opportunity to study the disease early in fetal development (1). This paper will describe some of the chemical features
of three cases of fetal Tay-Sachs disease (2). It will also include some preliminary studies on enzyme replacement with cultured fetal Tay-Sachs disease fibroblasts.

MATERIAL AND METHODS

Of the 11 high-risk pregnancies, four were aborted. In one
of the four, the pregnancy was terminated 12 weeks from the last
menstrual date for psychiatric reasons. The other three pregnancies were aborted when absent hexosaminidase A activity in
amniotic fluid and/or amniotic cells indicated that there was a
high probability that the fetus had Tay-Sachs disease. Acrylamide gel electrophoresis was used to determine the percent of
hexosaminidase A in the amniotic fluid and cells (3). Two were
aborted by saline infusion at 16 and 19 weeks from the last menstrual date respectively, and the third by hysterotomy 22 weeks
from the last menstrual date. The tissue from the 22-week old
fetus obtained by hysterotomy was immediately frozen at $-40°$, and
was used as the basis for most of the biochemical and morphological
studies of prenatal Tay-Sachs disease. The three control fetuses,
aged 16, 18 and 20 weeks from the last menstrual date were also
aborted by hysterotomy. Biochemical studies of brain, liver and
adrenal gland were performed by combined column, thin layer and

* Supported by a grant from the National Tay-Sachs and Allied
Diseases Association, Inc.

gas liquid chromatography. The details of the methods used have
been described in previous publications (4). Quantitative spectrophotometric analysis of DNA and RNA was performed according to the
technique of Santen and Agranoff (5).

RESULTS

There were only two chemical abnormalities detected in the
Tay-Sachs disease fetuses. One was the absence of hexosaminidase
A activity in all tissues analyzed (brain, liver, adrenal, kidney,
cultured skin fibroblasts and in the cultured fragments from the
12 week abortus). The second abnormality was the increase in the
percentage of cerebral G_{M2}-ganglioside. Although there was no
significant difference in the total lipid bound sialic acid in
brain, liver and adrenal (Table I), the percentage of G_{M2}-ganglio-
side in fetal brain was four times that found in the control fetal
brain, and six times that found in control infant brain (Fig. 1,
Table II). The water content, total protein, DNA, RNA, sterols
and phospholipids were essentially similar in the fetal control
and the Tay-Sachs disease brains (Table III).

Gas liquid chromatography confirmed that the ganglioside fraction with an Rf value similar to G_{M2}-ganglioside had an oligosaccharide composition identical to authentic G_{M2}-ganglioside or
Tay-Sachs disease ganglioside, fetal ganglioside had only C_{16}^{18}
sphingosine in the ceramide moiety, and the percentage of C^{16}
fatty acid was much higher than that found in postnatal brain
(Table IV). No qualitative or quantitative abnormalities of
gangliosides were seen in the Tay-Sachs disease liver or adrenal.
The finding that the lipid bound sialic acid in human fetal and
newborn adrenal is exclusively n-acetylneuraminic acid, is further
confirmation that in human tissue, n-acetylneuraminic acid is the
predominant type of sialic acid (6). Ultrastructurally abnormal
cytosomes were present in the Tay-Sachs disease fetal neurons
(Fig. 2) (7). These differed from the membranous cytoplasmic
bodies found in postnatal Tay-Sachs disease brain. No abnormal
cytosomes were seen in the fetal Tay-Sachs disease liver.

A series of experiments were undertaken to determine whether
the in vitro addition of purified hexosaminidase A enzyme would
modify the metabolism of G_{M2}-ganglioside of cultured fetal Tay-
Sachs disease fibroblasts. Four roller culture flasks of Tay-
Sachs disease fetal fibroblasts were cultured in Eagle's minimal
essential medium with 10% Tay-Sachs disease serum. Tay-Sachs
disease serum was used in order to eliminate the possibility that
hexosaminidase A, present in fetal calf serum, would influence the
metabolism of the G_{M2}-ganglioside. C^{14}-glucosamine was added to
the media in order to label the ganglioside. After the gangliosides were labeled, hexosaminidase A, purified 1000-fold by

Dr. J. Friedland, was added to two of the four culture flasks. After three days of incubation with the hexosaminidase A enzyme, the fibroblasts were harvested and analyzed. The experimental procedure employed is summarized in Fig. 3.

Part of the hexosaminidase A incubated with the cells in Tay-Sachs disease media was converted to hexosaminidase B and a third fraction C (Fig. 4). There was no detectable hexosaminidase A activity in the cultured cells that were incubated with the purified hexosaminidase A enzyme. The percentage of labeled G_{M2}-ganglioside in the cells cultured with hexosaminidase A activity were similar to that found in the cultured cells without the enzyme (Table V). These findings indicate that parenteral enzyme replacement is unlikely to significantly modify the disease process. Preliminary studies also suggest that there is no significant difference in the percent of labeled G_{M2} in control and Tay-Sachs disease fetal cultured fibroblasts (8).

SUMMARY

There is no hexosaminidase A activity in the Tay-Sachs disease fetus as early as 12 weeks from the last menstrual date. Besides the absence of hexosaminidase A activity, the only other detectable abnormality was an increase in the percentage of cerebral G_{M2}-ganglioside. Biochemical and morphological changes are already present during the second trimester. The addition of hexosaminidase A to cultured fetal Tay-Sachs disease fibroblasts did not significantly alter the percentage of labeled G_{M2}-ganglioside. Since the nervous system already has pathologic, biochemical and ultrastructural changes at the time of amniocentesis is practical, prenatal or postnatal treatment does not seem feasible. An effective way to control this disorder would be the indexing of high-risk marriages and the monitoring of high-risk pregnancies.

REFERENCES

1. Schneck, L., Friedland, J., Valenti, C., Adachi, M., Amsterdam, D. and Volk, B.W.: Prenatal diagnosis of Tay-Sachs disease. Lancet, 1, 582, 1970.

2. Schneck, L., Adachi, M. and Volk, B.W.: Fetal aspects of Tay-Sachs disease. Pediatrics. In press.

3. Friedland, J., Perle, G., Saifer, A., Schneck, L. and Volk, B.W.: Screening for Tay-Sachs disease in utero using amniotic fluid. Proc. Soc. Exp. Biol. Med., 136:1297, 1971.

4. Schneck, L., Adachi, M. and Volk, B.W.: Congenital failure of myelinization (Pelizaeus-Merzbacher disease?). Neurology, 21:817, 1971.

5. Santen, R.J. and Agranoff, B.W.: Studies on the estimation
    of deoxyribonucleic acid and ribonucleic acid in the rat
    brain. Biochem. Biophys. Acta, 72:251, 1963.

6. Gottschalk, A.: The Chemistry and Biology of Sialic Acids
    and Related Substances. Cambridge, University Press, 1960,
    p. 30.

7. Adachi, M., Torii, J., Schneck, L. and Volk, B.W.: The fine
    structure of fetal Tay-Sachs disease. Arch. Path., 91:48,
    1971.

8. Schneck, L., Feldman, N., Brooks, S., Amsterdam, D. and
    Volk, B.W.: Ganglioside metabolism in cultured Tay-Sachs
    disease fibroblasts. To be published.

TABLE 1

CHEMICAL COMPOSITION OF FETAL BRAINS

% Dry Weight

	TSD Fetus (22 wks)	Control Fetus (16 wks)	Control Fetus (18 wks)	Control Fetus (20 wks)
H_2O	91.00	91.00	92.00	91.00
Total Protein	53.50	42.10	44.50	44.50
DNA	1.10	0.93	1.10	1.00
RNA	1.11	1.15	1.50	1.46
Cholesterol	4.23	2.90	3.00	3.50
(% of total sterols)				
Cholesterol Ester	trace	trace	trace	trace
Desmosterol	8.80	———	———	
Phospholipids	15.75	10.43	12.35	12.50
(% of total phosphorus)				
Phosphatidic Acid	6.20	1.60	1.00	1.00
Phosphatidyl Serine	4.00	10.00	7.50	6.50
Phosphatidyl Inositol	6.20	1.00	1.50	2.60
Sphingomyelin	7.60	4.10	7.80	7.00
Phosphatidyl Choline	40.00	49.10	48.60	47.20
Phosphatidyl Ethanolamine	33.80	31.00	33.50	38.10
Origin	3.00	———	———	———

TABLE II

LIPID BOUND SIALIC ACID
(mg./gm. Dry Weight)

	TAY-SACHS DISEASE			CONTROL		
AGE IN WEEKS	16	19	22	16	18	20
Fetal Brain	2.35	2.40	2.39	1.87	2.00	2.37
Fetal Liver	——	0.33	0.37	0.30	0.30	0.36
Fetal Adrenal	——	——	1.28	1.20	1.40	1.81

TABLE III

CEREBRAL GANGLIOSIDE PATTERNS
(Expressed as % of Total NANA)

	TSD Fetus (16 wks)	TSD Fetus (22 wks)	Control Fetuses (3) Mean	Range	TSD Infant	Control Infant
G_{M3}	trace	trace	trace	trace	2.0	3.4
G_{M2}	26.4	28.0	6.3	(5.8-6.5)	84.2	4.7
G_{M1}	18.7	23.7	21.5	(19.5-24.5)	3.3	21.7
G_{D1a} + G_{D1b}	46.5	56.7	65.2	(63.2-67.0)	8.0	52.1
GT	7.6	11.1	7.0	(6.5-7.3)	2.5	17.9

TABLE IV

BRAIN GANGLIOSIDE CERAMIDE,
FATTY ACID AND SPHINGOSINE
(% of Total

Fatty Acid	TSD Fetus (22 wks)	Control Fetus (16 wks)	TSD Infant	Control Infant
C^{14}	4.38	5.7	----	----
C^{16}	34.05	45.7	4.08	2.44
C^{18}	53.90	27.5	93.25	90.56
C^{20}	5.00	12.6	2.72	7.31
C^{22}	2.58	6.9	----	----
C^{24}	----	----	----	----
Sphingosine				
C^{18}	100.00	100.00	84.00	50.00
C^{20}	0.00	0.00	16.00	50.00

TABLE V

GANGLIOSIDE IN CULTURED FIBROBLASTS

Zone	F.T.S.D. C.P.M.	% Total	F.T.S.D. + Hex A C.P.M.	% Total
$1-G_{M3}$	571	9.70	409	5.90
$2-G_{M2}$	968	16.50	1183	17.20
$3-G_{M1}$	2877	47.50	2814	40.90
$4-G_D$	1382	23.60	2094	30.30
$5-G_T$ + Origin	153	2.10	398	5.80

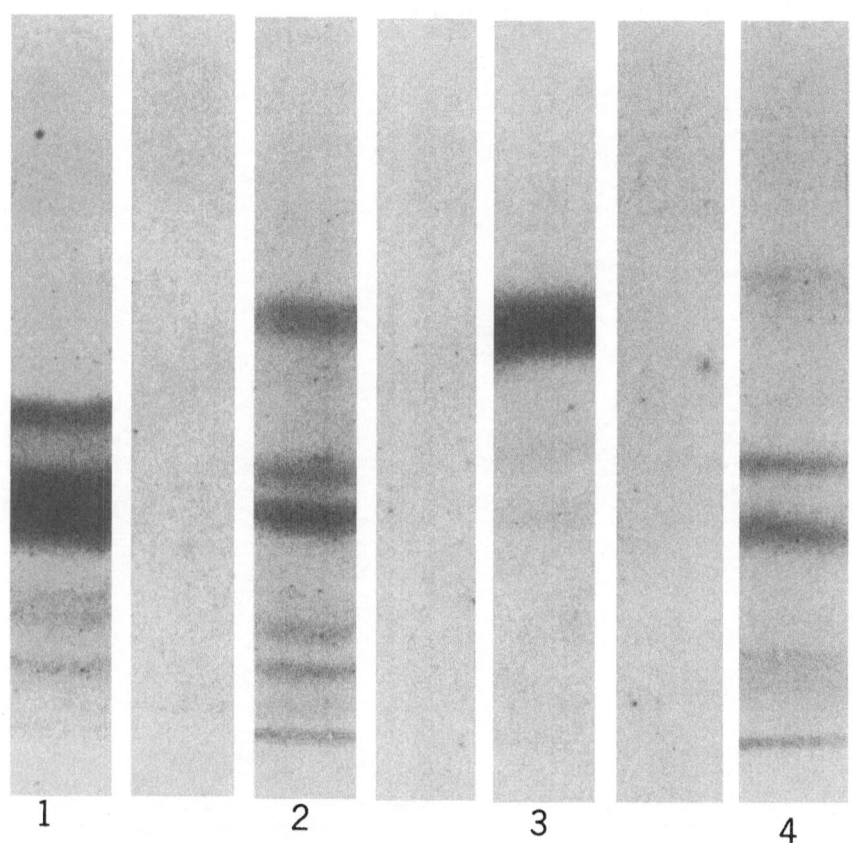

FIGURE 1: Thin Layer Chromatogram - Brain Gangliosides
Column 1: Normal Infant
Column 2: Fetal Tay-Sachs Disease
Column 3: Post-natal Tay-Sachs Disease
Column 4: Normal Fetus

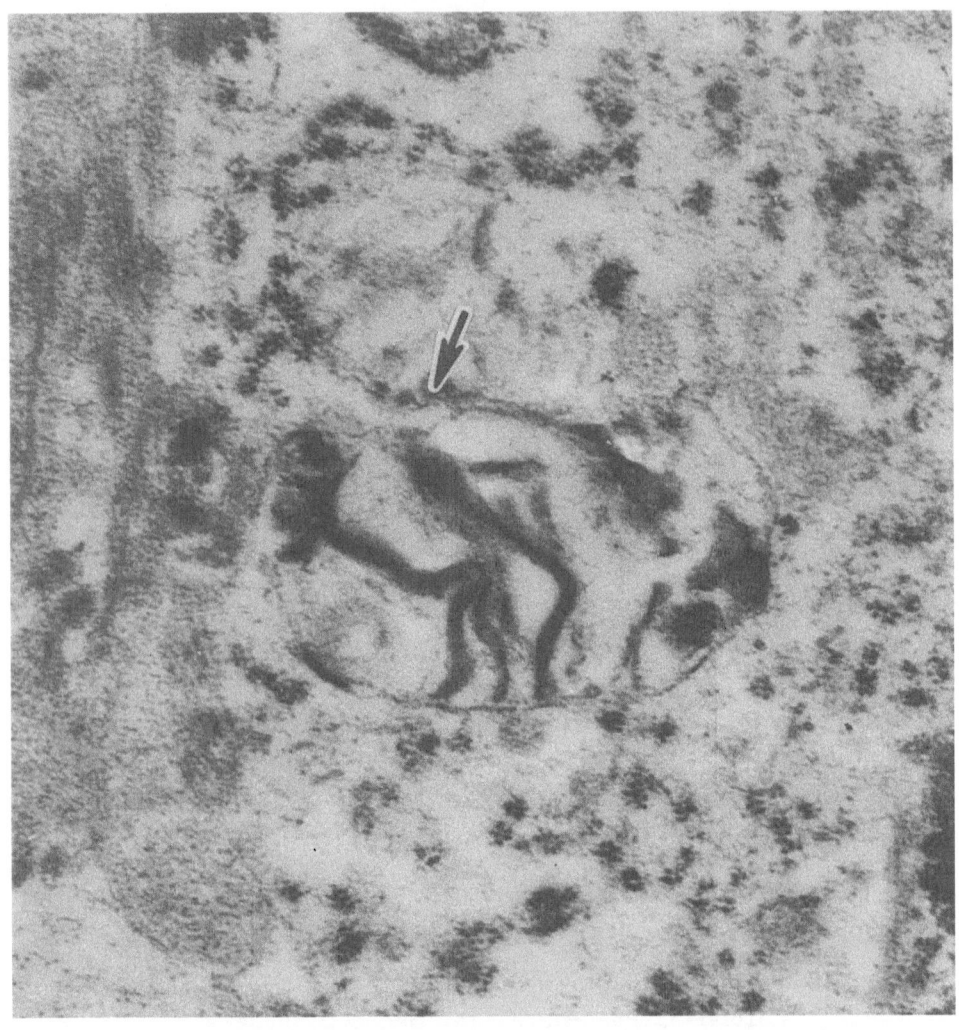

FIGURE 2: Electron microphotograph of cerebellum. Arrow
indicates abnormal lipid cytosome contiguous with
endoplasmic regiculum.

Enzyme Replacement
Fetal TSD Fibroblasts

Grow to subconfluency in roller cultures in
MEM + 10% FCS

Transfer to MEM + 10% TSD serum for 4 days

Maintain for 2 days in serum-deficient MEM with
C^{14}-glucosamine (0.5 uC/ml)

   No Hex A   Hex A (3.5×10^{-5}M/hr/ml)
(MEM + 10% TSD)   daily for 3 days
                                  (MEM + 10% TSD)

HARVEST FOR ANALYSES OF LABELLED GANGLIOSIDES

Lipids extracted and partitioned (Folch)

Alkaline hydrolysis of phospholipids (Marinetti)

Enzyme hydrolysis to remove nucleotide sugars (Kanfer)

TLC and scintillation counting of resorcinol + bands

FIGURE 3: Experimental outline for enzyme replacement of
fetal Tay-Sachs disease fibroblasts.

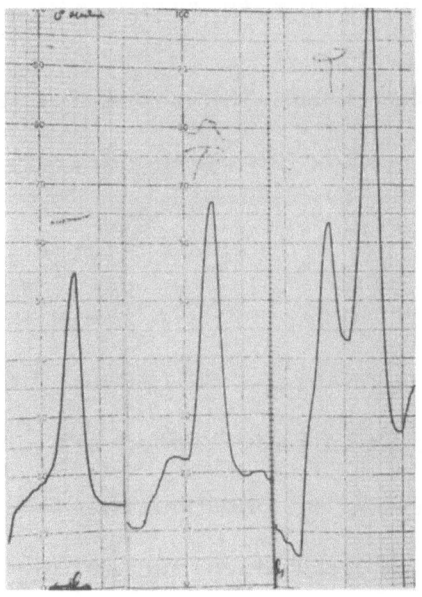

FIGURE 4: Acrylamide gel electrophoresis of hexosaminidase A
           added to fibroblast culture.
           Column 1: 0 time. Single peak represents hexosamini-
                      dase A.
           Column 2: 48 hours incubation, 3 peaks. Extreme left
                      hexosaminidase B, center peak hexosamini-
                      dase A and extreme right unknown.
           Column 3: 7 days incubation. Significant percent of
                      hexosaminidase B now apparent.

GLYCOSPHINGOLIPID ABNORMALITIES IN LIVER FROM PATIENTS WITH

GLYCOSPHINGOLIPID AND MUCOPOLYSACCHARIDE STORAGE DISEASES

GLYN DAWSON

Depts. Pediatrics and Biochemistry, Joseph P. Kennedy
Jr. Mental Retardation Research Center, University of
Chicago, Chicago, Illinois 60637

INTRODUCTION

The lipid and mucopolysaccharide storage diseases were first detected by characterizing the material which accumulated in liver or brain. In the case of the glycosphingolipidoses, these abnormal accumulations have been shown to be the result of specific inherited lysosomal hydrolase deficiencies. Normal human liver contains five major glycosphingolipid components, glucosylceramide (GL-1a), lactosylceramide (GL-2a), trihexosylceramide (GL-3), globoside (GL-4) and hematoside (G_{M3}) (4,15) together with smaller amounts of disialohematoside (G_{D3}) and galactosylceramide (GL-1b) (Fig. 1). Human liver also contains trace amounts of sulfatide (GL-1bS), gangliosides such as G_{M1}, and fucoglycosphingolipids (blood group substances). Further, liver has been shown to contain most of the lysosomal glycosyl hydrolases associated with the catabolism of glycosphingolipids. Therefore, the determination of glycosphingolipid levels in this organ (which can be readily biopsied) should be useful in understanding the biochemical defects in a wide range of storage diseases.

In Fabry's disease, an X-linked inherited α-galactosyl hydrolase deficiency (2,14) with only visceral manifestations, the concentration of the accumulating GL-3 (31) is about 200 times normal (22) or approximately 6 μmoles/g. fresh wt. of tissue. In contrast, exhaustive analysis of liver from patients with a neurological disease such as G_{M2}-gangliosidosis Type 1 (Tay-Sachs disease) (18) has revealed either small amounts (30) or the total absence (32) of the asialo-G_{M2} and G_{M2} which accumulate in the brain of such patients. In G_{M2}-gangliosidosis Type 2 (Sandhoff's disease) (21) visceral abnormalities are found and the accumulation of asialo-G_{M2} and globo-

395

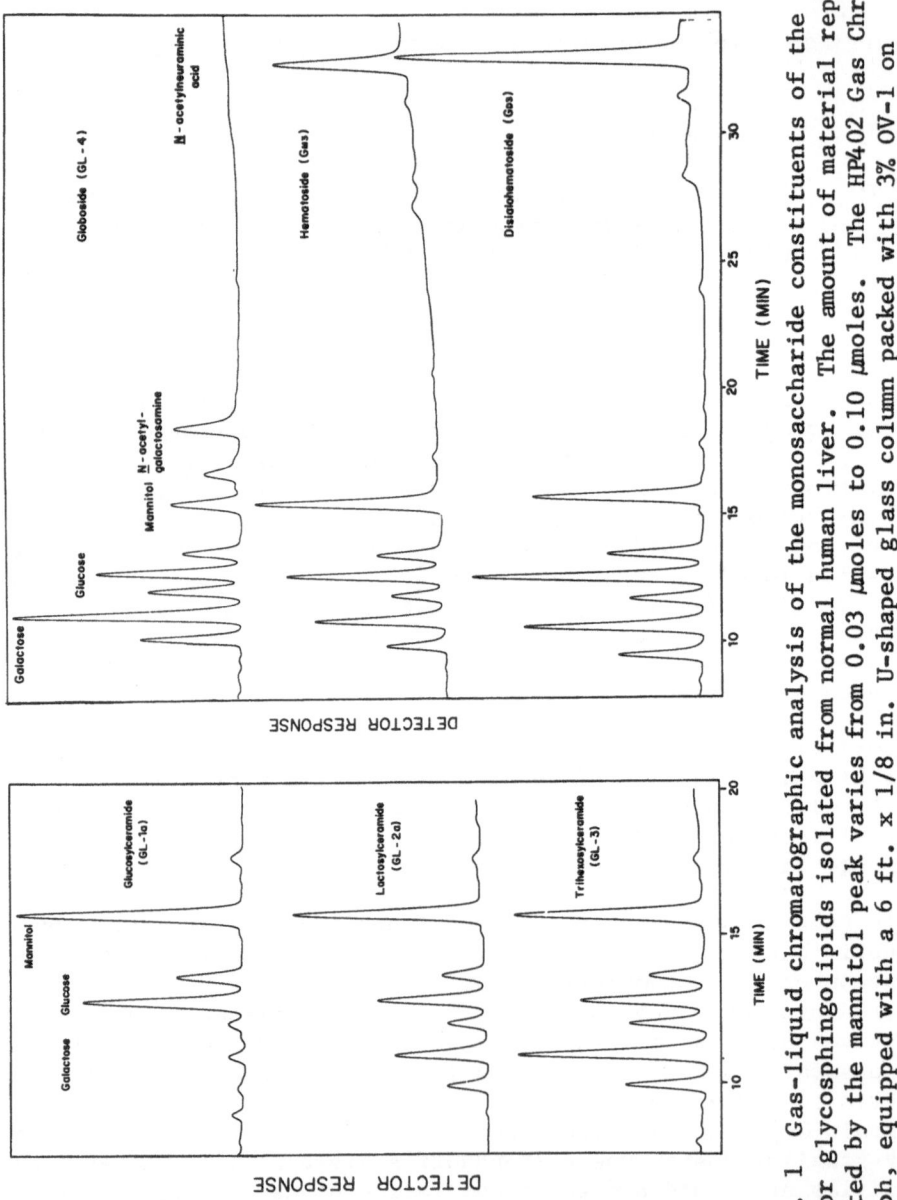

Fig. 1 Gas-liquid chromatographic analysis of the monosaccharide constituents of the six major glycosphingolipids isolated from normal human liver. The amount of material represented by the mannitol peak varies from 0.03 μmoles to 0.10 μmoles. The HP402 Gas Chromatograph, equipped with a 6 ft. x 1/8 in. U-shaped glass column packed with 3% OV-1 on Supelcoport (100–120 mesh), was temperature-programmed from 160° to 240° at 2°C/minute.

side (GL-4) in liver can be readily demonstrated (21,23,27). This
massive accumulation is presumably the result of the insoluble
nature of glycosphingolipids and the absence of alternative pathways for their metabolism (with the exception that G_{M2} could be
converted to asialo-GM2 rather than G_{M3}, and G_{M1} could be converted
to asialo-G_{M1} instead of G_{M2}). Such alternative pathways do appear
to occur in both G_{M1}- and G_{M2}-gangliosidoses.

This study investigates the glycosphingolipid levels in liver
from patients with glycosphingolipid storage diseases, presents
evidence that Fucosidosis is a glycosphingolipidosis, and indicates
that glycosphingolipid abnormalities are found in the mucopolysaccharidoses.

METHODS OF ANALYSIS

Gas-liquid chromatography (GLC) is extremely useful in the
study of glycosphingolipids because of its sensitivity and the fact
that all the constituent monosaccharides can be estimated and
identified from a single chromatographic analysis of 30 minute
duration (Fig. 1). Although trimethylsilyl ether derivatives of
0-methyl-glycosides may give as many as 3 peaks for a single sugar,
these are well resolved and, since the ratio of isomers and anomers
is constant, this affords an unambiguous identification of each
sugar.

Samples of liver, usually obtained at autopsy, were washed
with 0.15 M NaCl to remove as much blood as possible, blotted dry,
and the fresh weight determined. Approximately 1 g. (where available) was minced and homogenized in ten volumes of 0.15 M NaCl.
Methanol (300 volumes) was added, followed by chloroform (600 volumes). After extraction for 4 hours at room temperature, using a
magnetic stirrer, the mixture was filtered, the residue re-ex-
tracted, and 0.2 volumes of water added; the biphasic system was
left overnight.

The upper aqueous phase was evaporated to dryness and subjected to alkaline methanolysis with 0.3 $\underline{N}$ NaOH in chloroform-
methanol (1:1) for 1 hour at room temperature. The mixture plus
washings (chloroform-methanol, 2:1) was transferred to a tube,
neutralized with 0.05 ml. conc. HCl, and dialyzed exhaustively
against distilled water. The dialysate was then concentrated to
dryness and applied to a silica gel thin-layer chromatographic
(TLC) plate, good resolution being obtained with two sequential
developments in chloroform-methanol-2.5 N NH4OH (60:40:9). The
gangliosides were visualized with iodine and since comparison of
their Rf value to that of cerebral ganglioside standards is an
unreliable method of identification, they were scraped, eluted
with chloroform-methanol and water (10:4:0.5) and prepared for

GLC analysis. Mannitol (0.02-0.20 μmoles) was added to the glycolipid and methanolysis was carried out at $80°$ for 16 hr. in 1.0
N HCl in dry methanol (2.0 ml.). After neutralization with silver
carbonate, re-N-acetylation with acetic anhydride (0.05 ml.) and
removal of fatty acid methyl esters with n-hexane, the methyl
glycosides were trimethylsilyated and subjected to gas-liquid
chromatography (3,33) (Fig. 1).

The total lipid fraction was separated into neutral lipids,
glycosphingolipids and phospholipids (33) by silicic acid chromatography. The glycosphingolipid fraction was subjected to alkaline
methanolysis (as described above), TLC in chloroform-methanol-
water (110:40:6) and gas-liquid chromatographic analysis of the
monosaccharide constituents as described above.

RESULTS

1. Infantile Gaucher's Disease

Liver was obtained at autopsy from an infant with severe
hepatosplenomegaly, foam cells characteristic of Gaucher's disease
and severe mental retardation. An almost total deficiency of reactivity towards synthetic β-glucoside substrates at pH 4.5 was
found, confirming the clinical diagnosis of infantile Gaucher's
disease. Chemical analysis revealed a 200-fold elevation of
glucosylceramide (GL-1a) (Fig. 2) and a 4-fold elevation of GL-2a
and G_{M3} (Table 1); GL-3 and GL-4 levels were essentially normal.
This massive accumulation of GL-1a is consistent with many previous reports of analyses carried out on spleens (25) from the
adult form, where a 200 to 750-fold elevation of GL-1a is usually
found. In spleen from patients with the adult form of Gaucher's
disease, GL-2a and G_{M3} also show a 2 to 3-fold elevation and GL-3
and GL-4 levels are unaffected (4,25).

2. Lactosylceramidosis

This rare neurovisceral disease is documented by only one case
(6,7), although studies on formalin-fixed tissue suggest a previous
case (13,20). The age of onset (which may not be typical) was
2 1/2-years and the symptoms were primarily neurological such as
loss of motor skills and severe cerebral ataxia. Cerebral deterioration progressed to dementia and autopsy studies at age 4 revealed
extensive foamy infiltration of visceral organs with some hepatosplenomegaly. A liver biopsy had been used previously (7) to
demonstrate both the lactosylceramidase deficiency and lactosylceramide accumulation and this was confirmed by studies on autopsy
liver (Table 1). This 8-fold elevation of GL-2a was accompanied

TABLE 1 LIVER GLYCOSPHINGOLIPIDS IN PATIENTS WITH GLYCOSPHINGOLIPID STORAGE DISEASES

Glycosphingo-lipid	Control	Infantile Gaucher's Disease	Lactosyl-ceramidosis (S.H.)	α-Fuco-sidosis (M.S.)	G_{M1}-ganglio-sidosis (C.B.)	Globoid cell leuko-dystrophy (B.H.)
			μmoles/g. fresh wt.			
GL-1a	0.05 ± 0.02	11.40	0.39	0.07	0.04	0.05
GL-1b	<0.01	-----	-----	-----	-----	0.06
GL-2a	0.06 ± 0.01	0.26	0.45	0.09	0.05	0.15
GL-3	0.03 ± 0.01	0.05	0.08	0.07	0.01	0.04
GL-4	0.02 ± 0.01	0.04	0.02	0.09	0.02	0.04
Asialo-G_{M1}	-----	-----	-----	-----	0.09	-----
G_{M3}	0.18 ± 0.04	0.77	0.39	0.29	0.10	0.09
G_{M1}	-----	-----	-----	-----	0.15	-----
GL-F1*	-----	-----	-----	2.75	-----	-----
GL-F2+	-----	-----	-----	0.25	-----	-----

* Contains Fuc:Gal:Glc:GlcNAc in the ratio 1:2:1:1.
+ Contains Fuc, Gal, Glc and GlcNAc (no GalNAc) in non-integral amounts.

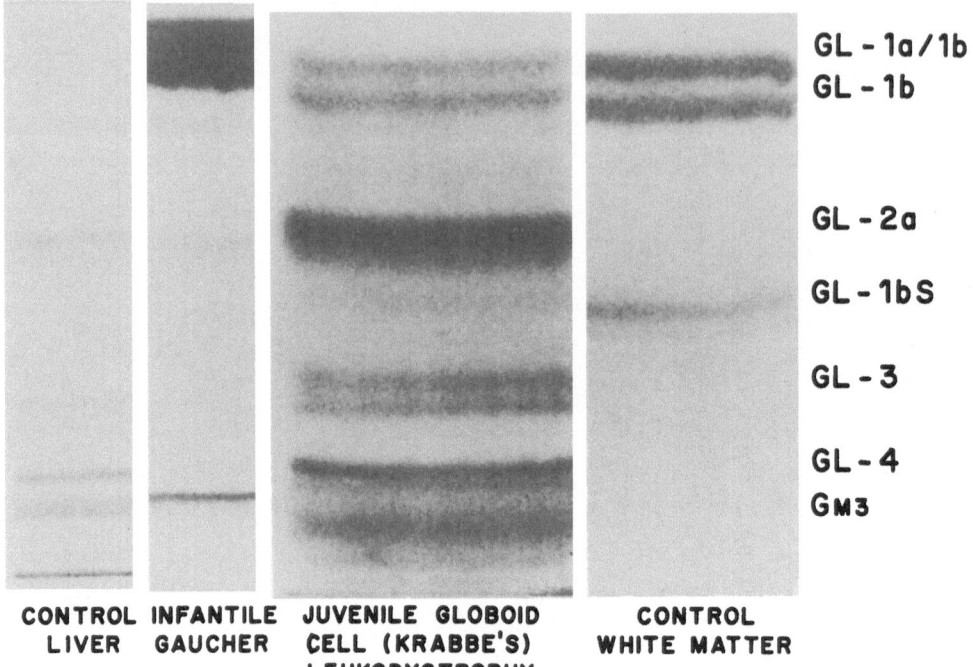

                                        GL - 1a / 1b
                                        GL - 1b

                                        GL - 2a

                                        GL - 1bS

                                        GL - 3

                                        GL - 4
                                        G M3

| CONTROL LIVER | INFANTILE GAUCHER | JUVENILE GLOBOID CELL (KRABBE'S) LEUKODYSTROPHY | CONTROL WHITE MATTER |

Fig. 2   Thin-layer chromatographic separation of glycosphingolipids from the liver of patients with Gaucher's disease and Globoid Cell Leukodystrophy, in the solvent system chloroform-methanol-water (110:40:6).

by a 6-fold elevation of GL-1a and a 2 to 3-fold elevation of G_{M3} (4), which are respectively the anabolic and catabolic precursors of GL-2a.

Despite these visceral abnormalities, Lactosylceramidosis is considered to be primarily a neurological disease. Chemical examination of autopsy gray matter from this patient (S.H.), in which the swollen apical dendrites appeared to contain considerable amounts of stored lipid, confirmed this and an accumulation of GL-2a (0.38 μmoles/g. fresh wt., compared to a total galactosylceramide level of 0.40 μmoles) was found. Accumulations of GL-1a (0.22 μmoles), G_{M3} (0.20 μmoles), asialo-G_{M2} (0.06 μmoles) and G_{M2} (0.20 μmoles/g. fresh wt.), were also found (4); these are extremely minor components of normal gray matter. White matter contained a more specific elevation of GL-2a (0.32 μmoles), the GL-1a level was normal, and the catabolic precursors (G_{M3}, asialo-G_{M2}, and G_{M2}) showed a much less dramatic increase. Cerebral GL-2a contained stearic acid (86.5%), which is characteristic of brain gangliosides and different from the fatty acid composition of the GL-2a which accumulated in liver, spleen, lymph node, adrenal gland and kidney, where $C_{22:0}$, $C_{24:0}$ and $C_{24:1}$ predominate (4). Although this disease manifests itself most clearly in the brain, the metabolism of liver glycosphingolipids was sufficiently altered to allow chemical confirmation of the enzymic defect. In addition, the concentration of GL-1a and G_{M3} was higher than normal in all tissues examined, but asialo-G_{M2} and G_{M2} were not detectable outside the brain.

This study of two rare diseases involving blocks in GL-1a and GL-2a catabolism respectively, has indicated that the rate of catabolism of GL-1a, GL-2a and G_{M3} is reduced in both diseases, whereas that of GL-3 and GL-4 is unaffected. It would be interesting to see if the rate of synthesis of GL-3 and GL-4 is sufficiently reduced in these diseases to a account for the findings.

3. Fucosidosis

A hepatic wedge biopsy was obtained from a 3 1/2-year old boy (blood group AB, c, d, e/c, Rh-) with the terminal stage of this disease (11), the fourth such case to be described. The absence of the lysosomal enzyme α-L-fucosidase suggested its affinity to other sphingolipidoses and previous reports (10,17) had suggested the

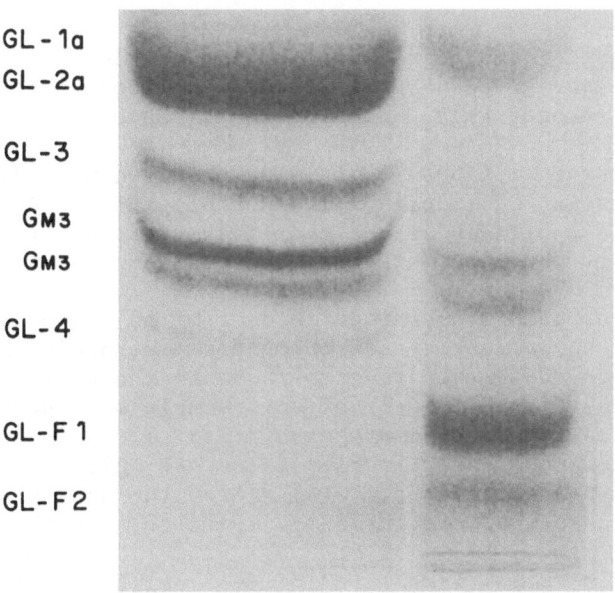

CONTROL   α-FUCOSIDOSIS
                      PATIENT

Fig. 3 Thin-layer chromatographic separation of glycosphingolipids from the liver of a patient (M.S.) with Fucosidosis. The solvent system was chloroform-methanol-water (110:40:6).

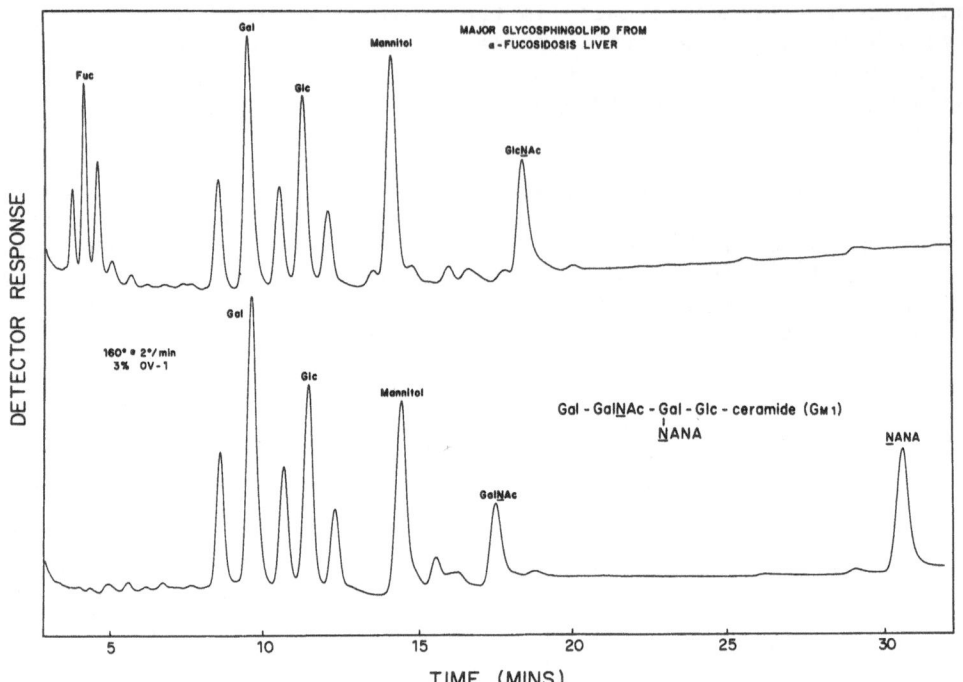

Fig. 4 Gas-liquid chromatographic analysis of the monosaccharides found in the major glycosphingolipid of Fucosidosis and G_{M1}-gangliosidosis liver respectively. Conditions are as described in Fig. 1.

widespread storage of fucose-containing glycosphingolipids and mucopolysaccharides in Fucosidosis. The neurological deterioration has progressed to dementia and since the liver continues to enlarge it is presumed that the same material is deposited in both organs.

    Analysis of the glycosphingolipids from an 0.063 g. liver biopsy, using the solvent system chloroform-methanol-2.5 N NH4OH (60:40:9), revealed a major abnormal band in the pentaglycosyl-ceramide region (Fig. 3). Half of this sample was subjected to quantitative gas-liquid chromatography (Fig. 4) indicating a penta-glycosylceramide-containing fucose, galactose, glucose and N-acetyl-glucosamine in the ratio 1:2:1:1 (8). From the work of Hakomori (12) two blood group-active substrates are known to have this composition:

H,   Fuc(1→2)Gal(1→3)GlcNAc(1→3)Gal(1→4)Glc-cer
Le^a,   Gal(1→3)GlcNAc(1→3)Gal(1→4)Glc-cer
$$\left(\begin{array}{c}4\\\uparrow\\1\end{array}\right)- \text{Fuc}$$

and their concentration in normal parenchymal organs is less than 1.0 μg (1.0 nmole)/g. fresh wt of tissue. The concentration of the

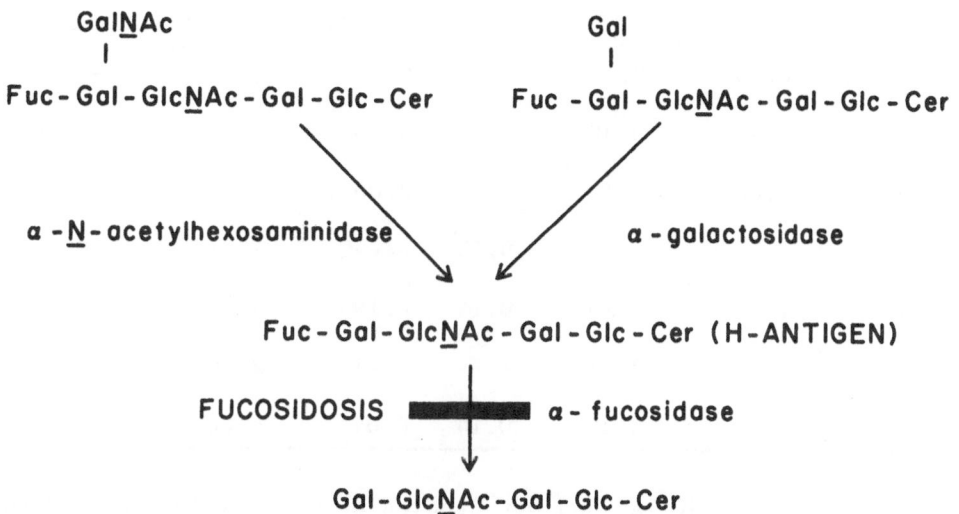

Fig. 5 Proposed site of the catabolic block in Fucosidosis.

major component was 2.8 μmoles/g. fresh wt. of tissue (Table 1)
which is comparable to the level found in other glycosphingolipid
storage diseases. Since the patient was blood group AB, both the
A and B glycosphingolipids should be synthesized; it is therefore
likely that the accumulating glycosphingolipid has the H structure
since this is a common catabolite of the A and B antigens (Fig. 5).
The Le^a glycosphingolipid has only been found in malignant tissue
(12) but the Le^b glycosphingolipid can be isolated from human red
cells (12). Patients with either gene could synthesize and store
these glycosphingolipids in addition to, or instead of, the H-anti-
gen. At present, the substrate specificity of α-fucosidases is
unknown and it was not possible to study the mucopolysaccharide or
glycoproteins in the biopsy sample available.

4. Leukodystrophies

Patients with metachromatic leukodystrophy (arylsulfatase A
deficiency) store sulfatide (GL-1bS) in brain and kidney but not
in liver (1). In globoid cell leukodystrophy (Krabbe's disease;
galactosylceramide galactosyl hydrolase deficiency) the lack of
accumulating galactosylceramide (GL-1b) has been explained (29) on
the basis of arrested myelination. Further, Suzuki et al. (26)
have shown that the moderate increase in kidney GL-1b is matched

TABLE 2 GLYCOSPHINGOLIPIDS AND "GLYCOPROTEINS"
IN G_{M1}-GANGLIOSIDOSIS (C.B.) LIVER

Sugar	CPC Supernatant	CPC Precipitate	G_{M1}	CPC Supernatant	Corneal Keratosulfate	G_{M1}
	μmoles/g. fresh wt.			molar ratio		
Fuc	0.25	0.11	----	0.05	0.05	----
Man	2.56	0.80	----	0.46	0.20	----
Gal	11.00	3.13	0.30	2.00	2.00	2.00
Glc	----	----	0.15	----	----	1.00
GalNAc	1.03	0.29	0.14	0.19	----	1.00
GlcNAc	9.40	2.01	----	1.71	2.16	----
NANA	0.23	0.23	0.14	0.04	0.06	1.00

by the increase in GL-la, and our studies on urine sediment confirm
this. However, we have recently studied formalin-fixed liver from
a patient diagnosed as having juvenile globoid cell leukodystrophy
(onset at age 4 years). Her twin sister is still alive (age 13
years) and shows the characteristic enzyme defect (28). Normal
liver contains less than 0.01 μmoles/g. fresh wt. but in the GLD
liver, the GL-1b level was greater than that of GL-la (Table 1)
(Fig. 2). Although one cannot rely completely on analyses carried
out on formalin-fixed material, the liver in GLD warrants further
investigation.

5. G_{M1}-gangliosidosis

Studies by O'Brien (19), Suzuki (30), Wolfe (34) and others
have established that the total β-galactosidase deficiency (pH 4.0)
characteristic of this disease results in the accumulation of G_{M1}
in brain and liver (Table 2) together with a "keratosulfate-like"
material which contains nearly equal amounts of galactose and N-
acetylglucosamine and lesser amounts of fucose, mannose, N-acetylgalactosamine and sialic acid (Table 2). If this material is indeed
structurally analogous to keratan sulfate, variations in the degree
of sulfation or nature of the protein moiety may explain its anomalous behavior with cetylpyridinium chloride and ion-exchange resins.

In addition to this Type 1 (infantile) form, a Type 2 (juvenile) form has been described in which skeletal abnormalities are
minimal and hepatomegaly much reduced. However, there is increasing

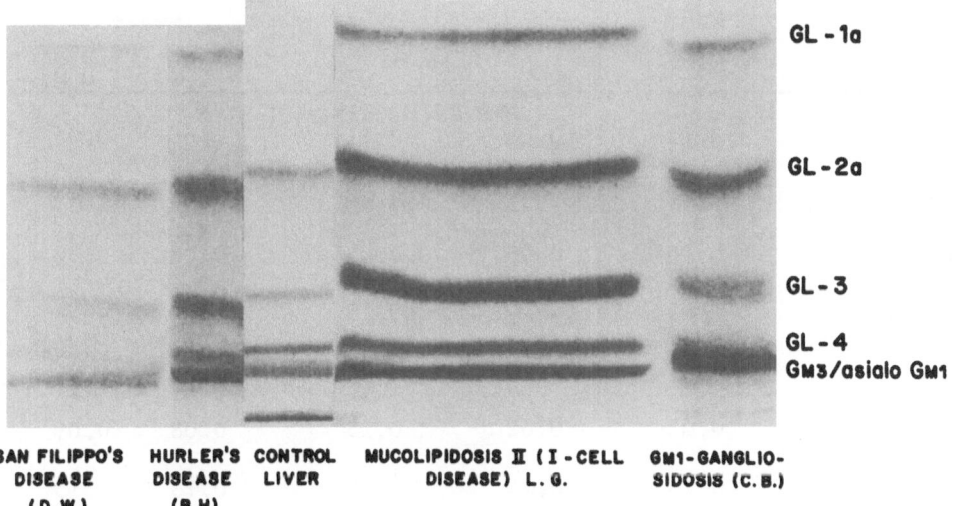

Fig. 6 Thin-layer chromatographic analysis of the glycosphingolipids isolated from liver of patients with diseases in which a
β-galactosidase deficiency has been reported. The solvent system
is chloroform-methanol-water (110:40:6).

evidence that biochemically diagnosed Type 1 patients with severe
hepatosplenomegaly, need not have the characteristic Hurler-like
appearance or bony abnormalities. We have examined two such
patients. Patient I (S.S.) died at age 14 months suffering from
severe neurological degeneration and showed the characteristic
accumulation of G_{M1} in formalin-fixed brain and liver. Fresh-
frozen liver was obtained from a second patient (C.B.) who was
severely retarded with a cherry red spot, hyperacusis and hepatosplenomegaly (but none of the facial or skeletal Hurler-like
features) and died at the age of 18 months. Glycosphingolipid
analysis of C.B. liver (Table 2) revealed the accumulation of both
asialo-G_{M1} (Fig. 6) and G_{M1}. This was anticipated from the total
absence of lysosomal β-galactosidase activity in the liver. Analysis of mucopolysaccharides by Dr. R. Matalon (Univ. of Chicago)
revealed no elevation of uronic acid-containing material and normal
amounts of material which behaved chromatographically on Dowex
resins as keratosulfate. However, both the cetylpyridinium chloride
(CPC) supernatant and CPC precipitate (of the papain-digested liver)
contained large amounts of material which corresponded to the keratosulfate-like material reported previously (19,30,34) in G_{M1}-

TABLE 3 <u>LIVER GLYCOSPHINGOLIPIDS IN PATIENTS WITH</u>
<u>MUCOLIPIDOSIS STORAGE DISEASES</u>*

Glycosphingo-lipid	Mucolipidosis I R.H.	V.H.	Mucolipidosis II ("I-Cell" Disease)		
			Type A O.W.	Type B L.G.	C.M.
			μmoles/g. fresh wt.		
GL-1a	0.15	0.08	0.11	0.06	0.06
GL-1b	----	----	0.03	0.01	----
GL-2a	0.09	0.08	0.03	0.06	0.06
GL-1bS	----	----	0.25	----	----
GL-3	0.04	0.04	0.10	0.08	0.09
GL-4	0.02	0.02	0.15	0.08	0.09
G_{M3}	0.15	0.14	0.19	0.18	0.15

* Control values for liver are given in Table 1.

gangliosidosis liver. The amount of macromolecular galactose (2600 μg./100 g. fresh wt.) was more than 20 times normal (Table 2) and corresponded closely to the amounts reported (30) for typical Type 1 patients. This material, which has not been further characterized, could be undersulfated keratosulfate or a complex carbohydrate as yet unidentified; the amount is sufficient to account for the hepatosplenomegaly. However, it appears that the facial features and skeletal abnormalities cannot be attributed to either this material or the G_{M1}- ganglioside accumulation.

6.   Inherited Diseases Involving Combined Storage of Lipid and Mucopolysaccharide Material

The study of G_{M1}-gangliosidosis inevitably leads one to consider the diseases grouped by Spranger (24) under the heading of "Mucolipidoses." Examination of liver biopsies from patients with Mucolipidosis I (MLI) revealed no gross abnormalities (Table 3) (Fig. 7) and no enzyme deficiencies have been associated with this disease. In contrast, "I-cell" disease (Mucolipidosis II), a variant of the Hurler syndrome, appears to be a generalized lysosomal glycosyl hydrolase disorder. It is much more severe than MLI, and in one patient we have found gross abnormalities. Patient O.W. is considered phenotypically similar (16,24) to the more characteristic "I-cell" patients (L.G. and C.M.) but the age of onset was much earlier and the hepatomegaly more pronounced. In

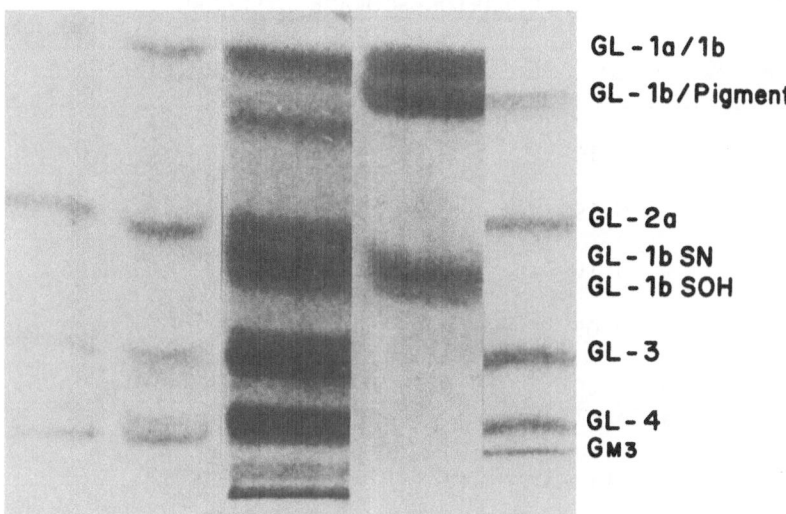

GL - 1a / 1b

GL - 1b / Pigment

GL - 2a

GL - 1b SN

GL - 1b SOH

GL - 3

GL - 4

G$_{M3}$

MUCOLIPIDOSIS I   MUCOLIPIDOSIS II ("I-CELL" DISEASE)

(R. H.)   (V. H.)   Type A   White matter   Type B

(O. W.)   (O. W.)   (L. G.)

Fig. 7 Thin-layer chromatographic analysis of the glycosphingolipids isolated from liver of patients with Mucolipidoses I and
II. White matter glycosphingolipids (GL-1b and GL-1bS) co-
chromatograph with components in liver from patient O.W. The
solvent system is chloroform-methanol-water (110:40:6).

O.W. liver, glycosphingolipids GL-3, GL-4 and sulfatide (GL-1bS)
were substantially elevated (Table 3) (Fig. 7) but the material
was not suitable for enzymatic study. Sulfatide is not normally
detectable in human liver (15). Liver from L.G. and C.M. showed
the characteristic (20% of normal) reduction in the level of
β-galactosidase activity and both GL-3 and GL-4 showed 2 to 3-fold
elevations when compared to normal (Fig. 6). No G$_{M1}$ could be
detected and the terminal galactose residue in the accumulating
GL-3 from L.G. liver was exclusively in the α-configuration. Therefore the β-galactosidase deficiency could not be confirmed chemically. However, the accumulation of GL-3, GL-4 and G$_{M3}$ was confirmed in skin fibroblasts from L.G. (5) as well as the generalized
lysosomal hydrolase deficiency which is characteristic of these
remarkable fibroblasts. It is probable that there are at least 2
types of "I-cell" disease, both of which involve some fundamental
defect in the structure or function of lysosomes.

TABLE 4   LIVER GLYCOSPHINGOLIPIDS IN PATIENTS WITH
          MUCOPOLYSACCHARIDE STORAGE DISEASES*

Glycosphingo-lipid	Hurler's Disease		Sanfilippo's Disease	
	(B.H.)	(D.H.)	(D.W.)	(R.H.)
	μmoles/g. fresh wt.			
GL-1a	0.14	0.12	0.08	0.07
GL-2a	0.19	0.28	0.06	0.07
GL-3	0.10	0.12	0.04	0.06
GL-4	0.05	0.09	0.02	0.03
G_{M3}	0.28	0.45	0.24	0.20

* Control values for liver are given in Table 1.

7. The Hurler-Hunter-Sanfilippo Syndrome

In contrast to "I-cell" disease, the reason for the hepatomegaly in Hurler's disease is well established since large amounts
(5-10 mg./g. fresh wt.) of dermatan sulfate and heparan sulfate
accumulate (9). As with "I-cell" disease, there is an unexplained
deficiency in β-galactosidase activity (as measured with synthetic
substrates) and it seemed of interest to determine if glycosphingolipid metabolism was also affected. It can be seen from Table 4
that liver from the two cases of "classical" Hurler's disease examined showed an overall 2 to 3-fold non-specific elevation of all
glycosphingolipids (Fig. 6). In contrast, liver from two patients
with Sanfilippo's disease (in which hepatomegaly is minimal) showed
normal levels of glycosphingolipids (Fig. 6) (Table 4) apart from a
slight increase in G_{M3}. As in "I-cell" disease, but in contrast to
G_{M1}-gangliosidosis, no G_{M1} could be detected in liver from either
Hurler or Sanfilippo patients.

Normal human liver glycosphingolipids differ from those of
brain in a number of important respects. Galactosylceramides and
hexosamine-containing "gangliosides" are virtually undetectable
(although it is clear from these and previous studies (19,30,34)
that such glycosphingolipids can be isolated from pathological
livers) and G_{M3}, GL-3 and GL-4 (the "visceral" glycosphingolipids)
are present in high concentration. Further, the intermediates in
G_{M3} and GL-4 metabolism, namely, GL-1a and GL-2a, are present in
relatively large amounts in liver whereas they are difficult to
detect in normal human brain, despite their apparent role in the
metabolism of G_{M1} and more complex "gangliosides." The presence
of G_{M1}, G_{M2}, GL-1b and GL-1bS in certain pathological livers indicates that glycosphingolipids typically associated only with nervous tissue, may be normal constituents of human liver and have
important biological activity.

The sensitivity and quantitative accuracy of gas-liquid chromatographic analysis of the constituent monosaccharides has enabled us to study, not only the diseases where there is massive glycosphingolipid accumulation in liver (Gaucher's disease and Fucosidosis), but also those diseases which are primarily neurological and in which smaller, but specific, changes are seen (Lactosylceramidosis, G_{M1}-gangliosidosis and Globoid Cell Leukodystrophy). Further, it has been possible to study the effect of these catabolic blocks on the concentration of other glycosphingolipids in the same pathway. Our major finding in this respect, is that in diseases affecting GL-1a and GL-2a catabolism, G_{M3} also accumulates but GL-3 and GL-4 do not. This is a somewhat surprising finding in view of the concept that GL-4 is synthesized from GL-1a by the sequential addition of monosaccharides. Analysis of liver from patients with mucopolysaccharidosis syndromes showed that Fucosidosis was a glycosphingolipidosis and that a number of glycosphingolipids (including in one case sulfatide) accumulated in both "I-cell" disease and Hurler's disease. The effect of glycosidase deficiencies on the metabolism of all complex carbohydrates (glycosphingolipids, mucopolysaccharides, glycoproteins and polysaccharides) should be the subject of further investigation in order to understand the mechanism of the disease process more fully. It is hoped that the study of metabolism in cultured cells (skin fibroblasts and possibly hepatocytes) from such patients, will facilitate these investigations.

ACKNOWLEDGEMENTS

I would like to thank Dr. Kunihiko Suzuki, University of Pennsylvania, Philadelphia, Pa., for the sample of infantile Gaucher liver; Dr. A.O. Stein, University of Chicago, for the Lactosylceramidosis liver; Dr. J. W. Spranger, University of Kiel, Germany, for liver from patients with Fucosidosis, G_{M1}-gangliosidosis, "I-cell" disease, mucolipidosis I, and Sanfilippo's disease; Dr. H. Müller, Basle, Switzerland, for the sample (C.B.) of G_{M1}-gangliosidosis liver; Dr. J. Sensenbrenner, Johns Hopkins University, Baltimore, for the "I-cell" disease liver biopsy (C.M.); Dr. R. Matalon, Dept. of Pediatrics, University of Chicago, for samples of liver from patients with Hurler's disease, for preparing the CPC fractions from G_{M1}-gangliosidosis liver, and for carrying out the enzymic assays with synthetic glycosides; Dr. A. J. Cifonelli, University of Chicago, for the sample of corneal keratosulfate; and Mr. John Oh for excellent technical assistance. This work was supported by United States Health Service Grant HD-04583 and Grant (RR-305) from the General Clinical Research Centers Program of the Division of Research Resources, National Institutes of Health. G. D. is a Joseph P. Kennedy, Jr. Scholar.

ABBREVIATIONS

Cer, ceramide (2-N-acylsphingosine); Gal, galactose; Glc, glucose; GalNAc, N-acetylgalactosamine; GlcNAc, N-acetylglucosamine; NANA, N-acetylneuraminic acid; Fuc, Fucose (6-deoxy-L-galactose); GL-1a, Glc-cer; GL-1b, Gal-cer; GL-2a, Gal-(1→4)-Glc-cer; GL-1bS, (SO$_3$H→3)-Gal-cer (sulfatide); GL-3, Gal-(1→4)-Gal-(1→4)-Glc-cer; GL-4, GalNAc-(1→3)-Gal-(1→4)-Gal-(1→4)-Glc-cer; G$_{M3}$, G$_{M2}$ and G$_{M1}$ are the standard Svennerholm nomenclature.

REFERENCES

1.   Austin, J. H.   Metachromatic form of diffuse sclerosis. III.
     Significance of sulfatide and other lipid abnormalities in
     white matter and kidney.   Neurol. (Minneap.) 10: 470 (1960).

2.   Brady, R. O., Gal, A. E., Bradley, R. M., Martensson, E.,
     Warshaw, A. L., and Laster, L.   Enzymatic defect in Fabry's
     disease: Ceramide trihexosidase deficiency.   New Engl. J. Med.,
     276: 1163 (1967).

3.   Clamp, J. R., Dawson, G., and Hough, L.   The simultaneous
     estimation of 6-deoxy-L-galactose (L-fucose), D-mannose, D-
     galactose, 2-acetamido-2-deoxy-D-glucose (N-acetyl-D-glucosa-
     mine) and N-acetylneuraminic acid (sialic acid) in glycopep-
     tides and glycoproteins.   Biochim. Biophys. Acta, 148: 342
     (1967).

4.   Dawson, G. Glycosphingolipid levels in an unusual neurovis-
     ceral storage disease characterized by lactosylceramide
     galactosyl hydrolase deficiency: Lactosylceramidosis.   J.
     Lipid Res., 13: 000 (1972).

5.   Dawson, G., Matalon, R., and Dorfman, A.   Glycosphingolipids
     in cultured human skin fibroblasts: II.   Characterization and
     metabolism in fibroblasts from patients with inborn errors of
     glycosphingolipid and mucopolysaccharide metabolism.   In
     preparation.

6.   Dawson, G., Matalon, R., and Stein, A. O.   Lactosylceramidosis:
     Lactosylceramide galactosyl hydrolase deficiency and accumula-
     tion of lactosylceramide in cultured skin fibroblasts.   J.
     Pediat., 79: 423 (1971).

7.   Dawson, G., and Stein, A. O.   Lactosylceramidosis: Catabolic
     enzyme defect of glycosphingolipid metabolism.   Science, 170:
     556 (1970).

8.   Dawson, G., and Spranger, J. W.   Fucosidosis: A glycosphingo-

lipidosis. New Engl. J. Exp. Med. 285: 122 (1971).

9. Dorfman, A. Heritable Diseases of Connective Tissues: The
    Hurler Syndrome. In, The Metabolic Basis of Inherited Disease.
    J. B. Stanbury, J. B. Wyngaarden, and D. S. Fredrickson,
    editors. McGraw-Hill, New York, 1966, p. 698.

10. Durand, P., Borrone, C., and Della Cella, G. Fucosidosis.
    J. Pediat., 75: 665 (1969).

11. Freitag, F., Kücheman, K., Blümcke, S., and Spranger, J. W.
    Hepatic ultrastructure in Fucosidosis. Virchows Arch. Abt.
    B. Zellpath., 7: 99 (1971).

12. Hakomori, S.-I. Glycosphingolipids having blood group ABH
    and Lewis specificities. Chem. Phys. Lipids, 5: 96 (1970).

13. Jørgenson, L., Blackstad, W., Harkmark, W. and Steen, J. A.
    Niemann-Pick's disease: Report of a case with histochemical
    evidence of neuronal storage of acid glycolipids. Acta
    Neuropathol., 4: 90 (1964).

14. Kint, J. A. Fabry's disease: Alpha-galactosidase deficiency.
    Science, 167: 1268 (1970).

15. Kwiterovich, P. O., Sloan, H. R., and Fredrickson, D. S.
    Glycolipids and other constituents of normal human liver.
    J. Lipid Res. 11: 322 (1970).

16. Leroy, J. G., Spranger, J. W., Feingold, M., Opitz, J. M.,
    and Crocker, A. C. I-cell disease: A clinical picture.
    J. Pediat., 79: 360 (1971).

17. Loeb, H., Tondeur, M., Jonneaux, G., Mockel-Pohl, S., and
    Vamos-Hurwitz, E. Biochemical and ultrastructural studies
    in a case of mucopolysaccharidosis "F" (Fucosidosis).
    Helv. Paed. Acta, 24: 519 (1969).

18. Okada, S., and O'Brien, J. S. Tay-Sachs disease: Generalized
    absence of a beta-D-N-Acetylhexosaminidase component.
    Science, 165: 698 (1969).

19. Okada, S., and O'Brien, J. S. Generalized Gangliosidosis:
    Beta-Galactosidase Deficiency. Science, 160: 1002 (1968).

20. Pilz, H., Sandhoff, K., and Jatzkewitz, H. Eine gangliosid-
    stoffwechselstorung mit Anhaufung von Ceramidlactosil,
    Monosialoceramid-Lactosid und Tay-Sachs-Gangliosid im
    Gehirn. J. Neurochem. 13: 1273 (1966).

21. Sandhoff, K., Andreae, U., and Jatzkewitz, H. Deficient hexosaminidase activity in an exceptional case of Tay-Sachs disease with additional storage of kidney globoside in visceral organs. Life Sci., 7: 283 (1968).

22. Schibanoff, J. M., Kamoshita, S., and O'Brien, J. S. Tissue distribution of glycosphingolipids in a case of Fabry's disease. J. Lipid Res. 10: 515 (1969).

23. Snyder, P. D., Krivit, W., and Sweeley, C. C. Generalized accumulation of neutral glycosphingolipids with G_{M2} ganglioside accumulation in the brain (Sandhoff's disease). II. Biochemical description. J. Lipid Res., 13: 000 (1972).

24. Spranger, J. W., and Wiedemann, H.-R. The genetic mucolipidoses. Humangenetik, 9: 113 (1970).

25. Suomi, W. D., and Agranoff, B. W. Lipids of the spleen in Gaucher's disease. J. Lipid Res. 6: 211 (1965).

26. Suzuki, K. Renal cerebroside in Globoid Cell Leukodystrophy (Krabbe's disease). Lipids, 6: 433 (1971).

27. Suzuki, Y., Jacob, J. C., Suzuki, K., Kutty, K. M. and Suzuki, K. G_{M2}-Gangliosidosis with total hexosaminidase deficiency. Neurol. (Minneap.), 21: 313 (1971).

28. Suzuki, Y., and Suzuki, K. Krabbe's Globoid Cell Leukodystrophy: Deficiency of galactocerebrosidase in serum, leukocytes and fibroblasts. Science, 171: 73 (1971).

29. Suzuki, K., and Suzuki, Y. Globoid Cell Leukodystrophy Krabbe's disease): Deficiency of galactocerebroside-β-galactoside. Proc. Natl. Acad. Sci., U.S.A., 66: 302 (1970).

30. Suzuki, K., Suzuki, K., and Kamoshita, S. Chemical pathology of G_{M1}-gangliosidosis (generalized gangliosidosis). J. Neuropathol. Exptl. Neurol., 28: 25 (1969).

31. Sweeley, C. C., and Klionsky, B. Glycolipid lipidosis: Fabry's disease: In, The Metabolic Basis of Inherited Disease. J. B. Stanbury, J. B. Wyngaarden, and D. S. Fredrickson, editors. McGraw-Hill, New York, 1966, p. 620.

32. Taketomi, T., and Kawamura, N. Cerebral and visceral glycolipids in a case of Tay-Sachs disease. J. Biochem., Tokyo, 66: 165 (1969).

33. Vance, D. E., and Sweeley, C. C. Quantitative determination

of the neutral glycosyl ceramides in human blood. $\underline{J}$.
$\underline{Lipid}$ $\underline{Res}$., $\underline{8}$: 621 (1967).

34. Wolfe, L. S., Callahan, J., Fawcett, J. S., Andermann, F.,
and Scriver, C. R. G_{M1}-Gangliosidosis without
chondrodystrophy or visceromegaly. $\underline{Neurol}$. $\underline{(Minneap}$.),
$\underline{20}$: 23 (1970).

RECENT ADVANCES IN METACHROMATIC LEUKODYSTROPHY

Neuwelt, E., Stumpf, D., Austin, J., and Kohler, P.,

University of Colorado Medical Center

Divisions of Neurology and Clinical Immunology,
Denver, Colorado

INTRODUCTION

Metachromatic leukodystrophy (MLD) is a fatal neurolipidosis characterized pathologically by both central and peripheral demyelination. It is genetically-determined as an autosomal recessive. MLD is caused by a deficiency of cerebroside sulfatase (arylsulfatase A;E.C.3.1.6.)(3), a lysosomal hydrolase responsible for the catabolism of sulfatide. Its substrate, cerebroside sulfate (sulfatide), is one of the key glycolipids in the myelin sheath.

There appears to be, at present, four genetically consistent forms of MLD (Table I).

TABLE I.

FORM OF MLD	USUAL AGE OF ONSET	ENZYME DEFICIENCY
Late Infantile	12-18 months	arylsulfatase A
Juvenile	3-10+ years	arylsulfatase A
Adult	After age 21	arylsulfatase A
Multiple Sulfatase Deficiency (MSA-MLD)	1-2 years	arylsulfatase A,B & C
		steroid sulfatase
		β-galactosidase

415

RECENT IMMUNOLOGICAL STUDIES IN MLD

One can prepare an antibody to sulfatase A by injecting highly purified enzyme into the popliteal lymph nodes of rabbits.(19) The antibody was rendered monospecific (as measured by immunodiffusion studies) by absorption with liver fractions which were isoelectrically focused next to the enzyme. This precipitating antibody had two unusual properties; 1) it increased the rate (as much as 3-4 fold) at which the normal enzyme hydrolyses its artificial substrate (nitrocatechol sulfate), 2) it stabilized the normal enzyme against inactivation by heat.

Liver obtained from MLD patients at autopsy contained a protein which was indistinguishable from the normal enzyme both by immunodiffusion and immunoelectrophoresis. The MLD enzyme precipitin line yielded no activity, however. In contrast, there was sulfatase activity in the precipitin line containing the normal enzyme and the antibody (19)

We have recently prepared a goat antibody to human sulfatase A by a similar method. Goat serum drawn 6-8 weeks after immunization inhibits enzyme activity when undiluted. But as one dilutes the serum, the inhibitory effect is lost. Thus, there are dilutions at which enzyme activity is precipitated, but not inhibited. These observations suggest that the enzyme is inhibited in antibody excess and/or that there is more than one class of antibody (one of which inhibits enzyme). Since the serum can be divided into markedly-inhibitory and non-inhibitory fractions by isoelectric focusing there seem to be at least two antibody classes. However, titration studies suggest that an excessive antibody : enzyme ratio may also be partially responsible for the inhibition.

THE PHYLOGENY OF SULFATASE A

Many of the classical experiments were performed on sulfatase A derived from the ox (30) Several lines of evidence suggest, however, that human and beef enzyme are substantially different. Thus, they differ in electrophoretic mobilities (16) and in isoelectric points (ox pI=3.4-3.6, human pI = 4.8).(19) Moreover, the ox enzyme is not inhibited by sulfhydryl reagents, (10) whereas the human enzyme is irreversibly inhibited. (8) This latter observation suggests that the environment of the active site might be different in these two species.

Immunological studies were performed using rabbit and goat anti-human sulfatase A (Table II). The antibody to the human enzyme cross-reacted with enzyme from the pigtail monkey and the dog. (Cross-reaction was defined either by precipitation of activity or by specific inhibition of enzyme activity). However, the antibody

Table II. IMMUNOLOGICAL COMPARATIVE STUDY OF ARYLSULFATASE - A

Source of Unfractionated Liver Supernatant***	Normal Goat Serum (1:8 dil)		Goat Antibody (1:8 dil)		Normal Rabbit Serum (1:8 dil)		Rabbit Antibody (1:8 dil)		0.1M Tris-HCl Buffer pH 7.35
	% Activity in Precipitate*	% Of Control**	% Activity in Precipitate*	% Of Control**	% Activity in Precipitate*	% Of Control**	% Activity in Precipitate*	% Of Control**	% Activity in Precipitate
Human	6	96	98	144	4	92	75	155	4
Pig-Tail Monkey	42	104	78	79	28	92	75	85	38
Dog	10	122	80	205	4	91	58	168	4
Beef	22	102	24	98	19	88	29	110	16
Sheep	10	98	16	101	8	89	19	93	9
Mouse	5	101	6	96	2	87	18	106	2

Each value represents the mean of 4 determinations

* The serum was reacted with enzyme for 90 minutes at 37°C, centrifuged at 30,000 g for 30 minutes, and the activity in the supernatant and pellet was assayed as described previously (19). Thus % activity in precipitate = activity in precipitate divided by activity in supernatant + activity in pellet.

** $\dfrac{\text{(activity in pellet + activity in supernatant)}}{\text{(total activity when buffer was added instead of serum)}}$ x100

*** Liver was homogenized 1:1 w/v in .02 M Tris-HCl, pH 7.35, centrifuged at 30,000 g for 30 minutes and the supernatant was used as the enzyme source.

to the human enzyme did not cross-react with sheep, beef or mouse enzyme. Thus, there are substantial antigenic differences between beef and human sulfatase A. It seems clear that one can extrapolate only with great caution between results obtained with sulfatase A in other species and those obtained in man.

The possibility was raised that the sulfatase A deficiency in MLD might be caused by a deficiency of a sialotransferase. This was based on studies with rat sulfatases which suggested that sulfatase B might be sulfatase A minus sialic acid groups. (8) However, there was no cross-reaction between human sulfatases A and B. (33) One wonders whether sialic acid groups per se could account for this negative observation.

SULFATASE ACTIVITY AGAINST NITROCATECHOL SULFATE IN PELLET FRACTIONS

It was surprising to find that pellet fractions obtained from classical MLD tissues seemed to have apparently normal levels of "sulfatase A."(3)(32) In contrast, pellet fractions in multiple sulfatase deficiency (MSD-MLD; the MLD variant) had low levels of this pellet activity. (32) Little attention has been given to this sedimentable arylsulfatase activity in the past. (.29).

We recently studied this aspect of arylsulfatase activity in normal human liver. (34) The sulfatase activity, though bound in sediment despite numerous water washes, is readily eluted into a supernatant phase by washing with 0.1M Tris-HCl pH 7.35. In fact, the activity associated with the sediment and that eluted from it both resemble sulfatase B, not sulfatase A. This conclusion is based on the effects of various inhibitors, on the inactivation by heat, and on the effect of pH. Furthermore, the eluted activity is precipitated at the same ammonium sulfate concentrations at which sulfatase B is precipitated. Finally, the eluted activity is not precipitated by the antibody to sulfatase A. All these studies show that the pellet sulfatase which is active against nitrocatechol sulfate is distinct from sulfatases A and C. Indeed, it closely resembles soluble sulfatase B in all parameters tested. It thus appears likely that essentially the same protein may be responsible for both pellet and supernatant sulfatase B activity.

THE CARRIER STATE IN MLD

Tissue Culture Studies of the Carrier

Our studies support the findings of Kaback and Howell (12) in that the mean level of sulfatase activity in the skin fibroblasts

of obligate heterozygotes seems to be intermediate between that of
normal controls and of patients with MLD (Table III). However, we
continue to have certain problems in detecting individual carriers
of MLD. Thus, on a single determination, we have not yet been
able to say with certainty that a given individual must be a carrier. Neither the specific activity of sulfatase A in fibroblasts
nor the ratio between arylsulfatase A activity and acid phosphatase activity has been helpful. Basically, there has been too
much overlap between the specific activity of our control cells
and those of our obligate heterozygote cells. We have found this
overlap both in late infantile and in juvenile MLD. The methods
used were very similar to those of others. (12) Even using monospecific antibodies to arylsulfatase A (Table III) (33) we have
not been able to positively identify individual carriers by differences in specific activity in fibroblasts. (activity/h/mgm immune
precipitate) (Table II). Other laboratories have also had this
same problem in detecting the heterozygote in fibroblasts. (13)

We would suggest that this problem may, in part, be an inherent limitation of the tissue culture system used. At least two
factors may be identified: 1) the enzyme level in fibroblasts
varies with the gestational age of the person from whom the primary
explant was taken, (12) and 2) the enzyme level varies markedly
with the time in subculture (see Figs. 1 and 2). For example, our
studies show there is a 3-4 fold difference between the enzyme
level of cells harvested two days post subculture and those harvested ten days post subculture (enzyme activity is related here
both to the amount of protein and to the number of cells). The transition period between low and high cellular enzyme levels seems to
be correlated with contact inhibition. Fibroblasts from different
people vary greatly in the time (±2-3 days) at which they show contact inhibition. This variation occurs even though the cell count
of the initial inoculum is the same. Possibly harvesting cells before contact inhibition occurs (i.e. when enzyme activity is more
stable) would alleviate this problem. Miedema and Kruse have shown
that alkaline phosphatase levels also change markedly with contact
inhibition. (17)

The use of fresh leukocytes may very well avoid the problems
noted above in the use of fibroblasts. The heterozygote state has
been successfully detected in leukocytes by Bass, et. al., (4) and
Taniguchi and Nanbu (35) Their methods may represent an improvement over those used by Percy and Brady (23) and by Kihara (13) who
have been unable to detect individual carriers using leucocytes.
However, leukocytes do present other problems. The differential
count of leukocytes does vary from person to person. The several
different kinds of leukocytes do not form, when pooled, a completely homogeneous population in terms of sulfatase A activity and protein levels. Indeed, in the case of pseudocholinesterase defi-

Table III. IN VITRO STUDIES OF ASA-A SPECIFIC ACTIVITIES WITH AND WITHOUT ANTIBODY

Condition Studied**	Family Studied	Mean ASA-A Specific Activity±S.D. (units/h/mgm Protein)	Range of Specific Activities	Mean ASA-A Specific Activity±S.D. (units/h/mgm Immune Precipitate)	Range of Specific Protein Activities
Late Infantile					
5 year old male	F	1.8	15±5	15±5	8-21
3 year old female	F	1.1±.63			
Juvenile MLD					
13 year old male	M	0.78	0.78	13±6	5-19
9 year old female	M	0.90±.3	.77-1.02	13±3	9-17
Late Infantile MLD Obligate Heterozygote					
33 year old male	F	44±8	52-37	143±110	25-291
29 year old female	F	61±31	29-92		
Juvenile MLD Obligate Heterozygote					
44 year old female	M	50±4	46-55	280-226	41-582
59 year old male	M	77±27	50-104	266-129	137-395
Juvenile MLD Siblings					
18 year old female	M	72±39	34-111	491±58	419-562
5 year old female	M	103±32	135-71	379±173	153-408
Controls					
3 year old		97±47	53-187		197
5 year old					584-1392
16 week old					397
35 year old		137±69	67-207		
Newborn		58±17	42-81		
Pooled Controls		89±59	52-207	638±456	197-1392

** Fibroblasts were obtained from forearm biopsies. Cells were grown in Falcon flasks or roller bottles and harvested 1-2 days following contact inhibition. ASA-A activity was measured as described previously (19), proteins were measured by the method of Lowry, et al.

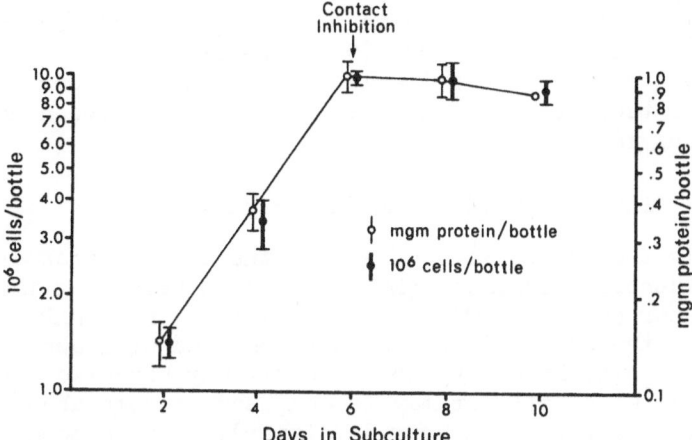

Fig. 1.   Cessation of growth and protein level in fibroblasts
at the time of contact inhibition. Note the log
scale on the vertical axis. The standard deviations
are indicated. Cells were obtained from a forearm
skin biopsy of a 3 year old.

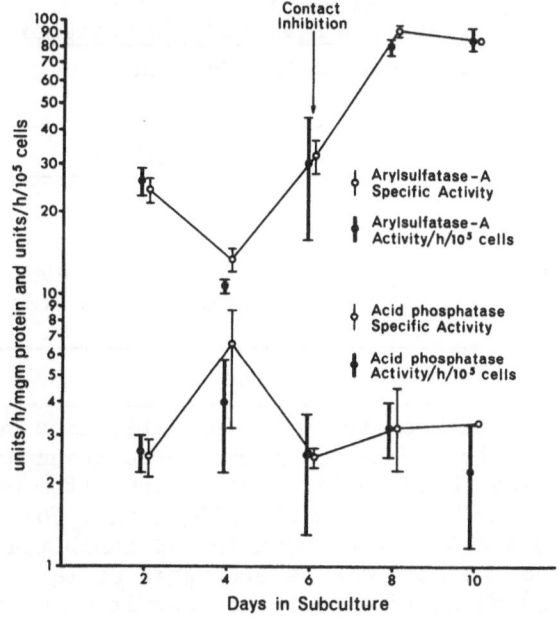

Fig. 2.   Variation of fibroblast enzyme levels during a single
subculture. Note the 3-4 fold increase in ASA-
activity (upper line). In contrast, acid phosphatase
activity changes much less (lower line). Cells used
are the same as those in Fig. 1. Standard deviations
are indicated.

ciency, as in other diseases, the variation in specific activity
is too great to allow the detection of a heterozygote individual
irregardless of the tissue used. (9) However, the use of an inhibitor very effectively distinguishes carriers from controls in
this disorder because of qualitative differences between normal
and mutant enzyme.

Biochemical Studies of the Carrier

Normally the sulfatase A enzyme of the ox is composed of four,
presumably identical monomers (MW 100,000) gathered together to
form a tetramer (MW 400,000). (20) Similarly, in an MLD patient
(homozygote), the enzyme is presumably composed of 4 abnormal mutant monomers. The heterozygote, however, may have two possible
structures: 1) each tetramer may be composed of both abnormal and
normal monomers (i.e., be a hybrid polymer). For purposes of illustration, this might be designated N-N-A-A, where N = normal
monomer, and A= abnormal monomer. 2) On the other hand, tetramers
might also be composed of two distinct, homogeneous classes of
enzyme (e.g., some might be NNNN, and others might be AAAA).
(Table IV).

TABLE IV.
Human Arylsulfatase-A M.W. 400,000 Tetramer
Assume 4 Identical Monomers

Normal	NNNN
Carrier	1. NNNN and AAAA (two distinct species)
	2. AAAA, NAAA, NNAA, NNNA, NNNN (hybrid polymer)
MLD	AAAA

To distinguish between these two possibilities we used a sulfhydryl group inhibitor, PHMB (p-hydroxymercuribenzoate). PHMB, in
earlier studies, was found to be a potent inhibitor of the normal
enzyme but not of the late infantile MLD enzyme. For example, the
urinary sulfatase A activity of normals was inhibited 93.8%; whereas, PHMB inhibited the obligate heterozygote of late infantile MLD
42-78.7%. (8) (12) We would expect this result only if the heterozygote enzyme were a hybrid polymer (e.g., N-N-A-A). If, on the
other hand, two enzyme classes were present, then the activity in
the carrier should be inhibited just as much as that in the normal
enzyme preparation. The reason is that completely abnormal tetramers (AAAA) would have only negligible catalytic activity to begin with. Hybrid proteins are known to exist in a number of other
heterozygous conditions (see review in ref 9).

The presence of a hybrid polymer in the heterozygote may also
contribute to our difficulties in detecting the carrier. That is,
a hybrid polymer might have a specific activity perhaps 75% of
normal (for example), rather than the 50% of normal activity one
might expect if both normal enzyme molecules (NNNN) and abnormal
enzyme molecules (AAAA) were present. Inborn errors of metabolism
have been reported in which the specific activity of carriers is
consistently above (1) or below (5) the 50% value.

Immunological Studies in the Carrier

Our immunochemical studies are based on the finding that the
rabbit antibody to sulfatase A precipitates both the MLD and the
normal human enzyme. One might expect that the method of immune
precipitation would yield reasonable values for enzyme specific
activity (i.e., enzyme activity/mgm immune precipitate)(See Table
II). However, even this method has not yet enabled us to consistently distinguish the individual carrier from normals on a single
determination either in fibroblasts or in urine.(33) However, immune
precipitation is only a secondary measurement of the interaction
of antigen with antibody. That is, it does not directly measure
the primary antigen-antibody interaction. Other methods are now
under investigation.

SOME GENETIC, PATHOGENIC AND THERAPEUTIC CONSIDERATIONS IN MLD

One can now ask some new questions regarding the correlations
between the genetic, biochemical and clinical features of MLD.
Clearly, the primary abnormality in MLD resides at the genome
level. At least two genes appear to be involved in controlling
sulfatase A activity. One genome (presumably a structural one) is
concerned only with sulfatase A. It is abnormal in classical MLD.
Another genome is responsible for a process common to several sulfatases. This is abnormal in that form of MLD with multiple sulfatase deficiencies (MLD-MSD; late infantile MLD variant).

In classical MLD, there are qualitative differences in biochemical behavior between the sulfatase A found in the late infantile form and that found in the juvenile form. These findings
suggest that the enzyme molecule in the one form is disabled by a
somewhat different chemical lesion than that in the other form.(31)
(32)

Several lines of evidence suggest that clinical differences
between these forms might also be a reflection of differences in
the function of different mutant enzymes. Thus, more substrate
accumulates (as measured at autopsy) in the earlier onset late
infantile form.(11) Correspondingly, sulfatide accumulates more

rapidly in cultured fibroblasts in this same form.(26) Sulfatase A
activity is also lower in the urine of patients with late infantile
MLD in our experience.(31)(32) The simplest explanation for the
above, for which there is precedent in humans,is multiple mutant
alleles involving a single structural genome. Thus, various mutations of this single structural genome may underlie the clinical
differences found in the different forms of classical MLD.

We have thus postulated a structural mutation in classical
MLD, the result of which would be normal amounts of sulfatase A
protein but deficient enzyme activity. What could be wrong with the
structure of the enzyme molecule? Surely, a precise chemical definition of this point will be helpful in designing rational modes
of therapy. First, the active site of the enzyme could be abnormal
For example, a crucial amino acid substitution might prevent binding
of the substrate or catalysis by the enzyme. To correct for this
kind of abnormality, one would have three alternatives: 1)alter the
genome, 2) alter the activity of the enzyme against its substrate,
or 3) add more normal enzyme (replacement therapy). Results with
the latter approach in MLD have not been encouraging.(2)(7) However,
replacement therapy in the presence of a stabilizing antibody, or
other stabilizing factor, which may also direct the enzyme to the
lysosome, remains to be attempted. It is of interest that in the
recent work by Porter, et. al., normal enzyme not only gained access
to the inside of a fibroblast, but also once there, was much more
stable than the enzyme left in the tissue culture medium.(25)
Certainly a major, possibly unsurmountable, problem with this
approach, at least in central nervous system lipid disorders, is the
risk of repeatedly putting purified human antibody or other stabilizing agents into the CSF. Those dealing with systemic lipidoses
which do not involve the nervous system are in a much better therapeutic position.

In what other ways could the enzyme molecule be abnormal?
Fortunately, only a relatively few amino acids are normally present
in the active site. Therefore, a mutation involving another region
of an enzyme protein may be statistically more likely. It is of note
that this kind of a point mutation has been amenable to "antibody
therapy" in bacterial models. Thus, an antibody to the normal enzyme
restores significant amounts of activity to point mutants deficient
in β-galactosidase or penicillinase activity.(24)(28)

Point mutations, not involving the active site, may also cause
an unstable molecular conformation, the enzyme activity of which is
very labile. Thus, it is possible that the late infantile MLD protein
might be the most labile and the adult MLD protein the most stable.
Such an hypothesis might also explain differences in the rate of
hydrolysis of sulfatide in fibroblasts among the various forms of
MLD.(26) If proven true, one might then be able to correlate an
earlier age of onset with a greater lability of the enzyme reflecting

this particular MLD allele. Indeed, in glucose-6-phosphate dehydrogenase deficiency young erythrocytes have normal amounts of activity, whereas older RBC's are markedly deficient in activity.(36) Thus, in this disorder deficient enzyme activity appears to be attributable to the increased lability of the mutant protein even though, initially, it can function at normal capacity.

An abnormally labile enzyme is also amenable to antibody therapy, as shown by the excellent work of Feinstein, et al.(6) He demonstrated that catalase deficiency in a certain strain of mice is due to an instability of the mutant enzyme. He was able to stabilize in vitro the residual activity of the abnormal enzyme with antibody, even though he could not restore the lost activity of the mutant enzyme back to normal. We have not been able to do this with sulfatase A in MLD, but this might reflect the fact that we have not yet obtained the enzyme in vitro soon enough. Indeed, Porter, et. al., have only detected sulfatide hydrolysis in intact MLD fibroblasts. (26) The observation that the normal sulfatase A can be stabilized (19) raises the possibility that an appropriate stabilizing agent may someday have a therapeutic role in MLD or in other enzyme deficiency diseases.

SUMMARY

The sulfatase A enzyme protein is present in metachromatic leukodystrophy but the enzyme protein is deficient in activity. An antibody to human sulfatase A does not cross-react with the sheep, beef or mouse enzyme. The pellet fractions obtained from human liver contain a nitrocatechol sulfatase activity which closely resembles soluble sulfatase B in all parameters tested.

There may be problems inherent in fibroblast metabolism that make it difficult to detect the MLD heterozygote in these cells. The reason is that the sulfatase A level in fibroblasts varies with the gestational age of the person. Moreover, the enzyme level also varies markedly during the time it is in subculture. The transition period between low and high cellular enzyme levels seems to coincide with the period of contact inhibition.

The response to a sulfhydryl group inhibitor (PHMB) suggests that the MLD heterozygote may have sulfatase A in the form of a hybrid polymer. Present evidence suggests that a structural genome carries the abnormality in classical MLD. A spearate genome is responsible for that form of MLD with multiple sulfatase deficiencies. (MLD-MSD).

The observation that the activity of normal sulfatase A can be stabilized by an antibody raises the possibility that an appropriate stabilizing agent may someday have a therapeutic role in MLD or in other enzyme deficiency diseases.

References

1) Aebi, H., Bossi, E., Cantz, M., Matsubara, S., and Suter, H.,
    Acatalas(em)ia in Switzerland, In, Hereditary Disorders of Ery-
    throcyte Metabolism, ed. E. Beutler, Grune & Stratton, New
    York, 1968, p. 48.

2) Austin, J., Some Recent Findings in Leukodystrophies and in
    Gargoylism, In, Inborn Errors of Sphingolipid Metabolism,
    Pergamon Press, Ltd., Oxford, 1967, p. 359-387.

3) Austin, J., Armstrong, D., and Shearer, L., Metachromatic
    Leukodystrophy V. The Nature and Significance of Low Sulfatase
    Activity: A Controlled Study of Brain, Liver and Kidney in Four
    Patients with Metachromatic Leukodystrophy, Arch Neurol,
    13:593-614, 1965.

4) Bass, N., Witmer, E., and Dreifuss, F., A Pedigree Study of
    Metachromatic Leukodystrophy, Neurology, 20:52-62, 1970.

5) Fallon, H., Smith, L., Graham, J., and Burnett, C., A Genetic
    Study of Hereditary Orotic Aciduria, N Engl J Med, 270:878,1964.

6) Feinstein, R., Jaroslow, B., Howard, J., and Faulhaber, J.,
    Stabilization of Mutant Catalase by Complex Formation with Anti-
    body to Normal Catalase, J Immunol, 106:1316-1322, 1971.

7) Greene, H., Hug, G., and Schubert, W., Metachromatic Leuko-
    dystrophy. Treatment with Arylsulfatase A, Arch Neurol,
    20:147-153, 1969.

8) Goldstone, A., Konecny, P., and Koenig, H., Lysosomal Hydro-
    lases: Conversion of Acidic to Basic Forms by Neuraminidase,
    F.E.B.S. Letters,13:68-72,1971.

9) Harris, H., The Principles of Human Biochemical Genetics,
    American Elsevier Co., New York, 1970, p. 32-35.

10) Jerfy, A., and Roy, A., The Sulfatase of Ox Liver. XII. The
    Effect of Trypsin and Histidine Reagents on the Activity of
    Sulfatase A. Biochim Biophys Acta, 175:355-364, 1969.

11) Jatzkewitz, H., Pilz, H., and Hollander, H., Biochemistre und
    vergleichende Histochemische in umschriebenen Gebieten das
    Gehirns bei Fallen von adulki und infantiler metachromatischer
    Leukodystrophie, Acta Neuropath, 4:75-89, 1964.

12) Kaback, M., and Howell, R., Infantile Metachromatic Leuko-
    dystrophy. Heterozygote Detection in Skin Fibroblasts and Poss-
    ible Applications to Intrauterine Diagnosis, N Eng J Med,
    282:1336-1340, 1970.

13)   Kihara, H., Personal Communication, 1971.

14)   Mahita, T., and Sandbom, E., Ultrastructural Localization of
      Arylsulfatase B in Mitochondria of Epithelial Cells of the
      Proximal Convoluted Tubules of the Rat Kidney, Experientia,
      27:187-189, 1971.

15)   McConahey, P., and Dixon, F., A Method of Trace Iodonation of
      Protein for Immunologic Studies, Int Arch Allergy,29:185-189,
      1966.

16)   Mehl, E., and Jatzkewitz, H., Cerebroside 3-sulfate as a
      Physiological Substrate for Arylsulfatase A., Biochim Biophys
      Acta, 151:619-627, 1968.

17)   Miedema, E., and Kruse, P., Effect of Prednisolone and Contact
      Phenomena on the Alkaline Phosphatase Activity of Hep-2 Cells,
      B.B.R.C., 26:704-711, 1967.

18)   Minden, P., Farr, R., The Ammonium Sulfate Method to Measure
      Antigen Binding Capacity in D.M. Weir (Ed), Handbook of
      Experimental Immunology, Philadelphia, Davis, 1967, Chap. 13.

19)   Neuwelt, E., Stumpf, D., Austin, J., and Kohler, P., A
      Monospecific Antibody to Human Sulfatase A: Preparation and
      Characterization and Significance, Biochim Biophys Acta,
      236:333-346, 1971.

20)   Nichol, L., and Roy, A., The Sulfatase of Ox Liver. IX. The
      Polymerization of Sulfatase A, Biochemistry (Wash), 4:396-401,
      1965.

21)   Nichol, L., and Roy, A., The Sulfatase of Ox Liver. X. Some
      Observations on the Intermolecular Bonding in Sulfatase A,
      Biochemistry (Wash), 5:1379-1388, 1966.

22)   Percy, A., and Kaback, M., Infantile and Adult Onset of Meta-
      chromatic Leukodystrophy, N Eng J Med, 283:785-787, 1971.

23)   Percy, A., and Brady, R., Metachromatic Leukodystrophy: Dia-
      gnosis with Sample of Venous Blood, Science, 161:594, 1968.

24)   Pollock, M., Fleming, J., and Petrie, S., The Effects of
      Specific Antibodies on the Biological Activities of Wild-Type
      Bacterial Penicillinases and their Mutationally Altered
      Analogues, In, Antibodies to Biologically Active Molecules,
      Ed., B. Cinader, Pergamon Press, Oxford, 1967.

25)   Porter, M., Fluharty, A., Kihara, H., Correction of Abnormal
       Cerebroside Sulfate Metabolism in Cultured Metachromatic
       Leukodystrophy Fibroblasts, Science, 172:1263-1364, 1971.

26)   Porter, M., Fluharty, A., Trammell, J., and Kihara, H., A
       Correlation of Intracellular Cerebroside Sulfatase Activity
       in Fibroblasts, Biochim Biophys Res Common, 44:660-666, 1971.

27)   Porter, M., Fluharty, A., Harris, S., and Kihara, H., The
       Accummulation of Cerebroside Sulfates by Fibroblasts in
       Culture from Patients with Late Infantile Metachromatic
       Leukodystrophy, Arch Biochem & Biophys, 138:646-652, 1970.

28)   Rotman, M., and Celada, Antibody Mediated Activation of A
       Defective β-D-galactosidase Extracted from an Eschericia coli
       Mutant, Proc Nat Acad Sci, U.S.A., 60:660-667, 1968.

29)   Roy, A., The Sulfatase of Ox Liver. 7. The Intracellular
       Distribution of Sulfatase A and B., J Biochem, 77:380-386,
       1960.

30)   Roy, A., and Trudingen, P., The Biochemistry of Inorganic
       Compounds of Sulfur, Cambridge Univ. Press, 1970.

31)   Stumpf, D., and Austin, J., Metachromatic Leukodystrophy (MLD)
       IX. Qualitative and Quantitative Differences in Urinary
       Arylsulfatase A in Different Forms of MLD, Arch Neurol,
       24:117-124, 1971.

32)   Stumpf, D., and Austin, J., Qualitative and Quantitative
       Differences in Sulfatase A in Different Forms of Classical
       Metachromatic Leukodystrophy, Lipid Storage Diseases

33)   Stumpf, D., Neuwelt, E., Austin, J., and Kohler, P., Meta-
       chromatic Leukodystrophy (MLD) X. Immunological Studies of
       the Abnormal Sulfatase A., Arch Neurol, In press.

34)   Stumpf, D., Austin, J., and LaFrance, M., In preparation.

35)   Taniguchi, N., and Nanbu, I., Enzymatic Abnormality of the
       Carrier State in Metachromatic Leukodystrophy, Clin Ch Acta,
       29:375-379, 1970.

36)   Yoshida, A., Stamatoyannopoulos, G., and Motulsky, A., Negro
       Variant of Glucose-6-phosphate Dehydrogenase Deficiency (A-)
       Science, 155:97-99, 1967.

LIVER GLYCOLIPIDS, STEROID SULFATES AND STEROID SULFATASES IN A FORM OF METACHROMATIC LEUKODYSTROPHY ASSOCIATED WITH MULTIPLE SULFATASE DEFICIENCIES

H. W. Moser, M. Sugita, M. D. Harbison, and M. Williams

The Eunice Kennedy Shriver Center at the Walter E. Fernald State School, Waverley, Massachusetts 02178

Austin et al. (4) and Mehl and Jatzkewitz et al. (14,22) have shown that metachromatic leukodystrophy (MLD) is associated with deficient activity of arylsulfatase A. This enzyme, in combination with a heat-stable complementary factor, cleaves sulfate from sulfatide.(22,23) Arylsulfatase A deficiency thus causes the sulfatide accumulation which is pathognomic of this disease.

In most cases of MLD, sulfatide is the only substance which accumulates in substantial amounts, and arylsulfatase A is the only defective enzyme.(24) However, in ten patients with this disease, one or more additional substances have been shown to accumulate. (18,25,26,28,30,36,37) (Table 1) The clinical manifestations and histopathological abnormalities have been reasonably consistent. The main points of difference from classical late infantile MLD are: (1) The presence of Alder-Reilly granulations in peripheral white blood cells. These have been observed in all of the seven patients in whom this abnormality was looked for.(2,3,26,30,36,37) (2) Increased urinary polysaccharide excretion was observed in five of six patients.(2,30,36,37) (3) Moderate hepatosplenomegaly was observed in five patients. (2, 26, 30) (4) In all of the four patients in whom postmortem studies were performed, the cortical neurones were distended with material with histochemical properties similar to those of the ganglio-sides.(2,3,18,25,26,28)

Since this constellation of abnormalities has been observed ten times in six separate families, it seems unlikely, on a statistical basis, that it is due to the chance association of rare entities such as classical late infantile MLD, a mucopoly-saccharidosis, and/or a lipidosis. Most authors have concluded

Table 1

Variant Form of Metachromatic Leukodystrophy
Pattern of Substrate Accumulation

Author	Sulfatide	Polysaccharide	Steroid Sulfates	Ganglioside Accumulation in Cortical Neurones
Mossakowski et al. (25)	+	?	?	+
	+	?	?	+
	+	?	?	+
Austin (2, 3)	+	+	±	+
	+	+	?	+
Thieffry et al. (36,37)	+	+	?	?
Luthy et al. (18, 28, 30)	+	+	?	+
Rampini et al. (30)	+	+	?	?
	+	+	?	?
Murphy et al. (26)	+	+	+	+

that it represents a distinct, genetically determined disease entity. This supposition is strengthened by enzymatic studies in three patients. Unlike the specific arylsulfatase A deficiency in classical MLD, their tissues showed a deficiency of arylsulfatases A, B and C, and in two patients a deficiency of steroid sulfatases was also demonstrated. (4, 26) This pattern of defects is unique.

No consistent name has as yet been agreed upon for this form of metachromatic leukodystrophy. Lüthy used the term "amaurotic idiocy with metachromatic change in the white matter", at a time when the mucopolysaccharide accumulation was not yet recognized. (18) The designation "metachromatic leukodystrophy associated with mucopolysaccharidosis" by Thieffry et al. (36,37) suggests a chance association which is no longer believed to be the case. Rampini's designation "mucosulfatidosis" implies a distinct entity and makes reference to the two main storage substances.(30) The only drawback, in our view, is the lack of precision of the prefix "muco". We prefer the designation "multiple sulfatase deficiency", for those cases (Austin's "M family" and our patient "G.L.") in which enzymatic studies are available.

We will present here data concerning the glycolipid and steroid sulfate levels, and additional data about the steroid sulfatases in the liver from two patients with multiple sulfatase deficiency. For comparison we have used postmortem materials from four patients with classical MLD, four patients with various forms of mucopolysaccharidoses, and from age matched controls.

LIVER GLYCOLIPIDS

Methods

Extraction of Lipids. A frozen sample of liver tissue was thawed, then homogenized in a Waring blendor and lyophilized. The dry tissue (from 1 to 3 g) was mixed with 20 volumes of chloroform-methanol (2:1, v/v). The mixture was stirred with a magnetic bar for 5 minutes at room temperature and filtered, and the residue on the filter paper was re-treated with 1/5 the original volume of chloroform-methanol (2:1, v/v). The combined extracts from liver were evaporated to dryness in vacuo in a rotating evaporator at + 40°C.

Mild Alkali-Catalyzed Hydrolysis. The extracted lipids were dissolved in a small amount of chloroform-methanol (2:1, v/v) and subjected to mild alkaline hydrolysis to remove glycerolipids by the modified method of Dawson described previously.(7, 12)

After acidification to pH 4 the lipids were extracted from
the hydrolysate by adding 4 vol. of chloroform-methanol (2:1, v/v),
shaking vigorously for 1-2 min., and then centrifuging at 3000 rpm
for 15 min. After discarding the upper phase the lower phase was
dialyzed against water for 20 hrs. The contents of the tube were
lyophilized.

Column Chromatography. The lyophilized material (50-100 mg)
was dissolved in a minimal amount of chloroform-methanol (2:1,v/v)
and then applied to a column (2.5 x 20 cm) packed with 15 g of
activated Florisil (Floridin Co., 60-100 mesh preheated at 100°C
for 6 hrs.). The elution was carried out successively with:
(a) 100 ml of chloroform; (b) 300 ml of chloroform-methanol
(2:1, v/v); (c) 100 ml of methanol. The fraction eluted with
solvent (b) contained all the neutral glycolipids and the
sulfatides.

Preparative Thin Layer Chromatography. The fraction eluted
with solvent (b) was subjected to preparative thin-layer chromatography on glass plates coated with Silica Gel G (Analtech Inc.
0.25 mm x 20 cm). The chromatograms were first developed with
chloroform-methanol-water (24:7:1, v/v). The lipids were visualized with iodine vapor. The gel containing the separated lipids
was scraped from the plates, packed into a column (1 x 10 cm) and
the lipids were recovered by elution with 150 ml of chloroform-
methanol-water (100:50:7.5, v/v). The eluate was evaporated to
dryness in vacuo. Preparative thin-layer chromatography was then
repeated with the solvent system n-propanol-water-15 M-NH$_3$ (6:2:1,
v/v). This solvent system separates sulfatides from the neutral
glycolipids.

Methanolysis. Methanolysis of the glycolipids was carried
out in methanolic HCl. Reaction mixtures containing 2 ml of 1.0 N
HCl in methanol were heated at 80°C for 18-20 hrs. in sealed tubes.
After cooling, the tubes were opened and 0.2 μmole (100 μl) of
mannitol was added as internal standard. Methyl esters of fatty
acids were partitioned into n-hexane by three extractions with
equal volumes of this solvent and the acidic methanol-solution
was treated with AG 1-X8 resin (OH⁻). Methanol was removed from
this solution under a stream of N$_2$ at 40°C.

GLC. The TMSi derivatives of methyl glycosides were prepared
from the above dry residue by the addition of 100 ul of pyridine-
hexamethyldisilazane-trimethylchlorosilane (9:3:1). After heating
at 60° for 5 min. an aliquot of the reaction mixture was injected
into a column containing OV-1 at 160°C. The areas of the GLC
peaks were estimated by planimetry.

Results

Table 2 shows the liver glycolipid levels in patients with classical MLD and in multiple sulfatase deficiency. To our knowledge no quantitative studies of liver glycolipids in MLD have previously been reported. No sulfatides were demonstrated in 5 gm samples of the control livers. The sulfatide levels in classical MLD and multiple sulfatase deficiency were approximately the same. It is of interest that in classical MLD, the levels of dihexoside sulfate are nearly the same as those of sulfatide. This differs from the data in normal and in MLD kidney, where monohexoside sulfate levels exceed those of the dihexoside sulfate by a factor of 2.6 to 8. (20) In the multiple sulfatase deficiency patient G.L., the relationship between mono- and dihexoside sulfate levels resembles that in control and MLD kidney. Table 2 also shows the levels of non-sulfated glycolipids. The pattern in the four classical MLD tissues was relatively consistent. They appear to have less cer-glu and cer-glu-gal than the control patients. Patient G.L. has a higher level of ceramide trihexoside, and lower levels of globoside than the control or classical MLD patients.

STEROID SULFATE LEVELS

To measure steroid sulfates these conjugates were: (1) separated from free steroids; (2) converted to free steroids by mild acid hydrolysis and (3) quantitated by gas liquid chromatography. Cholesteryl sulfate, unlike many of the more polar steroid sulfates, is poorly soluble in aqueous solvents. For this reason, the procedure used for separating this steroid sulfate differed from that for the other steroid conjugates.

To measure cholesteryl sulfate, the tissue was extracted with 20 volumes of chloroform-methanol (2:1, v/v) as described by Folch et al. (9) One ml of the extract was dried under a stream of nitrogen and dissolved at room temperature with 0.5 ml chloroform and 0.25 ml 0.2 N NaOH in methanol. After 30 minutes 0.25 ml of 0.2 N acetic acid in methanol was added. This mild alkaline hydrolysis eliminates certain substances, probably glycerophosphatides, which were found to interfere with subsequent steps of the analysis. The neutralized solution was again taken to dryness under a stream of nitrogen. The lipids were redissolved in 0.1 ml of 2:1 chloroform:methanol (v/v), 50 mg of Unisil was added and mixed thoroughly with the lipids with a sonicator. The solution was then dried again under nitrogen, taking care not to disturb the Unisil with too heavy a flow of nitrogen.

Table 2

Liver Glycolipids in Classical and Multiple Sulfatase Deficiency
Metachromatic Leukodystrophy (patient G.L.)

(µg/g dry weight)

	cer-glu	cer-glu-gal	cer-glu-gal-gal	Globoside	Sulfatide	Dihexoside Sulfate	Total
Control (2 cases)	185.2 ± 21.2	222.5 ± 51.7	54.2 ± 6.6	52.8 ± 7.0	< 20	< 20	514.8 ± 30.1
Classical MLD (4 cases)	106.9 ± 24.5	80.4 ± 18.7	40.6 ± 11.9	59.2 ± 17.7	279.9 ± 34.1	208.1 ± 53.8	774.9 ± 86.2
G. L.	174.9	265.6	124.4	22.9	234.9	57.1	879.8

The sample was then ready for transfer to a Unisil column. We found it convenient to prepare these columns in disposable Pasteur pipettes which contained a layer of glass wool and sand. 100 mg of Unisil suspended in chloroform was added to the column, the lipid sample was quantitatively transferred to the column with 4.5 ml of chloroform:methanol (97:3, v/v), and the column was rinsed with another 4.5 ml of the same solvent. These two eluates, which contained all of the free and fatty acid esterified cholesterol, were discarded. Cholesteryl sulfate was shown to be eluted quantitatively with 4.5 ml of chloroform:methanol (85:15, v/v). This fraction was collected in a test-tube (13 x 100 mm) fitted with a Teflon-lined screw top. The solvents were evaporated under a stream of nitrogen, 1 ml of ether and 5 μl of 1.0 N HCl were added, the test tube was capped, and placed overnight on a magnetic stirrer at room temperature. Authentic cholesteryl sulfate was quantitatively converted to cholesterol under these conditions.

Following the solvolysis 0.2 ml of $Na_2 CO_3$ was added, and thoroughly mixed with the ether solution. The ether upper phase was then removed, the sodium carbonate solution was rinsed twice with 1 ml of ether, and the ether upper phases were combined. The ether was evaporated and the cholesterol isolated on thin layer chromatography plates which were developed in Benzene:ethyl acetate (8:2, v/v). The plate was dried and sprayed lightly with brom thymol blue to visualize the cholesterol. The area of gel which contained the cholesterol was then transferred to a test tube, ground to a fine powder with a glass rod, dissolved in a small amount of freshly distilled ether and sonicated for 2 minutes. This material was then transferred to a disposable Pasteur pipette column, prepared as described above, which contained a 2 mm layer of Unisil. The lipid sample was passed through this Unisil column with 30 ml of freshly redistilled ether. This procedure removed contaminants introduced during thin layer chromatography.

The ether eluates were transferred to a screw - cap test tube, dried down, and saponified by heating for 1 hour at 80°C with 0.45 ml 95% ethyl alcohol and 50 microliters of 40% KOH. After the sample had cooled to room temperature it was mixed with 1.5 ml of water. Lipids were extracted 4 times with 0.5 ml of ether. The combined ether phases were taken to dryness, and 10 micrograms of cholestane was added as an internal standard. 30 microliters of TMS mixture were added and cholesterol was quantitated by gas liquid chromatography with a GLC-DEG column.

To measure dehydroepiandrosterone sulfate levels total lipids were extracted with 20 volumes of 2:1 chloroform:methanol (v/v) as described by Folch. (9) 0.4 ml of 0.1 N. NaOH were mixed with two ml of the total lipid extract, and the phases separated by centrifugation. The upper phase was removed and the lower phases

washed twice with 0.4 ml of a 1:1 mixture of methanol and 0.9 NaCl.
The combined upper phases were washed once with 1 ml of chloroform:
methanol:water (86:14:1 v/v). The washed upper phase was then
removed and taken to dryness.

The sample was then dissolved in 1 ml of water and placed on
an Amberlite XAD-2 column which had been washed several times
alternately with water and methyl alcohol. The sample was passed
through the column at a rate of approximately 1 drop per second,
and the column was rinsed with 30 ml of water. The water eluates
were discarded. DHEAS was quantitatively eluted with 30 ml of
methanol. This fraction was collected in a round bottom flask,
taken to dryness on a rotary evaporator, and then transferred to
a screw-capped test tube and subjected to solvolysis as described
for cholesteryl sulfate. The liberated free sterol was quantitated
by gas liquid chromatography using an 0.V -17 column, with copro-
stanol as the internal standard.

Results

Table 3 shows the results of these studies. The most striking
feature is the accumulation of cholesteryl sulfate in the liver of
patient G.L. The levels of free cholesterol and of fatty acid
esterified cholesterol in G.L. are somewhat reduced: the ratio of
cholesteryl sulfate to total cholesterol in patient G.L. is 0.27.
This is 50 to 100 times higher than that in the control and classical MLD tissues. Cholesteryl sulfate levels in Austin's "M" family
patient were increased to a smaller extent than those of patient
G.L. It is of interest that the levels of dehydroepiandrosterone
sulfate (DHEAS) were not at all increased, even though, as will be
shown below, the activity of DHEAS sulfatase in the livers of these
patients was deficient to the same extent as that of cholesteryl
sulfatase. We have not yet determined the steroid sulfate levels
in organs other than the liver. Our previous qualitative data
indicate that the kidney of patient G.L. did contain an excess of
cholesteryl sulfate.(26)

STEROID SULFATASE ACTIVITIES

Austin and his co-workers reported in 1965 that the tissues
of the "M" family patient showed deficient activities of arylsulfatase A and C. (4) We have confirmed these findings in
patient G.L. (26) Arylsulfatase B activity appears also to be
diminished, but not to the same extent as the two other enzymes.
However, in the kidney and brain of all three patients arylsulfatase B was clearly diminished.

Table 3

Liver Lipids in Multiple Sulfatase Deficiency (G.L. and "M Family") and Classical MLD

(mg/g dry weight)

	Total Lipid	Phospholipid	Cholesterol Free	Cholesterol Fatty Acid Esters	Cholesterol-SO_4	DHEA-SO_4	$\dfrac{\text{Cholesterol } SO_4}{\text{Total Cholesterol}}$
Control (10 cases)	106.4	77.5	8.0	2.0	.061	.012	.006
Classical MLD (4 cases)	274.7	103.0	6.0	4.9	.016	.004	.002
G. L.	157.7	100.0	3.0	1.0	1.45	.012	.266
"M" Family					.112	.000	
Mucopoly-saccharidoses (4 cases)					.038	.009	

We will focus here on the activities of the steroid sulfatases. As substrates we have used cholesteryl sulfate, DHEAS, and estrone sulfate. The structures of cholesteryl sulfate and of DHEAS differ only in respect to the side chain: they are both 3β - $\Delta 5$ steroids. However, estrone sulfate differs from the other two in that ring I of the steroid nucleus is phenolic.

Methods

Cholesterol Sulfatase. ^{35}S-Cholesterol sulfate with a specific activity of 9.2 mc/mmole was purchased from Amersham-Searle Corp. To a 15 ml test tube was added 0.05 ml of a liver tissue homogenate which represented 0.5 mg of fresh tissue and which was prepared by homogenizing frozen tissue in 0.25 M sucrose. To the tube was then added 0.3 ml of 0.5 M Tris-HCl (pH 7.4) containing 5.94×10^{-8} moles of the ^{35}S-cholesteryl sulfate. The mixture was incubated for two hours at 37°C. The reaction was stopped by adding 2.5 ml of 2:1 chloroform-methanol (containing 0.5 mg of non-radioactive cholesterol) and 0.5 ml of 0.1 M pyridine sulfate. The solutions were mixed on a vortex mixer and centrifuged at 1000 x g for 10 minutes at 4°C. The upper phase, which contains the ^{35}S-inorganic sulfate released from the cholesterol sulfate, was collected. The lower phase was mixed with 1.0 ml of a solution containing methanol and 0.1 M pyridine sulfate in equal proportions. The mixture was again centrifuged in the same way and the second upper phase was added to the first. The combined upper phases were evaporated to dryness, 10 ml of Triton X-100: toluene (1:2, v/v), containing 0.5% PPO and 0.03% POPOP (w/v), and one ml of water were added to each sample and the radioactivity content was measured with a Packard Tri-Carb Scintillation counting system with an efficiency of 90%. Results were expressed as n moles of substrate released per mg protein per hour.

Dehydroepiandrosterone Sulfatase. ^{14}C-DHEA-SO$_4$ and ^{3}H-DHEA-SO$_4$ were purchased from New England Nuclear Company. The specific activity was 58.5 μc/μm and 25.1 c/mm respectively. To a 15 ml culture tube was added 0.05 ml of the liver homogenate, 0.25 ml 0.5 M Tris-HCl (pH 7.6) and 0.05 ml of DHEAS in the same buffer at a concentration of 2.3×10^{-7} moles per ml. The mixture was incubated at 37°C for two hours. The reaction was stopped with 0.5 ml of 0.1 M NaOH. Three ml of ethyl ether was added and the tube was vortexed 35 times. The water and ether phases were allowed to separate and the tubes were put in a dry ice methanol bath. After the water phase was frozen, the ether extracts were poured into counting bottles. The ether was evaporated to dryness under a stream of nitrogen, and 10 ml of toluene-ethanol (19:1, v/v) containing 0.5% PPO and 0.03% POPOP (w/v) were added. The radio-activity content was measured with a Packard Tri-Carb Scintillation counting system with an efficiency of 90% for ^{14}C and 70% for ^3H. Results were expressed as n moles of substrate released per mg protein per hour.

Estrone Sulfatase. ^3H-Estrone sulfate with a specific activity of 41.7 mc/mM was purchased from New England Nuclear Company. To a 15 ml culture tube was added 0.05 ml of the liver homogenate and 0.3 ml of 0.5 M imidazole-HCl (pH 6.6) buffer containing estrone sulfate at a concentration of 2.9×10^{-6} moles per ml. The incubation and the assay for products were carried out as described above for dehydroepiandrosterone sulfatase, except that 1 ml of 0.1 M sodium carbonate rather than 0.1 M NaOH was used to stop the reaction.

Results

Most of the reported studies about steroid sulfatases have been conducted in human placenta, animal liver or testis. (10, 32, 27) Since our work has been concerned with human postmortem liver, we have examined the properties of these enzymes in this organ.

Table 4 lists the Michaelis constant (K_M) and maximum reaction velocity (V_{max}) for the desulfation of three steroid sulfates in homogenates of postmortem human liver. The K_M's for cholesteryl sulfatase and DHEA sulfatase are virtually identical to those reported for the corresponding reactions in rat testis. (27) Kinetic studies indicated that each of the three steroid sulfates was a competitive inhibitor for the desulfation of the other two. We used the graphic method of Dixon to estimate the inhibitor constants (K_i's).(8) The experimental data for one of these studies are shown in Figure 1. Table 4 lists all of the inhibition constants.

The K_M and V_{max} for estrone sulfate are considerably higher than those for the other two steroid sulfates. Cholesteryl sulfate is a relatively weak inhibitor for the desulfation of estrone sulfate. Other lines of evidence (see Discussion) suggest that estrone sulfatase is not the same enzyme as that which catalyzes the desulfation of 3β hydroxy 5α steroids.

Table 5 shows the activities of five "control" lysosomal enzymes in the liver of two patients with multiple sulfatase deficiency. The activities of four of the five "control" enzymes were normal or increased. This suggests that the sulfatase deficiencies cannot be attributed to general deterioration of the tissues. The diminution of β galactosidase activity is comparable to that which has been reported for the Hunter and Hurler syndromes. (19)

Table 4

Properties of Steroid Sulfatases in Postmortem Human Liver

Substrate	Optimum pH	V_{max} (n moles/hour)	K_M (Moles)	K_i (Moles)		
				DHEAS	CS	ES
DHEAS	6.6, 7.6*	1.43	1.64×10^{-5}		4.17×10^{-5}	5.84×10^{-5}
Cholesterol Sulfate	7.4	1.41	5.23×10^{-5}	5.94×10^{-6}		8.24×10^{-5}
Estrone Sulfate	6.6	20.0	1.39×10^{-4}	5.55×10^{-5}	2.16×10^{-4}	

*Kinetic studies done at pH 7.6.

Figure 1

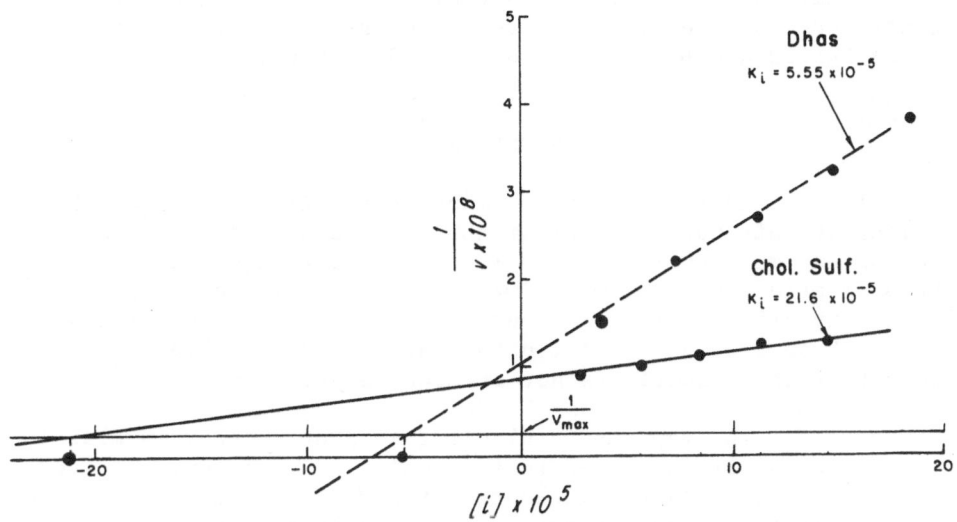

INHIBITION of ESTRONE SULFATASE
by
Dha. Sulf. and Chol. Sulf.

Table 5

Activities of Various Acid Hydrolases in
Postmortem Liver of Two Patients with
Multiple Sulfatase Deficiency

	G.L.	"M Family"	Control
Beta galactosidase	34.6	10.9	69.1
Alpha mannosidase	89.3	47.7	35.5 ± 14
Acid phosphatase	3,500	1,740	2070 ± 683
Alpha fucosidase	105	124	29.8
Hexosaminidase	13,230	1,400	1505 ± 457

Table 6 demonstrates that the desulfation of all three steroid sulfates was deficient in the liver of both patients with multiple sulfatase deficiency. Normal steroid sulfatase activities were demonstrated in the liver from patients with classical MLD, the Hunter and Hurler syndromes, and in age matched controls.

DISCUSSION

Table 7 lists the sulfatases whose activities are or may be deficient in this unusual form of MLD. Because of the considerable number of enzymes involved,it is important to rule out possible sources of artefact. The most immediate cause of concern is that all the enzymatic studies were performed with postmortem tissues which had been stored in the frozen state for up to 8 years. We believe that the results are not artefactual because:

1. Except for the expected arylsulfatase A deficiency in classi-MLD, normal or increased enzyme activities were demonstrated in the classical MLD and control tissues which had been stored under identical conditions for comparable time periods. Furthermore, arylsulfatase A, B and C and steroid sulfatase activities in fresh postmortem tissues were comparable to those in tissue samples which had been kept frozen for 1 - 8 years.

2. The multiple sulfatase deficiency tissues had normal or increased levels of acid phosphatase, mannoside, fucosidase and hexosaminidase activity.

3. Multiple substrate accumulation (sulfatide, mucopolysaccharides and cholesteryl sulfate) was present only in those tissues in which multiple sulfatase deficiencies were demonstrated.

For the reasons already cited in the introduction, we consider it likely that multiple sulfatase deficiency involves an abnormality of a single gene. If this is indeed the case this disorder joins the relatively small number of "single gene diseases" associated with deficiency of more than one enzyme. This list includes orotic aciduria (13), maple syrup urine disease, Sandhoff disease (33), possibly certain patients with glycogen storage disease (1), and possibly I-cell disease.(16,38)

It is not known exactly how many sulfatases are deficient. All the sulfatases which we have studied do appear to have deficient activities, but enzymes such as pregnenolone sulfatase, serine-o-sulfatase, tyrosine sulfatase and the glycosulfatases have not been examined. In addition, knowledge about the

Table 6

Steroid Sulfatase Activities in Two Patients with "Multiple Sulfatase Deficiency" MLD (G.L. and "M Family")

(Postmortem Liver)

	Cholesterol Sulfatase	Dehydroepiandrosterone Sulfatase	Estrone Sulfatase
		(n mole substrate released per mg protein/hr)	
G. L.	0.05	0.07	0.8
"M Family"	0.13	0.13	1.5
Classical MLD (4 cases)	1.67 ± 0.30	2.30 ± 0.54	29.8 ± 3.2
Mucopolysaccharidoses (4 cases)	----	2.67 ± 0.50	29.6 ± 8.8
Age Matched Controls (10 cases)	1.15 ± 0.32	1.66 ± 0.56	24.8 ± 5.7

Table 7

Sulfatases Which are or May be Deficient in

Multiple Sulfatase Deficiency

Enzyme	pH Optimum	Subcellular Localization	Test Substrate	Natural Substrate
Arylsulfatase A (Cerebroside Sulfatase)	4.7	lysosome	p-nitrocatechol sulfate	sulfatide
Arylsulfatase B	5.7	lysosome	p-nitrocatechol sulfate	?
Arylsulfatase C	7.3	microsome	nitrophenyl sulfate	?
3 β Steroid Sulfatases	7.4, 7.6	microsome	DHEAS,Cholesteryl sulfate	3 β sulfates of 5 α steroid series
3 β Estrone Sulfatase	6.6	microsome	ES	ES
? Polysaccharide Sulfatases	?	?	none available	MPS?

sulfatases which have been examined, is fragmentary. Only arylsulfatase A has been purified in substantial amounts, and it is
also the only one of the three arylsulfatases for which at least
one natural substrate (sulfatide) has been identified.

Arylsulfatase C and the steroid sulfatases are difficult to
solubilize, and have not been purified to any appreciable extent.
It is uncertain how many separate membrane bound sulfatases exist.
It is likely, but not proven, that arylsulfatase C, estrone
sulfatase, and dehydroepiandrosterone (DHEA) sulfatase are
separate enzymes. Thus, human fetal tissues have arylsulfatase C,
but lack DHEA sulfatase activity.(29) Kidney microsome preparations were found to cleave DHEAS but not estrone sulfate. (39) In
studies with placental enzymes nitrophenyl sulfate (the substrate
of arylsulfatase C) was found not to inhibit DHEA or estrone
sulfatase.(10) Furthermore, the pattern of heat denaturation,
and the effects of ribonuclease and of butanol were different
for each of these three enzyme activities.(10) It appears likely
that 3 β OH 5 α steroid sulfates, such as cholesteryl sulfate
and DHEA sulfate, are cleaved by the same enzyme.(32) However,
the recent demonstration that rat brain preparations could cleave
DHEA sulfate but not cholesteryl sulfate suggests that, even here,
separate enzymes may be involved.(15)

The supposition that there is also a polysaccharide sulfatase
deficiency in this form of MLD is based upon circumstantial evidence:

1.   Tissue and/or urinary polysaccharide levels have been elevated
     in all of the 7 patients in whom these substances have been
     measured. The degree of accumulation is comparable to that
     found in the mucopolysaccharidoses. Two types of polysaccha-
     rides appear to be present in excess: One has a composition
     consistent with that of dermatan sulfate, and the other with
     that of heparan sulfate.(26,30)

2.   In vivo turnover studies in our patient G.L. indicated that
     polysaccharide degradation was impaired.(26)

More direct studies of polysaccharide sulfatase have been hampered
by the difficulty of demonstrating polysaccharide desulfation in
vitro in normal tissues. Matalon and Dorfman have recently
demonstrated polysaccharide desulfation in normal human cultured
skin fibroblasts.(21) Unfortunately, no cultured cell lines are
available either from patient G.L. or from Austin's "M" family,
but it is hoped that skin fibroblasts cultured from other patients
with this disorder will soon become available.

Even though much remains unknown about the nature and even the number of sulfatases, there is little question that this unusual form of MLD is associated with multiple enzyme defects. In speculating about the origin of this phenomenon, we would first like to mention three mechanisms which we consider unlikely:

(a) The tissues of these patients contain a factor which inhibits all of the enzymes whose activities appear deficient. This is unlikely, since studies in which normal and MLD variant homogenates have been mixed have failed to demonstrate an inhibition of the normal enzyme activity.(26)

(b) The defect involves a regulator gene. This is unlikely because the immunological studies of Stumpf et al. indicate that the multiple sulfatase deficiency tissues contain approximately normal amounts of a protein which closely resembles enzymatically active arylsulfatase A.(35) If the defect involved a regulator gene, the affected protein would presumably not be produced.

(c) The abnormality involves a particular organelle, such as the lysosome. A "leaky" lysosomal membrane has been postulated to account for multiple enzymatic defects in I cell disease. (38) Such a hypothesis is not applicable to multiple sulfatase deficiency, since both lysosomal and microsomal enzymes are deficient. Furthermore, the activity of at least four lysosomal enzymes is normal or increased. (Table 5)

The multiple enzyme sulfatase deficiency could be due to lack of an activating factor required by all of these enzymes. Such a possibility is difficult to rule out. However, there is, at present, no evidence to support it. The heat stable complementary factor which Mehl and Jatzkewitz have shown to enhance the rate of the desulfation of sulfatide, (23) does not affect the activity of arylsulfatase A, one of the enzymes which is not functioning in this disease. No other sulfatase activating factors have as yet been identified.

Another possibility is that certain identical polypeptide chains are present in all of the sulfatases and that the mutation in multiple sulfatase deficiency involves the structure of one of these chains. An analogous hypothesis has been advanced to account for the deficiencies of hexosaminidase A and B in Sandhoff's disease. The work of Robinson and Stirling suggested that these two enzymes differed mainly in respect to the number of sialic acid residues.(31) A single lesion which affects the formation of a common protein moiety thus could lead to deficient activities of both enzymes.

Goldstone and Koenig have proposed that the same relationships may apply to several other lysosomal hydrolases which exist
in multiple forms. They suggest that these multiple forms differ
mainly in respect to the number of sialic acid residues which they
contain.(11) One of the points in support of this contention was
their demonstration that incubation with neuraminidase appeared
to lead to a partial conversion of arylsulfatase A to B. It will
be of great interest to repeat these studies with more highly
purified preparations of arylsulfatase A.

While Goldstone and Koenig's hypothesis could readily account
for the simultaneous inactivity of arylsulfatases A and B, there
is at this time no basis for extending it to membrane bound
enzymes such as arylsulfatase C or the steroid sulfatases. Except
for the fact that both arylsulfatase C and dehydropiandrosterone
sulfatase have been shown to cleave the O-S bond (17, 34) the only
other feature which these enzymes appear to have in common is that
they are both inactive in multiple sulfatase deficiency. Clarifi-
cation of these problems requires detailed knowledge about the
structure and mechanism of action of the sulfatases.

ACKNOWLEDGEMENTS

We wish to thank Dr. James Austin for making available the
postmortem tissues of the "M family" patient and Dr. Yasuo
Kishimoto for his advice in developing the steroid sulfate assay.
This work was supported in part by Grants NB-02672 and HD-05515
from the U.S. Public Health Service.

REFERENCES

1. Auerbach, V.H. and DiGeorge, A.M.: Genetic mechanisms producing multiple enzyme defects, a review of unexplained cases
   and a new hypothesis. Am. J. Med. Sci. 249: 718-747, 1965

2. Austin, J.H.: Recent studies in the metachromatic and globoid
   body forms of diffuse sclerosis. In: Brain Lipids and Lipoproteins, and the Leucodystrophies. Edited by J. Folch-Pi
   and H. Bauer, p. 120. Elsevier Publishing Company, N. Y.,
   1963

3. Austin, J.H.: Mental retardation metachromatic leucodystrophy
   (sulfatide lipidosis, metachromatic leucoencephalopathy). In:
   Medical Aspects of Mental Retardation, Charles Carter, Ed.,
   Charles C. Thomas Publisher

4.   Austin, J.H., Armstrong, D., and Shearer, L.: Metachromatic
     form of diffuse cerebral sclerosis. V. The nature and signifi-
     cance of low sulfatase activity: a controlled study of brain,
     liver and kidney in four patients with metachromatic leuko-
     dystrophy (MLD). Arch. Neurol. 13: 593-613, 1965

5.   Bischel, M., Austin, J., and Kemeny, M.: Metachromatic Leuko-
     dystrophy (MLD). VII. Elevated sulfated acid polysaccharide
     levels in urine and postmortem tissues. Arch. Neurol. 15:
     13-28, 1966

6.   Bischoff, A., and Ulrich, J.: Amaurotic idiocy connected with
     metachromatic leukodystrophy: transitional form or combination.
     Electron microscopic and histochemical finding. Acta. Neuro-
     path., 8: 292-308, 1967

7.   Dawson, R.M.C.: A hydrolytic procedure for the identification
     and estimation of individual phospholipids in biological
     samples. Bioch. J. 75: 45, 1960

8.   Dixon, M. and Webb, E.C.: Enzymes, 2nd Edition, p 329, New
     York Academic Press, Inc., 1964

9.   Folch, J., Lees, M. and Sloane Stanley, G.H.: A simple
     method for the isolation and purification of total lipids
     from animal tissue. J. Biol. Chem. 226: 497, 1957

10. French, A.P. and Warren, J.C.: Properties of steroid
     sulphatase and arylsulphatase activities of human placenta.
     Biochem. J. 105: 233, 1967

11. Goldstone, A., Konecny, P. and Koenig, H.: Lysosomal
     Hydrolases: Conversion of acidic to basic forms by neura-
     minidase. FEBS letters 13: 68, 1971

12. Hori, T., Sugita, M. and Itasaka, O.: Isolation of a sphingo-
     lipid containing 2 monomethylaminoethylphosphonic acid from
     shellfish. J. Biochem. 65: 451, 1969

13. Howell, R.R.: Inborn errors of metabolism: Some thoughts
     about their basic mechanisms. Pediatrics 45: 901, 1970

14. Jatzkewitz, H., and Mehl, E.: Cerebroside-sulphatase and
     arylsulphatase. A deficiency in metachromatic leukodystrophy
     (ML). J. Neurochem. 16: 19-28, 1969

15. Kishimoto, Y. and Sostek, R.: Activity of sterol-sulfate
     Sulfohydrolase in rat brain "Characterization, localization
     and change with age". J. Neurochem. In press

16. Leroy, J.G., Spranger, J.W., Feingold, M., Opitz, J.M. and
    Crocker, A.C.: I cell disease: A clinical picture. J. of
    Pediatrics 79: 360, 1971

17. Logan, C. and Warren, J.C.: Hydrolysis of dehydroepiandro-
    sterone sulfate by human placenta steroid 3β sulfatase in
    ^{18}O H_2O. Bioch. J. 114: 707, 1969

18. Luthy, F., Ulrich, J., Regli, F., and Isler, W.: Amaurotic
    idiocy with metachromatic change in the white matter? Proc.
    5th Int. Congress Neuropath. Int. Congress Series No. 100.
    Excerpta Medica Foundation, p. 125, Zurich, 1965

19. MacBrinn, M., Okada, S., Woollacott, M., Patel, Vimal, Ho,
    M. E., Tappel, A.L., and O'Brien, J.S.: Beta-galactosidase
    deficiency in the Hurler syndrome. N. Eng. J. Med. 281:
    338-342, 1969

20. Martensson, E., Percy, A. and Svennerholm, L.: Kidney
    glycolipids in late infantile metachromatic leukodystrophy.
    Acta Paed. Scand. 55: 1, 1966

21. Matalon, R.: Personal communication

22. Mehl, E., and Jatzkewitz, H.: Evidence for the genetic block
    in metachromatic leucodystrophy (ML). Biochem. & Biophys.
    Res. Commun. 19: (4) 407-411, 1965

23. Mehl, E., and Jatzkewitz, H.: Eine cerebrosidsulfatase aus
    Schweineniere. Ztschr. Physiol. Chem., 339: 260-276, 1964

24. Moser, H. W.: Sulfatide lipidosis. In: The Metabolic Basis
    of Inherited Disease. J. B. Stanbury, J. B. Wyngaarden and
    D. S. Fredrickson (Editors)3rd Edition, McGraw-Hill Book Co.,
    1972

25. Mossakowski, M., Mathieson, G., and Cumings, J.N.: On the
    relationship of metachromatic leucodystrophy and amaurotic
    idiocy. Brain 84: 585-604, 1961

26. Murphy, J.V., Wolfe, H.J., Balazs, E.A., Moser, H.W.: A
    patient with deficiency of arylsulfatases A, B, C and
    steroid sulfatase, associated with storage of sulfatide,
    cholesterol sulfate and glycosaminoglycans. In: Lipid
    Storage Diseases: Enzymatic Defects and Clinical Implica-
    tions. Academic Press, New York, J. Bernsohn and H. J.
    Grossman, Editors, 1971, pp. 67-110.

27.   Notation, A.D. and Unger, F. :   Regulation of rat testis
      steroid sulfatase. A kinetic study. Biochemistry $\underline{8}$: 501,
      1969

28.   Pilz, H., and Jatzkewitz, H.:   Biochemical evaluation of a
      combined sulfatidosis and gangliosidosis (glycolipidosis)
      of the brain. Path. Europ., $\underline{3}$: (2-3), 409-415, 1968

29.   Pulkkinen, M.:   Arylsulphatase and the hydrolysis of some
      steroid sulphates in developing organism and placenta.
      Acta Physiol. Scand. $\underline{52}$: Suppl. 180, 1961

30.   Rampini, S., Isler, W., Baerlocher, K., Bischoff, A.,
      Ulrich, J. and Plüss, H.J.:   Die Kombination von metachro-
      matischer Leukodystrophie und Mukopolysaccharidose als
      selbstandiges Krankheitsbild (Mukosulfatidose). Helvetica
      Paediatrica Acta $\underline{5}$: 436, 1970

31.   Robinson, D. and Stirling, J.L.:   N-acetyl-β-glucosamini-
      dases in human spleen. Bioch. J. $\underline{107}$: 321, 1968

32.   Roy, A.B.:   The sulphatase of ox liver,6:Steroid sulphatase.
      Biochem. J. $\underline{66}$: 700, 1957

33.   Sandhoff, K., Andreae, U. and Jatzkewitz, H.:   Deficient
      hexosaminidase activity in an exceptional case of Tay-Sachs
      disease. Path. Europ. $\underline{3}$: 278, 1968

34.   Spencer, B.:   Studies on sulphatases 20. Enzyme cleavage
      of arylhydrogen sulphates in the presence of H_2 ^{18}O.
      Bioch. J. $\underline{69}$: 155, 1958

35.   Stumpf, D., Neuwelt, E., Austin, J. and Kohler, P.:
      Trans. Am. Neurol. Assoc. $\underline{96}$: 1971. In press

36.   Thieffry, S., Lyon, G., and Maroteaux, P.:   Leucodystrophie
      metachromatique (sulfatidose) mucopolysaccharidose associees
      chez un meme malade. Rev. Neurol. $\underline{114}$: 193, 1966

37.   Thieffry, S., Lyon, G., and Maroteaux, P.:   Metabolic
      encephalopathy associating mucopolysaccharidosis and
      sulfatidosis. Arch. Franc. Pediat., $\underline{24}$: 425-32, 1967

38.   Wiesmann, U. N., Lightbody, J., Vassella, F. and Herschkowitz,
      N. W.:   Multiple lysosomal enzyme deficiency due to enzyme
      leakage? New Engl. J. Med. $\underline{284}$: 109, 1971

39.   Zuckerman, N.G., and Hagerman, D.D.:   The hydrolysis of
      estrone sulfate by rat kidney microsomal sulfatase. Arch.
      Biochem. & Biophys. $\underline{135}$: 410-415, 1969.

IN VITRO STUDIES IN SULFATIDE LIPIDOSIS

Michael M. Kaback, M.D., Alan K. Percy, M.D.
and Alfred G. Kasselberg, M.D.

Departments of Pediatrics and Neurology, Johns
Hopkins University School of Medicine,
Baltimore, Maryland 21205

Certain of the authors' studies cited were
supported by The John F. Kennedy Institute Tay-Sachs
Disease Fund, a Grant from the National Foundation --
March of Dimes, and the John A. Hartford Foundation, Inc.

INTRODUCTION

Recent developments in human somatic cell genetics now
permit the detailed in vitro evaluation of many mutant genotypes of man. Large, relatively uniform populations of diploid
human cells can be cultivated from a simple skin biopsy. For
prolonged periods, these fibroblastic cells reflect the chromo-
somal composition and many parameters of biochemical function
of the individual from whom the skin sample was obtained. The
biochemical abnormality associated with many recessive genetic
disorders and particularly those defects associated with the
sphingolipidoses and related conditions can now be demonstrated
in this in vitro system with easily obtained material with
little morbidity, and with minimal expense. Previously such
studies could only be achieved in post mortem tissues or in
material obtained by surgical biopsy of liver, nerve, brain,
etc.

In addition to its usefulness in diagnosis of the disease
state, the somatic cell system has proven of considerable
value in the determination of heterozygosity for several recessive disease-related genetic loci. (1) This becomes a
critical tool in appropriate genetic counseling to family
members when an affected individual has been identified.

The extention of this approach to the cultivation
and evaluation of somatic fetal cells (amniotic fluid
cells) obtained by amniocentesis in the early second trimester of pregnancy has been a most important recent development. Applications of this approach to high risk
pregnancies have provided an accurate mechanism for antenatal detection of several severe, untreatable genetic
disorders and have assumed an important role in genetic
counseling of couples at risk for such conditions in their
offspring. (2)

The cultivated somatic cell system also has application as an important tool in the elucidation of pathogenetic mechanisms of human genetic disorders. Moreover,
the availability of growing populations of human cells
with single gene mutations, may provide a prototype in
vitro system for the initial evaluation of possible therapeutic approaches to a number of these conditions.(3)

We wish to describe some of our recent somatic cell
studies in sulfatide lipidosis or metachromatic leukodystrophy (MLD). Before beginning this discussion, it is
perhaps most appropriate to point out some of the critical
considerations which must be raised in applying somatic
cell studies to human genetic disease. It is clear from
the work of many investigators that the in vitro human
cell culture is a dynamic system which may be affected by
a number of recognized variables and perhaps by an equal
or greater number of as yet undefined ones. Certainly,
such factors as the type and batch of media and serum in
which the cells are grown, the growth phase of the culture
at which time the cells are harvested (logarithmic, early,
or late confluency), the number of subcultures through
which a particular line has been passed, the presence of
contaminants (particularly mycoplasma organisms) may have
critical effects on any given parameter of cellular phy-
siology or function. In addition, such variables as the
use of trypsin or other proteolytic enzymes and/or chelating agents in subcultivation and harvesting of cells,
the method of cell disruption, and the particular methodology applied in assessing any cellular or subcellular
function might critically affect the results obtained as
well. For these reasons, it is essential that rigid control and consistency be paramount with regard to as many

of these variables as possible.

In all of the studies reported in this paper, skin fibroblasts were developed, maintained, and evaluated as previously described (4,5). The methods for amniotic fluid cultivation and study have also been indicated. (4, 5)

Care was taken to use early confluent cultures in all cases before the 8th subculture and less than 3 months after culture initiation. Negative mycoplasma screening was ascertained in representative cultures from each line studied.

The studies described deal mainly with sulfatase determinations in various cell lines. In all cases, cell sonicates of appropriate cultures were also assayed for other lysosomal hydrolase activities:

> arylsulfatase B
> β-D-N-Acetylglucosaminidase
> β-galactosidase

In each of the cultures studied, these enzyme specific activities fell into the range previously determined in control cells. (4)

Where heterozygote detection was performed using cultured cells, duplicate assays were performed on at least 3 independent cultures derived from each individual. Importantly statistical comparisons regarding heterozygote designation should be made with cultures from adult controls. Reasons for this will be apparent in the subsequent discussion.

HETEROZYGOTE DETECTION IN INFANTILE MLD

The apparent ubiquity of lysosomal hydrolases and particularly arylsulfatase A in many human tissues and the previously described deficiency of activity of this enzyme in MLD permits the evaluation of this disorder in fibroblast cells growing in vitro. Our laboratory, along with several others, has recently extended the finding of deficient arylsulfatase A activity in tissues and urine

from individuals with MLD to the in vitro skin fibroblast
system. (6, 7, 11) Figure 1 illustrates our cumulative
experience to date in cultured fibroblasts from individuals
with infantile MLD, obligate heterozygotes for this condition, and appropriate controls. A dramatic deficiency
of arylsulfatase A activity is found in individuals with
the infantile form of MLD. Each of these patients had a
typical history and clinical course and in 8 of the 10
cases illustrated, where peripheral nerve and/or brain
biopsy was performed, positive metachromasia with cresyl
violet or toluidine blue staining was noted.

In the evaluation of obligate heterozygotes, a distinct mid-range activity of arylsulfatase A is found in
skin fibroblasts developed from 16 of the parents of these
affected children. This evidence strongly supports the
autosomal recessive mode of inheritance for this condition.

It is of interest that heterozygote detection for
this condition by leukocyte analysis has not been uniformly successful. (8, 9) This may reflect differential ARA activity in different cell types of the leuko-
cytic series (10) and that fibroblasts under carefully
controlled culture conditions are more uniform and thereby more accurate in reflecting the genotype.

Urinary ARA determinations, while useful in disease
diagnosis, has not been found sufficiently quantitative
to be applicable to carrier detection. Other methods
such as quantitative urinary sulfatide excretion or rectal or sural nerve biopsy would seem excessively difficult
or unwarranted. It is of interest that heterozygotes in
fibroblasts have a mean arylsulfatase A activity of about
30% of that found in adult control cells. This has been
alluded to by other authors as well. (11)   The exact
explanation for why less than 50% ARA activity is found
in heterozygous individuals, as would be expected, is not
entirely clear at this point.

APPLICATIONS OF SOMATIC CELL STUDIES TO PRENATAL DETEC-
TION OF METACHROMATIC LEUKODYSTROPHY

If one is to extend the diagnostic capabilities as

ascertained in postnatal somatic cells to antenatal diagnosis, it is essential that quantitative data be developed
in normal amniotic fluid cells obtained at midtrimester
and cultured not longer than 6-8 weeks. The importance
of this point is shown in Table 1 which indicates that
normal midtrimester amniotic fluid cells, after 5-6 weeks
in culture, reflect a range of arylsulfatase A activity
considerably less than that found in control postnatal
skin fibroblasts. Since the <u>relationship</u> of heterozygous
to normal individuals in skin fibroblasts would be expected to apply in somatic fetal cells, (it is implicit that
the genotype is reflected by the relative amount of enzyme activity), one would then expect from these studies
that the heterozygous fetus for MLD would have relatively
low arylsulfatase A levels in cultured amniotic fluid cells.
In fact, these findings suggest possible difficulties in
the detection and differentiation of the heterozygous from
the homozygous recessive fetus based on amniotic fluid cell
analysis. However, being cognizant of this potential difficulty, it should be possible, in most cases, to distinguish the affected from the heterozygous fetus. We do
feel, however, that in certain instances such a distinction may be difficult and that parents should be fore-
warned of this problem before embarking on amniocentesis.
A recent pregnancy has been monitored in our facility in
which the amniotic fluid cell culture showed a specific
activity for arylsulfatase A of 80 units. This has been
interpreted to indicate a heterozygous fetus and the pregnancy is currently continuing.

The finding of diminished arylsulfatase A activity
in amniotic fluid cells and in cultivated fetal skin fibroblasts has led us to suggest that arylsulfatase A is
a "developmental enzyme". (7)   This has previously
been suggested in the mouse and rabbit and most recently,
in the small intestine of man. (12,13,14) With skin fibroblast cultures developed from fetal skin, neonatal fore-
skin, and adult skin biopsy, we have compared the specific
activity of arylsulfatase A in these cells and evaluated
some of the physicochemical properties of the enzyme from
these sources. This is shown in Table 2. There is an apparent increase in specific activity of arylsulfatase A
from fetal to neonatal to adult cells. The apparent
Michaelis-Menten constant for nitrocatechol sulfate in

these three cell types is not significantly different.
In addition, comparisons of electrophoretic mobility
using acrylamide gel electrophoresis indicates no clear
differences in the electrophoretic properties of arylsulfatase A from these three cell types. (15)   These
data suggest, therefore, that arylsulfatase A is, in
fact, quantitatively developmental in man and thereby
raises important questions as to the feasibility of early
intrauterine diagnosis of this disorder. It is for this
reason that we believe amniotic fluid cell data from pregnancies at risk for MLD must be interpreted with great
care if one is to avoid the mistake of incorrectly diagnosing an affected fetus in one who is actually heterozygous for this locus.

     If intrauterine detection of this disorder is to be
attempted, it is essential that corroborative studies be
applied in fetal tissues. Some have suggested that hysterotomy or hysterectomy be used in order that fetal tissues be obtained in optimal condition for corroborative
evaluation. It is important to emphasize that hysterotomy may clearly increase the risk that such a woman might
be unable to complete a subsequent pregnancy because of
complications resulting from that surgical procedure.
(16) Therefore, it is of greatest value to the families
in question that termination of pregnancy be done, should
it be indicated, in a way that would be least likely to
jeopardize subsequent pregnancies. Accordingly, we have
evaluated tissues obtained from saline aborted control
fetuses in order to ascertain whether significant levels
of fetal enzymes can be measured in such material. If
this be the case, then saline-aborted fetuses could certainly be utilized for corroborative studies and hysterotomy thereby avoided. Our findings are shown in Table 3.
Clearly measurable activities of arylsulfatase A and beta
galactosidase are found in liver homogenates from hypertonic saline-aborted fetuses. As seen in the fetus with
GM_1 gangliosidosis, the diagnostic specificity of such
tissues still applies. This also is true for hexosaminidase levels (both A and B forms) which are not shown but
are readily evident in the non-Tay-Sachs disease fetus
and totally absent (the A isozyme) in the two with Tay-
Sachs disease.

In addition, we have quantitatively evaluated sulfatide concentrations in the brains of human fetuses in
order to ascertain whether sulfatide levels are affected
by saline abortion. This is shown in Table 4. Sulfatide
levels in midtrimester control and sphingolipidosis affected fetuses show no significant difference when compared with non-saline-aborted fetuses from a slightly
earlier period. In addition, the sulfatide levels in
these midtrimester fetuses did not significantly differ
from the sulfatide content of cerebral tissue obtained
from 32-38 week live born fetuses who subsequently died
of unrelated causes.

We can conclude from these studies that cultivated
skin fibroblasts can accurately be applied to the diagnosis of MLD and detection of the heterozygous condition
for this genetic locus. Moreover, in light of the apparent developmental nature of arylsulfatase A activity
in human tissues, it is suggested that considerable caution be applied in attempts to detect this disease in
utero by amniocentesis in the second trimester of pregnancy. With appropriate precautions, however, it is
felt that for most cases accurate antenatal detection
should be achievable. However, certain heterozygous fetuses may show very low ARA specific activity in cultivated amniotic fluid cells thereby leading to the difficult question, "Is this an affected fetus?" The counseling of parents should alert them to this danger. Perhaps the probability of a successful pregnancy in a couple
at risk for this disease would, instead of being 75% if
heterozygous distinction were totally accurate, be
on the order of 60-65% since couples might well elect to
terminate pregnancies even if it were not clear based on
amniotic fluid cells whether the fetus was heterozygous
or affected. In addition, it would appear that hysterotomy is not a required means for termination of pregnancy.
Since saline-aborted tissues can effectively be utilized
for corroborative studies and since it would appear that
saline injection has a lesser hazard than hysterotomy,
both enzymologic and quantitative cerebral lipid studies
can be carried out if an MLD fetus is detected.

COMPARATIVE STUDIES IN INFANTILE AND ADULT-ONSET META-
CHROMATIC LEUKODYSTROPHY

We have recently had the opportunity to evaluate
dizygotic twins with adult-onset MLD. Absence of arylsulfatase A activity in both individuals in urine and
leukocytes plus metachromasia in sural nerve biopsies
from both sibs substantiated the diagnosis. Skin fibroblast preparations from these individuals were evaluated
for arylsulfatase A activity and for cerebroside sulfatase activity using an improved assay method for cerebroside sulfatase. (17, 18)   The results of these
studies are shown in Table 5. Both by arylsulfatase A
and cerebroside sulfatase determinations, no quantitative
distinction could be made between the adult-onset and infantile form of this disease. Because of the very minimal
residual enzyme activity found in cells from both the infantile and adult form, attempts to evaluate physicochemical properties of this miniscule enzyme activity have not
been successful to date. It is of interest that the parents
of the adult onset MLD twins showed heterozygous fibroblast levels comparable to that seen in parents of children with the infantile form. (18)

In addition, we have evaluated the siblings of these
two individuals and found a 16 year old younger sib who
was actively attending high school with no deficits and
who showed total absence of arylsulfatase A and cerebroside sulfatase in both leukocytes and skin fibroblasts.
This individual has subsequently gone on to develop early
symptoms of MLD. During the time he was symptom free, he
demonstrated increased sulfatide excretion in the urine
as well as delayed nerve conduction time.

It is quite obvious that these two distinct age-re-
lated variants of MLD must, in fact, have some inheritant
difference in the nature of the genetic defect. Experiments attempting to evaluate these variant forms of the
disease in vitro have been attempted. Porter, et al.
have recently shown physiological differences in the
ability to cleave ^{35}S-sulfatide (added to the growth media)
between fibroblast cultures from individuals with infantile versus adult-onset MLD. As contrasted with control
cultures, adult MLD cells cleave clearly less sulfatide

but significantly more than that achieved by the infantile MLD cells. No difference in the deficiency of cerebroside sulfatidase activity could be detected however
in lysates from the two mutant cell types on direct analysis. (19).

Others have attempted to characterize physicochemical differences in partially purified urinary ARA activity prepared from patients with infantile and adult-
onset MLD in contrast with normal urinary enzymatic activity. Preliminary studies suggest differences in inhibitor and other kinetic properties of the ARA activity from
the two disease forms. (20). Studies in our laboratory
however, have been unable to define such differences with
fibroblast enzymes. Since arylsulfatase B is also lysosomal in origin and soluble, one is plagued with the possibility that residual sulfatase activity may represent
the B form of the enzyme. Attempts to evaluate the pH
optimum and heat inactivation characteristics of residual
sulfatase A activity in infantile MLD cells would indicate a pattern comparable to arylsulfatase B rather than
arylsulfatase A. (21) .

Since it is likely that these two disorders represent different alleles or perhaps two distinct mutant
genes, we have attempted to evaluate the possibility of
interalelic complementation between the adult and infantile forms. With cultured skin fibroblasts, we first
studied the unlikely but possible presence of soluble
factors which might "correct" the deficiency of enzyme
activity in a manner similar to that shown by Fratantoni
and Neufeld for the mucopolysaccharidoses. (22). Mixed
cell culture experiments were done secondly to evaluate a
conceivably more intimate requirement for cross correction
and thirdly, heterokaryon experiments were initiated in
which cytoplasmic complementation could be evaluated.

In Table 6, the effects of conditioned media on respective fibroblast lines is shown. No correction of
either the infantile or the adult MLD fibroblast is obtained with media from either adult or infantile control
cells and similarly, no apparent correction or increase
in enzyme activity is evident in infantile cells grown in
the presence of conditioned media from adult cells or
the reverse.

Data from the mixed cell experiments are seen in
Table 7. Cells from adult controls, infantile and adult
MLD patients were grown in mixed culture in all possible
permutations. No stimulation of enzyme activity was found
when adult and infantile cells were grown together nor was
there any stimulation of enzyme activity evident in either
MLD/control mixes. No apparent inhibition of control activity is evident by mixed mutant control lines thereby
suggesting that a soluble inhibitor is not present in MLD
cells. This has also been corroborated in sonicate mixes
in which no loss of control enzyme activity is apparent
when MLD sonicate is added.

In Table 8, preliminary results of heterokaryon formation between infantile and adult MLD cells are shown.
Fusion of parent to parent and adult to infantile cells
was achieved by innoculation of mixed cell suspensions
with β-proprionolactone-inactivated Sendai virus at 4°
for 10-60 minutes. At 24 hours after addition of virus,
microscopic evaluation revealed 6-10% of the cells present
in culture were multi-nucleated heterokaryons. Sequential
enzymatic evaluation of the treated cultures, both parent-
parent crosses and mixed crosses, revealed no obvious stimulation of arylsulfatase A activity. However, it is important to emphasize that in these experiments, the parent
mononuclear cells would not be inhibited from growth so
that both parental cell types which lack arylsulfatase A
activity would continue to divide during the period of
these studies. It might be calculated that the increase
in enzyme activity in heterokaryons would necessarily be
quite extraordinary in order to pick up significant increases in a mixed culture experiment such as this.

This does point out, however, the importance of development of hybridization techniques applicable to these
cell types such as reported in galactosemia. (23)
To achieve outgrowth of hybrids with simultaneous inhibition of the non-hybridized parent cells, one would have to
develop a selective medium in which only ARA positive cells
(hybrids) could give rise to clones of dividing cells. We
have recently been exploring this possibility.

Porter et al. previously demonstrated that sulfatide
added to the medium (20μg/ml) in which MLD cells are

growing will result in the development of positive metachromasia in the cells and that they do incorporate large
amounts of sulfatide. (24)   Using this concept,
we have increased the concentration of added sulfatide
to the growth medium to evaluate possible growth inhibition in cells unable to metabolize or catabolize the added
sulfatide. (Table 9) Initial experiments in one control
and one adult-MLD line indicate that differential inhibition of the MLD line is evident when sulfatide is added
in increased concentrations. Although some inhibition is
apparent in control cells, the effect is clearly more
striking in the ARA deficient cells. It is conceivable
that with an approach such as this, successful hybridization studies could be carried out, which, in turn, may
be of considerable importance in resolving several of the
important genetic questions raised by these two disorders.

In summary, the development of somatic cell genetics
in recent years and the extension of these approaches to
the human organism have provided an added dimension in the
study of genetic disorders. In the sulfatide lipidoses,
these techniques now can be appropriately applied to diagnosis, to counseling (carrier detection), to prevention
(antenatal diagnosis), and to the further study and elucidation of the basic nature of these conditions. It is also
likely that therapeutic or even curative approaches will
(and already have begun) first be evaluated in this in
vitro system.

REFERENCES

1.   Kaback, M.M. and Howell, R. R., Heterozygote Detec-
tion and Prenatal Diagnosis of Lysosomal Diseases, in:
Lysosomes and Storage Diseases, H. G. Hers and F. Van Hoof
(Eds.), Chapter 26, Academic Press, New York, in press.

2. Nadler, H.L., Prenatal Detection of Genetic Defects,
J. Pediat. 74: 132 (1969).

3. Porter, M.T., Fluharty, A.L. and Kihara, H., Correction of Abnormal Cerebroside Sulfate Metabolism in Cultured Metachromatic Leukodystrophy Fibroblasts, Science
172: 1263 (1971).

4.   Kaback, M.M. Leonard, C. O., Parmley, T.H., Intrauterine Diagnosis: Comparative Enzymology of Cells Cultivated from Maternal Skin, Fetal Skin, and Amniotic Fluid
Cells, Pediat. Res. 5: 366 (1971).

5.   Kaback, M.M. andLeonard, C.O., Morphological and
Enzymological Considerations in Antenatal Diagnosis, in:
Antenatal Diagnosis, A. Dorfman (Ed.), University of Chi-
cago Press, in press, 1971.

6.   Porter, M.T., Fluharty, A.L., and Kihara, H., Metachromatic Leukodystrophy: Arylsulfatase-A Deficiency in
Skin Fibroblast Cultures, P.N.A.S. 62: 887 (1969).

7.   Kaback, M.M. and Howell, R.R., Infantile Metachromatic
Leukodystrophy: Heterozygote Detection in Skin Fibroblasts
and Possible Applications to Intrauterine Diagnosis, New
Eng. J. Med. 282: 1336 (1970).

8.   Percy, A. K. and Brady, R.O., Metachromatic Leukodystrophy: Diagnosis with Samples of Venous Blood, Science
161: 594 (1968).

9.   Bass, N.J., Witmer, E.J., Dreifuss, F.E., A Pedigree
Study of Metachromatic Leukodystrophy: Biochemical Identification of the Carrier State, Neurology (Minneap) 20: 52,
(1970).

10. Tanaka, K.R., Valentine, W.N., and Fredericks, R.E.,
Human Leukocyte Arylsulphatase Activity, Brit. J. Haemat,
8: 86, (1962).

11. Leroy, J.G., Dumon, J., and Radermecker, J., Deficiency of Arylsulphatase A in Leucocytes and Skin Fibroblasts in Juvenile Metachromatic Leucodystrophy, Nature,
226: 553 (1970).

12. Percy, A.K. and Yaffe, S.J., Sulfate Metabolism During
Mammalian Development, Pediatrics 33: 965 (1964)

13. Jatzkewitz, H., Cerebral Sphingolipidoses as Inborn
Errors of Metabolism, in: Some Inherited Disorders of
Brain and Muscle, J. D. Allan and D.N. Raine (Eds.), E &
S. Livingstone Ltd., Edinburgh and London, 1969, p. 114.

14. Heringova, A., Koldovsky, O., Yaffe, S.J., Jinsova, V., and Uher, J., Sulfatase Activity in Placenta, Liver, and Small Intestine of Human Fetuses, Biol. Neonat. 14: 265 (1969).

15. Kasselberg, A.G. and Kaback, M.M., unpublished observations.

16. Wilson, J.R., Beecham, C.T. and Carrington, E.R., Obstetrics and Gynecology, 4th Edition, C.V. Mosby Co., St. Louis, 1971, p. 466.

17. Percy, A.K., Farrell, D.F., and Kaback, M.M., Cerebroside Sulfatase: An Improved Assay Method, J. Neurochem. (in press).

18. Percy, A.K. and Kaback, M.M., Infantile and Adult-Onset Metachromatic Leukodystrophy, New Eng. J. Med. 285: 785 (1971)

19. Porter, M. T., Fluharty, A.L., Trammell, J. and Kihara, H., A Correlation of Intracellular Cerebroside Sulfatase Activity in Fibroblasts with Latency in Metachromatic Leukodystrophy, BBRC 44: 660 (1971).

20. Stumpf, D. and Austin, J., Metachromatic Leukodystrophy (MLD) XI. Qualitative and Quantitative Differences in Urinary Arylsulfatase A in Different Forms of MLD., Arch. Neurol. 24: 117 (1971).

21. Kaback, M.M., unpublished observations.

22. Neufeld, E.F. and Fratantoni, J.D., Inborn Errors of Mucopolysaccharide Metabolism, Science 169: 141 (1970).

23. Nadler, H., Chacko, C., and Rachmeler, M., Interallelic Complementation in Hybrid Cells Derived from Human Diploid Strains Deficient in Galactose-1-phosphate Uridyl Transferase Activity, PNAS 67: 976 (1970).

24. Porter, M.T., Fluharty, A.L., Harris, S.E., and Kihara, H., The Accumulation of Cerebroside Sulfates by Fibroblasts in Culture from Patients with Late Infantile Metachromatic Leukodystrophy, Arch. Bioch. Biophys., 138: 646 (1970).

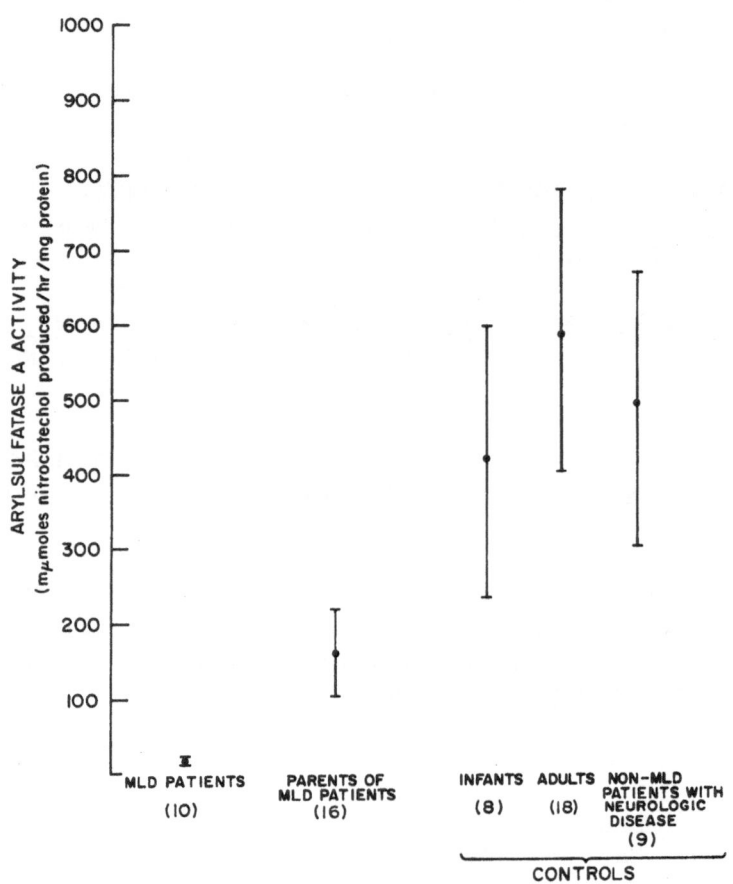

Figure 1.

Fibroblast arylsulfatase A specific activities in
infantile MLD, obligate heterozygotes, and appropriate
controls. The mean ± one standard deviation for each
group is illustrated.

TABLE 1

METACHROMATIC LEUKODYSTROPHY HETEROZYGOTE DETECTION IN FIBROBLASTS

AND IMPLICATIONS FOR ANTENATAL DIAGNOSIS

CELL TYPE	NO. LINES	NO. DETERMINATIONS	ARA ACTIVITY		
			Mean	SD	Range
Skin Fibroblasts					
MLD-infantile	10	48	18.0	6.7	6.9-34.5
Obligate heterozygotes	16	64	166.4	53.7	65.0-304.6
Control adults	18	54	581.5	180.0	320.4-982.5
Control Amniotic Fluid Cells (midtrimester)	24	60	215.3	63.8	90.1-360.2
Expected mean ARA activity in amniotic cell culture from heterozygous fetuses			65-80		

TABLE 2

ONTOGENY OF ARYLSULFATASE A (ARA) IN CULTURED SKIN FIBROBLASTS

FIBROBLAST SOURCE	NO. LINES	ARA ACTIVITY *	APPARENT K_m **
Fetal skin (16-22 wks.)	7	143.0 ± 60.8	$4.2 \times 10^{-3} M$
Neonatal foreskin	8	414.0 ± 181.0	$3.7 \times 10^{-3} M$
Adult skin	18	581.5 ± 180.0	$3.2 \times 10^{-3} M$

*   Mean ± SD expressed as n-moles nitrocatechol produced per hour per mg. soluble cell protein

**   Michaelis-Menten constants determined by Lineweaver-Burke analysis of enzyme activity over a 50-fold range of 4-nitrocatechol sulfate concentrations

TABLE 3

ARYLSULFATASE A (ARA) IN LIVER HOMOGENATES FROM HYPERTONIC SALINE-ABORTED FETUSES (17-23 WEEKS)

FETUS	ARA*	β-GAL**
Control 1	114.9	677.5
Control 2	128.9	140.8
Control 3	373.0	665.3
Tay-Sachs disease 1	131.1	959.4
Tay-Sachs disease 2	83.7	214.5
GM$_1$ gangliosidosis	136.0	10.1

* n-moles product released per hour per mg. soluble protein (homogenates spun 1000 gm. x 15 min. at 0° C)

**acid β-galactosidase, units as above

TABLE 4

CEREBRAL SULFATIDE CONCENTRATIONS IN HUMAN FETUSES AND NEONATES

SOURCE OF TISSUE	NO.	SULFATIDE*
Fetal Cerebrum		
Saline-aborted:		
control (16-26 wks.)	3	0.5-0.8
Tay-Sachs (22-24 wks.)	2	0.45-0.5
GM$_1$ gangliosidosis (22 wks.)	1	0.5
Non-saline aborted:		
control (12-14 wks.)	3	0.2-0.4
Live Births		
control (32-38 wks.)	3	0.4-0.6

*mg. per gm. dry weight brain

TABLE 5

COMPARISON OF ARYLSULFATASE A (ARA) AND CEREBROSIDE SULFATASE (CS) ACTIVITIES

IN PATIENTS WITH INFANTILE AND ADULT-ONSET METACHROMATIC LEUKODYSTROPHY

FIBROBLAST SOURCE	NO. OF PATIENTS	ARA*	CS*
Infantile MLD	3	9.6-26.8	0.83-1.3
Adult MLD	2	8.0-28.7	0.87-2.0
Control Adult	12	375.3-751.8	80.0 - 130.0

*Expressed as n-moles product released per hour per mg. protein

TABLE 6

EFFECT OF CONDITIONED MEDIA ON FIBROBLAST ARYLSULFATASE A (ARA) ACTIVITY

CELL TYPE	CONDITIONED MEDIA ADDED	NO. DETERMINATIONS	CELLULAR ARA ACTIVITY (RANGE)*
1. Control (adult)	--	6	380.1-460.8
	infant control	3	unchanged
	infantile MLD	4	"
	adult MLD	4	"
2. Control (infant)	--	5	240.2-375.7
	adult control	3	unchanged
	infantile MLD	4	"
	adult MLD	4	"
3. MLD (infantile)	--	5	12.8-31.8
	adult control	4	unchanged
	infant control	4	"
	adult MLD	4	"
4. MLD (adult)	--	6	10.6-28.4
	adult control	4	unchanged
	infant control	4	"
	infantile MLD	4	"

*ARA activity expressed as n-moles nitrocatechol released per hour per mg. soluble cell protein

TABLE 7

ARYLSULFATASE A (ARA) ACTIVITIES IN MIXED FIBROBLAST CULTURES

CELL TYPE	LINES	NO. DETERMINATIONS	ARA ACTIVITY (MEAN)
Control (adult)	A_1; A_2	6	A_1 = 406.2; A_2 = 388.0
MLD (infantile)	B_1; B_2	11	B_1 = 17.6; B_2 = 24.9
MLD (adult)	C_1; C_2	10	C_1 = 18.1; C_2 = 26.4

MIXED CULTURES	NO. DETERMINATIONS	ARA ACTIVITY (RANGE)
1. Parental Lines		
A_1 + A_2	4	383.0–465.4
B_1 + B_2	4	13.2– 28.6
C_1 + C_2	4	12.6– 31.9
2. Mixed Mutant Lines		
B_1 + C_1; B_1 + C_2	6	14.6– 29.3
B_2 + C_1; B_2 + C_2	6	12.8– 32.6
3. Control–Mutant Mix		
A_1 + B_1 or B_2; A_2 + B_1 or B_2	12	180.6–240.9
A_1 + C_1 or C_2; A_2 + C_1 or C_2	12	168.2–239.0

*Equal numbers of each cell type innoculated. All cultures terminated after 5 days (confluent)

TABLE 8

EFFECT OF HETEROKARYON FORMATION ON ARYLSULFATASE A (ARA) ACTIVITY

IN INFANTILE (A) AND ADULT (B) FIBROBLASTS

CELL LINE	ARA ACTIVITY (MEAN)
A. S.A.: Infantile MLD	16.8
B. G.B.: Adult MLD	18.3

DAYS AFTER VIRAL FUSION*	NO. DETERMINATIONS (each cross)	ARA ACTIVITY (RANGE)		
		A x A	A x B	B x B
3	2	9.4-18.6	14.6-20.2	13.0-21.4
5	4	12.0-21.1	14.0-34.3	14.8-31.7
7	4	11.2-17.1	7.8-35.0	20.1-29.6

*Fusion induced with β-propionolactone-inactivated Sendai virus. 6-10% heterokaryons seen in all cultures at 24 hours.

TABLE 9

EFFECT OF ADDED SULFATIDE ON GROWTH OF NORMAL AND METACHROMATIC LEUKODYSTROPHY CELLS

SULFATIDE*(μg/ml)	CONTROL	MLD
0	2.1×10^6	1.7×10^6
20	1.8×10^6	1.1×10^6
50	1.4×10^6	0.7×10^6
100	1.4×10^6	0.6×10^6
200	1.3×10^6	0.4×10^6
500	0.9×10^6	0.4×10^6

*Cultures grown in standard medium supplemented with sulfatide at indicated concentrations. 1.5×10^5 cells innoculated in each culture in duplicate. Media changed every third day. All cultures were terminated after 12 days in respective media and counted in duplicate. Average cell count from duplicate cultures are indicated.

FACTORS AFFECTING THE METABOLISM OF GALACTOCEREBROSIDE AND GLUCO-CEREBROSIDE

Norman S. Radin

Mental Health Research Institute

University of Michigan

Our laboratory has been studying the factors which affect brain cerebroside metabolism through two major approaches: (1) the comparison of enzyme specific activities with various substrates, and (2) the susceptibility of the enzymes to interference by synthetic lipids, analogous in structure to the substrates. The problem is complicated by the existence of the 2-hydroxy group in some of the fatty acids, and the existence of the two clusters of fatty acid chain lengths, around 18 and around 24 carbon atoms.

COMPARATIVE ENZYME ACTIVITIES

Let us first consider the acylation of sphingosine, which forms ceramide. This reaction was demonstrated in brain by Sribney (22), using microsomes, sphingosine, and palmitoyl-CoA. Pierre Morell, in my laboratory, investigated this acyl transferase with four different radioactive CoA derivatives: palmitoyl, oleoyl, stearoyl, and lignoceroyl (15). We used as acceptors the synthetic bases, DL-sphingosine and DL-dihydrosphingosine, coated on Celite diatomaceous earth. It proved to be a complicated comparison, as the optimal acyl-CoA concentrations were different for each derivative; however, the concentration of long chain base was not so critical. We compromised, for our comparison, on the use of 0.25 mg long chain base and 0.16 μmole of acyl-CoA, in a volume of 0.5 ml. Microsomes from young mouse brain served as enzyme source.

The acylations went quite nicely, in confirmation of Sribney's report, and TLC radioautographs confirmed the identities of the ceramides. The relative amounts of ceramide synthesized in

30 min turned out to be roughly proportional to the ratios of the natural occurrence in the nonhydroxy sphingolipids. Stearate was the best acyl donor; it is also the major fatty acid in sphingolipids. Lignocerate was next best; it is a less prominent acid quantitatively. Palmitate was somewhat poorer; it is only a minor acid percentagewise. Oleate was worst, and is one of the rarest. The relative conversions were 60:12:3:1. It is too bad we did not test nervonate, which is more common than lignocerate and should show a relative activity of about 20.

On the basis of this comparison one might guess that the acyltransferase is a controlling enzyme, deciding the relative amount of each fatty acid in the nonhydroxy sphingolipids. Of course this is a crude analysis of the problem; we don't even know the relative concentrations in brain of the different acyl-CoA's in the region of the acyl-transferring enzyme, and the assay conditions we used may not reflect the true conditions within the cells.

David Ullman has been making a similar comparison in my lab with the CoA derivatives of the alpha-hydroxy acids, using radioactive DL-hydroxystearate and hydroxylignocerate (cerebronate). In this study we used natural D-sphingosine, freed from dihydrosphingosine, as the acceptor base. Again the shorter acid proved to be the better substrate: the ratio was about 2 to 1. This was a surprise, as mice (and most animals) have very little hydroxystearate in their brain sphingolipids compared with cerebronate, which is a major fatty acid in galactocerebroside. Thus, this acyltransferase - assuming we are dealing with a different acyl transferase - does not seem to be the factor which controls the distribution of the different hydroxy cerebrosides.

There appear to be three different acyltransferases handling these acids. When labeled hydroxystearoyl-CoA is incubated with sphingosine, its conversion to hydroxy ceramide is not reduced by adding stearoyl- or lignoceroyl-CoA. The lack of competition for the transferase indicates that the hydroxy acid transferase does not utilize nonhydroxy acids. The reverse experiment, with labeled stearoyl-CoA, showed that hydroxystearoyl-CoA acts as an inhibitor. However, the inhibition was of the noncompetitive type, suggesting that there is an effector site on the nonhydroxy transferase that is sensitive to certain fatty acyl CoA's. Perhaps the hydroxy acids exert a controlling influence over the formation of very long chain ceramides, which I imagine are made in the same cell regions.

Our evidence for a third acylating enzyme comes from an age comparison. When we compared 8 day old mice, which are myelinating very slowly, and 16 day old mice, which are myelinating vigorously, Dr. Ullman found that the ceramide-synthesizing

activity with labeled stearate rose 31% with age. The activity
with lignocerate, however, rose 89%. Thus it looks as though
there is a transacylase which preferentially utilizes the very
long acids, and one which prefers the medium chain acids. It is
not surprising that the capability of forming lignoceroyl sphingosine should rise faster with age, as myelination is characterized
by the appearance of the sphingolipids containing the very long
chain acids.

Further evidence for the existence of these two enzymes comes
from Dr. Morell's study (15), in which we found that a crude
preparation of synaptosomes was able to utilize stearate, but not
lignocerate. This makes sense, since synaptosomes contain stearate
as their primary sphingolipid acid (9).

Another enzyme showing interesting specificity is the
galactosyltransferase which converts UDPGal and ceramide to
galactocerebroside. Pierre Morell and I worked this out with
mouse microsomes and labeled galactose-1-phosphate (14). (Later
experiments with labeled UDPGal gave the same results.) We found
that the microsomes formed some nonhydroxy cerebroside even without the addition of ceramide, evidently due to the presence in
microsomes of endogenous nonhydroxy ceramide. In different experiments we searched for hydroxy ceramide in brain, but were unable
to find any despite the report by Klenk and Huang (11) that some
does exist in human brain.

When we added exogenous nonhydroxy ceramide to the incubation
mixture, we found a small increase in the amount of nonhydroxy
cerebroside synthesis. However, when we added hydroxy ceramide,
the amount of hydroxy cerebroside formed was about 7 times the
control activity, and the formation of nonhydroxy cerebroside was
repressed. A later study, in collaboration with Drs. Morell and
Costantino-Ceccarini (13), showed that the synthesis with nonhydroxy ceramide could be stepped up moderately by the addition of
crude lecithin, but even then we found the hydroxy ceramide to be
a much better acceptor.

Following the same reasoning as before, one would expect that
brain cerebrosides contain primarily the hydroxy acids. Yet
hydroxy cerebrosides dominate the nonhydroxy cerebrosides only to
a small extent in the mouse (and a number of other higher animals).

Perhaps we have a partial answer to this matter of relative
lipid concentrations. When Dr. Ullman compared the rates of
ceramide synthesis in mouse microsomes with lignoceroyl-CoA and
cerebronoyl-CoA, he found relative rates of about 4 to 1. Thus it
appears likely that the brain makes hydroxy ceramide rather slowly,
compared with nonhydroxy ceramide. Indeed this might be inferred
from the relative amounts of the two ceramide families in brain.

To summarize our interpretation, it seems likely that non-hydroxy galactocerebroside is made at a rate controlled by the galactosylation step, and in the case of hydroxy cerebroside, the rate-controlling step is the acylation, not the galactosylation. We still don't know what controls the distribution of the fatty acids within the latter family; it seems likely that this is controlled at the hydroxylation step, that is, that the hydroxylase acts best on the very long fatty acids. (In cows, which contain a good deal of hydroxystearate, the hydroxylase may be less specific.) In the case of the nonhydroxy cerebrosides, it would appear that the distribution of the fatty acids is controlled by the specificity and relative concentrations of the two transacylases. It would not be surprising to find that the hydroxylase which forms 2-hydroxy acids is a rather slow enzyme.

Recently, Dr. Antoinette Brenkert and I examined the galactosyl- and glucosyltransferases that make galacto- and gluco-cerebrosides, using lyophilized whole rat brain as enzyme (3). We found that lyophilization greatly enhanced the apparent activities, probably because this permitted closer contact between enzyme and ceramide. You will be horrified, like the reviewers of our paper, to learn that we mixed the dried brain and ceramide in benzene, then evaporated them to dryness together. Actually, we took this idea from Wenger, Petitpas, and Pierenger (25), who found the technique helpful with a galactosyltransferase in brain which forms galactosyl diglyceride.

The two glycosyltransferases are rather similar in properties, both utilizing Mn^{++} or Mg^{++} as cofactors, although the glucosylating enzyme prefers Mn^{++}. The glucosylating enzyme, curiously enough, works equally well with hydroxy ceramide and nonhydroxyceramide. This point was noted also by Shah (21). Since Basu, Kaufman, and Roseman (2) have shown that glucocerebroside is the precursor of gangliosides, and since brain gangliosides do not seem to contain any hydroxy acids (10), one might have predicted that the glucosyltransferase could not utilize hydroxy ceramide. A likely explanation is that specificity of this sort is not required of the glucosyltransferase because it never encounters hydroxy ceramide. However, a very recent report by Hammarström (8a) has disclosed the occurrence of a small concentration in brain of hydroxy glucocerebroside, so evidently the enzyme does see some hydroxy ceramide. Perhaps this hydroxy glucocerebroside is not accepted by the enzyme which carries out the next step in the sequence leading to ganglioside (galactosylation to form lactosyl ceramide).

A long-standing question can now be considered: are ganglio-sides (and glucocerebrosides) made in neurons and galactocerebro-sides in glia? Support for a "yes" answer comes from some of the above considerations. It is likely that neurons contain the medium chain acyltransferase that makes the stearoyl sphingosine cluster of ceramides, the glucosyltransferase which makes gluco- cerebroside, and the other sugar transferases which yield ganglio- side. The glial cells, on the other hand, may contain the same acyltransferase, an additional transferase which handles the very long chain fatty acids, a third transferase which handles the hydroxy fatty acids, and the galactosyltransferase which makes galactocerebroside. According to this hypothesis, the small amount of hydroxy glucocerebroside occurring in brain is due to a small amount of intracellular transfer of hydroxy ceramide.

Dr. Antoinette Brenkert and I tested part of this hypothesis by assaying isolated glial and neuronal cell preparations for the presence of some of these enzymes. We obtained the neuronal preparations from Dr. Otto Sellinger, made by his new procedure (20) and the glial preparations from Dr. Arthur Flangas, made with the aid of his zonal centrifuge (7). Only the neuronal perikarya could make glucocerebroside, in agreement with our prediction. Of course a negative finding with a cell preparation cannot be taken as conclusive, as the glial cells may have been damaged in some vital way during the preparation. Temporarily, anyway, we can conclude that glia cannot carry out the conversion of nonhydroxy or hydroxy ceramide to glucocerebroside. If, then, glucocerebroside and gangliosides are made in neurons only, how do the gangliosides get into glia? Although a number of workers in this field have felt that gangliosides are primarily neuronal, more recent work has shown the presence of these lipids in glia and myelin (5, 17, 23). I am sure that the low values reported in some studies for the concentration of gangliosides in white matter were due to interference in the analytical method by myelin lipids. From our studies with the cells, we therefore propose the conclusion that the glia and myelin get their gangliosides by intracellular transfer.

We also assayed the cell preparations for the galactosylating enzyme and found it to be present in all cells studied. This finding is in agreement with a number of reports on galacto- cerebroside occurrence. The lipid has been found in isolated axonal (6) and neuronal (19) preparations. It has been shown that myelin is hardly the only site of galactocerebroside (9, 16). Moreover this lipid is distinctly present, albeit in lower concen- trations, in brain gray matter (12, 18). Thus there is every reason to believe that neurons make galactocerebroside, but I believe they are limited to the long chain nonhydroxy cerebro- sides (mainly stearoyl).

Dr. Ramesh Arora also evaluated the cell preparations for the galactosidase which degrades galactocerebroside. This enzyme too was present in every cell preparation. (Incidentally, the positive results with two enzymes in the glial preparations strengthens the

negative finding in the case of the glucosyltransferase.) It thus
appears that glia and neurons have the capacity to form and destroy
galactocerebroside. The higher concentration in white matter,
then, is simply due to the ability of glia to make the basic and
proteolipid proteins of myelin, which act to fixate galactocerebroside and protect it from rapid turnover.

These interpretations support very nicely an observation that
Amiya Hajra and I had made some years ago (8). We compared the
turnover rates of the various cerebrosides in young rats, following
the injection of tritium-labeled acetate. Of the various fatty
acids analyzed, stearic proved to have a relatively high turnover
rate, an observation we could not then explain. I think now that
a good part of the radioactivity must have arisen from stearoyl
cerebroside synthesized in neurons. Following the same line of
reasoning, I suggest that the relatively high proportion of
stearoyl cerebroside seen in young brain (24) is due to neuronal
synthesis. The same explanation applies to a number of brain
disorders which seem to produce cerebrosides that are deficient in
the long chain acids; the glial cells which make cerebrosides for
myelin may be quite sick but the neuronal synthetic mechanism may
still be working.

THE USE OF SYNTHETIC ANALOGS

Dr. Ramesh Arora and I have been engaged in this approach for
the past two years, in the hope that we could design compounds
which would interfere with the operation of specific sphingolipid
enzymes. Synthetic inhibitors have, of course, been of tremendous
value in many fields but they have received almost no attention in
the lipid field. We started with the simplest possible compounds,
keeping in mind some of the novel features of sphingolipids,
particularly the presence of the amide bond, the adjacent hydroxyl
groups, and the presence of lipoidal residues in the fatty acid
and sphingosine moieties. Fortunately for us, there is a
naturally occurring antibiotic, Chloramphenicol, which bears a
certain resemblance to ceramide:

$$O_2N-\!\!\!\bigcirc\!\!\!-CH-CH-CH_2$$
$$\quad\quad\quad\; OH \quad NH \quad OH$$
$$\quad\quad\quad\quad\quad\quad C{=}O$$
$$\quad\quad\quad\quad\quad\quad CHCl_2$$

Through the courtesy of chemists at Parke-Davis & Co., we were able to obtain a number of related amines which had been made as precursors of potential antibiotics. We acylated the amines with various fatty acids and halogenated or hydroxy acids, then tested the amides by drying solutions of the material to dryness in test tubes. The tests were carried out at a concentration of 0.3 mM, which might be considered a level at which a reasonably efficient inhibitor could be detected.

Most of our experiments have been done with cerebroside galactosidase, partially purified from rat brain. The enzyme, buffer, and emulsified substrate were added to the dry inhibitor and the mixture was incubated for 3 hr. We were pleased to find an inhibition by fatty acid amides of the Chloramphenicol base (p-nitro-3-phenyl-2-amino-1,3-propanediol). Removal of the nitro group enhanced the activity and removal of either one of the hydroxyl groups reduced the activity considerably. The best fatty acid was decanoate, or dodecanoate, and addition of an alpha-hydroxy group on the decanoate residue enhanced the activity. Several geometric isomers of the hydroxy amine were available: the D-threo and L-threo forms were inferior to the DL-erythro form. (Natural sphingosine has the D-erythro configuration.) Substituents on the benzene ring reduced the amide's effectiveness and replacement of the benzene ring with a methyl group or hydrogen destroyed the inhibitory effect (1).

In summary, our best inhibitor in this series was the amide formed from 2-hydroxydodecanoic acid and DL-erythro-3-phenyl-2-amino-1,3-propanediol. The inhibition at 0.3 mM was 69%; at 0.03 mM it was 43%. We assumed that this compound, which resembles ceramide in so many ways, went to the lipid-binding region of the substrate-active site in cerebrosidase but, to our surprise, kinetic analysis showed the compound to be a noncompetitive inhibitor. According to the general interpretation of non-competitive inhibition, this means that the amide is bound to some other region of the enzyme, not directly associated with the hydrolyzing site.

If such a region exists, does it serve a normal, functional role in the control of this galactosidase? What sort of compound in brain might exist that binds to this site? Ceramide itself does not seem to be the compound, as it has little effect on the enzyme's ability to hydrolyze cerebroside. Even the abnormally short chain ceramide, made synthetically from sphingosine and 2-hydroxydodecanoic acid, has little effect; the benzene ring seems crucial to the inhibitory effect.

When we evaluated some short chain galactocerebrosides, made from psychosine and short chain acids, we also found inhibition. The 2-carbon cerebroside, acetyl psychosine, inhibited 57% at

0.3 mM concentration. This, we thought, must surely act
competitively, at the substrate-active site. However, kinetic
analysis showed this behaved like a mixed-type inhibitor; that is,
some of the material went to the substrate-active site but some
went to a different site. It does not seem likely that this
second site of attachment is the same site which bound our
ceramide-like inhibitor, as the two inhibitors are structurally so
different.

We tested this question by the method of Woolfolk and
Stadtman (26), who pointed out that inhibitors acting on different
enzyme sites should show a cumulative type of inhibition when both
inhibitors are present. For example, if inhibitor A alone
combines with and deactivates 40% of the enzyme molecules present,
and inhibitor B alone deactivates 70% of the enzyme molecules
present, the mixture of the two inhibitors should produce an
inhibition of 40 + 70(1 - 0.40) = 82%. This reasoning process
assumes inhibitor B binds to a different site and that this
binding affinity is unaffected by the presence or absence of A in
the complex. If the two inhibitors compete for the same site, the
cumulative inhibition will be low.

In such an experiment we found 29% inhibition with the
aromatic hydroxy amide and 42% inhibition with acetyl psychosine;
the mixture of the two gave 55% inhibition. Since the calculated
cumulative inhibition was 59%, this indicates that the two
inhibitors act at independent sites (55% and 59% are the same,
within the error of our assay.) By this interpretation, there
must be two noncompetitive sites as well as the substrate-active
site. Similarly, when we tested galactonolactone, which is a
good inhibitor of lysosomal galactosidases (4), we found it to
act competitively with cerebroside, which means it acts at the
substrate-active site. It too gave the theoretical value in a
mixture with the inhibitory aromatic amide.

A curious observation was made with some very simple amides:
the decanoic acid amide of 2-amino-2-methyl-propanol-1 proved to
stimulate cerebrosidase. This compound, at 0.3 mM, gave about 55%
higher activity; at 2 mM, which is the saturating level, the
stimulation was 62%. The resemblance of this compound to cerebroside is somewhat reduced, compared to our inhibitors, since it
possesses only the amide grouping and one of the adjacent hydroxyl
groups. The branched methyl group is crucial to the effect, as
omission of this group produces a slightly inhibitory compound.
It is tempting to postulate that the amide fits into the same site
on cerebrosidase that holds our inhibitory aromatic amide. Some-
how the small distortion produced by the branched methyl group
makes the enzyme work faster, instead of more slowly. We know
from the Lineweaver-Burk plot that the compound does not affect
the binding constant between enzyme and substrate.

It will be interesting to see if adding a benzene ring on the propanol chain augments the stimulation.

We have done less work with the sugar transferases which make galacto- and glucocerebroside. In the case of the former, bromo-acetyl 3-phenyl-2-amino-propanediol-1,3 proved to be a good inhibitor, although it had no effect on the galactosidase. This amide behaved like a noncompetitive inhibitor, suggesting that the galactosyltransferase has an effector site too. Again we can only wonder if there is a naturally occurring effector substance which acts here. Some of our amides acted as acceptors, apparently making abnormal cerebrosides.

This part of our research program is continuing and we hope to make additional compounds of even higher inhibitory and stimulatory power. We must work out the details of the specificity toward the various sphingolipid enzymes. The compounds will be tested in vivo, as well as in cell cultures. Naturally occurring inhibitors will be sought. The possibility exists that such substances will be valuable in the treatment of the genetic diseases involving gluco- and galactocerebrosides. For example, Gaucher's disease might be controlled by intake of an inhibitor of glucocerebroside formation. Many experiments are left to be done.

REFERENCES

1. Arora, R. C. and Radin, N. S. Synthetic amides resembling ceramide which inhibit cerebroside galactosidase. J. Lipid Res., in press.
2. Basu, S., Kaufman, B. and Roseman, S. Enzymatic synthesis of ceramide-glucose and ceramide-lactose by glycosyltransferases from embryonic chick brain. J. Biol. Chem. 243, 5802, 1968.
3. Brenkert, A. and Radin, N. S. Synthesis of galactosyl ceramide and glucosyl ceramide by rat brain: assay procedures and changes with age. Brain Res., in press.
4. Conchie, J. and Levvy, G. A. Inhibition of glycosidases by lactones. Biochem. J. 65, 389, 1957.
5. Derry, D. M. and Wolfe, L. S. Gangliosides in isolated neurons and glial cells. Science 158, 1450, 1967.
6. DeVries, G. H. and Norton, W. T. Evidence for the absence of myelin and the presence of galactolipid in an axon-enriched fraction from bovine CNS. Federation Proc. 30, 1248Abs, 1971.
7. Flangas, A. L. and Bowman, R. E. Neuronal perikarya of rat brain isolated by zonal centrifugation. Science 161, 1025, 1968.
8. Hajra, A. K. and Radin, N. S. Isotopic studies of the bio-synthesis of the cerebroside fatty acids in rats. J. Lipid Res. 4, 270, 1963.

8a. Hammarström, S. Eur. J. Biochem. 21, 388, 1971.

 9. Kishimoto, Y., Agranoff, B. W., Radin, N. S. and Burton, R. M.
     Comparison of the fatty acids of lipids of subcellular brain
     function. J. Neurochem. 16, 397, 1969.

10. Kishimoto, Y. and Radin, N. S. Occurrence of 2-hydroxy fatty
     acids in animal tissues. J. Lipid Res. 4, 139, 1963.

11. Klenk, E. and Huang, R. T. C. Zur Kenntnis der Gehirn-
     ceramide und der darin vorkommenden Sphingosinbasen. Z.
     physiol. Chem. 349, 451, 1968.

12. Lewin, E. and Hess, H. H. Intralaminar distribution of
     cerebrosides in human frontal cortex. J. Neurochem. 12, 213,
     1965.

13. Morell, P., Costantino-Ceccarini, E. and Radin, N. S. The
     biosynthesis by brain microsomes of cerebrosides containing
     nonhydroxy fatty acids. Arch. Biochem. Biophys. 141, 738,
     1970.

14. Morell, P. and Radin, N. S. Synthesis of cerebroside by
     brain from uridine diphosphate galactose and ceramide
     containing hydroxy fatty acid. Biochemistry 8, 506, 1969.

15. Morell, P. and Radin, N. S. Specificity in ceramide
     biosynthesis from long chain bases and various fatty acyl
     Coenzyme A's by brain microsomes. J. Biol. Chem. 245, 342,
     1970.

16. Norton, W. T. and Autilio, L. A. The lipid composition of
     purified bovine brain myelin. J. Neurochem. 13, 213, 1966.

17. Norton, W. T. and Poduslo, S. E. Neuronal perikarya and
     astroglia of rat brain: chemical composition during
     myelination. J. Lipid Res. 12, 84, 1971.

18. Radin, N. S. and Akahori, Y. Fatty acids of human brain
     cerebrosides. J. Lipid Res. 2, 335, 1961.

19. Raghavan, S. and Kanfer, J. N. Compositional studies on
     ceramide galactoside of enriched glial and neuronal cell
     fractions from rat brain. Trans. Am. Soc. Neurochem. 2, 101,
     1971.

20. Sellinger, O. Z., Azcurra, J. M., Johnson, D. E., Ohlsson, W.
     and Lodin, Z. Independence of protein synthesis and drug
     uptake in nerve cell bodies and glial cells isolated by a new
     technique. Nature New Biol. 230, 253, 1971.

21. Shah, S. N. Glycosyl transferases of microsomal fractions
     from brain: synthesis of glucosyl ceramide and galactosyl
     ceramide during development and the distribution of glucose
     and galactose transferase in white and grey matter. J.
     Neurochem. 18, 395, 1971.

22. Sribney, M. Enzymatic synthesis of ceramide. Biochim.
     Biophys. Acta 125, 542, 1966.

23. Suzuki, K., Poduslo, S. E. and Norton, W. T. Gangliosides in
     the myelin fraction of developing rats. Biochim. Biophys.
     Acta 144, 375, 1967.

24. Svennerholm, L. and Ställberg-Stenhagen, S. Changes in the
     fatty acid composition of cerebrosides and sulfatides of human

nervous tissue with age. J. Lipid Res. 9, 215, 1968.

25. Wenger, D. A., Petitpas, J. W. and Pierenger, R. A.
     Biosynthesis of monogalactosyl diglyceride from uridine
     diphosphate galactose and diglyceride in brain. Biochemistry
     7, 3700, 1968.

26. Woolfolk, C. A. and Stadtman, E. R. Cumulative feedback
     inhibition in the multiple end product regulation of gluta-
     mine synthetase activity in <u>Escherichia coli</u>. Biochem.
     Biophys. Res. Commun. 17, 313, 1964.

FURTHER STUDIES ON GALACTOCEREBROSIDE β-GALACTOSIDASE

IN GLOBOID CELL LEUKODYSTROPHY

Kunihiko Suzuki and Yoshiyuki Suzuki

Department of Neurology
University of Pennsylvania School of Medicine
Philadelphia, Pa. 19104

and

Thomas F. Fletcher

Department of Veterinary Anatomy
College of Veterinary Medicine, University of Minnesota
St. Paul, Minn. 55109

The genetic cause underlying globoid cell leukodystrophy (Krabbe's disease) appears to be the deficiency of galactocerebroside β-galactosidase (galactosylceramide galactosyl hydrolase). Among postmortem organs, the deficiency was initially demonstrated in the brain, liver and spleen from three patients (11). This was later confirmed in the brain, liver and kidney of five additional patients (1, 13). Furthermore, the same deficiency has been demonstrated in peripheral leukocytes (5, 12), serum and cultured fibroblasts (12) from patients afflicted with this fatal neurological disorder. In addition to the diagnostic value of the galactocerebrosidase assay on these easily obtainable materials, our preliminary data indicated the possibility of heterozygous carrier detection utilizing these materials(12).

In addition to human globoid cell leukodystrophy, there is a canine form of the disease occurring in Cairn and West Highland terriers. The clinical parameters and morphological features of canine globoid cell leukodystrophy are quite similar to those of the human disease (3,4). Suzuki et al. (9) demonstrated that the canine form is also caused by the defect in galactocerebrosidase activity. The enzyme activity was deficient in the brain, liver and kidney of two affected dogs. It was expected,

therefore, that canine globoid cell leukodystrophy would be a useful model for study of the human disease.

The present report summarizes the study of galactocerebroside β-gal-
actosidase activities in leukocytes, serum and cultured fibroblasts from
patients, parents, and family members of patients with globoid cell leukodystrophy, indicating the feasibility of heterozygote detection, and results
of a recently accomplished in utero diagnosis of the disease. It also presents findings of galactocerebrosidase activities in canine leukocytes and
serum. The results on canine materials indicate strongly that the human
and canine forms of globoid cell leukodystrophy are enzymatically distinct.

MATERIALS AND METHODS

Serum was collected by simply letting untreated blood clot at room
temperature, followed by centrifugation at 1000 g for 10 minutes. Since
both galactocerebroside β-galactosidase and the control enzyme, 4-methyl-
umbelliferyl β-galactosidase, were unstable in serum (12), the assays were
always carried out within 48 hours after collection. For preparation of
leukocytes, approximately 10 ml of blood was drawn, anticoagulated with
either heparin or EDTA, and leukocytes were separated by differential
sedimentation by the addition of 1/4 vol of 6% dextran in physiological
saline, essentially according to Snyder and Brady (8). The final leukocyte
pellet was suspended in 1.0 ml of distilled water, sonicated for one min.
in a water-bath type ultrasonicator, frozen and thawed four times, and
finally centrifuged at 1000 g for 10 minutes. The supernatant was used
directly for assays of galactocerebroside β-galactosidase. For assays of
4-methylumbelliferyl β-galactosidase and the protein determination (6),
1 to 10 or 1 to 20 dilution of the original supernatant gave generally
satisfactory results.

All of the cultured fibroblast specimens were sent to us from other
laboratories, and, therefore, the conditions of the cultures varied considerably, including the nature of nutrient media, number of passages, and
the phase of cell growth. In most instances, cultured fibroblasts were
harvested from the monolayer with the use of a proteolytic enzyme, either
trypsin or pronase. The use of proteolytic enzymes did not appear to
affect the final results significantly. The same assay scales described
above for leukocytes were suitable for fibroblast pellets consisting of a
few million cells. The preparation of leukocytes and serum from dogs
was identical with those for human specimens.

Assay Procedure. The assay system for galactocerebrosidase was identical with the original system of Bowen and Radin (2) except that their partially purified enzyme fraction was replaced by 0.2 ml of serum or the supernatant of disrupted cells as described above. The substrate was natural bovine galactocerebroside specifically labelled at the galactose moiety according to Radin et al. (7), and had a specific activity of 4800 counts per minute per mμmole. At the end of 3–hr incubation at 37° with shaking, 100μg of unlabelled galactose in 0.1 ml were added as the carrier, and the reaction was stopped with the addition of 5 vols of chloroform–methanol (2:1, v/v). The tubes were shaken and centrifuged, and the lower chloroform phase was removed. The upper water–methanol phase was washed twice with chloroform, and an aliquot of the final upper phase was dried in a scintillation vial in an oven at 120°. When cooled, the material was dissolved in 0.5 ml of water, 12 ml of toluene–based scintillation solvent containing 10% Bio–Solv III (Beckman Instrument) added, and the radioactivity measured in a Packard Tricarb scintillation spectrometer. A blank tube without the enzyme source was carried through the entire procedure, and the sample counts were corrected for the blank counts.

4–Methylumbelliferyl β–galactosidase was assayed in a system in which 0.1 ml of the enzyme source was incubated with 0.3 ml of 1 mM 4–methylumbelliferyl β–D–galactopyranoside at 37° for 60 min. The substrate was in citrate–phosphate buffer, 0.1 M, pH 5.0 for leukocytes and fibroblasts, and pH 4.0 for serum. The selection of pH was based on the preliminary data on the pH optima of 4–methylumbelliferyl β–galactosidase in these materials. The reaction was stopped by the addition of 0.2 M glycine buffer, pH 10.7, and the liberated 4–methylumbelliferone was determined by fluorometry in Aminco SPF 125 spectrofluorometer with the excitation wave length 365 mμ and the emission wave length 448 mμ. Blank tubes were included in each assay and readings were corrected accordingly.

RESULTS

Galactocerebroside β–Galactosidase in Human Serum, Leukocytes, and Fibroblasts. (Table 1). Activities of galactocerebroside β–galactosidase were uniformly and profoundly deficient in sera, leukocytes and cultured fibroblasts from human patients with globoid cell leukodystrophy. The diagnosis of the disease can be established unequivocally utilizing any one of these three types of specimens. The arithmetic averages of enzyme activities in parents of patients, who are obligate heterozygotes, were all intermediate between the activities of patients and those of controls. Differences between patients and parents, and between parents

Table 1. Galactocerebrosidase in Human Serum, Leukocytes and
Fibroblasts.

Specimen	Galactocerebrosidase	Significance Test
SERUM		
Patients	0.13 ± 0.17 (n = 4)	] p < 0.01
Parents	5.09 ± 2.70 (n = 6)	
Controls	23.4 ± 7.83 (n = 12)	] p < 0.001
LEUKOCYTES		
Patients	0.11 ± 0.17 (n = 7)	] 0.01 < p < 0.02
Parents	1.07 ± 0.83 (n = 12)	
Controls	2.42 ± 1.13 (n = 44)	] p < 0.001
FIBROBLASTS		
Patients	0.30 ± 0.24 (n = 7)	] 0.05 < p < 0.10
Parents	1.53 ± 1.72 (n = 4)	
Controls	3.00 ± 2.38 (n = 38)	] not significant

Activities are expressed as mμmoles/hr/mg protein ± standard deviation,
except for serum activities which are mμmoles/hr/100 ml.

---

and controls were statistically highly significant in serum and leukocytes.
Due to the small number of carriers tested and the large variations observed
within each group, the difference in galactocerebrosidase activities in fibroblasts between patients and parents was barely significant, and that between
parents and controls was not significant statistically. The difference between patients and controls was, however, highly significant.

Not only were serum enzyme differences statistically highly significant, there was no overlap of enzyme activities in sera among the three
groups: patients, parents and controls. Apparently healthy family members
of patients, who are possible carriers, could be divided into the healthy
and heterozygous categories on the basis of galactocerebrosidase activities
in their sera (Fig. 1a). In leukocytes, on the other hand, there was
considerable overlap in enzyme activities between the obligate heterozygotes and the normal controls, despite the statistically significant difference
between the means of the two groups. As a consequence, identification
of heterozygous carriers among family members of patients was not as
certain as that based on the serum enzyme. A few individuals fell within
the overlapping area between the normal and heterozygous ranges (Fig. 1b),
thus making identification for these individuals impossible on the basis of
the leukocyte enzyme.

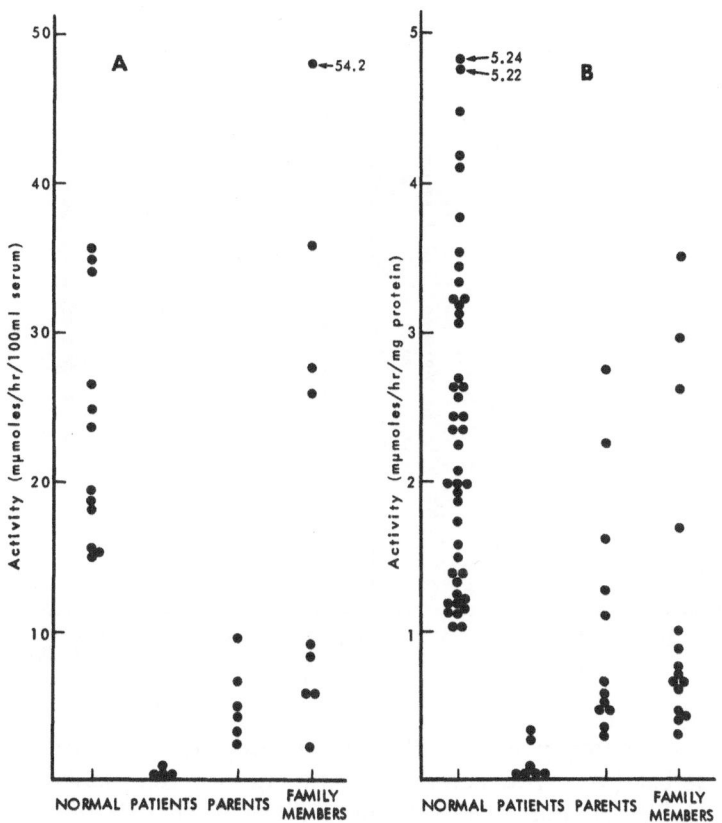

Fig. 1.   Galactocerebroside β-galactosidase activities in human serum
(a) and leukocytes (b).   Note the complete separation of the serum enzyme
activities between the normal and heterozygous groups, while there is
considerable overlap in leukocyte enzyme activities between the two
groups.

Galactocerebroside β-Galactosidase in Canine Leukocytes and Serum.
In a preliminary experiment, galactocerebroside β-galactosidase activities
were assayed in peripheral leukocytes from dogs affected with globoid cell
leukodystrophy, a known carrier, known normal dogs, and dogs for which
genotypic status was unknown.   The results indicated that, as in the human
disease, diagnosis of the canine disease is possible by the deficient activity of galactocerebroside β-galactosidase in leukocytes of affected dogs.
A heterozygous carrier dog exhibited lower activity than normal dogs,
suggesting that identification of carriers might also be possible on the basis

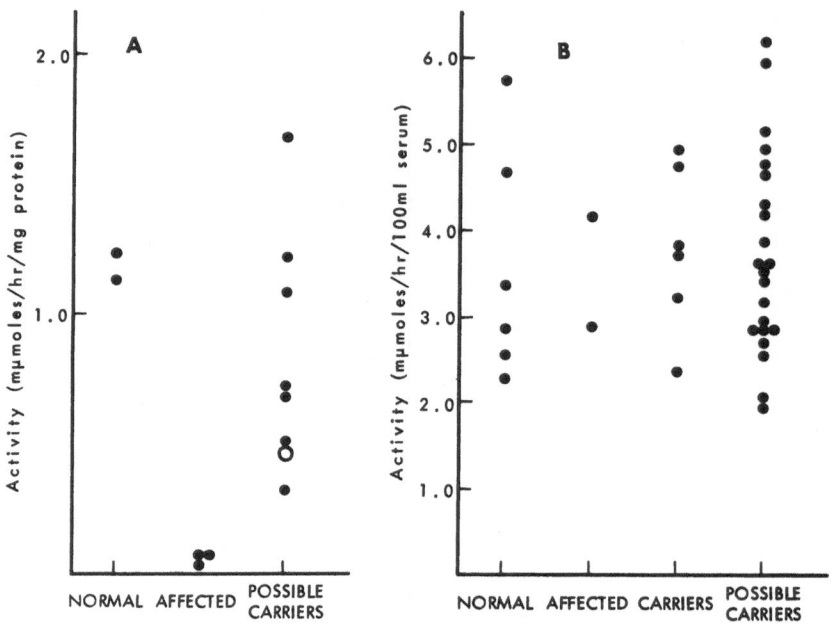

Fig. 2. Galactocerebroside β-galactosidase activities in canine leukocytes (a) and serum (b). The open circle in Fig. 2a represents a known
carrier dog. Unlike in the human disease, there is no difference in the
activities of serum galactocerebrosidase among the four genetically different categories.

of the leukocyte enzymes (Fig. 2a). The number of dogs examined in
this preliminary experiment was too low to permit statistical evaluation.

     In contrast, the findings on canine sera were completely different
from those of human sera (Fig. 2b). There was no difference in activities
of galactocerebroside β-galactosidase in sera among the three groups of
dogs, affected, heterozygous, and normal. The arithmetic averages of the
enzyme activities were essentially identical for all groups. These findings
present the first evidence that the human and canine forms of globoid cell
leukodystrophy are not identical enzymatically.

     In both human and canine globoid cell leukodystrophy, and in any
type of specimens, there was no difference in activities of the nonspecific

4-methylumbelliferyl β-galactosidase among the three groups, affected, heterozygous and normal.   These findings indicate the highly specific nature of the galactocerebrosidase deficiency in globoid cell leukodystropy.

DISCUSSION

The profound and specific deficiency of galactocerebroside β-galactosidase provides an unequivocal basis for the diagnosis of globoid cell leukodystrophy.   Since the first demonstration of the deficiency, we have examined, as of October 1, 1971, a total of 18 patients.   The deficiency of the enzyme was found in every single specimen, whether postmortem organs, serum, leukocytes, or cultured fibroblasts, of every patient studied. Furthermore, we have not observed such specific deficiency of galactocerebroside β-galactosidase in any specimens from normal individuals or from any patients with genetic or nongenetic neurological disorders other than globoid cell leukodystrophy.   Thus, definitive antemortem diagnosis of the disease is possible by assaying any of the three readily available specimens for activities of galactocerebroside β-galactosidase.

Among those we have studied, there were two patients who were older than the usual age category associated with globoid cell leukodystrophy. One was a seven-year old patient in whom the diagnosis had been established histologically by brain biopsy, and the other was a twelve-year old patient whose identical twin had died of histologically confirmed globoid cell leukodystrophy several years earlier.   Leukocytes of the former patient and fibroblasts of the latter also exhibited the specific deficiency of galactocerebroside β-galactosidase.   Therefore, the extremely rare older form of globoid cell leukodystrophy appears also to be caused by the same enzymatic defect as in the more common infantile form.

Careful consideration of advantages and disadvantages of each specimen type is necessary in the case of heterozygote detection.   The most reliable results were obtained with the use of serum as the enzyme source. The average levels of galactocerebrosidase activities in the normal and heterozygous groups were widely separated, and there was no overlap between the two groups.   Serum enzyme activities can be expressed on the basis of serum volume without protein determination, as required for other materials.   This eliminates another potential source of error.   The disadvantage of the serum enzyme assay is the relative instability of both galactocerebrosidase and nonspecific β-galactosidase in serum, either frozen or refrigerated (Fig. 3).   Serum enzymes are not only unstable, but rates of decrease in the enzyme activities vary from one specimen to another and also between galactocerebroside β-galactosidase and 4-methylumbelliferyl

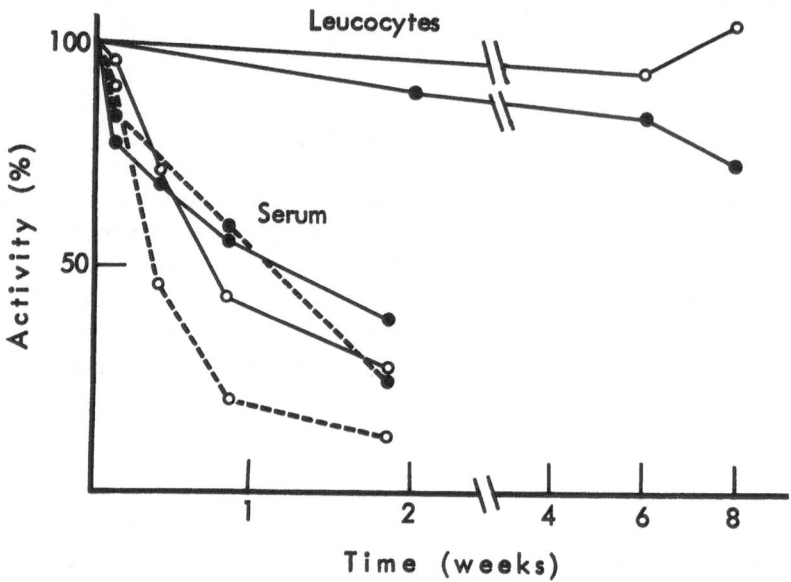

Fig. 3. Effect of storage on the activities of β-galactosidases. Serum
and leukocytes were prepared and stored either frozen or refrigerated for
designated period of time before enzyme assays. Closed circles, galactocerebrosidase; open circles, 4-methylumbelliferyl β-galactosidase. Solid
lines represent samples stored frozen at −20°, and dashed lines for samples
stored refrigerated at 4°. Reproduced from ref. 12 by permission. Copy-
right 1971 by the American Assoc. for the Advancement of Science.

β-galactosidase (Suzuki, unpublished). Therefore, it is not possible to
correct an observed activity for the loss of enzyme activities during
storage. It is important that assays be performed preferably within 24 hrs,
or at the latest within 48 hours after collection of serum. In our experience, it is usually possible to have serum collected anywhere within the
United States, shipped to our laboratory and assayed within 24 hours.
Despite the disadvantage of enzyme instability, we prefer serum as the
source for galactocerebrosidase assays to detect heterozygotes. Plasma is
unsatisfactory for this purpose, because commonly used anticoagulants,
heparin, EDTA and oxalate, are all moderately inhibitory to the enzyme.

While not as simple as serum collection, separation of leukocytes is
a relatively simple procedure; in fact, it has become a semi-routine procedure in many clinical laboratories. In activities of galactocerebroside
β-galactosidase in leukocytes, there was considerable overlap between

obligate heterozygotes and normal controls, when all of our data were combined and evaluated together. However, reliability of carrier detection by the leukocyte enzyme is actually greater than suggested by our combined data. To a significant degree, the overlapping of activities was the result of systematic variation in leukocyte preparations from different laboratories on different occasions. Determinations on series of leukocytes prepared simultaneously under identical conditions generally gave more consistent results, and heterozygous carriers could be identified with reasonable certainty. As we reported earlier (12), however, we have had a few obligate heterozygous individuals who showed activities of leukocyte galactocerebrosidase within the range of controls prepared and assayed simultaneously. Since galactocerebroside β-galactosidase in leukocyte is stable and can be stored frozen for at least a few months, leukocytes are the specimen of choice when immediate enzyme assays on freshly obtained serum are not possible. Whenever detection of carriers is involved, it is imperative to include at least two, preferably more, samples of control leukocytes, prepared simultaneously.

Cultured fibroblasts can be used reliably for diagnosis of affected infants. For detecting heterozygous carriers, however, cultured fibroblasts gave the least reliable results in our series. Since the number of fibroblast samples from obligate heterozygotes was small (four), rigorous evaluation of these data is difficult. The major difficulty appears to be the multitude of variables which potentially affect activities of enzymes, such as the composition of nutrient media, number of passages, phases of cell growth, and means of harvesting cells. All of the fibroblast samples were contributed from other laboratories, since our own laboratory presently lacks the facility for fibroblast culture. It is difficult to control all potential sources of variation when many different laboratories are involved, more so than in the case of leukocyte preparation. If all of the conditions of fibroblast culture can be rigorously controled in a single laboratory, cultured fibroblasts might give more consistent data, not only for diagnosis of globoid cell leukodystrophy, but also for heterozygote detection.

Cultured amniotic fluid cells possess activities of galactocerebroside β-galactosidase comparable to those in cultured skin fibroblasts. This finding predicted the feasibility of in utero diagnosis of globoid cell leukodystrophy. This prediction has been recently borne out in our laboratory in collaboration with Drs. Edward L. Schneider and Charles J. Epstein (10). Cultured amniotic fluid cells from a fetus at risk showed activities of galactocerebroside β-galactosidase which were only 5% of the control values. This specific deficiency of the enzyme was confirmed in the brain and liver tissues of the fetus following a therapeutic abortion. The activities of galactocerebroside β-galactosidase in these organs were 1% or less of the control tissues.

Our preliminary series of assays on galactocerebroside β-galactosidase in canine leukocytes gave data anticipated from those on human leukocytes. There is little doubt that affected dogs can be diagnosed by assaying leukocytes for the activity of galactocerebroside β-galactosidase. The degree of reliability with which carrier dogs can be identified remains to be evaluated, when we have a sufficient amount of data for detailed statistical treatment. An investigation is in progress to determine variability of leukocyte galactocerebrosidase activities in dogs in relation to age, sex, breed, family line, storage time of leukocyte pellets, etc.

The finding on galactocerebroside β-galactosidase in canine serum came as a shocking surprise, because the analogy between human and canine globoid cell leukodystrophy had appeared perfect. Both are similar clinically and have identical morphological alterations and the same specific deficiency of galactocerebroside β-galactosidase in tissues as well as in peripheral leukocytes. Activities of serum galactocerebrosidase were essentially identical in affected, heterozygous and normal dogs. This observation provides the first evidence that the human and canine forms of globoid cell leukodystrophy are not identical.

There are several possibilities for explaining this discrepancy between globoid cell leukodystrophy in the two species. Our present working hypothesis is as follows. Galactocerebroside β-galactosidase may consist of two subcomponents, major and minor. In human globoid cell leukodystrophy, both components are absent, while in canine globoid cell leukodystrophy, only the major component is missing but the minor component is preserved. In tissues and leukocytes, both components are normally present, and therefore, affected dogs show deficient activities of galactocerebrosidase in these materials. Only the minor component may be excreted normally into serum. If the minor component of galactocerebrosidase is not deficient in canine globoid cell leukodystrophy, there would be no difference in the enzyme activities in serum among affected, heterozygous and normal dogs. An investigation is in progress to prove or disprove this hypothesis.

ACKNOWLEDGEMENT

Cooperation of numerous colleagues throughout the United States, who provided us with sera, leukocytes, and cultured fibroblasts from patients with globoid cell leukodystrophy and their family members, made this investigation possible. This study was supported by research grants, NS-08420 and NS-06756, from the United States Public Health Service, and 670-B-2 from the National Multiple Sclerosis Society.

REFERENCES

1. Austin, J., Suzuki, K., Armstrong, D., Brady, R. O., Bachhawat, B. K., Schlenker, J. and Stumpf, D.: Studies in Globoid (Krabbe) Leukodystrophy (GLD) V. Controlled Enzymatic Studies in Ten Human Cases. Arch. Neurol., 23:502, 1970.

2. Bowen, D. M. and Radin, N. S.: Cerebroside Galactosidase: A Method for Determination and a Comparison with Other Lysosomal Enzymes in Developing Rat Brain. J. Neurochem., 16:501, 1969.

3. Fletcher, T. F., Kurtz, H. J. and Low, D. C.: Globoid Cell Leukodystrophy (Krabbe Type) in the Dog. J. Am. Vet. Med. Assoc., 149:165, 1966.

4. Fletcher, T. F., Lee, D. G. and Hammer, R. F.: Ultrastructure of Globoid Leukodystrophy in the Dog. Am. J. Vet. Res., 32:177, 1971.

5. Malone, M. J.: Deficiency in a Degradative Enzyme System in Globoid Leukodystrophy. Abstr. First Meeting of the Am. Soc. Neurochem., Albuquerque, N.M., 1970, p. 56.

6. Lowry, O. H., Rosebrough, N. J., Farr, A. L. and Randall, R. J.: Protein Measurement with the Folin Phenol Reagent. J. Biol. Chem., 193:265, 1951.

7. Radin, N. S., Hof, L., Bradley, R. M. and Brady, R. O.: Lacto-sylceramide Galactosidase: Comparison with Other Sphingolipid Hydrolases in Developing Rat Brain. Brain Res., 14:497, 1969.

8. Snyder, R. A. and Brady, R. O.: The Use of White Cells as a Source of Diagnostic Material for Lipid Storage Diseases. Clin. Chim. Acta, 25:331, 1969.

9. Suzuki, Y., Austin, J., Armstrong, D., Suzuki, K., Schlenker, J. and Fletcher, T.: Studies in Globoid (Krabbe) Leukodystrophy: Enzymic and Sphingolipid Findings in the Canine Form. Exp. Neurol., 29:65, 1970.

10. Suzuki, K., Schneider, E. L. and Epstein, C. J.: In Utero Diagnosis of Globoid Cell Leukodystrophy (Krabbe's Disease). Biochem. Biophys. Res. Commun., in press.

11. Suzuki, K. and Suzuki, Y.: Globoid Cell Leukodystrophy (Krabbe's Disease): Deficiency of Galactocerebroside β-Galactosidase.

Proc. Nat. Acad. Sci. (U. S. A.), 66:302, 1970.

12. Suzuki, Y. and Suzuki, K.: Krabbe's Globoid Cell Leukodystrophy:
    Deficiency of Galactocerebrosidase in Serum, Leukocytes and
    Fibroblasts.   Science, 171:73, 1971.

13. Suzuki, K., Suzuki, Y. and Eto, Y.: Deficiency of Galactocerebro-
    side β-Galactosidase in Krabbe's Globoid Cell Leukodystrophy.
    In Lipid Storage Diseases: Enzymatic Defects and Clinical Implications,
    edited by J. Bernsohn and H. J. Grossman, Academic Press, New
    York, 1971, pp. 111-136.

BRAIN GANGLIOSIDES IN KRABBE DISEASE[1]

Lars Svennerholm and Marie-Thérèse Vanier[2]

Department of Neurochemistry, Psychiatric Research

Centre, University of Göteborg, Göteborg, Sweden

Infantile globoid cell leucodystrophy (GLD) or Krabbe disease is considered to be a rare genetic disease, but in Scandinavia at the present time it is the most common form of the sphingolipidoses. In 1963 we published clinical, neuro-pathological, and biochemical studies of six cases (Hagberg et al., 1963) and more recently Hagberg et al. (1969) reported clinical and genetic studies of 32 Swedish cases collected during a 15-year period. Autopsy material from 12 representa-tive cases from this study, and from 5 new cases, has been used in the present biochemical study.

In 1961 (Svennerholm, 1963) we reported on the diminished sulfatide:cerebroside quotient in GLD, and subsequent studies by Austin (Austin, 1963) confirmed this finding. By intra-cerebral injection of normal brain cerebrosides Austin and Lehfeldt (1965) induced the formation of globoid elements in brain, a finding which was also shown in later studies by us (Olsson et al., 1966), and further confirmed in cultures of nervous tissue (Sourander et al., 1966). It was thus possible to classify Krabbe disease as a galactosylceramidosis (Svennerholm, 1969). Recently Suzuki and Suzuki (1970) demonstrated a generalized deficiency of galactocerebroside β-galactosidase in the disease.

[1]Supported by grants from the Swedish Medical Research Council (Projects nos: B70-13X-627-06B, B71-13X-627-07C, B72-13X-627 08A) and by Expressens Prenatal forskningsnämnd.

[2]Permanent address: Hôpital Sainte-Eugénie, Lyon, France. On a special fellowship from Comité Lyonnais de l'Enfance.

In 1967 we reported a profound change in the ganglioside composition in Krabbe brain; this was found mainly in the white matter (Svennerholm, 1967). There was an increase of di- and triglycosylgangliosides and a relative decrease of the normal tetraglycosylgangliosides. In a attempt to elucidate the pathogenesis of the ganglioside disturbance in Krabbe disease we have made further studies on the chemistry of the gangliosides and the neutral glucosylceramides, and some enzymes which play a key role in their biosynthesis and degradation. The structure and composition of the brain sphingoglycolipids in one case of Krabbe disease have recently been reported by Eto and Suzuki (1971).

MATERIALS AND METHODS

Brain autopsy material was available from 17 cases of Krabbe disease aged from 7 to 32 months. All cases had the clinical diagnosis of Krabbe disease which had been established from the clinical signs and symptoms (Hagberg et al., 1969), laboratory diagnosis (Hagberg et al., 1963), peripheral nerve or brain biopsy (Sourander and Olsson, 1968), and in addition, in five cases, by determination of the cerebroside β-galacto-sidase activity (Suzuki and Suzuki, 1970). The diagnosis was verified by histological examination of the autopsy material in all cases.

Normal human brain tissue was obtained from 20 subjects, newborn up to 2 years of age, who had died from accidents or diseases not primarily affecting the central nervous system or the blood circulation. Brain tissue was also available from three cases with infantile Gaucher disease and from two cases of classical Tay-Sachs disease.

Quantitative Determination of Gangliosides and Other Sphingoglycolipids

In all cases a total lipid extract of the brain tissue was prepared as described previously (Vanier et al.,1971). A crude ganglioside fraction was isolated by partition, and the individual gangliosides were determined by the resorcinol method after separation on thin-layer chromatography (TLC) plates, developed with propanol-water, 3:1 (v/v) as solvent system (Vanier et al., 1971). G_{D3} was also determined by running two-dimensional TLC plates with chloroform-methanol-water, 60:32:7 (v/v) and chloroform-methanol-4 M ammonia, 60:35:8 (v/v). Large scale isolations of gangliosides were

performed on silica gel columns as recently outlined by
Svennerholm (1971).

The lower phase from the ganglioside isolation was
subjected to mild saponification. Preliminary separation of
the sphingoglycolipids was conducted by silicic acid and
DEAE-cellulose chromatography and the individual sphingolipids
were further purified by preparative TLC (Svennerholm and
Svennerholm, 1963). The amount of glycosphingolipid was
determined by the orcinol reaction (Svennerholm, 1964), and
by gas-liquid chromatography (GLC) of sugar alditol acetates
and fatty acid methyl esters.

Fatty Acid and Carbohydrate Analysis

Acid methylation of the fatty acids was performed with
5% sulfuric acid in dry methanol with 17:0 as internal standard
for all glucosylsphingolipids, and with normal and hydroxy-
methyl-isoheneicosanoate for cerebrosides and sulfatides
(Svennerholm and Ställberg-Stenhagen, 1968).

The sugars were converted to alditol acetates and
determined according to published methods (Sawardeker, Sloneker
and Jeanes, 1965; Crowell and Burnett, 1967). Acid hydrolysis
was performed with 2 M HCl at 100° for 16 hours. The alditol
acetates were analyzed on 3% ECNSS-M with mannose acetate as
internal standard (Månsson, Vanier, Svennerholm, in preparation).
Hexosamine was also analyzed by a modified Elson-Morgan
procedure (Svennerholm, 1956). Sialic acid was determined by
the resorcinol reaction (Svennerholm, 1964) and as trimethylsilyl derivative by gas-liquid chromatography (Yu and Ledeen,
1971).

Assay of Glycohydrolase and Transferase Activities

Sialidase was determined with ganglioside G_{D1a} (Öhman
and Svennerholm, 1971) and unspecific glycohydrolases with p-
nitrophenyl glycosides as substrates (Vanier and Svennerholm,
in preparation). Cerebroside β-galactosidase was determined
as described by Radin and Arora (1971). Assay of UDP-
galactose : ganglioside G_{M2} galactosyltransferase and CMP-NAN :
lactosylceramide sialyltransferase were performed as described
by Roseman and coworkers (Kaufman, Basu and Roseman, 1967)
but with isolation of the products by TLC on silica-impregnated
paper (Whatman SG 81, Angel and Reeves Ltd.,London).

TABLE 1. PHOSPHOLIPIDS AND GALACTOSPHINGOLIPIDS IN CEREBRAL WHITE MATTER OF NORMAL AND KRABBE BRAIN

COMPOUND	NORMALS (n=6) 10 - 25 months		KRABBE DISEASE (n=15) 7 - 32 months	
	Range		Mean	S.D.
	(μmoles/g fresh tissue weight)			
Phospholipids	66 - 105		34.2	5.4
Cerebrosides	15.5 - 36.7		3.2	1.5
Sulfatides	3.2 - 7.2		0.4	0.2
Cerebrosides : Sulfatides	3.0 - 5.7		8.8	5.4

RESULTS AND DISCUSSION

Galactosylceramides

The total amount of phospholipids, cerebrosides, and sulfatides of white matter in normal and Krabbe brains are given in Table 1. Since in the controls these lipids increased throughout the period of study (6 to 25 months), mean figures have not been calculated, and the range of results are given. In the Krabbe brains the concentration of these lipids did not show any correlation with age, and was of the same magnitude in all cases. The figure for total phospholipids of white matter in Krabbe brains was much lower than in the control white matter, and also lower than in the grey matter of both Krabbe cases and controls. The very low content of phospholipids in white matter of Krabbe disease has been amply demonstrated previously and particularly stressed by Brante (1949) and Svennerholm (1963).

The concentration of the galactosylceramides, cerebrosides and sulfatides was even more reduced; usually the amount present was not more than 1/10th of that in control white matter, and the reduction was more pronounced for the sulfatides. It was notable that the individual variations in concentration were extremely small, in view of the major differences in the onset and duration of the disease. The

TABLE 2. SPHINGOGLYCOLIPIDS IN KRABBE, INFANTILE GAUCHER, TAY-SACHS AND NORMAL NEWBORN BRAINS

COMPOUND	KRABBE		GAUCHER(infantile)		TAY-SACHS		NEWBORN
	Cerebral Cortex	White Matter	Cerebral Cortex	White Matter	Cerebral Cortex	Total	Total
	(nmoles/g fresh tissue weight)						
I. GALACTOSYLCERAMIDES							
Galactosylceramide	650 (270)	3700 (1700)	2660	8320	250	750	12
Galactosylceramide-sulfate	150 (190)	490 (400)	540	2170	280	610	13
II. GLUCOSYLCERAMIDES							
Monoglucosylceramide	16 (125)	32 (255)	300	360	180	130	12
Diglycosylceramide	36 (trace)	140 (150)	120	380	50	230	13
Triglycosylceramides							
Trihexoside	8	40 (60)	11	-	-	28	-
G_{A2}	3	trace	-	-	350	800	2
Tetraglycosylceramides							
Globoside	13	64 (250)	-	-	-	35	1
G_{A1}	25	15 (50)	-	-	20	10	-

The figures in parentheses are from Eto and Suzuki (1971).

ratio of cerebrosides to sulfatides in white matter was
constantly higher than in the controls, which we consider to
be a biochemical prerequisite for a typical Krabbe case.

Concentration of Glucosylceramides

In five representative cases of Krabbe disease the
neutral sphingoglycolipids were isolated by combined column
and thin layer chromatography. The results are compared with
those obtained from one case of infantile Gaucher disease
(Svennerholm, 1967), two cases of Tay-Sachs disease, and four
normal newborns, all isolated with the same procedures
(Table 2). The recovery varied between 80-95%. The concentration of each fraction was calculated from its fatty acid
and carbohydrate content determined by means of the internal
standards. In Krabbe disease lactosylceramide was the major
fraction in cerebral cortex and white matter. The concentration of glucosylceramide, trihexoside, and globoside was
approximately one-third of lactosylceramide. These figures
showed several differences from those reported by Eto and
Suzuki (1971), who found a several fold larger concentration
of glucosylceramide and globoside in their material. The
concentration of glucosylceramide in Krabbe brain was similar
to the amount that we found in infantile Gaucher disease and
Tay-Sachs disease. Eto and Suzuki (1971) assumed trihexoside
and globoside to be characteristic for Krabbe disease, but we
found these compounds in similar concentration in Tay-Sachs
disease. A small amount of globoside was also found in
normal newborn brains. The neutral tetrasaccharide G_{A1},
considered to be the asialoganglioside corresponding to G_{M1},
contained both galactosamine and glucosamine, not only in the
Krabbe brains but also in the Tay-Sachs brains.

Ganglioside Patterns

In order to establish the structure of the gangliosides,
large scale isolation of all the ganglioside fractions was
performed by combined column and thin layer chromatography
(Svennerholm, 1971). The chemical structure of the gangliosides was proven by analysis of the fatty acid, sphingosine,
and carbohydrate moieties, by sialidase and partial acidic
hydrolysis, and by periodic acid-borohydride treatment.
Quantitative figures for all the major gangliosides, expressed
in nanomoles per g of fresh tissue weight, are given in
Fig. 1. The concentration of total gangliosides in the
cerebral cortex was 1.29 (S.D. 0.23) µmoles per g of fresh
tissue weight compared to 1.37 (S.D. 0.07) in the controls.

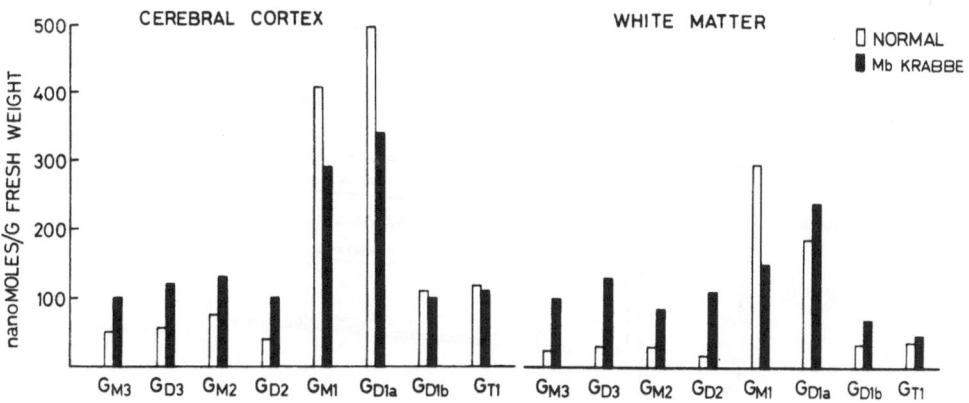

FIG. 1. THE CONCENTRATION OF INDIVIDUAL GANGLIOSIDES IN NORMAL AND KRABBE BRAINS.

However, the pattern of gangliosides differed; G_{M3}, G_{D3}, G_{M2} and G_{D2} were approximately 100% higher in Krabbe disease than in the controls, while the figures for G_{D1a} and G_{D1b} were significantly lower. In white matter, total gangliosides were higher in Krabbe disease compared to the controls, 0.93 (S.D. 0.20) and 0.65 (S.D. 0.17) μmoles per g, respectively. The difference in the pattern was even more pronounced than in the cerebral cortex; G_{M3}, G_{D3}, G_{M2} and G_{D2} were several-fold higher in Krabbe disease, whereas G_{M1} showed a marked reduction. In the white matter of Krabbe brains two other gangliosides were found, the chemical structure of which has not yet been elucidated. In neutral solvents they migrated with G_{M1}, but in ammonia-containing solvents between G_{D1a} and G_{D1b}. These results are in accordance with those previously reported for Krabbe disease by Svennerholm (1967). However, the sialosyllactosylceramide was not separated into G_{M3} and G_{D3} at this time.

A ganglioside pattern similar to that found in all our cases of Krabbe disease has also been reported in another form of leucodystrophy, MLD, (Suzuki, 1967; Svennerholm, 1967), although the magnitude of the changes was much less pronounced than in Krabbe disease. Similar types of changes in the ganglioside pattern have also been described in the white matter of cases with subacute sclerosing panencephalitis (Suzuki, 1967; Ledeen, Salsman and Cabrera, 1968).

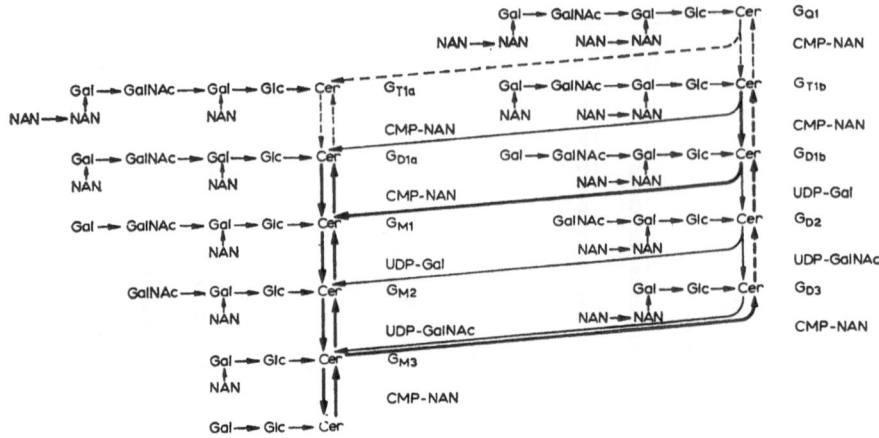

FIG. 2. METABOLISM OF BRAIN GANGLIOSIDES.

Thick line = major pathway, thin line = minor pathway, unbroken line = demonstrated pathway, dashed line = assumed pathway.

Determinations of Galactosyltransferase and Glycohydrolase Activities in Vitro

The increased concentrations of the four gangliosides G_{M3}, G_{M2}, G_{D3} and G_{D2} in the Krabbe brains could be caused by decreased activity of the galactosyltransferase system which catalyzes the formation of G_{M1} from UDP-galactose and G_{M2}, and G_{D1b} from UDP-galactose and G_{D2} (Fig. 2). In order to test this assumption the galactosyltransferase system was determined in whole homogenates and in the 8,500 x g - 100,000 x g fraction of cerebral cortex and white matter of control and Krabbe brains. Gangliosides G_{M2} and G_{D2} served as acceptors and the requirements for the reaction were tested as outlined by Kaufman et al., (1967). All the four sources of enzyme showed activity, but the specific activity varied with the age of the subjects, the duration of the storage of the brain, and the time between death and autopsy. Thus the quantitative data are uncertain, and exact figures will not be given. However, the specific activity was higher in the 8,500 x g - 100,000 x g fraction than in the homogenate. Under the experimental conditions, higher specific activity was obtained with G_{M2} than with G_{D2} as acceptor. In a study of three Krabbe brains and three control brains the ganglioside galactosyltransferase activity was 25% higher in the cerebral cortex and 100% higher in the white matter of the Krabbe than of the control brains. Thus, there were no indications for a diminished level of ganglioside G_{M2} and G_{D2} galactosyltransferase activities in the Krabbe brain.

TABLE 3. GLYCOHYDROLASE ACTIVITIES.

	CEREBRAL CORTEX				WHITE MATTER		
	Normals (n=11)		Krabbe (n=13)		Normals	Krabbe (n=13)	
	Mean	S.D.	Mean	S.D.		Mean	S.D.
	nmoles released/hr/mg protein						
β-Galactosidase pH 5.0	63	22	37	17	40	42	16
β-Galactosidase pH 3.6	101	40	52	15	-	82	35
β-Glucosaminidase	388	82	1451	614	150	2715	1388
Ganglioside sialidase	2.2	0.7	3.6	1.6	0.3	2.4	0.8

The CMP-NAN:lactosylceramide sialyltransferase activity was also determined in the same tissues. Very low and variable activities were found and no reliable quantitative figures were obtained.

It was possible that the increase in the levels of gangliosides might also result from a diminished activity of one or more glycolipid glycohydrolases. For instance, the reduced activity of ganglioside sialidase, ganglioside β-hexosaminidase, and lactosylceramide β-galactosidase would account for these results.

In normal individuals, ganglioside sialidase activity at birth was approximately the same in the cerebral cortex and in white matter, and the activity decreased as myelination of the white matter proceeded. It seems likely that the low activities of sialidase in white matter are due to the inhibitory effect of the myelin lipids, although this has not definitely been established (Öhman and Svennerholm, 1971). In Krabbe disease the ganglioside sialidase was slightly increased in the cerebral cortex, and in white matter the level was approximately the same (see Table 3).

P-Nitrophenyl hexosaminidase was strongly increased in grey and white matter, particularly in the latter. In storage diseases an increase of the glycohydrolases, especially hexosaminidase, has been interpreted to reflect lysosomal hyperactivity (Van Hoof and Hers, 1968). An increased level

was therefore expected in Krabbe disease. Since the hexosaminidase component A is lacking in G_{M2}-gangliosidosis, electrophoretic separation of the hexosaminidases was performed on
agarose gel (Öhman, Ekelund and Svennerholm, 1971). No
decrease in the amount of component A was found.

The p-nitrophenyl β-galactosidase activity was slightly
reduced in the cerebral cortex of the Krabbe brains when
compared to an age-matched control group. Suzuki and Suzuki
(1970) and Austin et al. (1971) reported normal activity for
p-nitrophenyl β-galactosidase activity, but their conclusions
were drawn from analysis of only a few age-matched controls.
The activity of lactosylceramide β-galactosidase was found
slightly higher in Krabbe disease than in the controls (Austin
et al., 1971).

Fatty Acid Composition of Gangliosides

In normal brain, stearic acid constitutes 80 to 95% of
the fatty acids in the major gangliosides. A lower percentage
of stearic acid with a concomitant increase of C_{16} and C_{22} to
C_{26} acids has been reported in G_{M3} (Svennerholm, 1967).
Lactosylceramide in normal brain has very similar fatty acids
to galactosylceramide, and no hydroxy fatty acids, which is
in complete agreement with Dr. Radin's hypothesis for the
biosynthesis of galactosylceramide. There were obviously some
characteristic features of the fatty acid patterns in Krabbe
brain. For example, in one group, which included G_{M2}, G_{M1}, and
G_{D1a}, stearic acid constituted 80% of the fatty acid, and the
pattern was the same in cerebral cortex and white matter. In
the other group, including G_{M3}, G_{D3}, G_{D2}, and $G_{D1b} + G_{T1}$, there
was a significant difference between the fatty acid composition
of the compounds in grey and white matter, with higher concentrations of C_{22} to C_{26} fatty acids in the gangliosides of white
matter. With increasing elongation of the carbohydrate moiety
the C_{18} concentration increased in both grey and white matter.
The interesting fact is that the gangliosides in the latter
group are all on the pathway suggested by Roseman and associates
(Kaufman, Basu, Roseman, 1968) for the biosynthesis of
gangliosides with a disialosyl group on the internal galactose
(Fig. 2). Arce et al. (1971) suggested that there was no
evidence for the existence of two different routes for the
formation of the disialogangliosides since it was shown that
both G_{D1a} and G_{D1b} were formed from G_{M1}. The present study of
the fatty acid composition of Krabbe brain gangliosides is in
favour of the hypothesis that, at least in white matter, two
different pathways exist. The results also indicate that a
certain cell type or particulate fraction might form gangliosides in the white matter.

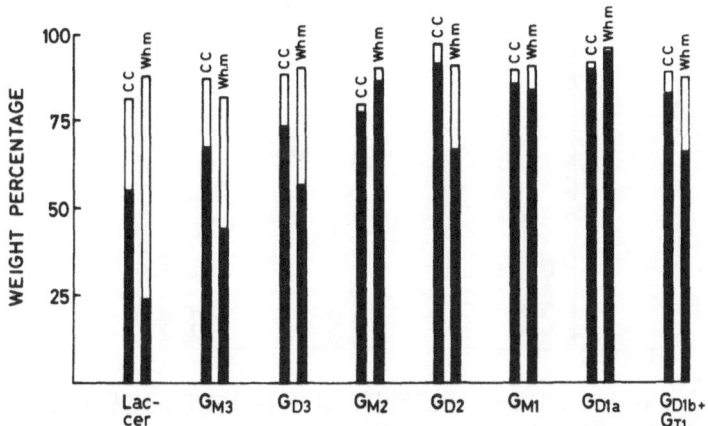

FIG.3. FATTY ACID COMPOSITION OF BRAIN GANGLIOSIDES IN KRABBE DISEASE.
C.C. = cerebral cortex, Wh.m. = white matter, ■ = $C_{18:0}$ ☐ = C_{22-26}.

Thus enzymatic studies did not support the theory that in Krabbe disease a disturbance in the levels of degradative enzymes was responsible for the change in ganglioside patterns.

A morphological feature of Krabbe disease is the severe gliosis of the white matter. It was therefore of interest to determine the normal concentration and composition of gangliosides in the glial cells. Neuron- and glial cell-enriched fractions were isolated from rabbit cerebral cortex (Hamberger and Svennerholm, 1971). The ganglioside concentration was very low in isolated neuron perikarya, only one-fifth of that in the synaptosomal fraction. The glial cells contained approximatively twice the concentration of that in the neurons. Similar results have been previously reported by Norton and Poduslo (1971). The ganglioside pattern was, however the same in the glial cells and the neurons. Further studies (Hamberger and Svennerholm, in preparation) have shown that the gangliosides are enriched in plasma cell membranes of the two cell types and that in these membranes and also in nerve-ending fractions the concentrations and patterns of the gangliosides are similar. It is thus evident that in the central nervous system gangliosides are not confined to the neurons but occur also in the glial cells. Similarly, cerebrosides occur in about the same concentration in the plasma membrane of neurons, glial cells, and white matter.

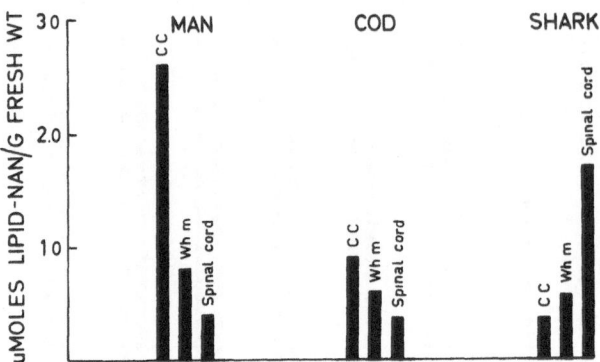

FIG. 4. THE GANGLIOSIDE CONCENTRATION IN THE CEREBRAL
CORTEX, WHITE MATTER AND SPINAL CORD OF MAN, COD AND
DOGFISH.
C.C. = cerebral cortex, Wh.m. = white matter.

Another example of the localization of the gangliosides
in cells other than the neurons in the nervous system is shown
by studies (Norén and Svennerholm, in preparation) of the
spinal cord of the dogfish (Squalus acanthias). In mammalian
brain the ganglioside concentration is 3-fold higher in grey
than in white matter, which in its turn has twice the concentration of the spinal cord. These differences were much
smaller in a bone-fish (cod), while dogfish spinal cord contained 4 times as much lipid-NAN as cerebral cortex. The
ganglioside pattern of the dogfish was very simple: G_{M2} and
G_{D2} constituted more than 75% of the lipid-NAN. Subcellular
fractionation showed these gangliosides to be enriched in the
myelin fraction and to have the same normal fatty acids as
galactosylceramides, $C_{22:1}$ and $C_{24:1}$.

The glial cell membranes isolated by us were derived
from the astrocytes and oligodendroglial cells, and myelin
of the central nervous system is also assumed to be derived
from plasma membranes of oligodendroglial cells. Thus, it is
evident that certain glial cells contain gangliosides
characteristic of the nervous system. In Krabbe disease the
number of oligodendroglial cells are reduced and the myelin
is replaced by astrocytic and microglial proliferation. A
similar morphological reaction is seen in subacute sclerosing
panencephalitis. The changes in the ganglioside pattern are
very similar in the two diseases. It is tempting to speculate
that the gangliosides G_{M2}, G_{D2}, G_{M3} and G_{D3} are mainly
localized in glial cells of mesenchymal origin.

ABSTRACT

The concentration and chemical structure of the ganglio-sides of 17 Krabbe cases have been determined. Both cerebral cortex and white matter had a highly abnormal ganglioside pattern with elevation of G_{M3}, G_{D3}, G_{M2} and G_{D2}. On the other hand G_{M1} and G_{D1a} were diminished in cerebral cortex and G_{M1} in white matter. The ganglioside concentration of white matter was about 50% higher than normal white matter. The altered ganglioside pattern could not be explained by any obvious enzymatic disturbance.

In G_{M2}, G_{M1}, and G_{D1a} the fatty acid pattern was the same in grey and white matter, and stearic acid constituted more than 80%. In G_{D3}, G_{D2}, and $G_{D1b} + G_{T1}$ the concentration of C_{22} to C_{26} fatty acids was much larger in the white matter than in cerebral cortex. These results were interpreted as supporting the assumption that G_{D1a} and G_{D1b} are formed by different pathways.

Some studies are presented which have demonstrated that gangliosides are not confined to the neurons but are com-ponents of the plasma cell membranes of neurons and glial cells in the central nervous system. It is suggested that the elevated gangliosides in Krabbe disease are derived from the glial cells.

REFERENCES

1. Arce A., Maccioni H.J. and Caputto R. The incorporation of galactose, N-acetylgalactosamine and N-acetylneuraminic acid into endogenous acceptors of subcellular particles from rat brain in vitro. Biochem. J.,121, 483, 1971.

2. Austin J.H. Studies in globoid cell leucodystrophy. Arch.Neurol.(Chic.), 9, 207, 1963.

3. Austin J.H. and Lehfeldt D. Studies in globoid(Krabbe) leucodystrophy III - Significance of experimentally produced globoidlike elements in rat white matter and spleen. J. Neuropath.exp.Neurol., 24, 265, 1965.

4. Austin J.H., Suzuki K., Armstrong D., Brady R., Bachhawat B.K., Schlenker J., Stumpf D. Studies in globoid(Krabbe) leukodystrophy (GLD) V - Controlled enzymic studies in ten human cases. Arch.Neurol., 23, 502, 1970.

5. Brante G. Studies on lipids in the nervous system. Acta physiol.Scand., 18, suppl. 63, 164. 1949.

6.   Crowell E.P., Burnett B.B.   Determination of the carbohydrate composition of wood pulps by gas chromatography of the
alditol acetates.   Anal. Chem., 39, 121, 1967.

7.   Eto Y. and Suzuki K.   Brain sphingoglycolipids in Krabbe's
globoid cell leucodystrophy. J. Neurochem., 18, 503, 1971.

8.   Hagberg B., Kollberg H., Sourander P. and Åkesson H.O.
Infantile globoid cell leucodystrophy. Neuropädiatrie 1, 74, 1969.

9.   Hagberg B., Sourander P. and Svennerholm L.   Diagnosis of
Krabbe's infantile leucodystrophy. J. Neurol. Neurosurg.Psych.
26, 195, 1963.

10.   Hamberger A. and Svennerholm L.   Composition of gangliosides and phospholipids in neuronal and glial cell enriched
fractions.   J. Neurochem., 18, 1821, 1971.

11.   Kaufman B., Basu S., Roseman S.   Studies on the biosynthesis
of gangliosides.   In Inborn disorders of sphingolipid metabolism,
Aronson S.M. and Volk B.W.(eds.), Oxford, Pergamon Press Ltd.
1967, P. 193.

12.   Kaufman B., Basu S. and Roseman S.   Enzymatic synthesis
of disialogangliosides from monosialogangliosides by sialyl-
transferases from embryonic chicken brain. J. Biol. Chem. 243,
5804, 1968.

13.   Ledeen R., Salsman K. and Cabrera M.   Gangliosides in
subacute sclerosing panencephalitis: isolation and fatty
acid composition of nine fractions.   J. Lipid Res. 9, 129, 1968.

14.   Norton W.T. and Poduslo S.E.   Neuronal perikarya and
astroglia of rat brain : chemical composition during myelination.
J. Lipid Res. 12, 84, 1971.

15.   Öhman R., Ekelund H. and Svennerholm L.   The diagnosis of
Tay Sachs disease.   Acta Paediat. Scand. 60, 399, 1971.

16.   Öhman R. and Svennerholm L.   The activity of ganglioside
sialidase in the developing human brain.   J. Neurochem. 18,
79, 1971.

17.   Olsson Y., Sourander P. and Svennerholm L.   Experimental
studies on the pathogenesis of leucodystrophies I – The effect
of intracerebrally injected sphingolipids in the rat's brain.
Acta neuropath.(Berl.) 6, 153, 1966.

18. Radin N.S. and Arora R.C. A simplified assay method for galactosylceramide β-galactosidase. J.Lipid Res. 12, 256, 1971.

19. Sawardeker J.S., Sloneker J.H. and Jeanes A. Quantitative determination of monosaccharides as their alditol acetates by gas liquid chromatography. Anal. Chem. 37, 1602, 1965.

20. Sourander P., Hansson H.A., Olsson Y. and Svennerholm L. Experimental studies of the pathogenesis of leucodystrophies II - The effect of sphingolipids on various cell types in cultures from the nervous system. Acta neuropath. 6, 231, 1966.

21. Sourander P. and Olsson Y. Peripheral neuropathy in globoid cell leucodystrophy(Morbus Krabbe). Acta neuropath. 11, 69, 1968.

22. Suzuki K. Ganglioside patterns of normal and pathological brains. In Inborn disorders of sphingolipid metabolism, Aronson S.M. and Volk B.V.(eds.), Oxford, Pergamon Press Ltd. 1967, p. 187.

23. Suzuki K. and Suzuki Y. Globoid cell leucodystrophy (Krabbe's disease) : Deficiency of galactocerebroside β-galactosidase. Proc.Nat.Acad.Sci. USA 66, 302, 1970.

24. Svennerholm L. The determination of hexosamines with special reference to nervous tissue. Acta Soc. Med. Ups. 61, 287, 1956.

25. Svennerholm L. Some aspects of the biochemical changes in leucodystrophy. In Brain lipids and lipoproteins and the leukodystrophies, Folch-Pi J. and Bauer H.J.(eds.), Amsterdam, Elsevier Publ. Co., 1963, p. 104.

26. Svennerholm L. The distribution of lipids in the human nervous system. I - Analytical procedure. Lipids of foetal and newborn brain. J. Neurochem. 11, 839, 1964.

27. Svennerholm L. The metabolism of gangliosides in cerebral lipidoses. In Inborn disorders of sphingolipid metabolism, Aronson S.M. and Volk B.V. (eds.), Oxford, Pergamon Press Ltd. 1967, p. 169.

28. Svennerholm L. New principles for the classification of glycolipidoses. Metabolismo, 5, 61, 1969.

29. Svennerholm L. Ganglioside metabolism. In Comprehensive Biochemistry, vol. 18, Florkin M. and Stotz E.M.(eds.), Amsterdam, Elsevier, 1970, p. 201.

30. Svennerholm L. Isolation of gangliosides. In Methods in Carbohydrate Chemistry, vol. 6, Whistler R.L. and Wolfrom M.L. New York, Academic Press, in press.

31. Svennerholm L. and Ställberg-Stenhagen S. Changes in the fatty acid composition of cerebrosides and sulfatides of human nervous tissue with age. J. Lipid Res., 9, 215, 1968.

32. Svennerholm E. and Svennerholm L. The separation of neutral blood-serum glycolipids by thin-layer chromatography. Biochem. Biophys.Acta 70, 432, 1963.

33. Van Hoof F. and Hers H.G. The abnormalities of lysosomal enzymes in mucopolysaccharidoses. European J. Biochem. 7, 34, 1968.

34. Vanier M.T., Holm M., Öhman R. and Svennerholm L. Developmental profiles of gangliosides in human and rat brain. J. Neurochem. 18, 581, 1971.

35. Yu R.K. and Ledeen R.W. Gas-liquid chromatographic assay of lipid-bound sialic acids: measurement of gangliosides of brain in several species. J. Lipid Res. 11, 506, 1970.

PHYTANIC ACID STORAGE DISEASE

Daniel Steinberg and David Hutton

Department of Medicine, School of Medicine, University of

California, San Diego, La Jolla, California 92037

Phytanic acid storage disease (Refsum's disease) has presumably been included in the present Symposium under the rubric "...and Allied Disorders." In that it is an inherited lipidosis and, like so many of them, affects the nervous system, it is to that extent "allied". However, the differences are several and important. First, phytanic acid storage disease is due to a defect in an oxidative enzyme system, not a hydrolase; second, it is a disease in which a particular fatty acid accumulates (and in essentially all lipid classes), rather than a particular subclass of lipids as in the hydrolase deficiencies; and, finally, the accumulated lipid is of exogenous rather than endogenous origin. This last difference is especially important since it affords in theory the opportunity to arrest (and possibly reverse) the storage and to determine whether that alters the progression of the disease. Methods are being actively sought to do this in the sphingolipidoses, as reported elsewhere in this Symposium, but the approaches are difficult and results remain equivocal. Thus, it may be of interest to report in some detail our encouraging experience with dietary treatment of phytanic acid storage disease. First, let us briefly review the biochemical basis of phytanate accumulation, add some recent results on the normal pathway for its oxidation and then finally summarize the clinical responses to diet observed to date.

The Clinical Syndrome in Relation to Phytanic Acid Storage

Sigvald Refsum first recognized the syndrome as a neurologic entity (heredopathia atactica polyneuritiformis) and his classical description in

PROMINENT CLINICAL FEATURES OF
HEREDOPATHIA ATACTICA POLYNEURITIFORMIS
OR
REFSUM'S SYNDROME

1. Familial pattern; recessive

2. Retinitis pigmentosa (night blindness;
    constriction of visual fields)

3. Hypertrophic peripheral neuropathy
    (motor and sensory losses)

4. Ataxia

5. Elevated cerebrospinal fluid protein
    (without cells)

6. Nerve deafness

Table I.   Prominent clinical features of Refsum's syndrome.

1946 has required very little modification (Table I)(23).   The association
between Refsum's syndrome and phytanic acid storage was made by Klenk
and Kahlke in post-mortem analysis of tissue from a child who had had
the clinical syndrome and who showed gross fatty infiltration of liver and
kidney (15).   There was no increase in cerebroside or ganglioside concentration nor accumulation of any unusual complex lipid, but gas-liquid
chromatography revealed the presence of an abnormal fatty acid which was
characterized as phytanic acid (Fig. 1).   This branched-chain, fully saturated acid accounted for fully 50% of total fatty acids in liver and kidney.   It is now clear that, almost without exception, patients with the
bona fide clinical syndrome as described by Refsum also store phytanate
and diagnosis can be affirmed by serum analysis (12,32).   There are many
closely similar heredo-ataxic syndromes but almost all of them lack some
of the essential features of Refsum's syndrome; those near phenocopies do
not store phytanate.   Mention should be made of two cases in particular
that have had clinical pictures qualifying as Refsum's syndrome but in
whom phytanate storage was not found at autopsy and in whom careful
clinical studies failed to demonstrate defective oxidation of phytanic acid--
one described by Kolodny et al. (17) and one studied by Prior et al.

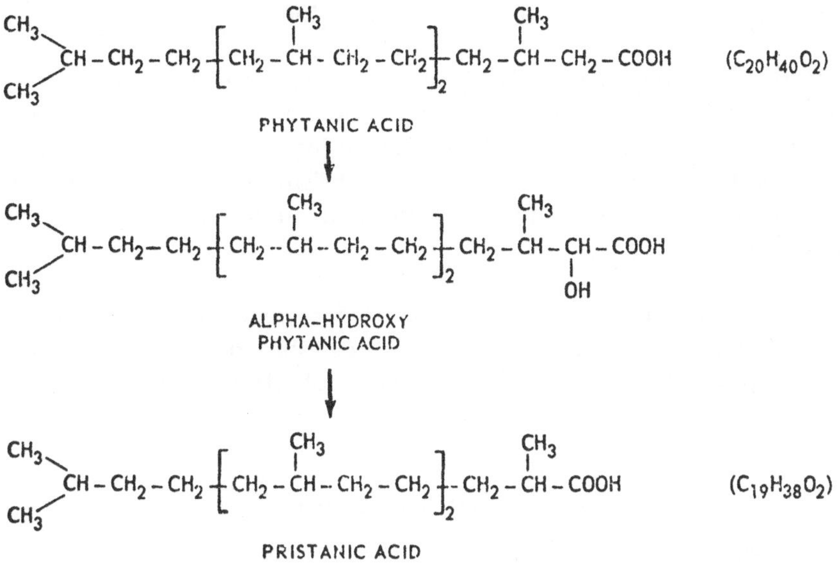

Fig. 1. Proposed pathway for conversion of phytanate to pristanate.

(Prior, Alexander, Steinberg, Mize and Herndon, in preparation). There may indeed be other entities that can mimic phytanic acid storage disease and until a defect in phytanate metabolism is explicitly demonstrated in a given patient the designation Refsum's syndrome is preferred (26). More extensive discussion of the clinico-pathologic features of the disease are available elsewhere (12,26,28).

Biochemical Basis

It is now well established that the defect lies in an inability to catabolize phytanic acid (29,30,32). Moreover, there is evidently no significant endogenous biosynthesis of phytanate either in patients with the disease or in experimental animals (30,31). Thus, the stored phytanate must have an exogenous origin. Phytol in free form is an excellent precursor of phytanate, both in man and in experimental animals (3,16,19, 27,28,30). However, the phytol moiety of the chlorophyl molecule is very poorly absorbed, remaining covalently bound to the tetrapyrrole ring during passage through the gastrointestinal tract (2,4). Phytanic acid itself, present notably in dairy products and ruminant tissues (7,8,25), is the major identified dietary precursor, as described later, but the possibility that other dietary components (e.g. tocopherols) contribute is not ruled out.

Phytanic Acid Oxidation

At the time phytanic acid storage was demonstrated there was no information available on the normal pathway for phytanate oxidation. Studies by our group at the National Heart Institute in Bethesda showed that alpha-oxidation to the (n-1) product, pristanic acid, was the major pathway, with alpha-hydroxyphytanic acid as an intermediate (Fig. 1) (1,18,21,33).

The further oxidation of pristanic acid appears to proceed via successive beta-oxidation steps, as inferred from the structures of identified degradation products (21)(Fig. 2). A series of clinical studies (20)

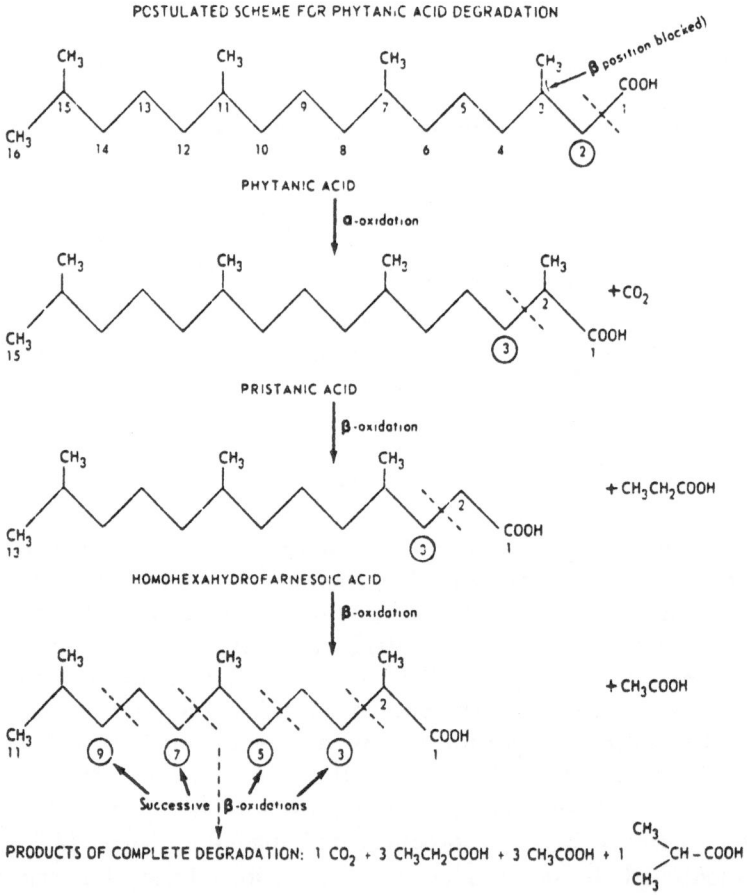

Fig. 2. Postulated scheme for phytanic acid degradation.

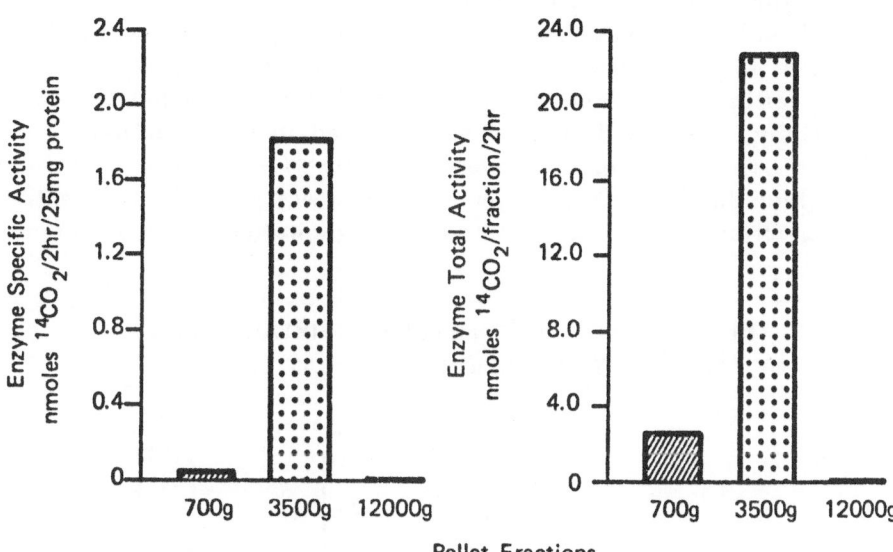

**$^{14}CO_2$ RELEASE FROM U-^{14}C-PHYTANIC ACID
BY RAT LIVER PARTICULATE FRACTIONS**

Fig. 3.   Release of $^{14}CO_2$ from U-^{14}C-phytanate by rat liver particulate preparations.   A 700 g supernatant fraction was prepared from homogenates by decantation after centrifuging 10 min, care being taken to exclude any of the red/brown pellet material but permitting inclusion of the
uppermost light tan colored layer.   Resuspension of the red/brown pellet
in buffer followed by a further 700 g 10 min centrifugation step, allowed
recovery of more tan colored particulate material from the pellet by decantation.   The combined 700 g supernatant fractions were then centrifuged
sequentially at 700 g, 3500 g and 12000 g to obtain the relevant particulate fractions.   Incubation in a final volume of 1 ml contained: 100
μmoles potassium phosphate buffer pH 7.7, 1 μmole ATP, 1 μmole NAD$^+$,
1 μmole MgCl$_2$, 1 μmole NADH, 1 μmole sodium fumarate, 21 mg BSA,
3 μmoles FeCl$_3$, 25 mg pellet fraction protein and 11 nmoles potassium
U-^{14}C-phytanate (47,300 dpm; albumin bound).   After incubation for 2 hr
at 37° reactions were terminated by acidification, the $^{14}CO_2$ evolved
collected in NCS solubilizer contained in plastic wells and radioactivity
determined conventionally (9).

and studies in fibroblast cultures (9) have established that the site of the
enzyme deletion is in the alpha-hydroxylation step.   Cultures from patients

oxidize phytanate at less than 2% of normal rates but oxidize alpha-hydroxyphytanate as well as do control cells. More recently it was shown
that fibroblasts from parents of cases (presumed heterozygotes) oxidize added
phytanate at rates about one-half of normal (10). Dr. Su-Chen Tsai has
studied the phytanic acid oxidation system in rat liver and found the activity predominantly in a mitochondrial fraction (33). There was an absolute requirement for O_2 and the reaction was stimulated by TPNH and,
interestingly, ferric ions. Recently Dr. Hutton has explored this system
further. Initially, mitochondrial fractions prepared in a conventional
manner showed very low rates of conversion of U-^{14}C-phytanate to $^{14}CO_2$.
It developed that the first 700 x g centrifugation was partially sedimenting
the active particles; when, instead of carefully aspirating the supernatant

$^{14}CO_2$ RELEASE FROM U-^{14}C-α-HYDROXYPHYTANIC ACID
BY PARTICULATE FRACTIONS FROM RAT LIVER

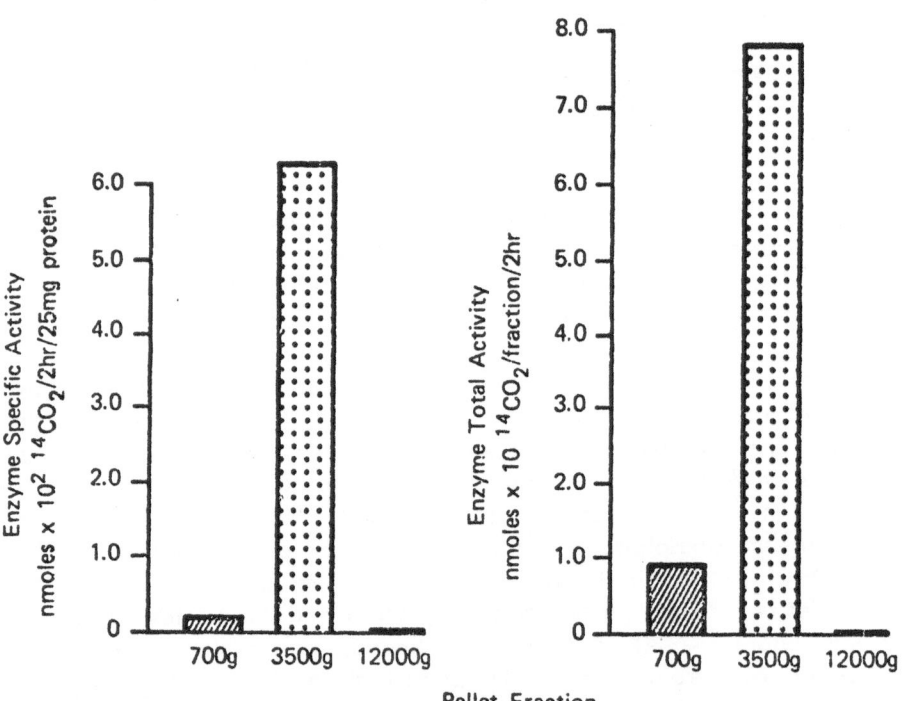

Pellet Fraction

Fig. 4. Release of $^{14}CO_2$ from U-^{14}C-α -hydroxyphytanate by rat
liver particulate preparations. Pellets prepared and incubations conducted
as outlined in legend to Fig. 3 with the exception that 0.44 nmoles of
potassium U-^{14}C-α -hydroxyphytanate (31,100 dpm; albumin bound) replaced phytanate.

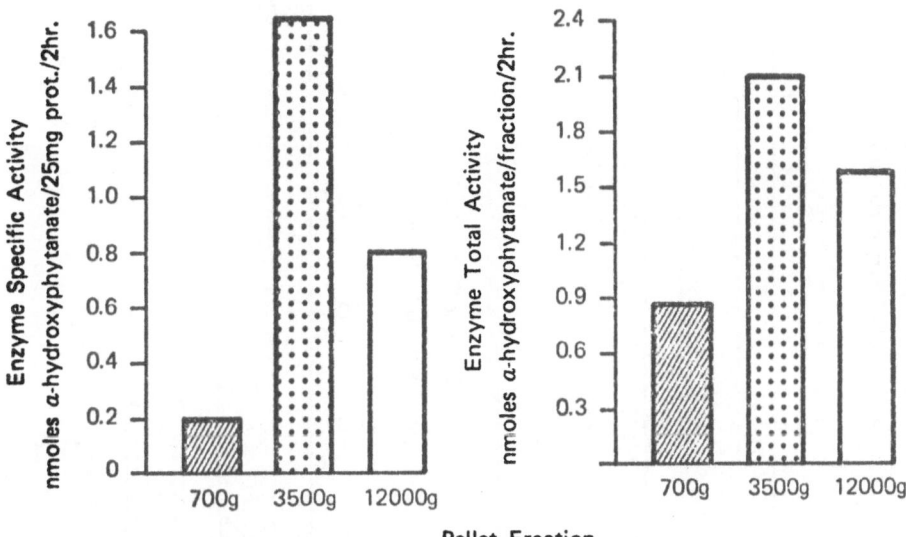

FORMATION OF U-^{14}C-α-HYDROXYPHYTANATE
FROM U-^{14}C-PHYTANIC ACID BY RAT LIVER
PARTICULATE FRACTIONS

Fig. 5. Formation of U-^{14}C- α -hydroxyphytanate by rat liver
particulate preparations. Pellets prepared and incubations carried out as
described in the legend to Fig. 3. Reactions were terminated by addition
of methanolic KOH followed by saponification for 1 hr at 80°. After
acidification and extraction of the free fatty acids with diethyl ether,
the dried extracts were chromatographed on Gelman ITLC SG media utilizing hexane/acetic acid/HCl (100:1:0.5) as solvent. The appropriate zones
for α -hydroxyphytanate and phytanate were cut out, immersed in scintillation fluid and radioactivity counted.

(leaving behind the layer just above the packed pellet), the supernatant
fraction was decanted (and thus included the "near-bottom" layer), good
rates of phytanate oxidation were obtained. Further studies showed that
the bulk of the phytanate oxidizing activity was recovered in particles
sedimenting at 3,500 x g (Fig. 3). The specific activity and total activity of the pellets obtained at 700 x g and at 12,000 x g were very low.
This same 3,500 x g particulate fraction also showed the highest activity
in oxidation of U-^{14}C-alpha-hydroxyphytanic acid (Fig. 4). Studies of
the formation of alpha-hydroxyphytanate showed highest activity again in
the 3,500 x g pellet but now there was considerable activity in the

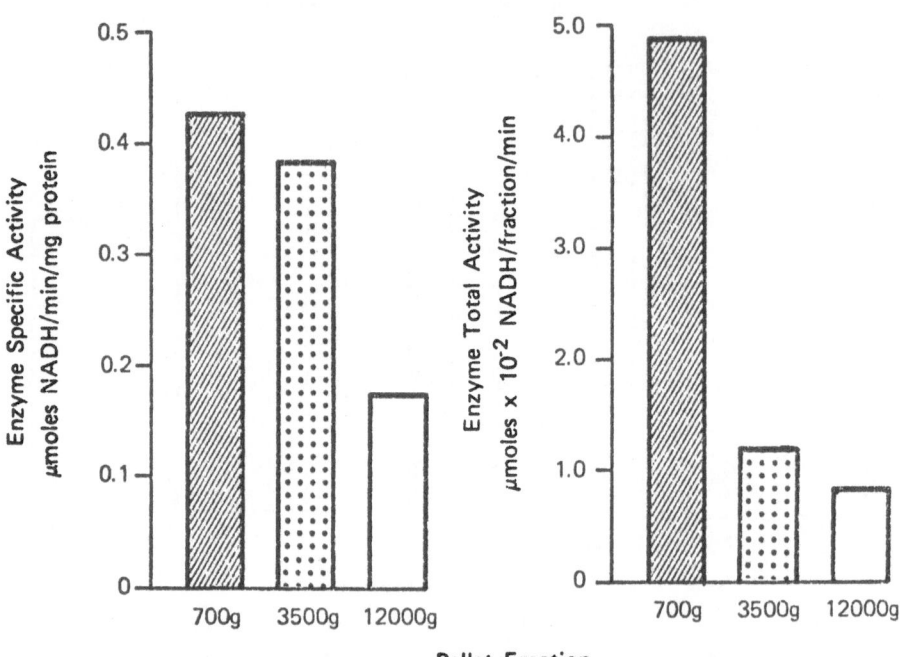

**β-HYDROXYACYL DEHYDROGENASE ACTIVITY
IN PARTICULATE FRACTIONS FROM RAT LIVER**

Fig. 6. Beta-Hydroxyacyl dehydrogenase activities in rat liver particulate fractions. Assays utilized the method of Overath et al. (22). Pellets were prepared as described in the legend to Fig. 3.

12,000 x g pellet as well (Fig. 5). The distribution of beta-hydroxyacyl-dehydrogenase, a mitochondrial marker, is shown in Fig. 6. These preliminary results provide the first suggestion that the introduction of the alpha-hydroxyl group may be catalyzed by a particle separate from that responsible for the later steps in phytanate oxidation. The particulate fractions prepared by successive centrifugal steps are almost certainly mixtures and attempts to further purify them are being undertaken. Unfortunately, density gradient procedures employing sucrose and ficoll tend to cause loss of activity for reasons not yet clear.

The proposed pathway for degradation of pristanic acid (Fig. 2) was inferred from the structure of identified products, compatible with successive beta-oxidative steps. If this proceeds as in classical beta-oxidation of straight-chain fatty acids, every other cleavage should give rise to pro-

$^{14}CO_2$ AND ^{14}C-PROPIONATE FORMATION FROM U-^{14}C-PHYTANATE BY A PARTICULATE FRACTION FROM RAT LIVER

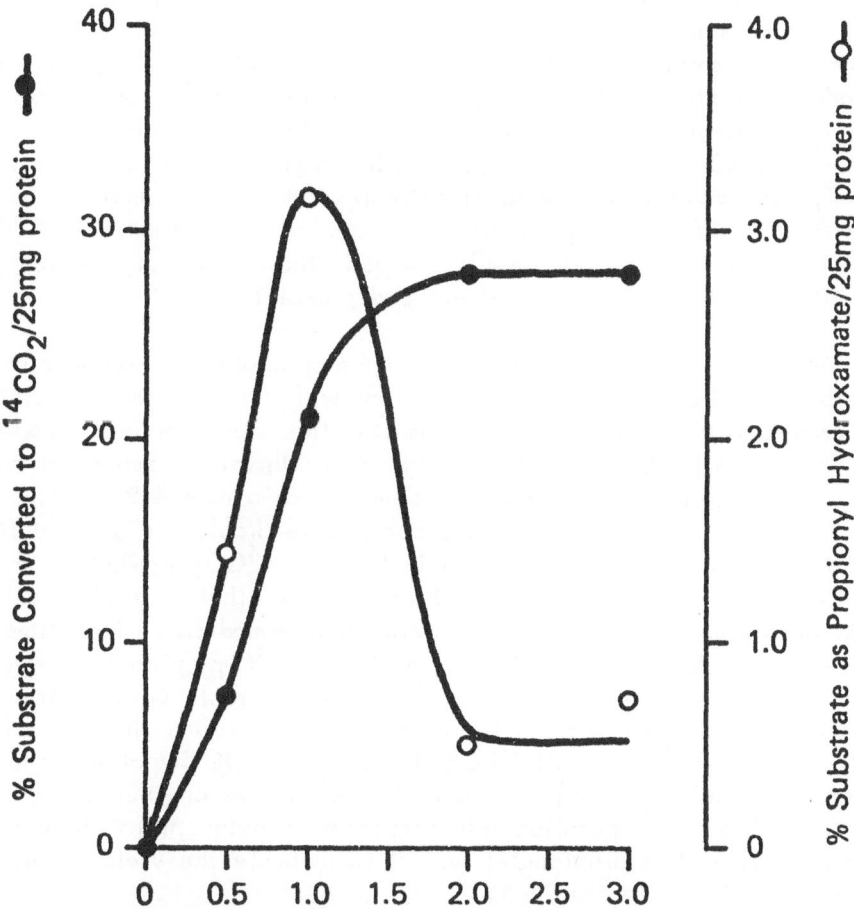

Fig. 7. ^{14}C-Propionate accumulation by a rat liver particulate preparation catabolizing U-^{14}C-phytanate. The pellet fraction utilized was a combined 3500 g, 12,000 g preparation obtained as outlined in Fig. 3. Incubations were conducted as described in Fig. 3 except that fumarate and BSA were omitted. After $^{14}CO_2$ had been collected, carrier propionic acid (10 μmoles) was added, the fatty acid extracted with diethyl ether and converted to hydroxamates according to the method of Giovanelli and Stumpf (6). The TLC hydroxamate zones were cut out and radioactivity counted conventionally.

pionyl CoA rather than acetyl CoA. Previous studies demonstrating significant incorporation of ^{14}C from $U-^{14}C$-phytanate into glucose provided indirect evidence compatible with this hypothesis (1) but did not rule out cleavage to yield lactate or other fragments that might be incorporated into glucose. Some labelled propionate accumulated during the mitochondrial oxidation of phytanate but in very low yield, possibly due to rapid further oxidation of propionyl CoA (1,21). We wish to report recent results that strengthen the proposal that propionate is a major product of phytanate oxidation. We have followed the time course for $^{14}CO_2$ release and ^{14}C-propionate accumulation during oxidation of $U-^{14}C$-phytanate by a 3,500 x g particulate preparation from rat liver. As shown in Fig. 7, the accumulation of labelled propionate was maximal at the time when the rate of $^{14}CO_2$ production was maximal. As the rate of $^{14}CO_2$ formation decreased and eventually stopped, the amount of labelled propionate accumulated fell off and dropped almost to zero.

A second approach to demonstrating propionate as a product utilized a fibroblast culture derived from a patient with an inherited defect in propionyl-CoA carboxylase (24). This cell line was generously made available to us by Dr. Leon Rosenberg, Yale University School of Medicine. These cells oxidized added propionate at a rate 4.9% of that seen in control cells and might therefore accumulate propionate derived from breakdown of phytanate. As shown in Fig. 8, $^{14}CO_2$ production by this cell line was considerably decreased compared to that in control cells, as would be anticipated if propionate were an intermediate. Furthermore, there was a highly significant accumulation of ^{14}C-propionate. Interestingly, there was some labelled propionate demonstrable with control fibroblasts as well but, in relation to the amount of $^{14}CO_2$, this was minimal. While these results are qualitatively in support of the hypothesis that propionate is a direct cleavage product, further studies are needed a) to rule out indirect incorporation into propionate subsequent to cleavage of a product other than propionate; and b) to estimate the yield of propionate per mole of phytanate oxidized.

Dietary Treatment

If phytanate arises exclusively from exogenous sources, it should be possible by appropriate modification of diet to at least arrest further accumulation and possibly, if mechanisms for degradation and excretion are not totally defective, to reduce body stores. The feasibility of dietary intervention was established in our early collaborative studies with the Oslo group (30), showing that plasma phytanate levels could be decreased almost to normal levels on a diet low in phytol and phytanate. Definite clinical

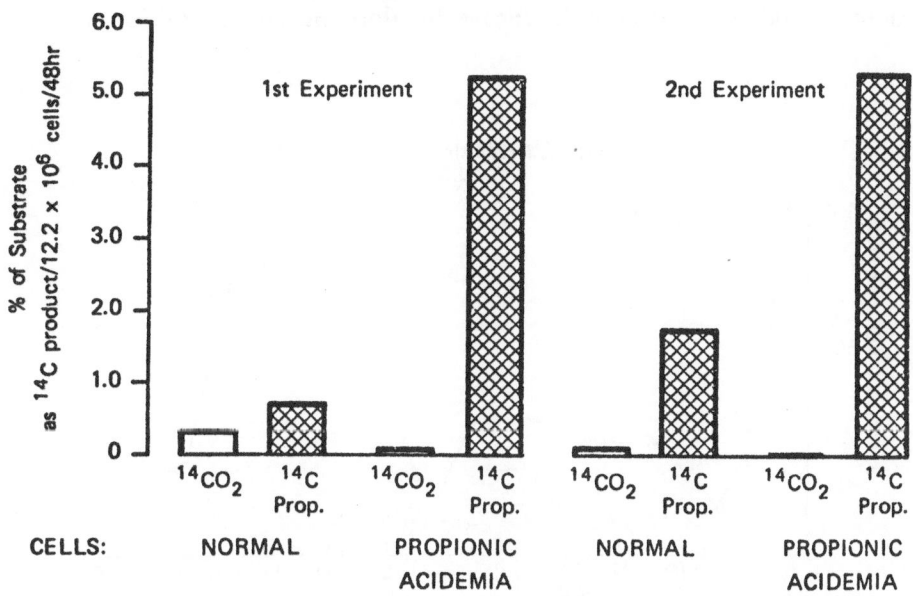

FORMATION OF $^{14}CO_2$ & ^{14}C-PROPIONATE
FROM U-^{14}C-PHYTANATE BY NORMAL AND PROPIONIC ACIDEMIA
FIBROBLAST CELL CULTURES

Fig. 8. Accumulation of ^{14}C-propionate in fibroblast cultures derived from normal and propionic acidemia patients exposed to U-^{14}C-phy-
tanate. Monolayer incubations were conducted in flasks containing 20 ml
MEM (Eagles) supplemented with 1% fetal calf serum. Radioactive phytanate was provided as previously described (9). After 48 hr incubation at
37° reactions were terminated by addition of 2N H_2SO_4 and $^{14}CO_2$
collected in NCS solubilizer contained in plastic wells. Contents of the
flasks were now made alkaline, carrier propionate (3 μmoles) and ^{3}H-pro-
pionate (2 x 10^6 dpm; 1.7 nmoles) added, the cells scraped off and the
total cellular debris and media freeze dried. Following acidification (1 ml
2N H_2SO_4), silicic acid was added until a smooth powder was obtained.
Propionate separation was achieved chromatographically following the procedure of Kesner and Muntwyler (14) and radioactivity determined on appropriate column eluate fractions.

improvement and an increase in nerve conduction velocities was noted in
one of the original cases treated; the second case was only mildly affected
and showed little improvement (5). Neither patient has relapsed over a
7 year interval on diet (Sigvald Refsum, personal communication). In 1970

we reported on two Irish siblings studied intensively over a 15 month period, 4 months of base-line observations on an ad libitum diet and 11 months
of observations on a special diet low in phytanate and phytol (31). Plasma phytanate concentrations and phytanate concentrations in subcutaneous
adipose tissue fell markedly in both patients. Objective evidence of improvement included significant increases in ulnar nerve conduction velocity

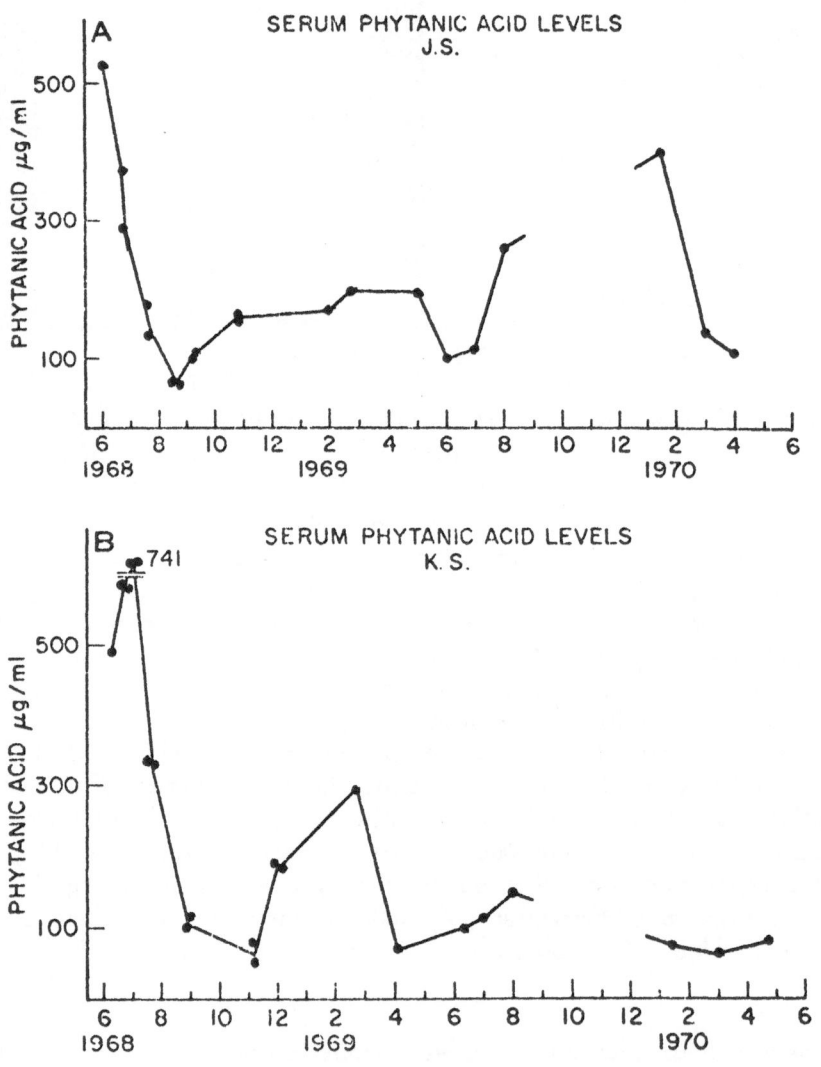

Fig. 9.   Serum phytanic acid levels, J.S. and K.S.

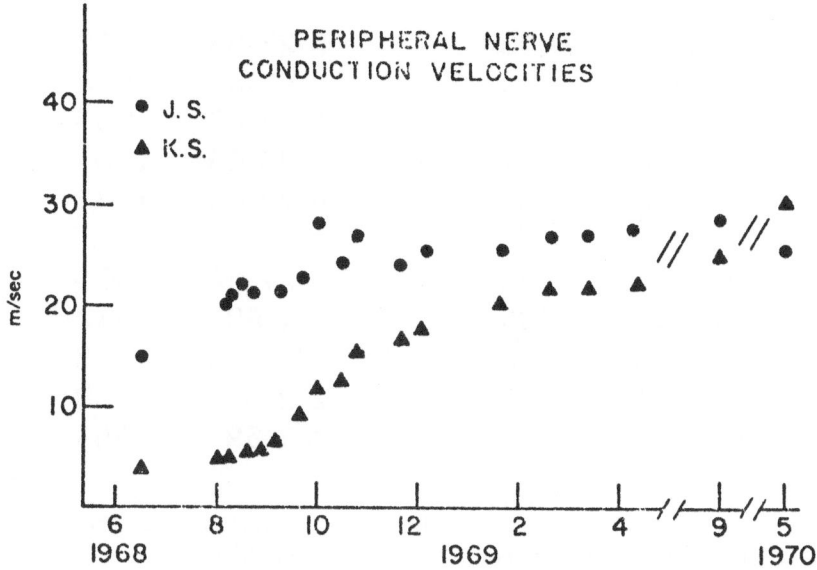

Fig. 10. Effect of diet treatment on ulnar nerve conduction velocity.

normalization of ST-T wave changes in ECG, return of previously unobtainable tendon reflexes, increase in strength of certain muscle groups (measured with a standardized transducer system) and improvement in objective timed tests of coordination. Both patients noted improvement in their gait, in their own impressions of muscle strength and ability to perform everyday tasks.

At the end of this prolonged study the patients returned to Ireland. Unfortunately, they were unable to continue the rather Spartan diet and over a period of months their plasma phytanate levels rose toward pretreatment values again. Concurrently they noted deterioration in their neurologic status. They were readmitted in June 1968 (13) and the deterioration was quite evident. K.S. was confined to a wheel chair by her weakness and ataxia. In both patients all deep tendon reflexes were once again unobtainable and muscle strength had decreased. Ulnar nerve conduction velocity, which had risen to about 25 m/sec in both cases by the time of discharge after the first dietary trial, had dropped back to 16 m/sec in J.S. and to less than 10 m/sec in K.S. In both cases the ST-T changes in ECG had reappeared. Both showed peripheral sensory losses to a greater extent than at discharge.

Now the diet used originally, even with deletion of ruminant fats, dairy products and green vegetables, still contained 21 mg phytanic acid

J.S.	7-19-66	363	6-27-68	649
	9-7-66	689	9-4-68	855
	3-14-67	743	11-7-68	933
	5-25-67	841	2-24-69	1061
	9-27-67	766	4-22-69	1143
K.S.	7-22-66	326	6-27-68	334
	11-16-66	468	9-4-68	417
	1-11-67	538	11-4-68	405
	3-15-67	519	2-25-69	633
	9-6-67	521	4-7-69	659

Table II.   Effect of diet on quantitative muscle tests.   First trial
of diet treatment 1966–1967; second trial, 1968–1969.

in a daily ration (versus 56 mg in the regular hospital diet)(31).   In view
of the serious deterioration of these patients it was decided (and they were
willing) to try an even more restricted diet, i.e. a liquid-formula diet
offering less than 3 mg phytanic acid and less than 1 mg phytol daily.
As shown in Fig. 9, plasma phytanate levels fell very rapidly on this
regimen and, except for several unexplained rebounds, were maintained at
low levels.   The changes in ulnar nerve conduction velocity are shown in
Fig. 10 and the changes in muscle strength (average values for selected
muscle groups) in Table II.   Timed tests of coordination showed marked
improvement.   By 2 months the ECG in both patients had reverted to normal.   Tendon reflexes began to appear again at 7 months and were normal
by 18 months.   K.S., confined to a wheel chair on admission, was walking
with the aid of leg braces by 2 months and unaided by 4 months.   On
admission she could hold a glass only using a flat "simian" grip; by 10
months she held it with opposed fingertips.   Both showed reduced light
touch and pin sensation in stocking-and-glove distribution on admission;
by 12 months this had totally regressed in J.S., and K.S. showed only
reduced light touch sensation over foot and ankle.   Vibration sense, absent or poor in hands and feet on admission, was virtually restored at 12
months.

Dr. Kark's conservative conclusion was: "...objective and subject-
ive findings indicate very significant improvement in both patients, on two
occasions each, while on the dietary therapy.   Evidence suggests the improvement is due to the diet.   Between the two courses of regimented

dietary therapy, the patients themselves failed to continue the diet. Each then had an exacerbation. At the present time (July, 1970), we are reluctant to confirm the dietary effect by stopping the diet to produce exacerbation of the neurologic involvement. Each month that the patients remain in remission on the diet makes it less likely that the remissions in both were spontaneous and merely coincidental with dietary therapy" (13).

REFERENCES

1. Avigan, J. et al.: Alpha-decarboxylation, An Important Pathway for Degradation of Phytanic Acid in Animals. Biochem. Biophys. Res. Commun. 24:838, 1966.

2. Baxter, J.H.: Absorption of Chlorophyll Phytol in Normal Man and in Patients with Refsum's Disease. J. Lipid Res. 9:636, 1968.

3. Baxter, J.H. et al.: Absorption and Metabolism of Uniformly ^{14}C-labeled Phytol and Phytanic Acid by the Intestine of Rat Studied with Thoracic Duct Cannulation. Biochim. Biophys. Acta 137:277, 1967.

4. Baxter, J.H. and Steinberg, D.: Absorption of Phytol from Dietary Chlorophyll in the Rat. J. Lipid Res. 8:615, 1967.

5. Eldjarn, L. et al.: Dietary Effects on Serum Phytanic Acid Levels and on Clinical Manifestations in Heredopathia Atactica Polyneuritiformis. Lancet 1:691, 1966.

6. Giovanelli, J. and Stumpf, P.K.: Fat Metabolism in Higher Plants. X. Modified β Oxidation of Propionate by Peanut Mitochondria. J. Biol. Chem. 231:411, 1958.

7. Hansen, R.P.: Occurrence of 3,7,11,15-Tetramethylhexadecanoic Acid in Ox Perinephric Fat. Chem. Industr. 7:303, 1965.

8. Hansen, R.P.: 3,7,11,15-Tetramethylhexadecanoic Acid: Its Occurrence in Sheep Fat. N. Zeal. J. Sci. 8:158, 1965.

9. Herndon, J.H., Jr., Steinberg, D., Uhlendorf, B.W. and Fales, H.M.: Refsum's Disease: Characterization of the Enzyme Defect in Cell Culture. J. Clin. Invest. 48:1017, 1969.

10. Herndon, J.H., Jr., Steinberg, D., Uhlendorf, B.W.: Refsum's Disease: Defective Oxidation of Phytanic Acid in Tissue Cultures Derived from Homozygotes and Heterozygotes. New Eng. J. Med. 281:1034, 1969.

11. Hutton, D. and Stumpf, P.K.: Fat Metabolism in Higher Plants. XLII. The Pathway of Rinoleic Acid Catabolism in the Germinating Castor Bean (Rinicus communis L.) and Pea (Pisum sativum L.) Arch. Biochem. Biophys. 142:48, 1971.

12. Kahlke, W.: "Heredopathia Atactica Polyneuritiformis (Refsum's Disease)", in Lipids and Lipidoses. Schettler, G. (ed) New York:

Springer-Verlag, pp. 352-379, 1967.

13. Kark, R.A.P., Engel, W.K., Blass, J.P., Steinberg, D. and Walsh, G.O.: Heredopathia Atactica Polyneuritiformis (Refsum's Disease): A Second Trial of Dietary Therapy in Two Patients. Nervous System. Birth Defects: Original Article Series 7:53, 1971.

14. Kesner, L. and Muntwyler, E.M.: "Separation of Citric Acid Cycle and Related Compounds by Partition Column Chromatography", in Methods in Enzymology. Colowick, S.P. and Kaplan, N.O. (eds) New York: Academic Press, Vol. XII, p. 415.

15. Klenk, E. and Kahlke, W.: Uber das Vorkommen der 3.7.11.15-Tetramethylhexadecansaure (Phytansaure) in den Cholesterenistern und anderen Lipoidfraktionen der Organe bei einem Krankheitsfall unbekannter Genese (Verdacht auf Heredopathia atactica polyneurififormis-Refsum's Syndrome). Hoppe Seyler Z Physiol. Chem. 333: 133, 1963.

16. Klenk, E. and Kremer, G.J.: Untersuchungen zum Stoffwechsel des Phytols, Dihydrophytols und der Phytansaure. Hoppe Seyler Z Physiol. Chem. 343:39, 1965.

17. Kolodny, E.H., Hass, W.K., Lane, B. and Drucker, W.D.: Refsum's Syndrome: Report of a Case Including Electron Microscopic Studies of the Liver. Arch. Neurol. 12:583, 1965.

18. Mize, C.E. et al.: A pathway for Oxidative Degradation of Phytanic Acid in Mammals. Biochem. Biophys. Res. Commun. 25:359, 1966.

19. Mize, C.E. et al.: Effects of Dietary Phytol and Phytanic Acid in Animals. J. Lipid Res. 7:684, 1966.

20. Mize, C.E. et al.: Phytanic Acid Storage in Refsum's Disease Due to Defective Alpha-Hydroxylation. Clin. Res. 16:346, 1968 (Abs).

21. Mize, E.C. et al.: A Major Pathway for the Oxidative Degradation of Phytanic Acid. Biochim. Biophys. Acta 176:720, 1969.

22. Overath, P., Raufuss, E.M., Stoffel, W. and Ecker, W.: The Induction of Enzymes of Fatty Acid Degradation in E. Coli. Biochem. Biophys. Res. Commun. 29:28, 1967.

23. Refsum, S.: Heredopathia Atactica Polyneuritiformis. Acta Psychiat. Scand. suppl. 38:1, 1946.

24. Rosenberg, L., Hsia, Y.E. and Scully, K.J.: Defective Propionate Carboxylation in Ketotic Hyperglycinaemia. Lancet 1:757, 1969.

25. Sonnevald, W., Begeman, P.H., van Beers, G.J., Keuning, R. and Schogt, J.C.M.: 3,7,11,15-Tetramethylhexadecanoic Acid, A Constituent of Butterfat. J. Lipid Res. 3:351, 1962.

26. Steinberg, D.: Phytanic Acid Storage Disease, in Metabolic Basis of Inherited Diseases. Stanbury, J.B., Wyngaarden, J.B. and Fredrickson, D.S. (eds) 3rd Edition. New York: McGraw-Hill Book Co., (in press).

27. Steinberg, D., Avigan, J., Mize, C.E., Baxter, J.H., Cammermeyer, J., Fales, H.M. and Highet, P.F.: Effects of Dietary Phytol and

Phytanic Acid in Animals. J. Lipid Res. 7:684, 1966.

28. Steinberg, D. and Herndon, J.H., Jr.: Refsum's Disease, in The Cellular and Molecular Basis of Neurologic Disease. Shy, G.M., Goldensohn, E.S. and Appel, S.H. (eds). Philadelphia: Lea and Febiger, 1971 (in press).

29. Steinberg, D., Mize, C.E., Avigan, J. Fales, H.M., Eldjarn, L., Try, K. Stokke, O. and Refsum, S.: On the Metabolic Error in Refsum's Disease. J. Clin. Invest. 45:1076, 1966 (Abs).

30. Steinberg, D. Mize, C.E., Avigan, J., Fales, H.M., Eldjarn, L., Try, K., Stokke, O. and Refsum, S. : Studies on the Metabolic Error in Refsum's Disease. J. Clin. Invest. 46:313, 1967.

31. Steinberg, D., Mize, C.E., Herndon, J.H., Jr., Fales, H.M., Engel, W.K. and Vroom, F.Q.: Phytanic Acid in Patients with Refsum's Syndrome and Response to Dietary Treatment. Arch. Int. Med. 125:75, 1970.

32. Steinberg, D. et al.: Refsum's Disease--A Recently Characterized Lipidosis Involving the Nervous System. Ann. Int. Med. 66:365, 1967.

33. Tsai, S.C. et al.: The Formation of Alpha-hydroxy Phytanic Acid from Phytanic Acid in Mammalian Tissues. Biochem. Biophys. Res. Commun. 28:571, 1967.

STUDIES ON A CASE OF LIPOGRANULOMATOSIS (FARBER'S DISEASE) WITH PROTRACTED COURSE

K. Samuelsson, R. Zetterström, and B. I. Ivemark

Departments of Neurology and Pediatric Pathology, Karolinska sjukhuset and of Pediatrics, S:t Görans sjukhus, Karolinska Instituet and the Department of Medical Chemistry, Royal Veterinary College, Stockholm, Sweden

INTRODUCTION

The first description of lipogranulomatosis was published by Farber in 1952 (8). On the basis of the findings in three children, two of whom were siblings he described the clinical and pathological features of this rare systemic disorder. At present eight additional cases, including the present one have been reported (1,3,4,6,7,17, 25). It has been suggested that the disease is inherited in an auto-somal recessive manner (7).

In nine out of 11 cases reported the course of the disease has been rather similar. Onset usually has been soon after birth, the disease has been progressive, and death from infection or inanition has occurred at ages between seven and 22 months. The major clinical features have been respiratory and nutritional difficulties, swollen tender joints and joint deformities, multiple subcutaneous nodules particularly over the joints, osteoporosis, and erosions of the bones. In addition, a marked retardation of psychomotor development and other manifestations of neurological involvement have been present.

However, in one of the cases of lipogranulomatosis reported the clinical course has been milder (7), and in another more protracted (25) than in the rest of them. At ages of six and 16 years, respectively, they were also free of apparent nervous system involvement. These findings point to the existence of phenotypes of lipogranulomatosis which are different from the ordinary one.

Pathological examinations of infantile cases have revealed gra-

533

nulomatous infiltrations of subcutaneous and synovial tissues,
lymph nodes, and of various viscera such as liver, spleen and
lungs; the most characteristic feature of these infiltrations being
the presence of "foam-cells". In the central nervous system severe
neuronal atrophy and distention of many of the neurons with PAS-
positive material have been found (16).

There is general agreement that lipogranulomatosis is a "storage" disease. Recently Moser and coworkers (16,17) demonstrated
accumulation of free ceramides in white cerebral matter and in
other tissues. An excess of gangliosides was also found in all
organs studied.

So far the only chemical analyses which have been presented in
a patient with lipogranulomatosis of the type without clinical
evidence of cerebral involvement are those in our earlier report
(25), demonstrating that there was no mucopolysaccharide accumulation in subcutaneous granuloma.

In this communication we present a case of lipogranulomatosis
with protracted course. Ceramides were analyzed in plasma and a
subcutaneous nodule while the patient was still alive. Various
tissues obtained at autopsy after he had expired one year later,
at an age of 16 years, have also been examined (21). Histochemical
studies on lipogranuloma and kidney have been performed (13).

CASE REPORT

The case history has earlier been reported in detail after the
patient had been followed for the first two years of life (25).

He was the second child in a Swedish family with two children.
Both parents and the brother are healthy. There is no known consan-
guinity between the parents.

A few days after birth severe vomiting started and he became
moderately dehydrated. His face was puffy, the large tongue pro-
truded and his cry was hoarse. Other major early clinical features
were failure to thrive, episodes of fever, laryngeal obstruction
from nodular infiltrations, pulmonary infiltrations, generalized
lymphadenopathy, swollen tender joints, and the appearance of contractures. At the age of 10 months the first subcutaneous granuloma appeared. There was a continuous involvement and at two years
of age he had abundant subcutaneous granulomas, particularly over
the joints, the scalp, the spine and the ribs. During his second
year tracheotomy had to be performed as an acute, life-saving procedure.

Physical examination at an age of two years did not reveal any neurological abnormalities. He was then able to stand with support but was unable to walk due to the contractures. Psychological examination at the same age revealed a normal mental development.

During the further course there was a slow continuous increase of the motor handicap. He was never able to walk but managed to use an electrically driven wheel chair. His growth was markedly retarded. At an age of 15 years his height was estimated to be about 110 cm after correction for the flection contractures in the hips and the knees. The trunk was very short due to compressions of the vertebrae. He developed severe osteoporosis and got several bone erosions around the joints. There was no obvious impairment of his sexual development.

New subcutaneous and submucous granulomas appeared continuously. After the age of eight years the granulomas were mainly localized over the joints on the dorsal side of the hands and to the face where they appeared on the eyelids, the external ears, around the nostrils and on the lips (Fig. 1). Nodular infiltrations also appear-

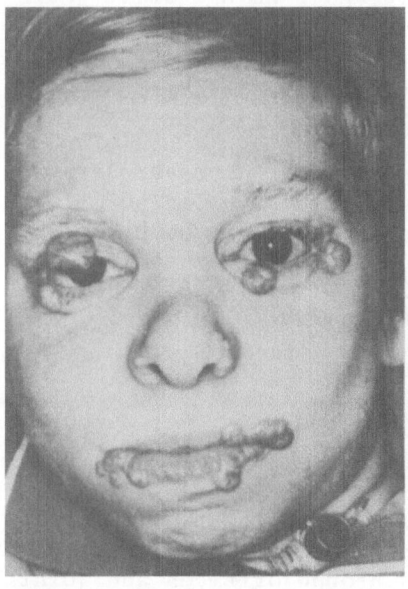
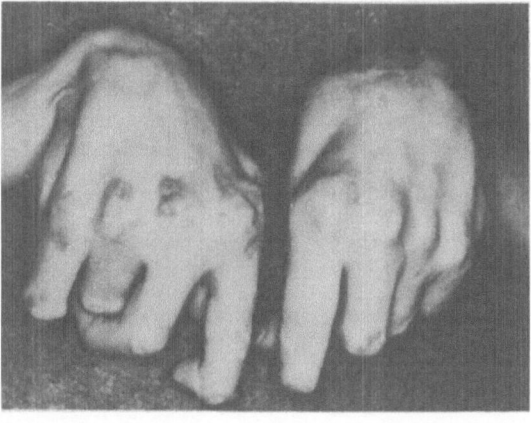

Fig. 1. The face and the hands of the patient with lipogranulomatosis one month before he died (at an age of about 16 years). As can be seen granulomas in the face were localized around the mouth and on the lips, on the eyelids, around the nostrils and on the external ears. On the hands they were found on the joints. Severe contractures in finger joints and wrists are evident. In the face there was, particularly on the forehead, a punctuate red rash. In the superficial layers over the granulomas dark red angiectasies could be seen.

ed on the tongue and the tonsils and at other sites in the mouth. He also got granulomas around the anus. From the age of 14 years he had a papulous red rash over the cheeks and on the forehead. Dark red angiectasies were seen over the granulomas (Fig. 1).

A psychological examination at an age of seven years had shown that his intellectual development most probably was normal. Because of the tracheotomy he was unable to speak. He had, however, learned to use an electric typewriter. His communication with other people then improved remarkably. He soon learned to read; his spelling was fairly good.

Granulomas were repeatedly removed due to handicapping or cosmetic reasons. Since prednisone gave him relief of the joint pains he was most of the time kept on a small dose. The tracheotomy cannula had to be kept until he died.

After the age of 13 years there was a continuous deterioration. The respiratory difficulties progressed after an age of 14 years. There was a total atelectasis of the left lung. He became more and more cachectic, his weight which was 30.0 kg at an age of 12 years had dropped to 20.3 kg shortly before he died at an age of almost 16 years. He expired in connection with an attack of heart arrest during general anesthesia given, when granulomas were being removed from the eyelids.

No proteinuria or hematuria was demonstrated. Repeated determinations of the urinary excretion of uronic acid revealed normal results. Thus, there was no evidence of an increase of the urinary excretion of mucopolysaccharides. There was neither azotemia nor any particular hematological abnormalities. Serum lipids (cholesterol, phospholipids and triglycerides) were normal.

PATHOLOGY

Summary of Gross Findings

The autopsy was performed in an outside hospital by Dr. Bengt Larsson. The body was severely emaciated, kyphoscoliotic, and there were numerous hard, subcutaneous nodules around orifices and joints as described above. They measured up to 3 x 2 x 1 cms., and presented a shiny homogenous yellowish cut surface. In the viscera, similar nodules were found in the tongue, in the submucosas of the epiglottis, larynx, trachea and bronchi. The kidneys were of normal size and showed no nodules. The spleen, lymph nodes, thymus and bone marrow and brain were unremarkable. The liver only weighed 610 g. The skeleton showed osteoporosis and the adrenals were atrophic (cortisone-effect).

Histologic Findings

Sections from paraffin embedded <u>nodules</u> presented the well-known picture of sclerosing granulomas containing thick bundles of collagen surrounding islands of mononuclear cells. These cells had bean-shaped or elongated nuclei and the cell boundaries were indistinct. The cytoplasm was slightly foamy. Some of these cells contained a PAS-positive substance. There was no birefringent material and no obvious trace of dissolved crystals in the form of empty spaces. In many subcutaneous nodules large areas of degeneration - without cells and collagen, but with mineral salt deposits - were found. Such areas were not seen in the visceral nodules. The <u>kidneys</u> presented minute, non-specific changes in paraffin-embedded material. There were occasional focal cortical scars, a slight, PAS-positive thickening of the glomerular basement membrane and very occasional basement membrane thickening of tubules, but no birefringent material or obvious PAS-positive material in the cells. All other organs, including brain, liver, spleen, the lymphoid apparatus, endocrine organs, lungs and vascular system were essentially normal.

Histochemical Findings (13)

Calcium formalin fixed specimens were sectioned on a thermoelectric microtome and the results were compared with gelatin suspended smears of synthetic ceramides, fixed and stained in the same manner as the frozen sections. Applying the lipid histochemical techniques of Adams (2) two substances were demonstrated in the <u>granulomas</u>, one with the tinctorial properties of ceramides and a second substance differing from ceramides, inasmuch as it was PAS-positive, non-refractile, easily removed by chloroform-methanol extraction and positive with the modified PAS-procedure for gangliosides. The ceramides in the smears and in the tissue was PAS-negative, birefringent, negative with the modified PAS-reaction, black in OTAN and easily removed by lipid extraction. The ceramides in the granulomas appeared as large (10-13 µ) crystals. It could not be determined in the frozen sections whether they were intra- or extracellular; however, no definite nuclei were present adjacent to the crystals. On the other hand, the PAS-positive substance appeared to be located within cells that often formed groups or long clusters. They probably corresponded to the PAS-positive cells of the paraffin sections, some of the glycolipid resisting the treatment with alcohols and xylol prior to embedding. The nature of this second substance is not entirely clear, but its tinctorial properties and its solubility in lipid solvents are consistent with a ganglioside.

Frozen sections from the <u>kidneys</u> contained birefringent crystals

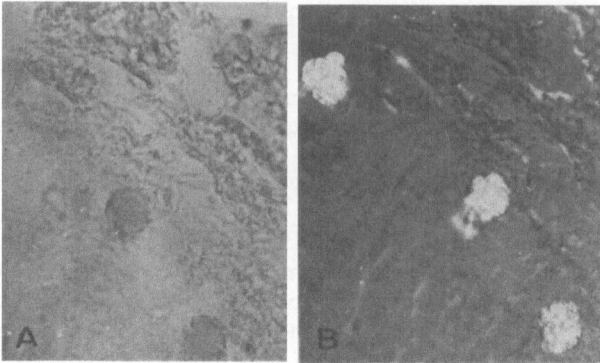

Fig. 2. Lipogranulomatosis. Frozen section from subcutaneous granuloma. A. The ceramide crystals are barely visible in ordinary light.
B. In polarized light they are obvious. Crystal violet-acetic acid
x 380.

of ceramide in proximal and distal tubular cells. They were invis-
ible in paraffin embedded sections. Other cells, often in the same
tubule, contained a PAS-positive substance which was non-refractile
in polarized light and showed the same staining properties as the
second substance - the probable ganglioside - of the granulomas. It
was not possible histochemically to differentiate the 2-hydroxy
fatty acid ceramides in smears from those with normal fatty acids.

CERAMIDE ANALYSES

Material and Methods

Ceramide analyses were carried out on plasma of the patient with
lipogranulomatosis 13 months before he died. At the same time a subcutaneous nodule was excised from the eyelid for ceramide analysis.
Plasma from an apparently healthy 16 year-old boy was used as control.

Samples of brain, lung, liver, spleen and kidney were obtained
at autopsy. All the material was stored at $-18°$ prior to use. None
of these samples contained any granulomas according to gross inspec-
tion. The brain samples (left frontal lobe) were divided into white
and grey matter for separate analyses. The kidney samples from the
patient and the control contained approximately the same proportions
of cortex and medulla. As control we used tissue samples from a 68
year-old man who died suddenly from coronary disease and who showed
no clinical or pathological evidence of other diseases. Autopsy was
performed at about the same time after death.

The ceramides were isolated and analyzed as trimethylsilyl (TMS) ethers by gas-liquid chromatography (GLC) and GLC-mass spectrometry. These methods have recently been published in detail (20,21).

Duplicate quantitative analyses were performed on the autopsy material (tissues) and the mean values are given in Tables I and II. Most of the GLC-fractions were identified by GLC-mass spectrometry (11,12,19). No thin-layer chromatographic (TLC) fractionation according to the degree of unsaturation was performed for these analyses.

Results

Subcutaneous nodule. The GLC analysis of free ceramides in the subcutaneous nodule is shown in Fig. 3 and the main molecular species as identified by GLC-mass spectrometry are indicated. The total amount was 11.9 mg/g wet weight. There was no evidence of ceramides containing hydroxy fatty acids. The major components were mainly due to N-palmitoyl sphingosine (LCB 18:1-16:0), LCB 18:1-22:0 and LCB 18:1-24:1. Sphingosine was the major long-chain base (LCB) also in the other GLC fractions. However, hexadeca sphingosine (LCB 16:1), LCB 17:1, LCB 18:0 and LCB 18:2 were also detected. No evidence for the presence of other major LCB or abnormal fatty acids was obtained.

Plasma. The concentration of ceramides in plasma as well as various GLC fractions quantitated were of the same order of magnitude in the patient and in the control and there was also good agreement with data obtained previously for normal subjects (20,21). Mass-spectrometric analyses were not obtained on the plasma ceramides of the patient. Ceramides containing hydroxy fatty acids were neither detected in the patient nor in the control.

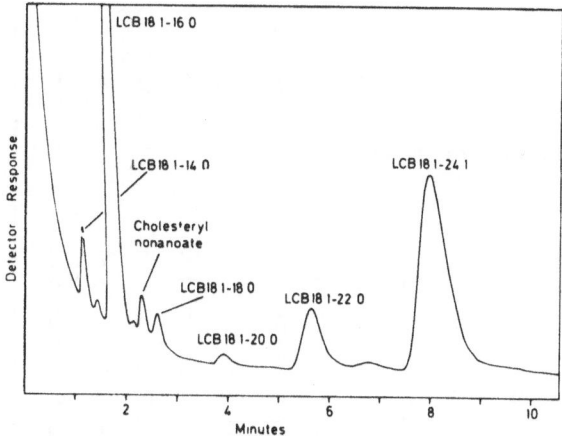

Fig. 3. GLC of TMS derivatives of ceramides from subcutaneous nodule from a patient with lipogranulomatosis. Column 1.4 m, 2% OV-1 at 320°.

Table I

Summary of GLC-Mass Spectrometric Analysis of TMS Derivatives of Ceramides from Spleen, Lung, Liver and Brain (grey and white matter) of a Patient with Lipogranulomatosis and Control[*].

Main constitutents	SPLEEN		LUNG		LIVER		BRAIN GREY MATTER		BRAIN WHITE MATTER	
	L[**]	C[**]	L	C	L	C	L	C	L	C
LCB 18:1-14:0	2	1	2	1	5	2	–	–	–	–
LCB 18:1-16:0	38	37	31	18	70	45	19	8	17	10
LCB 18:1-18:0	6	6	15	4	24	10	186	81	110	121
LCB 18:1-20:0	10	11	8	1	23	18	45	28	21	35
LCB 18:1-21:0	–	–	–	–	6	3	–	–	4	3
LCB 18:1-22:0	32	45	26	10	80	75	10	8	27	30
LCB 18:1-23:0	3	4	1	1	13	9	4	1	22	27
LCB 18:1-24:1	67	81	84	42	153	183	97	39	226	313
LCB 18:1-25:1	–	–	–	–	–	–	–	–	23	37
LCB 18:1-26:1	–	–	–	–	–	–	–	–	10	1
Total conc.	158	185	167	77	374	345	362	166	460	577

[*] Expressed as µg per gram of wet weight

[**] L, patient with Lipogranulomatosis; C, control

Spleen, Lung and Liver. The values for spleen, lung and liver
are shown in Table I. No major differences were found between the
patient and the control in the analyses of spleen and liver ceramides. The concentration of ceramides in the lungs of the patient, however, was higher than in the control but the composition according
to GLC-mass spectrometric analyses was quite similar in both samples. The main LCB of spleen ceramides was sphingosine. LCB 18:2 and
trace amounts of LCB 16:1 were also found. Ceramides containing the
fatty acids 16:0, 22:0 and 24:1 were the major components. The composition of ceramides in lung and liver was relatively similar to
that found for spleen ceramides. None of the mass spectra contained
fragments indicating any abnormal structure of the ceramides. No
ceramides containing 2-hydroxy fatty acids were seen in any of these
samples.

Brain. The ceramides of grey and white matter of brain were
analyzed separately. The results of the GLC and mass spectrometric
analyses of the TLC fractions corresponding to reference ceramides
with normal fatty acids are summarized in Table I.

The composition and concentration of brain ceramides of white
matter of the patient did not show any major differences from those
of the control. The level of ceramides of grey matter from the patient was moderately increased compared with the control. The composition was quite similar in the ceramides of the patient and of the
control whereas the difference in composition of ceramides from
grey and white matter was obvious. In the grey matter the major GLC
fraction consisted mainly of LCB 18:1-18:0. Ceramides with LCB 18:1
and long chain fatty acids were considerably less abundant than in
white matter.

In the ceramides of white matter the GLC fraction with LCB 18:1
-24:1 was the largest component.

Sphingosine was the major LCB in all the fractions. Evidence
for the presence of LCB 16:1, 17:1, 18:2, 18:0 and 20:1 was found
but they seemed to occur only in small amounts. Trace amounts of
ceramides with 2-hydroxy fatty acids were found in white matter but
the amounts were too low to allow reliable quantitations of the individual fractions.

Kidney. Thin-layer chromatograms of ceramides from kidney of
the patient with lipogranulomatosis gave two fractions with about
the same R_f values (0.55 and 0.61) as the references LCB 18:1-18:0
and LCB 18:1-24:0, respectively. These were seen in the analysis of
the control subjects as well. The samples from the patient also showed one fraction corresponding to N-2-hydroxy-myristoyl sphingosine
(LCB 18:1-14h:0) (R_f=0.33) and one with the R_f value 0.42 (corresponding tentatively to LCB 18:1-24h:0). The samples were recovered from

the plate in two fractions, one corresponding to the reference ceramides with normal fatty acids and one to the references containing 2-hydroxy fatty acids. The results of the GLC-mass spectrometric
analyses are shown in Table II and Fig. 4 and 5.

The total concentration of ceramides containing normal fatty
acids was more than two times higher in the patient than in the control. The increase was most prominent in the ceramides containing
long chain fatty acids (20:0 and higher homologues). According to
the mass spectrometric analyses the LCB 18:2 seemed to be somewhat
more abundant in the control ceramides as compared to those of the
patient. Moreover, the kidney of the patient did not seem to have
any detectable amounts of ceramides with oleic acid and the proportions between ceramides containing nervonic acid and lignoceric acid
in the patient seemed to be reversed compared with the control. Besides that, no major differences in the mass spectra were noted.

The thin-layer chromatographic fractions corresponding to the
2-hydroxy fatty acid ceramide references were analyzed in a similar
way. The kidney of the control patient did not contain any detectable amounts of ceramides with 2-hydroxy fatty acids. In the kidney
of the patient, however, a comparatively high concentration of ceramides with 2-hydroxy fatty acids was present. The GLC and mass spec-

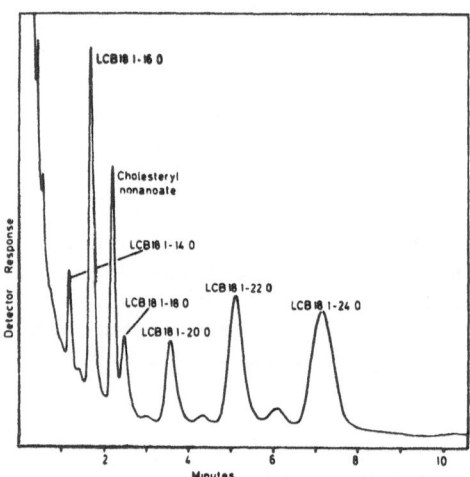

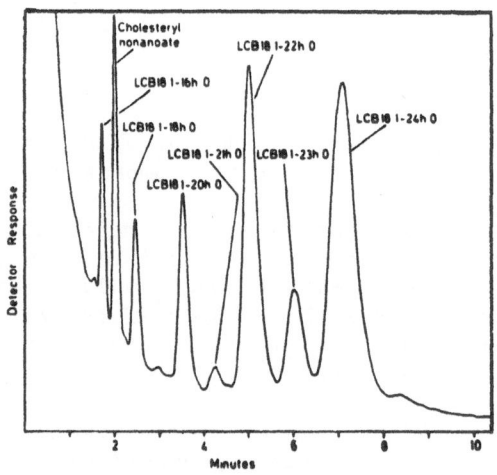

Fig. 4. GLC of TMS derivatives
of ceramides (normal fatty acid
fraction) of kidney from a patient with lipogranulomatosis.
Column 1.4 m, 2% OV-1 at 320°.

Fig. 5. GLC of TMS derivatives
of ceramides (hydroxy fatty
acid fraction) of kidney from
a patient with lipogranulomatosis. Column 1.4 m, 2% OV-1 at
320°.

Table II

Summary of GLC-Mass Spectrometric Analysis of TMS Derivatives of Ceramides from Kidney of a Patient with Lipogranulomatosis and Control*.

Normal fatty acid fraction

Main constituents	Patient	Control
LCB 18:1-14:0	6	2
LCB 18:1-16:0	70	46
LCB 18:1-18:0	26	12
LCB 18:1-20:0	26	4
LCB 18:1-21:0	3	–
LCB 18:1-22:0	76	15
LCB 18:1-23:0	12	–
LCB 18:1-24:1	139	49
LCB 18:1-24:0		
Total conc.	358	128

Hydroxy fatty acid fraction

Main constituent	Patient	Control
LCB 18:1-16h:0	18	–
LCB 18:1-18h:0	22	–
LCB 18:1-19h:0	3	–
LCB 18:1-20h:0	48	–
LCB 18:1-21h:0	9	–
LCB 18:1-22h:0	147	–
LCB 18:1-23h:0	49	–
LCB 18:1-24h:0	306	–
LCB 18:1-25h:0	7	–
Total conc.	608	–

* Expressed as µg per gram of wet weight

trometric data of the ceramides containing 2-hydroxy fatty acids
are shown in Table II and Fig. 5. Ceramides with short chain 2-
hydroxy fatty acids (19h:0 or less) were only minor components. LCB
18:1-24h:0 constituted about 50% of the 2-hydroxy fatty acid ceramides.

DISCUSSION

     Recently Moser et al. have demonstrated an accumulation of ce-
ramides in various tissues from an infant with lipogranulomatosis
who died at an age of 11 months (16). Ceramides were measured by
spectrometric determination of the sphingosine content (14) of a
fraction obtained by thin-layer chromatography. Compared with controls the ceramide levels were found to be markedly increased in
liver (60-fold), lung (30-fold), and kidney (10-fold). The ceramide
contents in a lymph node and a subcutaneous nodule were of the same
order of magnitude as in the liver. A moderate increase of ceramides was also demonstrated in cerebral white matter.

     The phenotype of the patient with lipogranulomatosis we have
studied was in some important respects different from that of the
case examined by Moser et al. (16). The disease of our patient had
a much more protracted course and the patient had no clinical signs
of central nervous system involvement whereas there was an acute
course and profound neurological abnormalities in the case of Moser
et al. (16). Furthermore, the postmortem examination only showed the
typical granulomatous infiltrations in subcutaneous and synovial no-
duli, the tongue and the respiratory tract. They were absent from
other viscera and the brain did not show any specific abnormality.
This finding contrasted distinctly from the infantile case, where
changes suggestive of lipid storage were found in most organs including brain.

     Although we have confirmed the findings of Moser et al. of an
excess of free ceramides in lipogranulomatosis there are definite
differences between our findings and those of Moser et al. (16) with
regard to the sites of accumulation of ceramides. In the granuloma
taken from an eyelid of our patient when he was 15 years old the content of ceramides was as high as 11.9 mg per g wet weight which means
about twenty times that found in any tissue from the control subject.
The concentration was comparable to that found by Moser et al. in
a granuloma (16).

     After autopsy the concentration of ceramides was determined
in various tissues from our patient. In kidney a sevenfold increase
of the total concentration of ceramides was found compared with the
control. However, in liver, spleen, lung and cerebral grey and white
matter the concentrations of ceramides were about the same as in

corresponding tissues from the control subject. This is at variance
with the results of Moser et al., who reported an excess of ceramides not only in the kidneys but also in the lungs, in liver and
in cerebral white matter. The definite biochemical differences between the phenotype of lipogranulomatosis reported by Moser et al.
(16) and that seen in the case we have studied may indicate that
they represent two different genotypes. The existence of various
phenotypes, each one corresponding to a particular genotype, has
earlier been suggested in other "cerebral" lipidoses like in Gaucher's disease (5).

Moser et al. from their studies of the products of hydrolysis
of ceramides from liver could not find any evidence for an abnormal
structure of the accumulated ceramides (16). However, since they did
not present any analyses of the composition of the ceramides of
other tissues it seemed of interest to study the ceramides which
accumulate in lipogranulomatosis in more detail.

In our patient the main molecular species of the ceramides
accumulated in a subcutaneous granuloma consisted of sphingosine
(LCB 18:1) with the fatty acids palmitic, behenic, and nervonic
acid. No ceramides containing hydroxy fatty acids were found. No
evidence for ceramides with abnormal long-chain bases or fatty acids
was observed during the analyses by thin-layer chromatography,
gas chromatography, or mass spectrometry. Especially the mass spectra were conclusive in this respect since all of the ions observed
on electron impact could be accounted for by ceramides with normal
constituents. In the kidney about two thirds of the excess ceramides contained hydroxy fatty acids, viz. 2-hydroxy-behenic acid (22h:
0) and cerebronic acid (24h:0). Of the ceramides with normal fatty
acids the increase was mainly confined to those containing arachi-
dic   acid (20:0), behenic acid (22:0), and lignoceric acid (24:0).
No ceramides containing 2-hydroxy fatty acids were detected in the
kidney from the control subject. There was no major differences between the composition of the ceramides from plasma, liver, spleen,
lung, cerebral white and grey matter in our patient with lipogranulomatosis and the control subject.

It is of interest that there were quite different patterns of
ceramides in the subcutaneous granuloma and the kidney in our patient. These findings may indicate that the accumulated ceramides are
formed locally. The fact that the concentration of ceramides in plasma was similar to that of the control of the same age supports such
a hypothesis.

Our histochemical studies demonstrated the presence of two substances in lipogranulomatosis. One was birefringent and PAS-negative,
the other showed no birefringence but was PAS-positive in frozen
sections. The first substance we have shown to be ceramide, while
the PAS-positive material is consistent with ganglioside. These

findings are somewhat at variance with the results of Moser et al., since they found the PAS-positivity and birefringence in the same cells.

Moser et al. discussed various metabolic defects which might be responsible for the accumulation of ceramides. Ceramides have been shown to be intermediates both in the biosynthesis and the catabolism of sphingolipids (10,15,23). Moser et al. had no evidence for deficient biosynthesis of sphingolipids (16). Furthermore, a block in the degradation of ceramides seemed unlikely since ceramidase activity of liver tissue was found to be normal. It was pointed out, however, that other ceramidases, which were not included in the assay, might exist (16). No determination of ceramidase activity has yet been carried out in the present case. However, in view of the normal level of ceramidase activity reported by Moser et al. and since sphingosine can be converted back to ceramides (10,22) impairment of the degradation of sphingosine (24) should also be considered as a cause of the accumulation of ceramides.

ACKNOWLEDGEMENT

This investigation has been supported by Svenska multipel skleros-föreningarnas riksförbund.

REFERENCES

1.   Abul-Haj, S.K., Martz, D.G., Douglas, W.F. and Geppert, L.J. Farber's disease. Report of a case with observations on its histogenesis and notes on the nature of the stored material. J. Pediat. 61: 221 (1962).

2.   Adams, C.W.M. Neurohistochemistry. Elsevier Publishing Co., Amsterdam, 1965.

3.   Azanza, X. Une Nouvelle Neurolipidose. La Maladie de Farber (Thesis). Editions Bergerel, Bordeaux, 1969.

4.   Bierman, S.M., Edgington, T., Newcomer, V.D. and Pearson, C.M. Farber's disease: A disorder of mucopolysaccharide metabolism with articular respiratory and neurologic manifestations. Arthr. and Rheum. 9: 620 (1966).

5.   Brady, R.O. Cerebral lipidoses. Amer. Rev. Med. 21: 317 (1970).

6.   Clausen, J. and Rampini, S. Chemical studies of Farber's disease. Acta neurol. scand. 46: 313 (1970).

7.   Crocker, A.C., Cohen, J. and Farber, S. The "lipogranulomatosis"
     syndrome; Review, with report of patient showing milder involve-
     ment. In: Aronson, S.M. and Volk, B.W. (eds) Inborn Disorders
     of Sphingolipid Metabolism. Pergamon Press Ltd., Oxford, 1967,
     pp. 485-503.

8.   Farber, S. A lipid metabolic disorder-disseminated "Lipogranu-
     lomatosis" - a syndrome with similarity to and important differ-
     ence from, Niemann-Pick and Hand-Schüller-Christian disease.
     Amer. J. Dis. Child. 84: 499 (1952).

9.   Farber, S., Cohen, J. and Uzman, L.L. Lipogranulomatosis. A
     new lipo-glyco-protein "storage" disease. J. Mt Sinai Hosp.
     24: 816 (1957).

10. Gatt, S. Enzymatic aspects of sphingolipid degradation. In:
     Sweeley, C.C. (ed) Chemistry and Metabolism of Sphingolipids.
     North Holland Publishing Co., Amsterdam, 1970, pp. 235-249.

11. Hammarström, S. Gas-liquid chromatography-mass spectrometry of
     synthetic ceramides containing phytosphingosine. J. Lipid Res.
     11: 175 (1970).

12. Hammarström, S., Samuelsson, B. and Samuelsson, K. Gas-liquid
     chromatography-mass spectrometry of synthetic ceramides con-
     taining 2-hydroxy acids. J. Lipid Res. 11: 150 (1970).

13. Ivemark, B.I. Lipid histochemical findings in juvenile lipo-
     granulomatosis (Farber). Proceedings of the 5th annual meeting
     of the Scandinavian Society of Pediatric Pathology in Helsinki,
     June 10-12, 1971. Acta paediat. scand. In press.

14. Lauter, C.J. and Trams, E.G. A spectrophotometric determination
     of sphingosine. J. Lipid Res. 3: 136 (1962).

15. Morell, P., Costantino-Ceccarini, E., and Radin, N.S. The bio-
     synthesis by brain microsomes of cerebrosides containing non-
     hydroxy fatty acids. Arch. Biochem. 141: 738 (1970). And refer-
     ences therein.

16. Moser, H.W., Prensky, A.L., Wolfe, H.J. and Rosman, N.P. Far-
     ber's lipogranulomatosis. Report of a case and demonstration
     of an excess of free ceramide and ganglioside. Amer. J. Med.
     47: 869 (1969).

17. Prensky, A.L., Ferreira, G., Carr, S. and Moser, H.W. Ceramide
     and ganglioside accumulation in Farber's lipogranulomatosis.
     Proc. Soc. exp. Biol. (N.Y.) 126: 725 (1967).

18. Samuelsson, B. and Samuelsson, K. Gas-liquid chromatographic separation of ceramides as di-0-trimethylsilyl ether derivatives. Biochim. biophys. Acta (Amst.) 164: 421 (1968).

19. Samuelsson, B. and Samuelsson, K. Gas-liquid chromatography-mass spectrometry of synthetic ceramides. J. Lipid Res. 10: 41 (1969).

20. Samuelsson, K. Identification and quantitative determination of ceramides in human plasma. Scand. J. clin. Lab. Invest. 27: 371 (1971).

21. Samuelsson, K. and Zetterström, R. Ceramides in a patient with lipogranulomatosis (Farber's disease) with chronic course. Scand. J. clin. Lab. Invest. 27: 393 (1971).

22. Sribney, M. Enzymatic synthesis of ceramide. Biochim. biophys. Acta (Amst.) 125: 542 (1966).

23. Sribney, M. and Kennedy, E.P. The enzymatic synthesis of sphingomyelin. J. Biol. Chem. 233: 1315 (1958).

24. Stoffel, W. Studies on the biosynthesis and degradation of sphingosine bases. In: Sweeley, C.C. (ed) Chemistry and Metabolism of sphingolipids. North Holland Publishing Co., Amsterdam, 1970, pp. 139-158.

25. Zetterström, R. Disseminated lipogranulomatosis (Farber's disease). Acta paediat. (Uppsala) 47: 501 (1958).

BIOCHEMICAL STUDIES ON BRAIN EXPLANTS AND FIBROBLAST CULTURES

IN BATTEN'S DISEASE

John H. Menkes, M.D. with Don R. Harris, B.S. and
Natalie Stein, B.A.
Division of Pediatric Neurology, University of Califor-
nia at Los Angeles and Brentwood V.A. Hospital

Batten's disease is a syndrome of mental, motor, and
visual deterioration having its onset between the second and
fifth year of life. Through combined ultrastructural and biochemical examinations at least five different entities are
currently known to assume a clinical course corresponding to
that described by Batten in 1914 (1).

In our experience the most common of these has been the
one characterized by an electron microscopic picture of cytoplasmic bodies having a granular and multiloculated appearance.
First described in 1963 by Zeman and Donahue (2), they were subsequently termed "curvilinear bodies" by Duffy and coworkers (3).
The chemical identity of the stored material is still obscure,
but one striking characteristic is the accumulation of lipofus-
cin-like pigments within affected neurons. The mechanism of
pigment accumulation is unknown, but a number of polyunsaturated fatty acids have been postulated to act as pigment precursors (4), undergoing peroxidation in the presence of divalent
cations. Polymerization of the peroxide has been demonstrated
experimentally; the reaction product having a fluorescence spectrum similar to that of the stored lipofuscin.

In 1968 Hagberg and coworkers (5) reported a patient with
a lipidosis that had its onset in late infancy, in whose grey
matter there was a pronounced reduction of fatty acids of the
linolenic acid (18:3ω3) series. Thus the percentages of 22:6 ω3,
and of 22:4 ω 3 were reduced, while arachidonic acid (20:4 ω 6)
concentration was normal. The concentrations of linoleic acid
(18:2), and linolenic acid (18:3) were not reported.

In view of these findings, the postulate that patients
with Batten's disease are unable to metabolize one or more
of the dietary polyunsaturated fatty acids seemed sufficiently attractive to warrant initiating a study of polyunsaturated
fatty acid metabolism in brain explants and fibroblast cultures
in patients with late infantile neurovisceral storage disease
and curvilinear bodies.

CASE REPORTS

Case 1, (M.S.): This Mexican-American girl was well until
four years of age when her gait became unsteady, and she began
having seizures. These consisted of episodes of staring with
extension and jerking of the upper extremities. She regressed
rapidly, and by 4 1/2 years of age she had lost all speech, the
ability to ambulate or sit, and bladder control. For about five
months thereafter there was some improvement in that she again
was able to walk, feed herself, and utter single words, but by
five years of age she again regressed.

On admission to the UCLA Center for the Health Sciences
at age 6 years, she was a profoundly retarded and bed ridden child
who had frequent, massive myoclonic seizures. Optic disks were
pale, and there was arteriolar narrowing, diffuse peripheral
pigmentary deposition and macular degeneration. She showed marked
spastic quadriplegia and truncal ataxia.

During this hospital admission a biopsy of the right frontal
lobe and a skin biopsy for fibroblast cultures were performed.

Case 2, (A.P.): A detailed case history of this patient has
already been reported (6; Case 2). In essence this white, non-
Jewish girl began having neurological symptoms at three years of
age. These included adversive and grand mal seizures, ataxia and
slurred speech. A frontal lobe biopsy was performed at the age
of four years. Since then deterioration has continued, despite
therapy with butylated hydroxy toluene, an antioxidant, and toco-
pherol at dosages of 600 mg and 900 mg per day, respectively.

Case 3, (T.P.): This four year old boy, the younger brother
of Case 2, was first seen at 2 and 3/12 years for a neurological
evaluation because of his delayed speech and intermittent right
esotropia. No neurological abnormalities were noted at that time.
One year later, however, he had definitely regressed, had
developed mild spastic diplegia and minor motor seizures. Despite
treatment with antioxidants and anticonvulsants he has continued

a downhill course. A skin biopsy for fibroblast cultures was
obtained at 3 and 4/12 years.

PATHOLOGICAL FINDINGS

The neuropathological findings in the two patients who underwent brain biopsy (Cases 1 and 2) revealed cytoplasmic inclusions
of curvilinear bodies. The findings on Case 2 have already been
reported in detail (6).

EXPERIMENTAL STUDIES

Metabolic Studies on Brain Tissue Explants

The procedures, currently used in our laboratory for the preparation and maintenance of brain tissue explants, have already
been described in detail (7,8).

In essence, tissue derived from the brain biopsies was maintained in serum-supplemented medium until good glial outgrowth
became evident. A lipid-free medium was then substituted, and
the labelled fatty acid was added.

Explants derived from Case 1 were separated into grey matter,
white matter, and mixed grey and white matter before the start of
culture. Each of these tissues was incubated for 48 hours with
stearic acid [1-^{14}C] (0.2 μCi) (48.4 mCi/mM) (Amersham-Searle,
Des Plaines, Ill.).

Explants from Case 2 were incubated for 48 hours with linoleic acid [1-^{14}C] (0.2 μCi) (52.9 mCi/mM) (Amersham-Searle) and
stearic acid [1-^{14}C] (0.2 μCi). Fatty acids were added in the form
of their albumin complexes prepared according to the method of
Fillerup, Migliore, and Mead (9). Molar ratios of added free
fatty acid: albumin of the order of 0.003 resulted in optimal
microscopic appearance of explants. Under phase microscopy the
explants showed outgrowths of multipolar glial cells which in some
instances had a cytoplasm filled with refractile bodies. Electron
microscopic examination of these is in progress (10). There
was no evidence of neuronal outgrowth.

Metabolic Studies on Fibroblasts

Skin biopsies were obtained from Cases 2 and 3, and from
six controls. They were grown in plastic Falcon flasks (30 ml)

using Minimum Essential Medium, containing Earle's buffered salt
solution (pH 7.0 to 7.2), and 1 ml antibiotic-antimycotic solution
per 100 ml medium. After good outgrowth was observed the cells
were trypsinized with 0.5 ml of 0.25% trypsin. Once monolayers
were obtained the contents of a small flask were used to inoculate
a large plastic Falcon flask (250 ml), containing 15 ml of medium.
The contents of four flasks were used for the biochemical studies.
Fibroblasts demonstrated a large number of refractile cytoplasmic
bodies. Initial electron microscopic examination revealed the presence of myelin figures and zebra-like bodies. More complete
studies are in progress (11). Linoleic acid [1-^{14}C] (1.0μCi)
(50 Ci/0.88 mM) (New England Nuclear Corp., Boston) was added to
each 15 ml of medium. The solution was heated briefly to 56.5°C,
to complex the fatty acid to the serum albumin in the medium. The
medium containing the labelled substrate was then added to the cells
in the flask, which were incubated at 37.7°C for 48 hours under an
atmosphere of 95% air - 5% CO_2.

Lipid Extraction and Fractionation

At the termination of the experiment tissue from the flasks
was combined, the cells were scraped off with a policeman, the
medium removed by centrifugation, and cells were washed three
times with 0.15 M NaCl. The tissue was homogenized in 3 ml of
chloroform: methanol (2:1, v/v), and aliquots removed for determination of total radioactivity and protein content (11).

The procedure for the lipid extraction and fractionation has
already been published in detail (7,8). For identification of the
labelled fatty acids, the lipid extract was dried under a stream
of nitrogen. Fatty acid methyl esters were prepared by heating
the dried sample at 100°C for 90 minutes with 14% (2/v) boron tri-
fluoride in methanol (13). The fatty acids were extracted into
hexane, and purified by TLC on Silica Gel G plates developed with
hexane-ether (9:1 w/v) under an atmosphere of nitrogen. Gas-liquid
chromatography of the fatty acids was carried out on a Barber-
Coleman Model 5000 gas chromatograph with an argon detector. The
column was packed with 15% diethylene glycol succinate on acid
washed Gas Chrom W as stationary phase. (Applied Science Laboratories,
State College, Pa.). The column was operated at 200°C and 19 lbs.
argon pressure. Peaks were identified by comparison with standard
mixtures of fatty acid esters, and after hydrogenation of the
fatty acids, using 35 lbs. hydrogen and platinum oxide catalyst.

Radioactive fatty acid methyl esters were collected from the
gas chromatograph by means of a glass U-tube (4 mm in diameter)
directly connected to the heated outlet, and cooled in a dry ice
mixture. The fatty acid esters were rinsed from the collection tubes
into a scintillation vial with 15 ml of scintillation mixture.

TABLE I

DISTRIBUTION OF RADIOACTIVITY IN FIGURES FROM BRAIN TISSUE EXPLANTS
AFTER INCUBATION WITH $1-{}^{14}C$ STEARIC ACID

	Case 1 Matter			Case 2 Matter Mixed G/W	Control (One 3 day old rat)	Controls (Five 3 day old rats)
	Grey	White	Mixed			
Total Radioactivity Uptake*	24.8	9.3	11.5	11.4	52.2	67-241
"Neutral Lipids"			74.5	94.5	78.3	74.9 ± 7.4
Free Fatty Acids			71.2	0.4	33.5	39.2 ± 10.1
Cholesterol			7.9	0.4	8.6	3.0 ± 1.3
Triglycerides			18.3	6.3	48.8	41.8 ± 10.9
Cholesterol Esters			1.8	0.5	6.4	---
Diglycerides + Fatty Acid Esters			0.9	92.0	2.6	---
Glycolipids			8.2	1.4	3.0	1.9 ± 0.7
Phospholipids			20.3	4.1	18.7	23.2 ± 7.8

* (cpm x 10^{-3}/mg protein)

Unless otherwise specified, figures represent the percentages of total radioactivity with each of the three principal lipid fractions, and the percent of fraction radioactivity within each lipid species. Control was run concurrently; the other five were obtained at a different time.

Approximately 90% of the radioactivity injected into the column
was recovered.

RESULTS

Fatty Acid Metabolism of Brain Explants

The incorporation of stearic acid by brain explants of Cases
1 and 2 is presented in Table 1. Total incorporation was greater
in grey than in white matter, and in mixed grey and white matter
of patients was less than was obtained on explants derived from
three day old rats, which served as controls. This finding was
consistant with previously reported data showing that incorporation
of stearate into explant lipids is maximal at 3 days of age (7).

However the patient incorporated less stearic acid into triglycerides than did the control animals. In Case 1 the major
amount of radioactivity remained as tissue-bound fatty acids, and
in Case 2 entered the diglyceride and fatty acid ester fraction.
This was considered to be a normal finding. With maturation the
relative amount of stearic acid incorporated into triglycerides
undergoes a striking reduction, while the amount remaining in
the form of tissue-bound stearic acid increases (Table 2).

TABLE 2

INCORPORATION OF 1-^{14}C STEARIC ACID INTO TRIGLYCERIDE
FRACTION IN BRAIN EXPLANTS OF VARIOUS AGES
AND IN TWO PATIENTS WITH BATTEN'S DISEASE

Age	% of Radioactivity in "Neutral Lipid" Fraction
3 day	60.4
6 day	58.1
10 day	2.3
17 day	0.9
22 day	0.3
Adult	0.1
Case 1 (6 years)	18.3
Case 2 (4 years)	6.3

TABLE 3
INCORPORATION OF 1-C^{14} LINOLEIC ACID BY BRAIN EXPLANTS

	Case 2 G/W Matter	Control (One 3 day old rat)
Total R.A. Uptake*	42.6	---
Neutral Lipids	51.2	92.2
Free Fatty Acids	3.3	70.3
Cholesterol	3.7	3.0
Triglycerides	75.0	14.5
Cholesterol Esters	4.3	6.7
Diglycerides & Fatty Acid Esters	11.3	1.2
Glycolipids	3.2	1.6
Phospholipids	45.6	6.1
PC	24.1	49.2
PE	73.4	7.7
PS + PI	1.7	13.8
Sphingomyelin	0.8	2.8

* cpm x 10^{-3}/mg protein. Unless otherwise specified, figures represent the percentages of total radioactivity in each of the three
principal lipid fractions, and the percent of fraction radioactivity
within each lipid species. R.A. = radioactivity, PE = phosphatidyl + phosphatidal ethanolamine, PS = phosphatidyl serine,
PI = phosphatidylinsitol, PC = phosphatidyl choline.

When the incorporation of [1-^{14}C] linoleic acid into brain
lipids was examined differences in the behaviour of explants derived from Case 2 and those obtained from control material were
noted.

In Case 2 a greater proportion of radioactivity entered the
triglyceride fraction than was observed in controls, in which the
majority of label remained in the form of tissue-bound free fatty
acids (Table 3). There also was a considerable increase in the
relative amounts of radioactivity incorporated into the phosphatidyl
and phosphatidal ethanolamine fraction by brain explants from Case 1.

Total linoleic acid incorporation into brain explants is
relatively less influenced by the age of the brain from which the
explant is derived than is the case for stearic acid incorporation.
In another experiment incorporation of linoleic acid by cultures
from 3 day old animals was 6500 cpm/mg protein; at 6 days, 9600
cpm/mg protein; at 15 days, 10,000 cpm/mg protein; at 22 days
18,000 cpm/mg protein; and in adult rats 11,000 cpm/mg protein.

TABLE 4
PATTERN OF LABELLED FATTY ACIDS IN BRAIN
TISSUE EXPLANTS FROM PATIENT WITH BATTEN'S DISEASE
IN PRESENCE OF LINOLEIC ACID [1-^{14}C]

Carbon Chain Lengths	Control			Case 2		
	% Wt.	% R.A.	R.S.A.	% Wt.	% R.A.	R.S.A.
16:0	33.5	4.4	0.13	16.7	---	---
18:0	16.0	1.1	0.07	19.5	2.0	1.0
18:1	14.0	1.3	0.09	22.5	1.8	0.08
18:2	1.2	56.3	46.9	4.6	64.2	13.9
18:3 to 20:2	tr.	9.0	---	tr.	20.3	---
20:4	12.1	19.9	1.65	5.9	2.8	0.47
22:4	3.6	1.7	0.47	2.0	1.7	0.85
22:5	4.2	1.1	0.26	2.8	0.8	0.29
22:6	9.4	0.6	0.06	19.1	1.4	0.07

Values represent fatty acid composition of neutral lipid fraction.

These variations with maturation are probably not significant.

There was a significant difference in the metabolism of linoleic acid by explants from Case 2, and control animals (Table 4).

In the neutral lipid fraction of control tissues linoleic acid (18:2) was converted to arachidonic acid (20:4) by way of 20:2. This was ascertained by hydrogenation of the labelled fatty acids, and demonstrating that little of the radioactivity collected in the fraction including 18:3 and 20:2 was due to 18 carbon fatty acids. Further chain elongation of 20:4 to 22:4 and dehydrogenation to 22:5 and 22:6 also occurred to a significant extent. A similar finding was observed in the phospholipid fraction.

In both neutral and phospholipid fractions of Case 2 the conversion of 18:2 to 20:4 proceded to a lesser extent. Interestingly enough, almost as much radioactivity was found in the fraction corresponding to 22:4 as was collected in 20:4, and the relative specific activity of the former was higher (Table 4).

Linoleic Acid Metabolism of Fibroblast Cultures

The studies conducted on brain explants were sufficiently suggestive of a defect in linoleic acid metabolism to warrant their extension to fibroblast cultures. The morphologic appearance of fibroblasts of patients with Batten's disease suggested that the same metabolic defect found within the brain was operative under

TABLE 5

PRODUCTS OF $[1-^{14}C]$ LINOLEIC ACID METABOLISM IN FIBROBLAST CULTURES

Carbon Chain Lengths	Case 1		Control I (3)		Case 3		Control II (3)	
	Wt.	R.A.	Wt.	R.A.	Wt.	R.A.	Wt.	R.A.
14:0	1.8	0.3	0.4– 1.2	0.2	2.7	0.2	0.5– 1.9	0.4
16:0	23.7	0.5	21.2–35.8	0.6	39.3	0.8	21.1–47.9	1.3
16:1	4.1	0.1	2.0– 4.5	0	4.9	0.4	2.4– 3.6	0.7
18:0	28.2	0.8	22.4–30.9	0.5	21.7	1.0	23.7–31.3	1.0
18:1	25.2	0.4	26.7–27.2	0.3	28.8	0.4	19.0–29.3	0.8
18:2	2.2	81.9	2.1– 3.6	85.7	2.5	76.9	1.7– 4.1	59.6
18:3	tr.	0.5	---	0.4	tr.	1.2	tr.	4.3
20:2	tr.	0.5	tr.	0.3	tr.	1.2	tr.	5.1
20:3	tr.	1.4	---	3.0	tr.	0.8	---	1.8
20:4	15.0	3.7	8.3–17.4	2.7	tr.	0.9	3.3–12.7	4.5
20:5	tr.	1.1	---	0.6	tr.	2.1	---	1.9
22:4	tr.	2.9	---	0.7	tr.	5.1	---	2.8
22:5	tr.	1.0	---	0.3	tr.	1.2	---	1.6
22:6	tr.	0.5	---	0.7	tr.	1.0	---	0.6

All amounts given are % of total. Figures in brackets indicate number of control strains. Culture conditions as indicated in text.

these circumstances.

The metabolism of linoleic acid in fibroblast cultures proceded less rapidly than in brain explants. Only 1.7 to 8.6 percent of radioactivity (mean 3.6 percent) was found in 20:4. The conversion of 18:2 to 20:4 by cultures from Cases 1 and 3 proceded to about the same degree (3.7 and 0.9 percent of total radioactivity, respectively). The amount of radioactivity in 22:4 ranged from 0.8 to 3.3 percent of total radioactivity (mean 1.8 percent) in controls, but was 2.9 and 5.1 percent in Cases 1 and 3 respectively. More significantly, 22:4 was more highly labelled than 20:4 in both patients (Table 5). Since the amount of 22:4 in patients and controls was too low for accurate quantitation using the argon detector, calculations of relative specific activities (R.S.A.) were not possible, except for one experiment with control cultures in which R.S.A.'s of approximately 1.5 and 1.8 were obtained for 20:4 and 22:4, respectively (Table 6).

DISCUSSION

In a study of linoleic acid metabolism in brain explants and fibroblast cultures of patients with late infantile amaurotic idiocy and storage of curvilinear bodies (Batten's disease), preliminary evidence points to a possible disorder in the metabolism of this essential fatty acid.

In the mammalian tissues the conversion of linoleic acid (18:2) to arachidonic acid (20:4) occurs mainly via gamma-linoleic

TABLE 6
RELATIVE SPECIFIC ACTIVITIES
OF FATTY ACIDS IN CONTROL FIBROBLAST CULTURE

Carbon Chain Lengths	Percentage of Total		R.S.A.
	R.A.	Fatty Acids	
16:0	3.5	10.2	0.3
18:0	4.2	15.6	0.3
18:1	0.3	18.9	0.02
18:2	46.5	8.8	5.3
18:3 + 20:0	9.3	6.9	1.3 (1.9)
20:2	1.6	1.1	1.5
20:3	2.6	9.0	0.3
20:4	12.0	7.7	1.5
22:0	2.1	7.1	0.3
22:4	4.4	2.4	1.8

The value in brackets for the R.S.A. of 18:3 + 20:0 assumes no labelling of 20:0. RA= radioactivity, RSA= relative specific activity.

acid (18:3) and its C-$_{20}$ homologue (20:3). In control brain explants the conversion appeared to bypass 18:3, and to procede via 20:2. In both brain and fibroblast cultures patients with Batten's disease converted 18:2 to 20:4 only to a limited extent. In brain explants the difference between patient and control was probably significant. In fibroblast cultures the control tissues also had only limited ability to undertake the linoleic to arachidonic acid conversion. In one fibroblast culture, in which quantitation of intermediates was possible, the conversion of 18:2 to 20:4 did not appear to procede via 20:3, which had a significantly lower relative specific activity than 20:4.

In both brain explants and fibroblast cultures a considerable proportion of the radioactivity added in the form of linoleic acid was found in the 22:4 fatty acid ester fraction. The relative specific activity of 22:4 in brain explants and fibroblast cultures of patients with Batten's disease was higher than that of 20:4, suggesting either that 22:4 was derived by desaturation of 22:3, or that the radioactivity in this fracture is due to another fatty acid. Studies to elucidate this problem are in progress.

Our data may serve as support for a tentative hypothesis concerning the defect in the curvilinear form of Batten's disease. If we assume an inability to metabolize 22:4 or a like dietary derived, long-chain unsaturated fatty acid, these compounds would accumulate to a certain level, then be subject to peroxidation, producing the variety of intracellular inclusions observed in this condition. Studies to obtain support for this hypothesis are in progress.

SUMMARY

Linoleic acid incorporation and metabolism was studied in brain explants and in fibroblast cultures of patients and the results contrast with that obtained from patients with late infantile amaurotic idiocy and curvilinear body storage. Conversion of 18:2 to 20:4 proceded to a greater extent in brain explants than in fibroblast cultures. Patients with Batten's disease showed little conversion of 18:2 to 20:4 in either tissue, but a significant proportion of radioactivity resided in the 22:4 fraction. The relationship of this finding to the symptomatology of Batten's disease is under investigation.

REFERENCES

1. Batten, F.E.: Family cerebral degeneration with macular
    change (so-called juvenile form of family amaurotic idiocy)
    Quart. Journ. Med. 7:444, 1914.

2. Zeman, W., and Donahue, S.: Fine structure of the lipid bodies
    in juvenile amaurotic idiocy. Acta Neuropath. 3:144, 1963.

3. Duffy, P.E., Kornfeld, M. and Suzuki, K.: Neurovisceral storage
    disease with curvilinear bodies. J. Neuropath. Exp. Neurol.
    27:351, 1968.

4. Zeman, W.: Second Conference on Batten's Disease, Proceedings,
    San Francisco, California, January 23, 1971.

5. Hagberg, B., Sourander, P. and Svennerholm, L.: Late infantile
    progressive encephalopathy with disturbed polyunsaturated
    fat metabolism. Acta Paediat. Scand. 57:495, 1968.

6. Andrews, J.M., Sorenson, V., Cancilla, P.A., Price, H.M. and
    Menkes, J.H.: Late infantile neurovisceral storage disease
    with curvilinear bodies. Neurology 21:207, 1971.

7. Menkes, J.H.: Lipid metabolism in brain tissue explants. J.
    Neurochem. 18:1433, 1971.

8. Menkes, J.H.: Lipid metabolism of brain tissue in culture.
    Ciba Foundation Symposium: Lipids and Developing Brain
    London, 1971 (In Press).

9. Fillerup, D.L., Migliore, J.C. and Mead, J.F.: The uptake
    of lipoproteins by ascites tumor cells. J. Biol. Chem.
    233:98, 1958.

10. Tellez-Nagel, I. and Menkes, J.H. (In Preparation).

11. Blass, J.P. and Menkes, J.H. (In Preparation).

12. Gornall, A.G., Bardawill, C.J. and David, M.M.: Determination
    of serum proteins by means of the biuret reaction. J. Biol.
    Chem. 177:751, 1949.

13. Morrison, W.R. and Smith, L.M.: Preparation of fatty acid
    methyl esters and dimethylacetals from lipids with boron
    fluoride-methanol. Journ. Lipid Res. 5:600, 1964.

POPULATION DYNAMICS OF TAY-SACHS DISEASE. II. WHAT CONFERS THE SELECTIVE ADVANTAGE UPON THE JEWISH HETEROZYGOTE?

Ntinos C. Myrianthopoulos and Stanley M. Aronson

National Institute of Neurological Diseases and Stroke, National Institutes of Health, Bethesda, Md., and Miriam Hospital - Brown University, Providence, R. I.

It is now well established that the birth incidence of Tay-Sachs disease (TSD) is a hundred times higher, and the gene frequency ten times higher among Ashkenazi Jews than among other Jewish groups and non-Jewish populations (Goldschmidt et al., 1956, Kozinn et al., 1957, Myrianthopoulos, 1962, Aronson, 1964). The present authors (Myrianthopoulos and Aronson, 1966) examined several possible mechanisms but found no evidence that differential breeding pattern, genetic drift or differential mutation rate could explain the difference in gene frequency distribution. We then tested the possibility of differential fertility of the heterozygote for the TSD gene by comparing the reproductive performance of the grand-parents of a large number of Jewish infants affected with TSD with that of an appropriate control group. The results suggested that the Jewish TSD heterozygote enjoys an overall reproductive advantage of about 6% over the presumed Jewish homozygous normal and that TSD sibships had significantly higher survival to age 21 than did control sibships. This advantage is of more than sufficient magnitude to have raised the frequency of the lethal TSD gene among the Ashkenazi Jews from a presumed frequency equal to that of non-Jews of 0.0013 at the end of the first century A.D. when the mass emigration of the Jews began, through 50 generations to the late 19th century, when TSD was recognized as occurring chiefly among Ashkenazi Jews with a gene frequency of 0.0126.

Our data have recently been re-analyzed by Shaw and Smith (1969) using more precise statistical methodology. These investigators confirmed our results and also suggested that the TSD gene frequency may be increasing. While there is no evidence for this suggestion, the confirmation of our findings provided a further incentive for a search for a selective agent which might have been operating among the east European Ashkenazi communities in the areas where the antecedents of the TSD cases lived for many generations. It would be reasonable to attribute differential survival, and thus increased fitness, to resistance to some adverse situation, e.g. some infectious or chronic disease, conferred by the TSD gene. Unfortunately, because of the recent genocide of the Jewish peoples during the second World War, the destruction of records, and the rapidly changing traditional Jewish way of life it is extremely difficult today to study such disease relationships.

Several bits and pieces of epidemiologic, demographic and medical data, however, made the search for a selective agent feasible. One of them was our demographic study of the east European Ashkenazi communities. Aronson (1964) showed that a greater proportion of antecedents of Jewish TSD cases in the U.S. came from the provinces neighboring upon the Baltic sea, namely the regions of South Lithuania (Kovno) and the adjacent provinces of Suwalki and Grodno, fewer from the Ukrainian and Moldavian regions and very few from the Western Balkan areas or Germany. Thus, some variation in Tay-Sachs frequency, as high as fivefold, existed between Ashkenazi communities of these areas, and this variation was not random but showed a definite geographic trend.

Another useful body of data came from the original questionnaires through which we collected information about the parents and grandparents of our TSD cases. These forms included sections on diseases in the family, deaths and causes of death. We reviewed the questionnaires of those grandparents who had died and for whom there was information on the likely cause of death. There were 306 of these and the stated causes of their deaths are given in Table I. Unfortunately we do not have comparable information from our control group nor is it possible to compute death rates from these figures. It is not difficult to see, however, that of the natural causes of death, cardiovascular and cerebrovascular diseases are the most frequent, followed by cancer, diabetes and respiratory infections, mainly influenza. (A review of the recorded illnesses of the TSD grandparents who are still alive also showed a preponderance of the same diseases.) These figures hold no surprises. Cancer, if anything, is a little more frequent than what one would expect and the distribution of cancer by site (Table II), is in accord with expectation (Krikler, 1970, Seidman, 1970). Diabetes is also high, and in agreement with findings of many studies from various countries (see Krikler, 1970, for review). What is surprising is the virtual absence of deaths due to tuberculosis (TBC), a disease quite prevalent in northeastern Europe, especially during the 19th and early 20th century.

Many early observers have commented on the relative infrequence

TABLE I

CAUSES OF DEATH OF 306 TSD GRANDPARENTS

| | Year of birth | | | | | | |
| | 1861-1885 | | 1886-1900 | | 1901+ | | Total |
	M	F	M	F	M	F	
Cardiovascular disease	28	11	37	24	3	2	105
Cerebrovascular disease	9	4	12	5	3	1	34
Senile cerebral disease	2	3	2	1	1	0	9
Encephalitis	0	0	1	0	0	0	1
Influenza, pneumonia	4	1	5	1	0	0	11
Pulmonary infarction	0	0	0	1	0	0	1
Emphysema	0	0	0	1	0	0	1
Tuberculosis	0	0	0	0	1	0	1
Colitis	0	1	0	0	0	0	1
Nephritis, uremia	1	1	1	2	1	2	8
Cirrhosis	2	1	1	0	0	1	5
Cancer	15	4	10	18	4	4	55
Diabetes	3	2	4	13	0	0	22
Parkinson's disease	0	0	0	1	0	0	1
Multiple sclerosis	0	0	0	1	0	0	1
Anaphylactic shock	0	0	0	0	0	1	1
Intestinal obstruction	0	0	0	0	0	1	1
Psychosis (institutionalized)	0	0	0	3	0	0	3
Post-operative complications	2	2	1	1	0	0	6
Concentration camp	2	0	9	12	3	3	29
Accident	2	0	5	0	0	1	8
Suicide	0	0	2	0	0	0	2
Totals	70	30	90	84	16	16	306

TABLE II

FATAL NEOPLASMS IN 55 TSD GRANDPARENTS

	Male	Female	Total
Cancer, site not specified	15	13	28
Lung	4	2	6
Liver	1	0	1
Breast	0	1	1
Stomach	2	1	3
Kidney	1	0	1
Esophagus	1	0	1
Uterus	0	2	2
Rectum, colon	0	3	3
Skin	0	1	1
Leukemia	4	0	4
Lymphoma	0	1	1
Myeloma	0	1	1
Brain tumor	1	1	2
Totals	29	26	55

of TBC among Jews and as early as 1928 Sir Humphry Rolleston drew attention to the fact that

> "the comparative resistance of the Jews to tuberculosis,
> in spite of adverse environment, life in towns, their
> narrow chest measurement which would be thought to
> dispose them to the disease, and their special liability
> to diabetes which may terminate with pulmonary tuberculosis,
> has been proved by statistics from various parts of the
> world by showing that their mortality rate is lower
> than that of their gentile neighbors."

A third source of most helpful information was the availability of medical records of a large number of Jewish TBC patients at the American Medical Center at Denver. It became possible now to test the hypothesis of TSD heterozygote resistance to TBC, albeit indirectly, by comparing the distribution of places of origin of the TSD grandparents with that of a group of patients with pulmonary TBC who also came from eastern Europe.

The American Medical Center at Denver was founded in 1904 as
the Jewish Consumptives' Relief Agency and for many years served as
a sanatorium for Jewish patients suffering mainly from pulmonary
TBC. Through the courtesy of its Director, Dr. Samuel Levine, we
were given access to the patients' records for the purpose of as-
certaining their place of origin from which they emigrated to the
United States. Patients were included in the study if they had
pulmonary TBC; were born outside the United States between 1860 and
1910 (a period during which most of the TSD grandparents and controls
were born); emigrated to the United States not later than 1920, i.e.
before x-ray evidence indicating absence of pulmonary TBC was required
by the immigration authorities; and if the town, city or region of
their birth could be identified from the record.

After a long and tedious search, 1466 records were selected as
satisfying all of these criteria. A large number of records **was**
excluded because the place of origin was not recorded or it referred
to very general geographic regions, such as Poland or Russia. It
is not possible to say how the exclusion of these records affected
the distribution of places of origin of the TBC patients. This
shortcoming may have been compensated for, or been compounded, by
the fact that a large number of TSD grandparents and of controls
had also been excluded from the distribution for the same reason.

In a considerable number of records, though the place of origin
was given, it could not be identified on present-day maps of these
areas. This is not surprising, for since the 1900's the geographic
boundaries of the northeastern European nations have been rather
fluid and the names of many towns and villages have changed more
than once. The situation was rescued with the aid of old gazetteers
and the help of the geographic divisions of the Department of the
Interior and the Library of Congress which provided us with the old
and new names of hundreds of villages and towns of northeastern
Europe. In some instances the place of origin could not be identified even after this exhaustive search. These records have also
been excluded.

Table III shows the distribution of TSD grandparents, TBC
patients and our original controls, by region of origin. (For
selection of TSD grandparents and controls see Myrianthopoulos and
Aronson, 1966.) There were 618 TSD grandparents, 1466 TBC patients
and 1675 controls. It should be remembered that a greater proportion
of the TSD ancestors came from the Baltic provinces than did the
ancestors of the non-TSD controls and that the reverse was true in
the southern regions. We tried, therefore, to assign these regions
into groups which would reflect, more or less, a north-south
gradient. One, of course, could take issue with these groupings but
there is no easy way of resolving the question of what region should
go into what group. We tried to take into account the possible

TABLE III

DISTRIBUTION OF TSD GRANDPARENTS, TBC PATIENTS
AND CONTROLS BY REGION OF ORIGIN

REGION	TSD		TBC		CONTROL	
	No.	%	No.	%	No.	%
Baltic provinces, NE Poland (Latvia, Suwalki, Kovno, Grodno)	146	23.6	122	8.3	204	12.2
NW Poland (Poznan, Silesia, Plock, Kalisz, Piotrkow)	32	5.2	6	0.4	40	2.4
North Central Russia (Byelorussia, Vilno, Wolyn)	103	16.7	196	13.4	316	18.9
Central SE Poland (Warsaw, Siedlce, Lublin, Lomzo, Radom, Kielce)	42	6.8	58	3.9	121	7.2
South Russia (Ukraine)	84	13.6	167	11.4	262	15.6
Galicia (Lwow, Krakow)	56	9.1	44	3.0	124	7.4
Rumania (Bucovina, Bessarabia, Moldavia)	42	6.8	187	12.8	150	8.9
Austria	22	3.5	351	23.9	91	5.4
Hungary	27	4.4	171	11.7	110	6.6
C. Europe (including Czechoslovakia, Germany)	60	9.7	155	10.6	236	14.1
Mediterranean	4	0.6	9	0.6	21	1.3
Totals	618	100.0	1466	100.0	1675	100.0

TSD-TBC heterogeneity X^2_{10} = 317.7, p $<$ 0.0005

$R_{CONT-TBC}$ = 0.261

$R_{TSD-TBC}$ = $-$ 0.181

variations in geographic names determined by historical events: thus Rumania, Bucovina, Bessaravia and Moldavia are all grouped together; similarly the neighboring province of Ukraine, which at one time may have incorporated a portion of Moldavia, is listed separately but next to the Rumanian group; Austria, which may have variously signified Rumania, Hungary, Austria, South Poland, Galicia or Lwow, has also been grouped in proximity to these variants. As it turns out, the TSD/Control ratio in the Kovno-Grodno region and Western Poland is approximately 2 and decreases gradually with the geographic gradient to 0.68 in Western Europe and 0.51 in the Mediterranean area.

We can now compare the distribution of places of origin of the TBC patients with that of the TSD grandparents and the controls. It is evident at a glance that the TSD and TBC data came from different populations. A heterogeneity test yields a chi-square of 317.7 and the probability of obtaining such a high chi-square if the data in these groupings came from the same populations is infinitesimal.

The first comparison is by means of rank correlation, a statistic which relates two sets of data, in this case our geographic groupings, on a hierarchical scale rather than on the basis of scores but does not take into account the magnitude of the differences. The rank correlation between the Control and the TBC data is 0.261 which means that the occurrence of TBC is higher with increasing population (Control) frequency. The rank correlation, however, between the TSD and the TBC data is negative, − 0.181 and, though small, it indicates that the frequency of TBC decreases with increasing TSD frequency, and vice versa. We hasten to warn that both correlations are too small to be significant and only suggest trends; besides, the observed linear relationship may not be meaningful since the TSD and TBC data are based on indirect estimates and not on actual prevalence figures for these diseases in each region.

A simpler and more meaningful way of examining the data is by grouping them in three major geographic groups representing the Northern, Central and Southern regions. This is shown in Table IV. As with the previous grouping, the heterogeneity is again enormous. But now it is clearly evident that TBC is almost 3 times higher in the Southern region where the TSD frequency is the lowest, than in the Northern region where the TSD frequency is the highest.

These results are consistent with the hypothesis of resistance to TBC on the part of the Jewish TSD carrier. We are very much aware of the fact that our data may be inadequate and unrepresentative and that the demonstrated negative correlation, so elegant in its simplicity, may well be spurious. We present, therefore, our data and results modestly and cautiously, with the suggestion that

TABLE IV

DISTRIBUTION OF TSD GRANDPARENTS AND TBC

PATIENTS IN THREE NORTH-SOUTH GEOGRAPHIC GROUPS

GEOGRAPHIC GROUP	TSD		TSD/CONT. ratio	TBC		TSD/TBC ratio
	No.	%		No.	%	
Northern	281	45.5	1.5	324	22.1	2.0
Central	182	29.4	0.9	269	18.4	1.6
Southern	155	25.1	0.7	873	59.5	0.4
Totals	618	100.0		1466	100.0	

$$x_2^2 = 221.1, \quad p < 0.0005$$

the hypothesis could be experimentally tested in a variety of ways. We would like, however, to add one further comment.

Aronson (1964) drew attention to the fact that while the TSD incidence in American or Israeli descendants of north Polish-Russian Jews is relatively high, there is nothing in the reports of European neurologists interested in the disease to indicate that the TSD incidence was also high in Jewish children born in the same regions of Poland and Russia. This discrepancy was noted even before the turn of the century and as one investigator observed, it seemed as though the disease waited until the carriers emigrated to America or England before appearing. Kowarski (1912) attributed this discrepancy largely to lack of recognition of the disease by local physicians. But it is peculiar that from 1890 until the destruction of the East European Jewish communities during the second World War, no medical report appeared from these northeastern European regions indicating anything other than occasional isolated cases of TSD.

Aronson suggested as remotely conceivable the possibility that the proportion of TSD carriers in the emigrating Jewish populations was higher than the proportion among those who did not emigrate. This explanation would actually be in line with the hypothesis of carrier resistance to TBC. During the early years of migrations only healthy and vigorous individuals, capable of withstanding the hardships and deprivations of a long journey to a new world, were able to emigrate; and later, when a health law required x-ray evidence of absence of pulmonary disease of all immigrants, only those providing such evidence were admitted to the United States. Presumably, among the immigrant Polish-Russian Jews a large proportion was free of pulmonary disease because they were carriers of the gene for TSD.

ACKNOWLEDGEMENTS

We gratefully acknowledge the help and cooperation of the Director and staff of the American Medical Center at Denver, and the manifold assistance of Dr. Herman Slatis and Mrs. Blanche Vincent.

REFERENCES

1. Aronson, S.M. Epidemiology. In Tay-Sachs' Disease. B.W. Volk ed., New York, Grune & Stratton, 1964, pp. 118-153.

2. Goldschmidt, E., Lenz, R., Merin, S. Ronen, A. and Ronen, I. The frequency of the Tay-Sachs gene in the Jewish communities of Israel. Abstract, 25th Annual Meeting of Genetics Society of America, 1956.

3. Kowarski, H. Sechs Fälle von Idiotica amaurotica progressiva familiaris infantilis. Arch. f. Kinderheilk. 76:59, 1912.

4. Kozinn, P.J., Wiener, H. and Cohen, P. Infantile amaurotic family idiocy. J. Pediat. 51:58, 1957.

5. Krikler, D.M. Diseases of the Jews. Postgrad. Med. J. 46: 687, 1970.

6. Myrianthopoulos, N.C. Some epidemiologic and genetic aspects of Tay-Sachs' disease. In Cerebral Sphingolipidoses: A Symposium on Tay-Sachs' Disease and Allied Disorders. S.M. Aronson and B.W. Volk eds., New York, Academic Press, 1962, pp. 359-374.

7. Myrianthopoulos, N.C. and Aronson, S.M. Population dynamics of Tay-Sachs disease. I. Reproductive fitness and selection. Amer. J. Hum. Genet. 18:313, 1966.

8. Rolleston, H. Some diseases of the Jewish race. Bull. Johns Hopkins Hosp. 43:117, 1928.

9. Seidman, H. Cancer death rates by site and sex for religious and socioeconomic groups in New York City. Environ. Res. 3:234, 1970.

10.   Shaw, R.F. and Smith, A.P.   Is Tay-Sachs disease increasing?
      Nature 224:1214, 1969.

EFFECT OF MATERNAL PROTEIN DEFICIENCY ON GANGLIOSIDE METABOLISM IN NEONATAL RAT BRAIN*

Robert S. Tyzbir and Joel A. Dain

Department of Biochemistry, University of Rhode Island

Kingston, Rhode Island   02881

Malnutrition induced by a severe dietary protein deprivation in early life can retard subsequent neurological development in both humans and experimental animals (1). Although several laboratories have demonstrated that protein undernutrition in the newborn decreases the lipid, phospholipid, cerebroside and DNA content of brain (2-6) as well as retard sulfatide synthesis (7), little attention has been devoted to the effects of protein undernutrition on ganglioside metabolism. Today I am going to discuss some effects on weanling rat brain ganglioside metabolism of severe maternal protein deprivation prior to and during gestation and lactation. Specifically, I will report the effects on the gangliosides, a representative ganglioside biosynthetic enzyme, UDP-galactose: G_{M2} galactosyl transferase and a representative ganglioside degradative enzyme, neuraminidase.

Maternal Protein Deficiency

Rats of the Sprague Dawley strain were given free access to the synthetic diet (8). The control diet contained 22% casein and the

---

*This work was supported in part by grant No. NS-05104 from the National Institute of Neurological diseases and Stroke, National Institutes of Health, U.S. Public Health Service. The authors would like to thank Dr. Henry A. Dymsza of the Department of Food and Nutritional Science at the University of Rhode Island for his suggestions on the formulation of the diets.

Abbreviations: Individual ganglioside abbreviations are those proposed by Svennerholm (23).

deficient diet containing 8% casein was made isocaloric to the
controls by increasing the sugar concentrations. Two groups of
adult female rats which had reared at least one litter were fed
either the control or the deficient diet ad libitum for a minimum
of one month. At the end of this time, rats from each group were
mated with adult rats fed a commercial laboratory ration. After
birth, the pups were nursed in litters of eight, weaned at 21
days and fed the same diet as their dam ad libitum. Maternal protein deficiency prior to and during gestation and lactation had
little effect on the birth weight of the newborn rat (Fig. 1) when
compared to the control. At 7 days the differences became

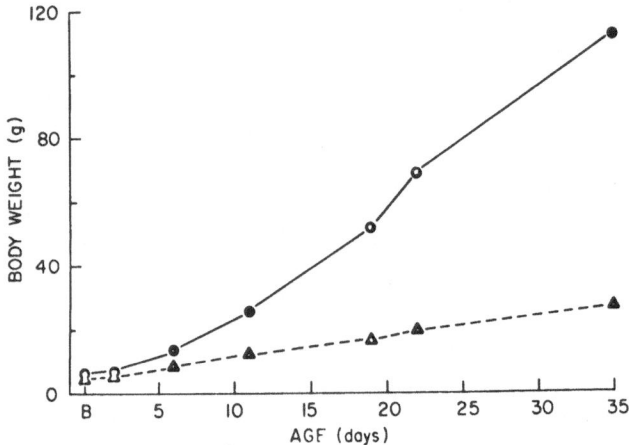

Fig. 1. Effect of maternal protein deficiency prior to and during
gestation and lactation on total body weight as a function of age
in days, Control, _____, deprived, _ _ _ _.

noticeable and appeared more dramatic with increasing age until at
35 days the deprived weighed only 23.5% of the controls. Brain
weight was slightly decreased at birth (Fig. 2), but as the animals
aged, it was not as severely affected as total body weight indicating a "sparing effect" on the brain at the expense of the
rest of the body. One possible reason for the drastic differences
in body weight between the deprived pups and the controls during
development may be the effect protein restriction has on the
quantity of milk produced (9). Another reason may be the inability
of deprived pups to suckle sufficiently to maintain the flow of
milk from the dam.

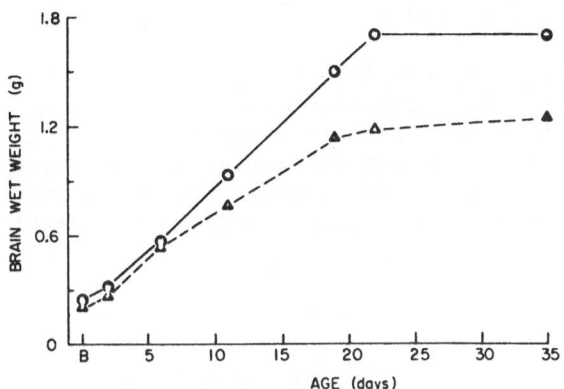

Fig. 2. Effect of maternal protein deficiency prior to and during gestation and lactation on brain wet weight as a function of age in days. Control, _____, deprived, _ _ _ _.

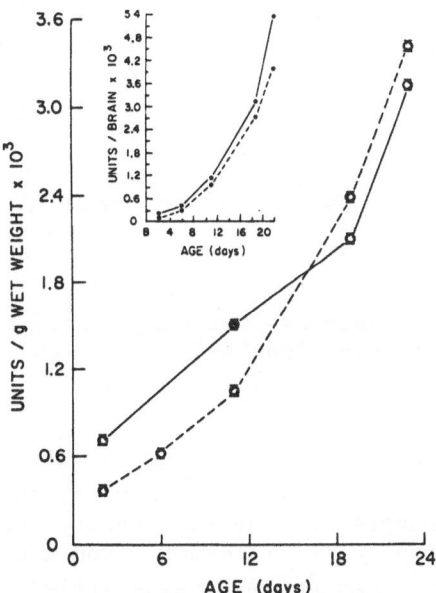

Fig. 3. Acetylcholinesterase activity expressed as units per gram wet weight of brain or per whole brain (insert) as a function of age in days. The method of Ellman et al. (13) was used in the assay. Control _____, deprived _ _ _ _.

Acetylcholinesterase

Acetylcholinesterase was chosen as a developmental marker enzyme because , along with the gangliosides (10) and two ganglioside biosynthetic enzymes (11, 12),it is concentrated in synaptic membranes. The developmental profile obtained (Fig. 3) showed no apparent differences between acetylcholinesterase activity in the control and deprived rat brain.

UDP-Galactose: G_{M2} Galactosyltransferase

UDP-galactose: G_{M2} galactosyltransferase (Reaction 4 of Scheme 1) has been demonstrated in chick (14), rat (12, 15, 16) and frog (17, 18) brain. Competition studies in our laboratory (12) with the substrates G_{M2} and Cer-Glc-Gal-GalNAc of reactions 4 and 6 respectively suggested that both reactions are catalyzed by the

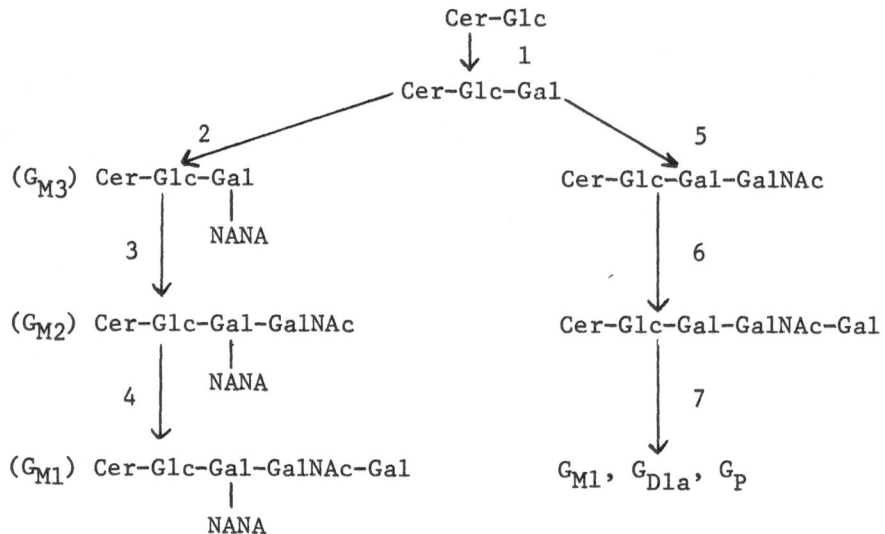

Scheme 1. Proposed pathways for ganglioside biosynthesis. Reactions 2-4 (14), Reactions 5-7 (19).

same galactosyltransferase. This enzyme activity is representative of the two pathways in Scheme 1. In contrast, these same types of competition studies suggested that the N-acetyl-galactosaminyl-transferase in reaction 3 is different from the one in reaction 5. The UDP-galactose: G_{M2} galactosyltransferase activity rose postnatally from birth to eleven days (Figure 4) and then declined slightly. The developmental profile in the protein deprived rats was similar to that of the controls and at twenty-two days the activity of both groups was the same. When the results are

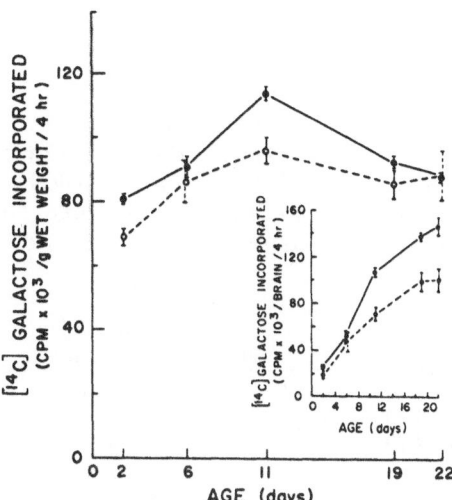

Fig. 4. The activity of UDP-galactose: G_{M2} galactosyltransferase
expressed as a function of gram wet weight of brain or whole brain
(insert). Each value represents the mean ± S.D. The assay has
been described (14,16) control, _____, deprived _ _ _ _.

expressed as (^{14}C) galactose incorporated per brain (Fig. 3, insert)
the galactosyltransferase activity increased steadily to 22 days
postpartum. The decrease in activity noted in deprived rats is
really a reflection of brain weight. We conclude that protein
deprivation has no significant effect on UDP-galactose: G_{M2}
galactosyltransferase activity in young rat brain.

Gangliosides from Control and Deprived Rats
     Ganglioside was isolated by the "Folch" (20) procedure from
brains of 35 day old control and deprived rats and NANA content
determined. The two experiments in Table 1 show that the
gangliosides isolated from the deprived rat brains were significantly
richer in NANA than the controls in both experiments. The NANA
was determined after acid hydrolysis by the Warren method (21). The
same conclusion was reached when the ganglioside in Experiment 2 of
Table 1 was treated with neuraminidase preparations (8) from three
different adult rat brains (Table 2). With each preparation, the
NANA released per mg protein per hour was significantly greater with
the deprived ganglioside preparation than with the control. We then
proceded to separate our mixed ganglioside preparations into their
components to determine which specie or species of ganglioside
was responsible for the increased NANA.

Table 1. N-acetylneuraminic acid content of gangliosides isolated
from deprived and control rat brains. The procedure of Warren
(21) was used after hydrolysis of the gangliosides with 0.1 N
H_2SO_4 for 2 hours at 80°. In the parentheses are the number of
pooled rat brains used in that experiment.

			nmoles NANA/ mg ganglioside	% control
Experiment 1	Control	(3)	305[1]	
	Deprived	(2)	367[1,2]	121
Experiment 2	Control	(10)	316[1]	
	Deprived	(10)	357[1,2]	113

[1]Mean of four determinations

[2]Significantly different from control, PL 0.01.

Table 2. Release of NANA from the ganglioside preparations used
in Experiment 2, Table 1 by neuraminidase. The enzyme source was
a 20,000 x g rat brain homogenate supernatent. Each assay tube (8)
contained 125 μg ganglioside, 0.65 mg protein, 20 n moles sodium
acetate-acetic acid buffer (pH 5.5) in a final volume of 0.2 ml.
Free NANA was determined after a one hour incubation at 37° by
the Warren method (21).

Rat brain	n moles NANA/ mg protein/hr Control	Deprived	% Control
1	7.55	9.70	128.5
2	6.62	7.54	114.0
3	7.23	7.84	108.5

[1]Mean ± Standard Deviation

Individual Ganglioside Patterns

Control and deprived ganglioside preparations (Experiment 2 of Table 1) were resolved into individual ganglioside species by ascending TLC with $CHCl_3-CH_3OH-2.5$ N NH_4OH (60:35:8 by vol) as the developing solvent and each ganglioside determined by the procedure of Suzuki (22). Both preparations contained the same amount of the monosialoganglioside G_{M1} and no heroic increase in any single major or minor ganglioside was noted. We did find that "NANA rich" gangliosides, G_{D1a}, G_{D1b} and G_{T1} were increased an average of 20% in the deprived over the control. We then proceeded to test the hypothesis that the increase in "NANA rich" species of ganglioside in the deprived could be due to a decreased ganglioside neuraminidase level.

Ganglioside Neuraminidase in Developing Rat Brain

Brain ganglioside neuraminidase activity increased slowly during the first week after birth in the young of control and protein deprived dams (Fig. 5). In both groups activity increased sharply

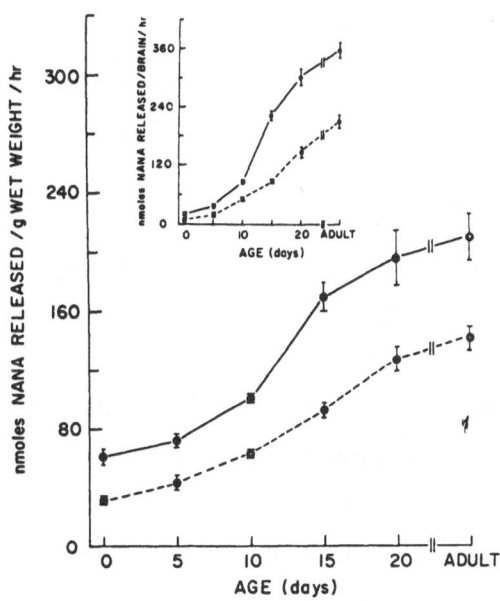

Fig. 5. Neuraminidase activity expressed as n moles NANA released per gram wet weight of brain or per whole brain (insert). Control, _____, deprived, _ _ _ _. Each value represents the mean ± S.D. The assay is described in the legend of Table 2, with the exception that bovine, instead of rat brain gangliosides, were used as substrate.

the beginning of the second week and approached the adult level by
the beginning of the third week. It must be emphasized that the
undernourished group had a neuraminidase activity at birth which
was 50% of the control and increased in the adult to 67% of the
control value. The decrease in neuraminidase activity in the
deprived is amplified when expressed as n moles NANA released
per brain per hour (Fig. 5 insert). This decrease in neuraminidase
activity in the deprived rat is probably reflected in our observed
increase in "NANA rich" gangliosides.

Conclusion

We would like to present our conclusions in the form of the
following question: Does the increase in the "NANA rich"
gangliosides and the decrease in ganglioside neuraminidase in the
protein deprived weanling rat brain induced by a severe maternal
protein deprivation represent a type of Sphingolipidoses?

References

1. M.B. STOCK and P.M. SMYTHE, in "Malnutrition, Learning and
        Behavior" (N.S. SCRIMSHAW and J.E. GORDON, Eds.), p.278.
        M.I.T. Press, Cambridge, Mass. (1968).

2. J. DOBBING, Ibid. p. 181.

3. W.J. CULLEY and R.O. LINEBERGER, J. Nutr. 96, 375 (1968).

4. N.J. BASS, M.G. NETSKY and E.Y. YOUNG, Arch, Neurol. 23, 289
        (1970).

5. R.L. GEISON and H.A. WAISMAN, J. Nutr. 100, 315 (1970).

6. S. ZAMENHOF, E. VAN MARTHENS and F.L. MARGOLIS, Science 160,
        322 (1968).

7. H.P. CHASE, J. DORSEY and G.M. MCKHANN, Pediatrics 40, 551
        (1967).

8. R.S. TYZBIR, "The Effect of Maternal Protein Deficiency on
        Ganglioside Accumulation in the Young Rat Brain," Ph.D.
        Thesis, University of Rhode Island, 1972.

9. J. PERISSE and E. SALMON-LEGAGNEUR, Arch. Sci. Physiol. 14,
        105 (1960).

10. E.G. LAPETINA, E.F. SOTO and E. DEROBERTIS, Biochim. Biophys. Acta. 135, 33 (1960).

11. J.L. DICESARE and JOEL A. DAIN, Biochim. Biophys. Acta 231, 385 (1971).

12. J.L. DICESARE and JOEL A. DAIN, J. Neurochem. In press (1972).

13. G.L. ELLMAN, K. G. COURTNEY, U. ANDRES and R.M. FEATHERSTONE, Biochem. Pharmacol. 1, 88 (1961).

14. S. BASU, B. KAUFMAN and S. ROSEMAN, J. Biol. Chem. 240, 4116 (1965).

15. J. HILDEBRAND, P. STOFFYN and G. HAUSER, J. Neurochem. 17, 403 (1970).

16. G.B. YIP and J.A. DAIN, Biochim. Biophys. Acta. 206, 252 (1970).

17. J.A. YIAMOUYIANNIS and J.A. DAIN, Lipids 3, 378 (1968).

18. M.C.M. YIP and J.A. DAIN, Biochem. J., 118, 247 (1970).

19. M.C.M. YIP and J.A. DAIN, Lipids 4, 270 (1969).

20. J. FOLCH, M. LEES and G.H. SLOANE-STANLEY, J. Biol. Chem 226, 497 (1957).

21. L. WARREN, J. Biol. Chem. 234, 1971 (1959).

22. K. SUZUKI, Life Sci., 3, 1227 (1964).

23. L. SVENNERHOLM, J. Lipid Res. 5, 149 (1964).

SPHINGOLIPIDOSES:

DETECTION OF HETEROZYGOTES AND HOMOZYGOTES

O'Brien, J.S., Ho, M.W., Okada, S., Zielke, K.,
Veath, M.L. and Tennant, L.

Department of Neurosciences, University of
California at San Diego School of Medicine,
La Jolla, California

INTRODUCTION

Recent progress has made it possible to detect homozygotes and heterozygotes for many of the sphingolipidoses by assays of specific enzymes in tissues and body fluids. These assays are of importance in the differentiation of disorders which are phenotypically similar. They are also of importance in detecting heterozygous family members for accurate genetic counselling. Finally, these assays provide a means for the prenatal diagnosis of affected fœtuses in utero in many instances. In this presentation we discuss enzyme assay for the diagnosis of homozygotes and detection of heterozygotes in Tay-Sachs disease, Sandhoff's disease, juvenile GM_2 gangliosidosis, juvenile GM_1 gangliosidosis, chronic Gaucher's disease, Fabry's disease, and fucosidosis.

Tay-Sachs Disease: The discovery of the absence of hexosaminidase A in tissues and body fluids of patients with Tay-Sachs disease (12) has made it possible to use enzyme assays to detect homozygotes for this disorder. The enzyme defect is present in all tissues and body fluids examined from patients with Tay-Sachs disease. One of the most useful diagnostic tests is serum hexosaminidase assay by the method we published previously (9). The results of our most recent experience are shown in Figure 1 in which 24 patients with Tay-Sachs disease were studied. The small activity for hexosaminidase A in the serum of these patients is very likely due to artefact in the heat denaturation test, since by starch gel electrophoresis and iso-electric focusing we are unable to detect activity for hexosaminidase A in this disease.

The serum assay has been useful to us in the clinical

diagnosis of Tay-Sachs disease, especially in atypical cases without cherry red spots, in non-Jewish patients and in the differentiation of Tay-Sachs disease from infantile Gaucher's disease,
metachromatic leucodystrophy, Niemann-Pick disease, Batten-
Spielmeyer-Vogt disease and Sandhoff's disease. We have reported
(10) that the enzyme is absent in serum from a Tay-Sachs fetus as
early as 18 weeks gestation.

Obligate heterozygotes have nearly normal values for serum
hexosaminidase B but reductions in the activity of hexosaminidase
A (Figure 1). Thusfar, we have carried out serum assays in 56
parents of Tay-Sachs children and compared their activity with 77
control subjects. The results demonstrate a small degree of overlap between heterozygotes and controls, which amounts to about 5%
of the controls and 5% of the heterozygotes. When subjects which
fall in the "indeterminate zone" are retested, the overlap diminishes to less than 1%.

We have found serum assay to be of great value in detecting
heterozygotes in families in which the disease has appeared. We
have carried out serum enzyme assays in 44 relatives of probands,
including grandparents, uncles and aunts, first cousins, and siblings. As can be seen (Fig. 1), 14 of these had activity of the
enzyme in the normal range and 30 had activity of the enzyme in
the range for heterozygotes. The mean and range of activity of the
enzyme in serum from presumptive heterozygotes is nearly identical
to the mean and range of activity of the enzyme in serum from obligate heterozygotes. This underscores the usefulness of the assay
for heterozygote detection. Thusfar, the proportion of heterozygotes among relatives is close to that expected for autosomal recessive inheritance, although the total number tested is still small.

In the past we demonstrated that hexosaminidase A is markedly
deficient in skin fibroblasts grown from many cellular generations
from patients with Tay-Sachs disease (13) (Fig. 2). We also demonstrated that cultured skin fibroblasts from heterozygotes have
intermediate reductions of hexosaminidase A throughout all stages
of a 30 day growth period after subculture (13). A large differential is apparent when the enzyme values obtained from controls,
heterozygotes, and affected patients are compared. We demonstrated
that the enzyme is present in normal cultured amniotic cells (12),
an indication that the prenatal diagnosis of Tay-Sachs disease is
possible by hexosaminidase A assay. We have monitored 24 pregnancies for Tay-Sachs disease by amniocentesis and assays of the
enzyme in amniotic fluid, uncultured amniotic cells, and cultured
amniotic cells as described previously (10) (Fig. 3). All subjects
were women who had one or more affected children with Tay-Sachs
disease, each with a 25% recurrence risk. Amniocentesis was carried
out between 16 and 18 weeks of pregnancy in most cases. Ten to 20
milliliters of amniotic fluid was obtained by sterile transabdominal

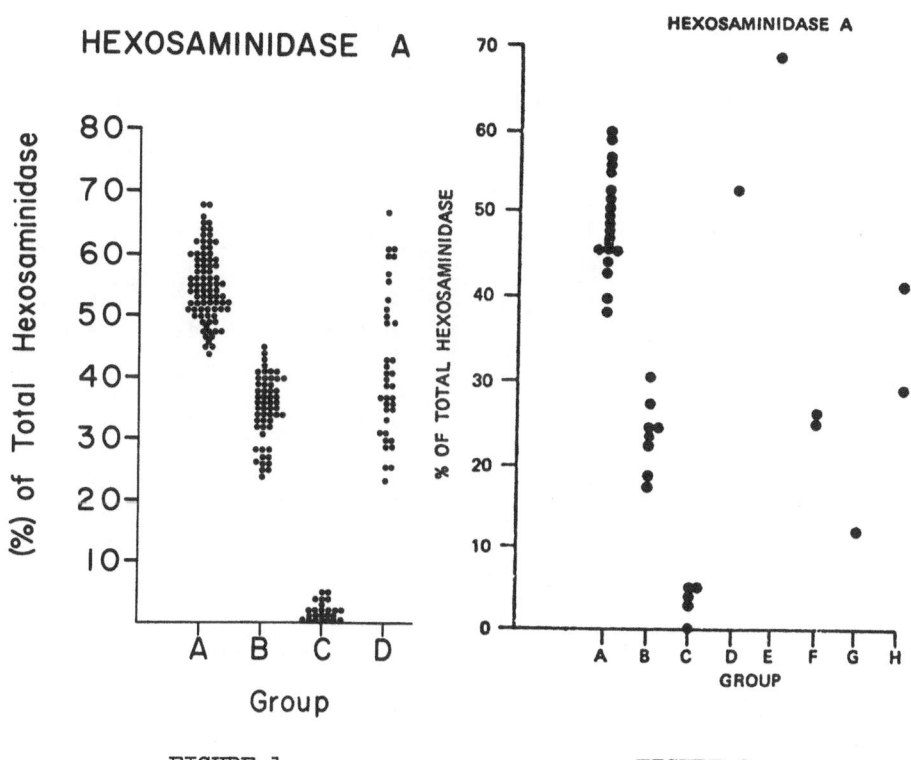

FIGURE 1

FIGURE 2

FIGURE 1: Activity of hexosaminidase A in serum from control subjects (A), parents of patients with Tay-Sachs disease (B), patients with Tay-Sachs disease (C) and relatives of probands (D).

FIGURE 2: Hexosaminidase A activity in skin fibroblasts three weeks or more after subculture, expressed as percent of total hexosaminidase. Values given are from controls (A), parents of children with Tay-Sachs disease (B), children with Tay-Sachs disease (C), patient with Sandhoff's disease (D), parent of child with Sandhoff's disease (E), parents of child with juvenile GM_2 gangliosidosis (F), child with juvenile GM_2 gangliosidosis (G), and her siblings (H). From Okada et al, 1971 (13).

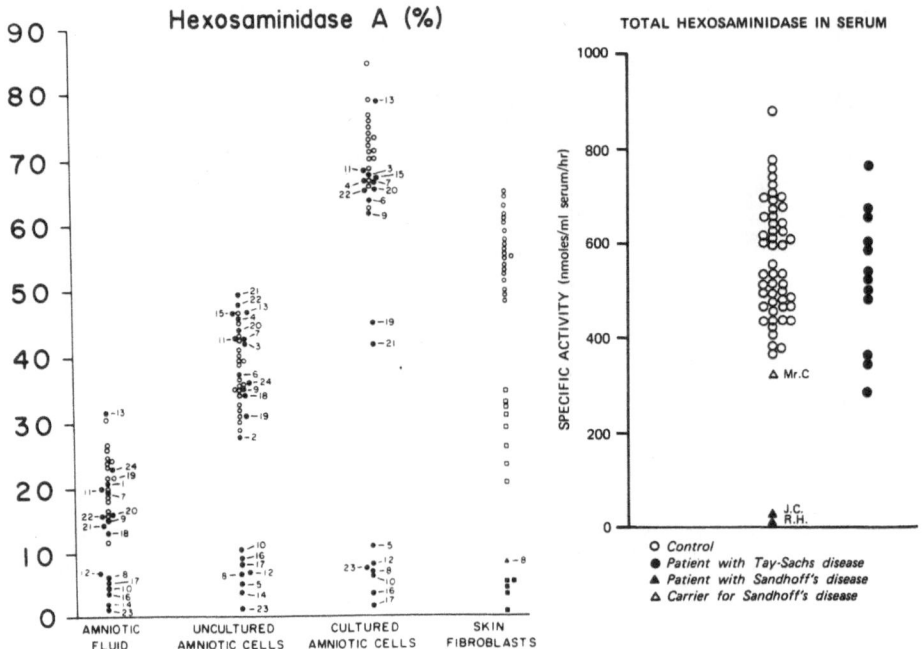

FIGURE 3:   Hexosaminidase A activity in high-risk pregnancies
            expressed as percent of total hexosaminidase. Values
            from the 24 high-risk pregnancies (closed circles) are
            compared with controls (open circles). Values from
            cultured skin fibroblasts from patients with Tay-Sachs
            disease (closed squares), their parents (open squares),
            controls (open circles), and an affected fetus with
            Tay-Sachs disease (case 8, closed diamond) are also
            shown.

FIGURE 4:   Total hexosaminidase (β-D-N-acetylglucosaminidase)
            activity in serum in Sandhoff's disease. Assayed as
            described previously (9).

TABLE 1

PRENATAL DIAGNOSIS OF TAY-SACHS (AUG. 1971)
      (BOTH PARENTS HETEROZYGOUS)

NUMBER MONITORED   24

HOMOZYGOTES   8

    ABORTED   7 (6 analyzed and diagnosis
                      confirmed, 1 still waiting
                      analysis)

    1 MONITORED TOO LATE (27 weeks),
    NOW 16 MONTHS, HAS TSD

NOT TAY-SACHS   16

    BORN   11 (All have adequate HEX A)

    IN UTERO   5

All diagnoses made by assays of amniotic fluid,
    uncultured cells and cultured cells.

technique. Amniotic fluid and uncultured amniotic cells were
assayed within days after the amniocentesis. Cultured amniotic
cells were assayed within two weeks to four weeks after growth in
tissue culture.

We diagnosed Tay-Sachs disease prenatally in eight of the 24
pregnancies. In each the results on amniotic fluid, uncultured
amniotic cells, and cultured amniotic cells agreed with respect to
the presence or absence of Tay-Sachs disease since marked deficiencies of the enzyme were found in each sample. The results obtained
on cultured amniotic cells and on uncultured amniotic cells were
more reliable than those in amniotic fluid due to a larger spread
of values between affected homozygotes and controls. In seven of
the eight cases, amniocentesis was carried out early enough to
safely terminate the pregnancy and these pregnancies were terminated.

The diagnosis of Tay-Sachs disease was confirmed in each fetus
by electron microscopy, ganglioside analysis, and enzyme assays
(10). In one instance amniocentesis was carried out at 27 weeks of
pregnancy, too late for safe termination. Hexosaminidase assay
indicated an affected girl and the prenatal diagnosis of Tay-Sachs
disease was made. This girl, now 16 months old, has bilateral
cherry-red spots, mental and motor deterioration, and absent
hexosaminidase A in serum, confirming the diagnosis of Tay-Sachs
disease.

In the remaining 16 pregnancies, prenatal assessment indicated the absence of Tay-Sachs disease. This was confirmed postnatally in all 11 infants who have been born by clinical examinations and enzyme assays of leucocytes, cultured skin fibroblasts,
or serum. Five fetuses have yet to be born. The summary of our
collected experiences with the prenatal diagnosis of Tay-Sachs
disease is presented in Table 1.

Sandhoff's Disease (GM$_2$ gangliosidosis Type II). We use the
term "Sandhoff's disease" for the disorder involving massive storage of ganglioside GM$_2$, GA$_2$ and globoside and absence of both
hexosaminidase A and B (15). In our experience thusfar, nine non-
Jewish families have been referred to us for the diagnosis of Tay-
Sachs disease. Sandhoff's disease was the diagnosis in four of
these families. Thusfar, we have not encountered Sandhoff's disease in Jewish families. In the non-Jewish population the incidence
of Sandhoff's disease may actually be equal to the incidence of
Tay-Sachs disease. Studies of a much larger population will be
necessary to ascertain its true frequency. In the experience of
one of us (J.S.O.) Sandhoff's disease is clinically identical to
Tay-Sachs disease with regards to the presence of cherry-red spots,
time of onset, absence of hepatosplenomegaly, rate and type of
neurological deterioration, progressive development of macrocephaly

and doll-like facial appearance.

The simplest and most reliable way to differentiate the two disorders is by enzyme assay. A striking deficiency of total hexosaminidase occurs in the serum of children with Sandhoff's disease which clearly differentiates them from Tay-Sachs disease (Fig. 4).

The serum assay is not reliable for the detection of hetero-zygotes for the gene for Sandhoff's disease. The variability and activity of total hexosaminidase from one subject to the other is too large. However, assays of total hexosaminidase in cultured skin fibroblasts from obligate heterozygotes for Sandhoff's dis-ease gives activity of the enzyme which is intermediate between controls and homozygotes (13) (Fig. 5). This then appears to be a reliable way to detect the heterozygote.

Since the enzyme defect persists in cultured skin fibroblasts over many cellular generations, it is likely that the prenatal diag-nosis of Sandhoff's disease is feasible. Thusfar, no homozygotes have been detected in utero. We have diagnosed one normal fetus by amniocentesis and enzyme assay; this was confirmed postnatally (Fig. 5).

Juvenile GM_2 Gangliosidosis. In 1969 we reported the partial deficiency of hexosaminidase A in juvenile GM_2 gangliosidosis (8) and this has been confirmed by others (16,18). The defect can be demonstrated in serum from homozygotes (13). The activity of the enzyme in the homozygote is clearly higher than the activity in serum from patients with Tay-Sachs disease, but it is considerably lower than controls or heterozygotes. This test becomes an impor-tant clinical means to differentiate juvenile GM_2 gangliosidosis from related juvenile lipidoses such as Batten-Spielmeyer-Vogt disease and juvenile GM_1 gangliosidosis.

The defect in juvenile GM_2 gangliosidosis also persists in cultured skin fibroblasts (13) and obligate heterozygotes have an intermediate reduction of the enzyme both in serum and in cultured skin fibroblasts (Fig. 2). In fact the degree of hexosaminidase reduction puts them within the range for obligate heterozygotes for Tay-Sachs disease. On the basis of activity measurements alone it is impossible to distinguish heterozygotes for juvenile GM_2 ganglio-sidosis from those for Tay-Sachs disease. More sophisticated means will be necessary to detect differences between the carrier states for the two diseases.

We have monitored one pregnancy for juvenile GM_2 gangliosi-dosis and predicted an unaffected girl. This prediction was con-firmed postnatally.

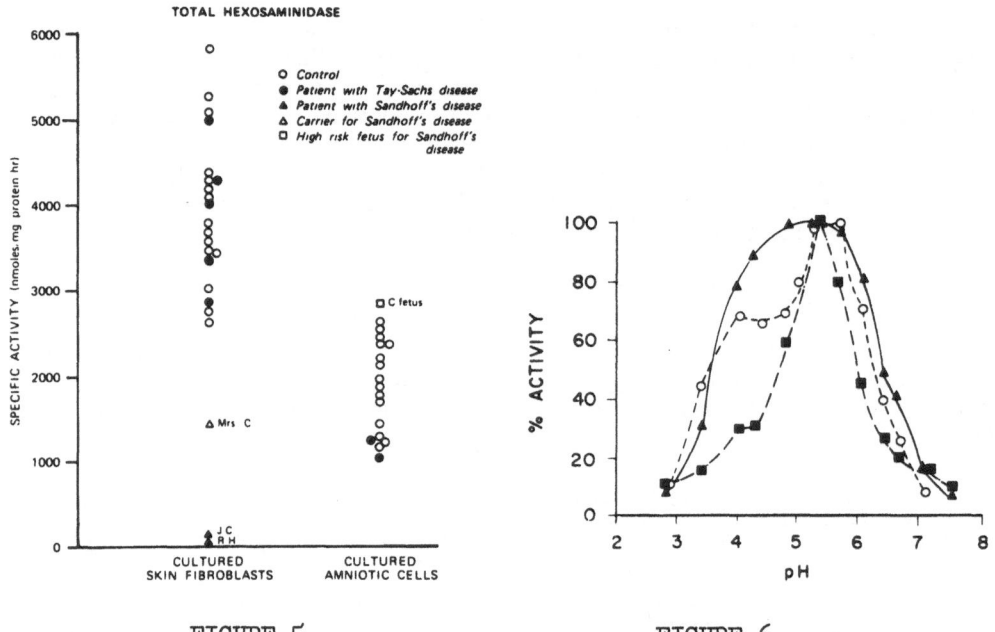

FIGURE 5   FIGURE 6

FIGURE 5: Total hexosaminidase (β-D-N-acetylglucosaminidase)
           activity in cultured skin fibroblasts and cultured
           amniotic cells in Sandhoff's disease. Enzyme assay
           was carried out as described previously (13).

FIGURE 6: β-glucosidase activity in cultured skin fibroblasts
           as a function of the pH of assay (the pH was measured
           at final buffer concentration of 20°C. ——▲——▲——
           Control; ——■——■——patient with Gaucher's dis-
           ease; ——○——○——parent of patient with Gaucher's
           disease. An activity of 100% represents the maximum
           activity found in each sample.

Juvenile GM₁ Gangliosidosis: The deficiency of β-galactosidase in juvenile GM₁ gangliosidosis can be demonstrated by assays of the enzyme in skin biopsies and in cultured skin fibroblasts from affected patients (Table 2) (11). Parents of children with this disease have an intermediate reduction of the enzyme in skin biopsies and in cultured skin fibroblasts (Table 2) (11). Ratios of one enzyme to the other such as β-galactosidase to β-N-acetylglucosaminidase are often helpful in distinguishing heterozygotes from normal homozygotes.

Although the enzyme is present in neglible quantities in human serum, it is present in leucocytes and leucocyte assay may be the simplest way to diagnose the homozygote (6,17). Thusfar, no homozygotes have been detected prenatally for this disease although there is good reason to believe that this is now feasible.

Gaucher's Disease: We have used cultured skin fibroblasts for diagnosing homozygotes and detecting heterozygotes for chronic Gaucher's disease. In agreement with Beutler et al. (1) we have found that the pH activity curve of β-glucosidase in control fibroblasts had two pH optima, one at pH 4.0 and the other at pH 5.0. Patients homozygous for the gene for Gaucher's disease were preferentially deficient in the peak of pH 4.0 (Fig. 6). We have worked out conditions to optimize the enzyme assay in the detection of heterozygotes and homozygotes. The assay conditions we use are given in Table 3.

The specific activities of β-glucosidase in skin fibroblasts from members of three kindreds (Fig. 7) gave a trimodal distribution. β-glucosidase activity in controls averaged 40.7 units with a range of 25-57. The activity in homozygotes averaged 2 units with a range of 1.1-3.0 units. The parents of patients averaged 12.3 units with a range of 5.2-15.5. No overlap values for β-glucosidase activity occurred when parents, patients and controls were compared (Table 4). Other family members in these kindreds also had an intermediate level of β-glucosidase, incidating that they are also heterozygotes. Activities of related lysosomal glycohydrolases including β-galactosidase and N-acetyl-β-D-glucosaminidase fell within the range of control values.

In kindred (a) the disease had appeared in two generations with an intervening generation being symptom free suggesting possible dominant inheritance with variable penetrance in II-2 or recessive inheritance with both II-1 and II-2 being heterozygous (Fig. 8). Clinical examinations of II-1 and II-2 (both over 50 years of age) revealed no splenomegaly. Bone marrow examination carried out on II-2 failed to demonstrate Gaucher-type histiocytes. The only reliable means to determine the mode of genetic transmission in kindred (a) appeared to be a thorough study of β-glucosidase activity in key family members.

TABLE 2

β-GALACTOSIDASE AND HEXOSAMINIDASE ACTIVITIES IN SKIN BIOPSIES
AND CULTURED SKIN FIBROBLASTS IN JUVENILE GM$_1$ GANGLIOSIDOSIS.

	β-Galacto-sidase	Hexosa-minidase	
Skin Biopsies - W. Family	(A)	(B)	B/A
Patient 1 (4 yrs.)	0.8	123	151
Patient 2 (3 yrs.)	0.6	120	210
Patient 3 (2 yrs.)	1.2	133	115
Father	14.2	149	10.5
Mother	16.9	193	11.4
Sister	21.7	136	6.3
Controls (12)	24.9	139	5.6
	(12.6-34.1)	(51-198)	(3.9-7.3)
Cultured Skin Fibroblasts - U. Family			
Patient 1 (4 yrs.)	32	3465	108
Patient 2 (7 mos.)	8	4714	589
Mother	243	3873	16
Brother	500	4082	8
Controls (6)	568	4841	8.5
	(414-675)	(4008-5838)	(7.6-10.0)

Both enzymic activities are expressed as m moles substrate
cleaved per mg protein per hour.

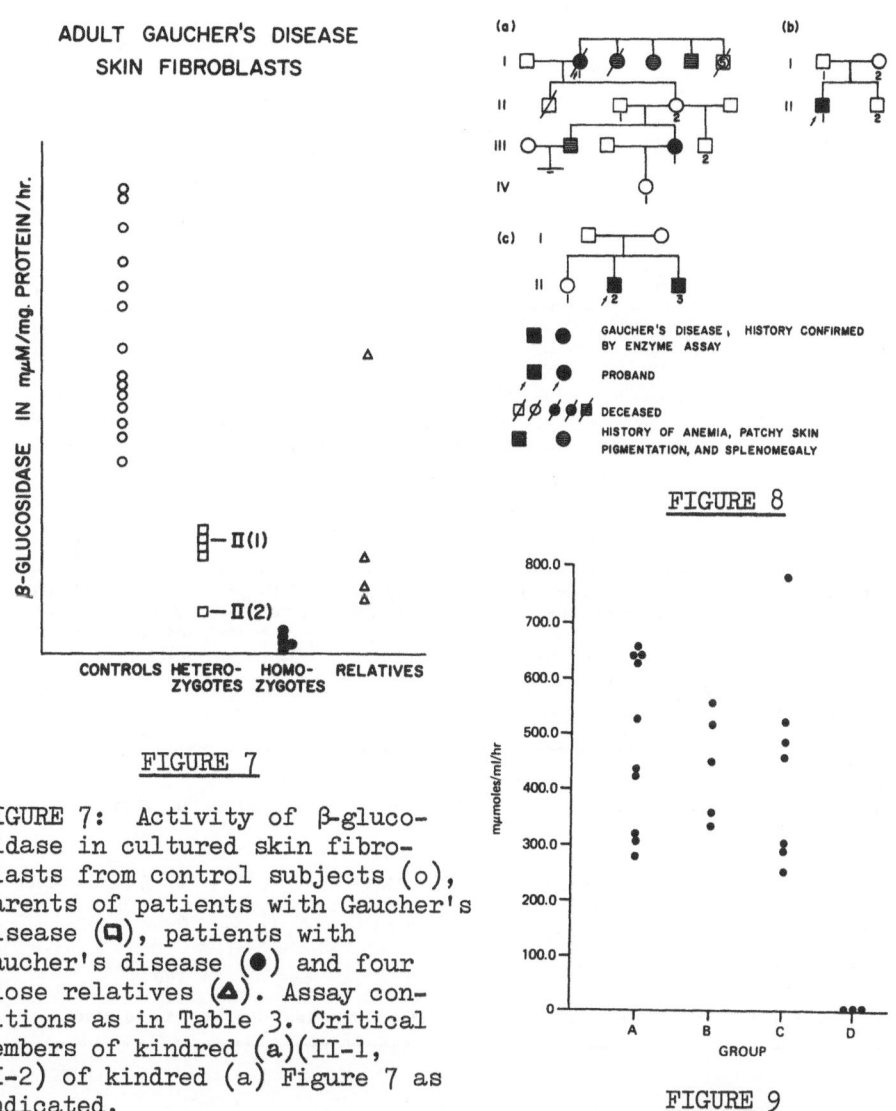

FIGURE 8

FIGURE 9

<u>FIGURE 7</u>

FIGURE 7: Activity of β-glucosidase in cultured skin fibroblasts from control subjects (o),
parents of patients with Gaucher's
disease (▫), patients with
Gaucher's disease (●) and four
close relatives (▲). Assay conditions as in Table 3. Critical
members of kindred (a)(II-1,
II-2) of kindred (a) Figure 7 as
indicated.

FIGURE 8: Partial pedigree of three kindreds with Gaugher's
disease.

FIGURE 9: α-L-frucsidase activity in serum from normal subjects
(group A), in plasma from normal subjects (group B), in
serum from the patients with Hurler's, Hunter's, Tay-
Sachs and other storage diseases (group C) and in serum
from three patients with fucosidosis (group D).

TABLE 3

Conditions for assay of acid glycosidases

	Enzyme		
	β-D-glucosidase	β-D-galactosidase	N-Acetyl-β-D-glucosaminidase
Substrate	4-methylumbelliferyl-β-D-glucopyranoside	4-methylumbelliferyl-β-D-galactopyranoside	4-methylumbelliferyl-2-acetamido-2'-deoxy-β-D-glucopyranoside
Buffer-Substrate mixture: Conc. of substrate	1mM	0.5mM	1mM
Buffer	------------------Citrate phosphate-----------------------		
Conc. of buffer (in terms of phosphate)	0.02M	0.022M	0.022M
pH	4.05	4.35	4.4
Additions	0.02% Triton X-100	0.1M NaCl	0.1% human albumin
μl Homogenate	10	10	5
μl Buffer-Substrate Mixture	50	50	100
Times of Incubation	30, 60 minutes	15, 30 minutes	15, 30 minutes

The two critical members in kindred (a), both had intermediate reductions of β-glucosidase activity demonstrating that both were heterozygous (Fig. 7). Recessive transmission of Gaucher's disease was confirmed in this kindred. Previous pedigree analyses based on clinical observations have suggested occasional dominant transmission of adult Gaucher's disease (4,5). In several kindreds the disease was present in two successive generations. Although statistically unlikely the presence of Gaucher's disease in successive generations in such kindreds may have resulted from heterozygotes (or homozygotes) marrying heterozygotes, as occurred in kindred (a) reported here. The assay of β-glucosidase in key members of such kindreds should reveal whether adult Gaucher's disease is ever transmitted as an autosomal dominant trait.

The persistence of the enzymic defect in cultured skin fibroblasts over many cellular generations indicates that it is now possible to diagnose the homozygous state for chronic Gaucher's disease prenatally by enzyme assays of cultured amniotic cells.

Fabry's Disease: Subsequent to Kint's work (7) in which he demonstrated the deficiency of α-galactosidase in serum and white cells from patients with Fabry's disease and an intermediate reduction of the same enzyme in female heterozygotes, we have used cultured skin fibroblasts to diagnose hemizygous males and detect heterozygous carriers for the gene for this disease. Thusfar, we have confirmed Kint's findings, as have others (14), of a deficiency of α-galactosidase in cultured skin fibroblasts of four patients with Fabry's disease. In our experience the activity of the enzyme in cultured fibroblasts from obligate heterozygotes ranges between 40 and 72% of controls. In one heterozygote studied by Romeo and Migeon (14) activity of the enzyme was within the normal range. This is not unexpected in view of the fact that these authors have demonstrated two-cell populations in heterozygous females, one normal and the other deficient in α-galactosidase activity, consistent with X-linkage of α-galactosidase and random inactivation of one of the X chromosomes in female carriers. The wide variation in α-galactosidase in heterozygotes is probably due to variations of the proportion of enzyme-deficient cells in the total population of cells studied. If the female at risk studied has markedly deficient levels of the enzyme, then one can feel confident that she is heterozygous. However, if she has normal levels, one cannot be sure she is not heterozygous since the proportion of mutant cells may be low, giving an average activity near normal. What is needed for accurate carrier detection here is a differential histochemical stain for α-galactosidase to demonstrate the two-cell populations in the heterozygous female.

Recently, assays of α-galactosidase have been used to prenatally diagnose Fabry's disease using amniotic cells (2). An

TABLE 4

Acid Glycosidases* in Skin Fibroblasts

	β-Glucosidase	Glucocerebrosidase	β-Galactosidase	β-Glucosaminidase
Patients**				
(a) I-1	1.98	6.3	482	6866
(a) III-1	1.10	8.9	356	4028
(b) II-1	3.00		283	3021
(c) II-2	2.10		557	3955
(c) II-3	1.90		447	3993
Mean ± S.D.	2.05 ± 0.78		419 ± 123	4467 ± 1663
Parents**				
(a) II-1	14.34		559	8873
(a) II-2	5.20	89.0	417	4403
(b) I-1	15.50		250	3849
(b) I-2	12.61		321	4120
(c) I-1	13.90		781	5310
Mean ± S.D.	12.3 ± 4.1			5311 ± 2066
Relatives**				
(a) III-2	8.82		273	3084
(a) IV-1	7.07	41.0	273	3377
(b) II-2	12.11		266	2331
(c) II-1	38.00		949	6331
Controls				
Mean ± S.D.	40.7 ± 11.2	218 ± 54	578 ± 138	4715 ± 974
Range	25.1 - 56.7 (n=14)	119 - 309 (n=9)	303 - 949 (n=29)	2427 - 6331 (n=27)

* Activity is expressed as mμM of substrate cleaved per mg. protein per hour.
** See Figure 8 for identification.

affected male has been detected in utero, the pregnancy terminated, and the diagnosis confirmed on analysis of fetal tissues. The prenatal diagnosis of Fabry's disease now appears to be feasible.

Fucosidosis: Alpha-L-fucosidase activity is present in normal human serum. The enzyme has a pH optima of 5.3, a Km of 0.156 mM and is stable in the frozen state. Using para-nitrophenyl L-fucoside as substrate, Drs. Klaus Zielke, Shintaro Okada and I devised an assay which requires 0.4 ml. of serum (19). Serum α-L-fucosidase activity in normal subjects averages 488 ± 153 nanomoles of substrate cleaved per milliliter of serum per hour at 37°.

Using this assay we have diagnosed fucosidosis in three children from two different families, a German family and an Italian family, both apparently unrelated to the original Italian family of Durand et al. (3). No activity for α-L-fucoside was found in the serum of these three patients (Fig. 9). When α-L-fucosidase activity was measured in the serum of patients with varying degenerative disorders, including some with Hurler's disease, Hunter's disease, and other sphingolipid storage diseases, normal α-L-fucosidase activity was found, demonstrating the differential diagnostic value of the assay (Fig. 9).

Previously the diagnosis of fucosidosis has been made by enzyme assays of organs and urine from suspected patients. The use of the serum assay described here should make it possible to diagnose fucosidosis simply during life and to differentiate it from related genetic mucopolysaccharidoses, including Hurler's syndrome, I-cell disease, lipomucopolysaccharidosis, generalized gangliosidosis, and juvenile GM_1 gangliosidosis, all of which have phenotypic features in common with fucosidosis.

REFERENCES

1. Beutler, E. and Kuhl, W.: Detection of the defect of Gaucher's disease and its carrier state in peripheral-blood leukocytes. Lancet, 1:612, 1970.

2. Brady, R.O., Uhlendorf, B.W. and Jacobson, C.B.: Fabry's disease: Antenatal detection. Science, 172:174, 1971.

3. Durand, P., Borrone, C. and Della Cella, G.: Fucosidosis. J. Pediatrics, 75:665, 1969.

4. Groen, J.J.: Gaucher's disease. Hereditary transmission and racial distribution. Arch. Int. Med., 113:543, 1964.

5. Hsia, D.Y.Y., Naylor, J. and Bigler, J.A.: The Genetic Mechanism of Gaucher's Disease in Cerebral Sphingolipidoses. A Symposium on Tay-Sachs Disease and Allied Disorders, Academic Press, New York, 1962, pp. 327-342.

6. Kint, J.A., Dacremont, G. and Vlietinck, R.: GM_1 gangliosi-
    dosis type 2. Lancet, 2:108, 1969.

7. Kint, J.A.: Fabry's disease: Alpha galactosidase deficiency.
    Science, 167:1268, 1970.

8. O'Brien, J.S.: Five gangliosidoses. Lancet, 1:805, 1969.

9. O'Brien, J.S., Okada, S., Chen, A. and Fillerup, D.L.: Tay-
    Sachs disease. Detection of heterozygotes and homozygotes
    by serum hexosaminidase assay. New Eng. J. Med., 283:15, 1970.

10. O'Brien, J.S., Okada, S., Fillerup, D.L., Veath, M.L., Adornato,
    B., Brenner, P.H. and Leroy, J.G.: Tay-Sachs disease: Pre-
    natal diagnosis. Science, 172:61, 1971.

11. O'Brien, J.S., Okada, S., Ho, M.W., Fillerup, D.L., Veath, M.L.
    and Adams, K.: Ganglioside storage diseases. Fed. Proc., 30
    (#3):956, 1971.

12. Okada, S. and O'Brien, J.S.: Tay-Sachs disease: Generalized
    absence of Beta-D-N-acetylhexosaminidase component. Science,
    165:698, 1969.

13. Okada, S., Veath, M.L., Leroy, J. and O'Brien, J.S.: Ganglio-
    side GM_2 storage diseases: Hexosaminidase deficiencies in
    cultured fibroblasts. Am. J. Human Genet., 23(31):55, 1971.

14. Romeo, G. and Migeon, B.R.: Genetic inactivation of the α-
    galactosidase locus in carriers in Fabry's disease. Science,
    170:180, 1970.

15. Sandhoff, K., Andreae, U. and Jatzkewitz, H.: Deficient hexo-
    saminidase activity in an exceptional case of Tay-Sachs dis-
    ease with additional storage of kidney globoside in visceral
    organs. Life Sciences, 7:283, 1968.

16. Suzuki, Y. and Suzuki, K.: Partial deficiency of hexosamini-
    dase component A in juvenile GM_2-gangliosidosis. Neurology,
    20:848, 1970.

17. Wolfe, L.S., Callahan, J., Fawcett, J.S., Andermann, F. and
    Scriver, C.R.: GM_1 gangliosidosis without chondrodystrophy
    or visceromegaly; β-galactosidase deficiency with ganglio-
    sidosis and the excessive excretion of a keratan sulfate.
    Neurology, 20:23, 1970.

18. Young, P., Ellis, R.B., Lake, B.D. and Patrick, A.D.: Tay-
     Sachs disease and related disorders: Fractionation of brain
     N-acetyl- β -hexosaminidase on DEAE-cellulose. FEBS Letters,
     9:1, 1970.

19. Zielke, K., Okada, S. and O'Brien, J.S.: Fucosidosis: Diag-
     nosis by serum assay of α-L-fucosidase. J. Lab. Clin. Med.
     In press.

PRE- AND POSTNATAL DETECTION OF TAY-SACHS DISEASE.

A COMPARATIVE STUDY OF BIOCHEMICAL SCREENING METHODS.

Abraham Saifer[*], Guta Perle[*], Carlo Valenti[**] and Larry Schneck[***]

Department of Biochemistry[*] Isaac Albert Research Institute of the Kingsbrook Jewish Medical Center, Department of Obstetrics and Gynecology[**] State University of New York, Downstate Medical Center and Department of Neurology[***]Kingsbrook Jewish Medical Center, Brooklyn, N.Y.

Tay-Sachs disease, an invariably fatal cerebral storage (G_{M2}-ganglioside) disorder inherited as an autosomal recessive trait, is presently the only such genetic disease which possesses all three criteria necessary to prevent the birth of homozygotes. These criteria are:- (a) The characterization of a well-defined, high risk group in the general population which carries the defective gene, e.g., Ashkenazi Jews in the United States (1). (b) A simple, quantitative biochemical test, preferably based upon the analysis of the deficient enzyme, which will permit the detection of the heterozygotes in the normal population and the isolation of the high-risk carrier-couples, e.g., the assay of hexosaminidase A in serum (2) or white blood cells (3,4) with fluorimetric procedures. (c) The prenatal diagnosis of the disease by enzymatic analysis of the amniotic fluid or cells obtained from the fetuses

of carrier-couples sufficiently early to give the
parents the choice of safely terminating the pregnancy(5).

Despite the small number of infants born in the
United States with this disorder, less than 50 per year,
the importance of developing suitable methods for its
detection and prevention reside in the potential application of similar techniques to other more frequently
occurring genetic disorders, e.g. sickle cell anemia.

In human body fluids and tissues two main N-acetyl-
β-D-hexosaminidases, A and B, have been found (6,7).
Previous investigators (8,9) have shown that the A component is missing or deficient in the fluids and tissues
of patients afflicted with Tay-Sachs disease. Kolodny
and coworkers (10) and Sandhoff (11) have shown that
the primary enzymatic defect in Tay-Sachs disease is
due to the absence of N-acetyl-β-D-hexosaminidase A
which normally converts the G_{M2}-ganglioside into G_{M3}-
ganglioside by cleaving the terminal N-acetylgalactosamine residue of the stored ganglioside. This enzyme
also acts upon a number of synthetic substrates such as
the Napthol-AS-BI-derivative of β-D-N-acetylhexosaminide
(8) and the sensitive fluorogenic substrate, 4-methyl-
umbelliferyl-N-acetyl-β-glucosamide (2,3,4).

Since these artificial substrates react almost
equally well with both the hexosaminidase A and B components, the reactivity of a biological fluid or tissue
containing the enzymes will measure total hexosaminidase.
The separate fluorimetric measurement of hexosaminidase
B activity of the fluid is based on the experimental
fact that hexosaminidase A is almost completely denatured by heating the sample at 50° for 3 to 4 hours
while the B fraction is relatively unaffected (2,3).
An alternative method for the separation of hexosaminidase A from B by means of acrylamide gel electrophoresis and their direct quantitative determination by
fluorimetric analysis has been described by Friedland
et al (4).

The present paper deals with a comparative study
of these two quantitative procedures for hexosaminidase
A and B as applied to the mass screening of heterozygotes for Tay-Sachs disease and to the prenatal detection of the disease "in utero".

MATERIAL AND METHODS

Leucocytes and amniotic cells (cultured and uncultured) were analyzed for their hexosaminidase A and
B content by the acrylamide gel electrophoretic technique described by Friedland et al (4) except that electrophoresis was carried out for 5 min at 1mA/tube and
then for 1 hr and 25 min at 3.0 mA/tube. Amniotic
fluids were run in the same manner except that after
electrophoresis for 5 min at 1mA/tube the run was continued for 1 hr and 40 min at 3.5 mA/tube. The gels
were then immersed in a covered shallow dish containing
the fluorogenic substrate and incubated for 1 hour at
37° (12).

These fluids, as well as blood sera from the same
subjects from which the leucocytes were obtained, were
analyzed for their hexosaminidase A content with the
heat denaturation method of O'Brien et al (2). Samples
analyzed included the following groups:- (a) normal
adult sera and leucocytes (male and female subjects 13
to 65 yr); (b) normal (non-neurological) childrens sera
and leucocytes (9 mo to 5 yr); (c) normal pregnancy
sera and leucocytes (20-38 yr); (d) Tay-Sachs children's
sera and leucocytes; (e) sera and leucocytes from Tay-
Sachs parents; (f)normal amniotic fluids; (g) normal
uncultured amniotic cells; and (h) amniotic fluids and
amniotic cells (uncultured and cultured) from pregnancies in which both parents were obligatory carriers.

RESULTS

Statistical analysis of the data obtained for serum
hexosaminidase A levels(as % of total hexosaminidase) is
illustrated in Fig. 1 for the various groups of subjects
that were tested with the heat denaturation method (2).
It can be seen that the sera of normal children yield
the same results as do the sera of normal adults so
they can be considered as a single group for statistical
purposes. The heat denaturation method also provides
clear-cut dufferentiation between the normal group, the
carrier(Tay-Sachs parents) group and the children with
Tay-Sachs disease. There is, however, a complete overlap of values between the normal pregnancy and the carrier groups which precludes the use of this technique
for the detection of heterozygotes in pregnant women.
It should also be noted that patients with the disease
show low but detectable hexosaminidase A values with
this method for reasons discussed by O'Brien et al (2).

The data obtained with the heat denaturation
method for leucocyte hexosaminidase levels (as % of
total hexosaminidase) are shown in Fig. 2. There is
again good statistical differentiation between the
adult control group, the carrier group and the Tay-
Sachs children. However, the normal (non-neurological)
children show a wider spread of values than was found
for serum. It should be pointed out that this group
consists of hospitalized children with non-neurological involvement some of whom may have had elevated
white blood counts. Conversely, the pregnant control
group shows only a small overlap, less than 20%, with
the carrier group. This finding permits one to deduce
that a pregnant woman whose leucocyte hexosaminidase
A values are in the normal range would most likely not
be a carrier of the Tay-Sachs gene.

The data obtained for leucocyte hexosaminidase A
levels (as % of total hexosaminidase) by acrylamide gel
electrophoresis are presented in Fig. 3. As is the
situation for the serum values by heat denaturation,
the normal children's range falls within that found
for adult normals so that the two groups can be combined
for statistical purposes. The spread of the adult control values is somewhat wider than those obtained for
serum (Fig. 1) or leucocytes (Fig. 2) with the heat
denaturation technique. This has resulted in about a
25% overlap between the adult normal and carrier groups.
As is the case for leucocyte hexosaminidase A values
with the heat denaturation method, there is a small
overlap, i.e., about 10%, between the pregnant controls
and Tay-Sachs parent groups. However, the acrylamide
gel electrophoretic technique gives zero hexosaminidase
A values for the Tay-Sachs children's leucocytes, as
only the B component is present in the gel, which fur-
nishes the best statistical indicator for the diagnosis
of this disease.

Statistical data for amniotic fluid and (cultured
and uncultured) amniotic cell hexosaminidase A levels,
which were determined by both the heat denaturation
and acrylamide gel electrophoretic techniques, are
given in Fig. 4. The mean values for amniotic fluid
hexosaminidase A obtained with the heat denaturation
and acrylamide gel electrophoretic methods are almost
identical although the latter method has a somewhat
broader normal range.

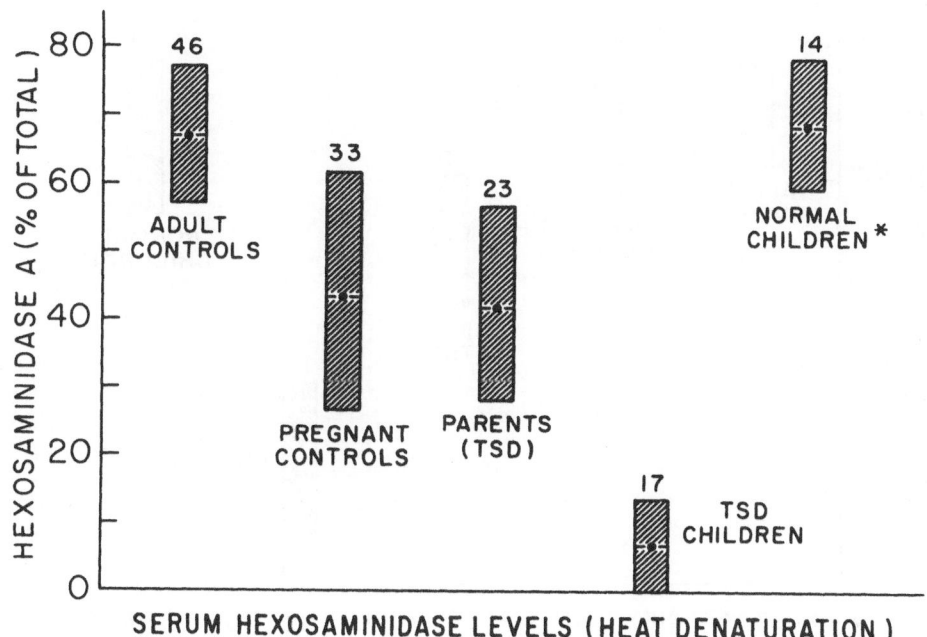

Fig. 1. Statistical data (Mean (–•–) ±2SD) of serum hexosaminidase A levels obtained by heat denaturation for: - adult (normal) controls (46), pregnant controls (33), Tay-Sachs parents (23), Tay-Sachs children (17) and normal (*non-neurological) children (14).

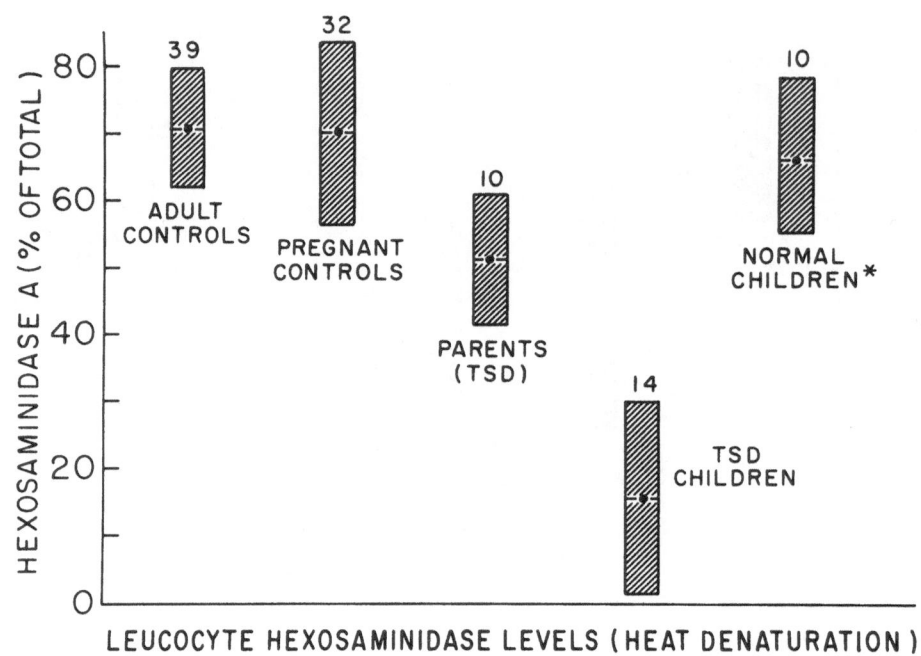

Fig. 2. Statistical data (Mean (—•—) ±2SD) of leucocyte hexosaminidase A levels obtained by heat denaturation for: - adult (normal) controls (39),
pregnant controls (32), Tay-Sachs parents (10), Tay-
Sachs children (14) and normal (*non-neurological)
children (10).

Amniotic fluids were also obtained from eleven pregnant women who had either given birth to previous Tay-Sachs infants or whose fetuses resulted from the mating of known carrier-couples. The acrylamide gel electrophoretic technique permitted a clear-cut separation of these 11 fluids into two groups, 8 of which fell within the normal range while 3 fluids (AF No's 26,28 and 81) showed no A component. The results obtained for these amniotic fluids with the heat denaturation method for hexosaminidase A were unsatisfactory. While all the predicted normal cases with the acrylamide gel method were also normal with the heat denaturation methods, one of the predicted abnormal fluids (AF26) fell within the normal range while another (AF81) gave a border-line value. Somewhat better differentiation between normal and affected fetuses was found when the heat denaturation method was applied to uncultured amniotic cells and the best differentiation is obtained only when cultured cells were analyzed with this method. On a strictly statistical basis there is no improvement in the differentiation of normal from diseased fetuses with the acrylamide gel electrophoretic method if uncultured and cultured cells are analyzed for their hexosaminidase A levels instead of the amniotic fluid. However, the uncultured cells since they can be analyzed at the same time as the amniotic fluid, provides additional assurance of the correctness of the result without further delay. Whereas, amniotic cell culture growth requires 2-3 weeks time.

DISCUSSION

The range of total hexosaminidase values as determined with the fluorimetric assay method of Leaback and Walker (13) has been found to be so wide as to be of no clinical significance. In addition, no significant differences were found between the control and abnormal groups which confirms the results reported by O'Brien and co-workers (2). Therefore, no total hexosaminidase values are included in this report.

The serum hexosaminidase A values reported by O'Brien et al (2) with the heat denaturation method are somewhat lower for the adult control, parent and Tay-Sach children groups than those given in Fig. 1 although there is a clear-cut statistical separation among the groups in both studies. These differences may be due to the fact that our assay was performed without blank corrections or to slight variations of temperature in the heating bath in which the denaturation of the A component is being carried out. At any rate it points out the necessity for each laboratory, that plans to use this method for the mass screening of heterozygotes, to set-up its own normal control and carrier group ranges. The detection of homozygotes with this test and the diagnostic differentiation of Tay-Sachs disease from infants with related disorders, e.g., Niemann-Pick disease, late infantile and juvenile amaurotic idiocy, Gaucher's disease and metachromatic leukodystrophy presents no difficulty since they give hexosaminidase A values in the normal range. Of more serious consequence is the fact that heterozygote detection with this method is not possible if the individual being tested has diabetes mellitus or other severe illnesses or is pregnant (2). The situation in pregnancy with respect to carrier detection (Fig. 1) is of the utmost importance if the father has been found to be a carrier and the mother was not tested prior to the pregnancy. Stirling (14) has reported the presence of a new form of N-acetyl-β-glucosaminidase, i.e., the P form, in pregnancy serum whose thermal stability is intermediate between that of forms A and B.

Since hexosaminidase P is not present to any appreciable extent in leucocytes, the possibility of determining whether a pregnant woman is normal or a carrier of the Tay-Sachs gene is considerably enhanced by its use (Figs. 2 and 3). The leucocyte hexosaminidase A values reported by Padeh and Naron (3) by the heat denaturation method show good separation among the normal control, Tay-Sachs parent and Tay-Sachs children groups similar to that illustrated in Fig. 2 although our absolute values are somewhat higher for all three groups. The leucocyte hexosaminidase A levels obtained for adult controls, pregnant controls and Tay-Sachs parents with the acrylamide gel electrophoretic technique (Fig. 3) is very close to those found with the heat denaturation method (Fig. 2). The major difference between the two methods lies in the zero hexosaminidase A values for the Tay-Sachs children obtained with the gel electrophoretic method as compared with values of 15.8 $\pm$ 7.1 for the heat denaturation method which are almost twice those found for Tay-Sachs serum (Fig. 1).

The main advantage of the acrylamide gel electrophoretic technique over the heat denaturation method for hexosaminidase A analysis lies in its ability to differentiate between a normal and Tay-Sachs fetus

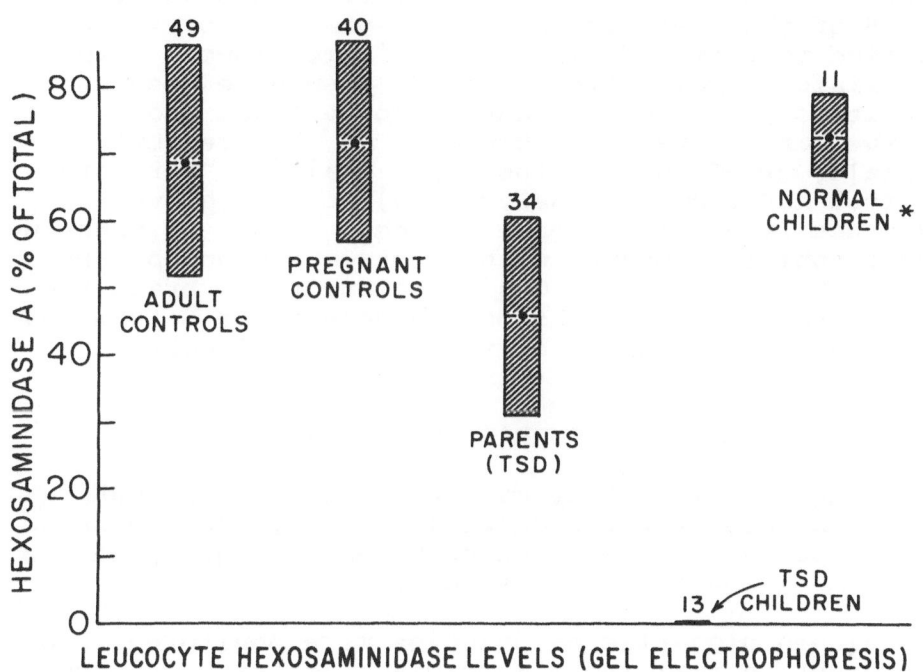

Fig. 3. Statistical data (Mean (—•—) ±2SD) of leucocyte hexosaminidase A levels obtained by acrylamide
gel electrophoresis for: - adult (normal) controls
(49), pregnant controls (40), Tay-Sachs parents (34),
Tay-Sachs children (13) and normal (*non-neurological)
children (11).

utilizing amniotic fluid and uncultured cells obtained
by amniocentisis (5), as is clearly evident in Fig. 4.
Cultured fibroblasts should, whenever possible, be
used to confirm the findings obtained on amniotic fluid
or uncultured cells. Of the eleven cases of potential
Tay-Sachs births, 8 were predicted normal and 3 were
predicted abnormal based on amniotic fluid analysis.
All 8 of the predicted normal pregnancies have been
carried to term and all these children appear normal
on clinical examination. Six of them have been tested
for leucocyte hexosaminidase A content and show values
in the carrier range or higher. Of the predicted ab-
normals, one of the 3 fetuses was available for pathological and chemical analysis (5) and was proven to
have had Tay-Sachs disease by the presence of membranous cytoplasmic bodies with electron microscopy, by
the marked increase in G_{M2}-gangliosides in brain tissue
and by the absence of hexosaminidase A, as determined
with gel electrophoresis, from various tissues.

SUMMARY

1. A comparative study was undertaken of two published methods for the detection of Tay-Sachs disease
heterozygotes and homozygotes based upon quantitative
hexosaminidase A determinations.

2. Eleven high-risk pregnancies were monitored, 8 of
which were normal and 3 were diagnosed as Tay-Sachs
fetuses. The results obtained suggest that amniotic
fluid can be used in the preliminary monitoring of a
fetus for Tay-Sachs disease when the acrylamide gel
electrophoretic method is utilized for the analysis.
However, conclusive supportive evidence for the prenatal diagnosis of the disease should be based, wher-
ever possible, on hexosaminidase A assay of cultured
amniotic cells.

3. Serum hexosaminidase A assays by heat denaturation
can be used for differentiation among normal (adults
and children), carrier (Tay-Sachs parent) and Tay-
Sachs children groups. There is, however, a complete
overlap of values between normal pregnant women and
carriers with this method.

4. Leucocyte hexosaminidase A determinations, by
either the heat denaturation or acrylamide gel electrophoretic procedures, considerably reduces but does

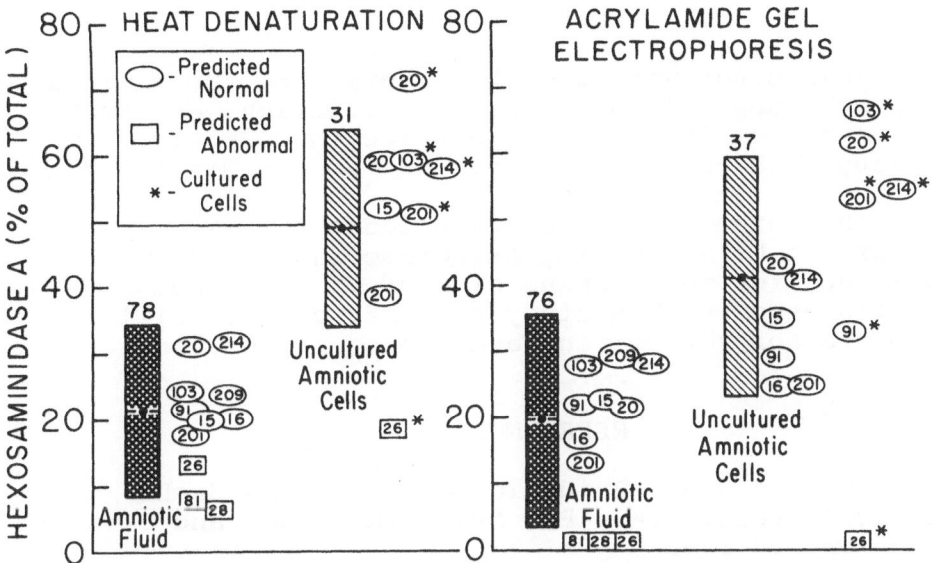

AMNIOTIC FLUID AND UNCULTURED CELLULAR HEXOSAMINIDASE LEVELS

<u>Fig. 4.</u> Statistical data (Mean (→) ±2SD) of normal amniotic fluid and uncultured amniotic cell hexosaminidase A levels obtained with the heat denaturation and acrylamide gel electrophoretic methods. Hexosaminidase A values are also given for all amniotic fluids and cells (uncultured and cultured) obtained from the fetuses of carrier-couples of which 8 (AF No's 15, 16, 20, 91, 103, 201, 204, 209, 214) were predicted normal and 3 (AF No's 26, 28, 81) were predicted as Tay-Sachs disease.

not eliminate this overlap.

ACKNOWLEDGEMENTS

This study was aided by grants from the National Tay-Sachs and Allied Diseases Association, New York, N.Y. and from the U.S.P.H. Service (NS00285-19) dealing with "Protein Studies in Chronic Diseases".

The authors wish to acknowledge the aid of Dr. Irving L. Moskowitz, Associate in Internal Medicine, for the drawing of many of the blood samples used in this study and that of Mrs. Lillian Salowitz for the editing and typing of the manuscript.

REFERENCES

1. Aronson, S.M., Epidemiology. In "Tay-Sachs Disease", Volk, B.W., Ed. New York, Grune and Stratton, 1964, pp 118-153.

2. O'Brien, J.S., Okada, S., Chen, A., and Fillerup, D.L., Tay-Sachs disease. Detection of heterozygotes and homozygotes by serum hexosaminidase assay. New Eng. J. Med. __283__, 15 (1970).

3. Padeh,B., and Navon,R., Diagnosis of Tay-Sachs disease by hexosaminidase activity in leukocytes and amniotic fluid cells. Israel J. Med. Sci. __7__, 259 (1971).

4. Friedland,J., Schneck,L., Saifer,A., Pourfar,M., and Volk,B.W., Identification of Tay-Sachs disease carriers by acrylamide gel electrophoresis. Clin. Chim. Acta __28__, 397 (1970).

5. Schneck, L., Valenti,C., Amsterdam, D., Friedland, J., Adachi,M., and Volk,B.W., Prenatal diagnosis of Tay-Sachs disease. Lancet __1__, 582 (1970).

6. Robinson, D., and Stirling,J.L., N-Acetyl-β-glucosaminidases in human spleen. Biochem. J. __107__, 321 (1968).

7. Sandhoff,K., Auftrennung der Säuger-N-Acetyl-beta-D-hexosaminidase in multiple Formen durch Elektro-

fokusserung. Z. Physiol. Chem. 349, 1095 (1968).

8. Okada, S., and O'Brien, J.S., Tay-Sachs disease: generalized absence of a beta-D-N-acetylhexosaminidase component. Science 165, 698 (1969).

9. Sandhoff,K., Variation of β-N-acetylhexosaminidase -pattern in Tay-Sachs disease. FEBS Letters 4, 351 (1969).

10. Kolodny, E.H., Brady,R.O., and Volk,B.W., Demonstration of an alteration of ganglioside metabolism in Tay-Sachs disease. Biochem. Biophys. Res. Commun. 37, 526 (1969).

11. Sandhoff,K., The hydrolysis of Tay-Sachs ganglioside (TSG) by human N-acetyl-β-D-hexosaminidase A. FEBS Letters 11, 342 (1970).

12. Friedland, J., Perle,G., Saifer,A., Schneck, L., and Volk,B.W., Screening for Tay-Sachs disease "in utero" using amniotic fluid. Proc. Soc. Exp. Biol. & Med. 136, 1297 (1971).

13. Leaback,D.H., and Walker,P.G., Studies on glucosaminidase. The fluorimetric assay of N-acetyl-β-glucosaminidase. Biochem. J. 78, 151 (1961).

14. Stirling,J.L., A new form of N-acetyl-β-glucosaminidase present in pregnancy serum. Biochem. J. 120, 11p (1971).

HETEROZYGOTE DETECTION IN TAY-SACHS DISEASE: A PROTOTYPE COMMUNITY SCREENING PROGRAM FOR THE PREVENTION OF RECESSIVE GENETIC DISORDERS

Michael M. Kaback, M. D., and Robert S. Zeiger, M. D., Ph.D.

Department of Pediatrics, Johns Hopkins University, School of Medicine, Baltimore, Maryland 21205

Supported by the John F. Kennedy Institute Tay-Sachs Fund, The Aaron and Lillian Strauss Foundation, and a grant from the Maryland State Department of Health and Mental Hygiene.

The previous Symposia on Sphingolipidoses serve as a chronicle of the increased interest and in-depth investigations which have been directed at these conditions over the past decade. Since this is the 4th International Symposium on Sphingolipidoses, it is appropriate that the results of the first mass community screening effort directed at prospective prevention of the prototype sphingolipidosis, Tay-Sachs disease (TSD), be presented.

The major breakthroughs in diagnosis, carrier detection, and intrauterine diagnosis of Tay-Sachs disease in the recent past now raise the possibility of total prevention of this fatal and currently untreatable disease of infancy. Tay-Sachs disease is the first recessive genetic disorder which meets three specific requirements thereby making this possibility tenable:

First, the disorder occurs in a defined population group. Tay-Sachs disease is 100 times more frequent in Jewish children of central and eastern European ancestry (Ashkenazim) as compared with other population groups. Since a finite population group is therefore at risk, this reduces the proportions for a program directed at prospective prevention.

Second, the definition of a total deficiency of
hexosaminidase A (Hex A) activity in tissues and
blood from children with Tay-Sachs disease (Okada
and O'Brien, 1969) provides the foundation upon
which such a program can be based (1). Their subsequent findings of a consistent and clear diminution of Hex A activity in serum from obligate
heterozygotes for the Tay-Sachs gene (parents of
affected children) as compared to other groups is
also of paramount significance (2).   This work
provides the basis for a simple, accurate, and inexpensive carrier detection test, a critical requirement of the prevention program.

Third, with the applications of second trimester
amniocentesis to genetic counseling, and the advances in human somatic cell genetics, the pro-
visions have become available for the detection
of Tay-Sachs disease in the fetus prior to the
18th week of gestation (3). This has been successfully achieved to date in a number of laboratories (4, 5, 6). Absence of Hex A activity in
amniotic fluid, its component cells, and in cultivated amniotic fluid cells has been consistently
found in fetuses proven to have Tay-Sachs disease.

These prerequisites provide the basis for the
mass prevention program. Application of the simple,
accurate, and inexpensive carrier-detection test to
married couples of child-bearing age in the defined
population should allow the identification of those
"rare" couples in that population (1 in 900 Jewish
couples: 1/30 x 1/30) in which both husband and wife
are heterozygous for the Tay-Sachs gene. Having been
so identified, these couples can be counseled appropriately as to the risks for Tay-Sachs disease in their
children. Because the disorder is autosomal recessive
in character (each pregnancy at 25% risk for an affected conceptus where both parents are carriers) and
because accurate intrauterine diagnosis is feasible,
these couples can be helped to have as many children

as they wish "selectively" none of whom will suffer
with this fatal, untreatable, disease. This is evident since couples, so informed after amniocentesis,
may elect to terminate pregnancies in which a Tay-
Sachs fetus is identified.

     There are a number of essential issues which
must be considered before attempting mass screening
for a genetic carrier-state in an adult population.
Serious consideration must be given to the feasibility,
costs, and conceivable deleterious genetic impact of
such a program. Each of these issues has been considered in depth prior to the outset of this program
(7). Suffice it to say that screening married adults
in a defined population is feasible if effective education can be delivered and if high volume screening
methods can be applied. Careful estimation of costs
versus benefits of such a program would indicate that
the economic benefits, solely in terms of the savings
in hospital costs which would otherwise be generated
by those children born with Tay-Sachs disease, exceeds
the cost of mass screening by at least a factor of 5.
This, of course, says nothing of the major costs, the
human ones. Lastly, calculations concerning deleterious genetic impact (increase in gene frequency),
indicate that such a program would have an extremely
minimal effect on increasing the heterozygote frequency in the defined population. Having made several
reasonable assumptions, we have calculated that it
would take more than 8,000 years to double the carrier
rate as the result of such a program if it were imple-
mented and effectively delivered, henceforth, in the
North American Jewish population.

METHODOLOGY

     Before any laboratory method is applied to popu-
lational screening, it is imperative that the method
first be critically and exhaustively evaluated. The
method must be accurate and extremely sensitive. In
fact, it is preferable that the screening method used
be overly sensitive, that is, rather than miss positives, to over-call them. The carrier detection

method as described by O'Brien et al. 1970 (2) appeared to be a highly accurate method which readily
lends itself to high-volume screening. However, prior
to widescale application, it was critical that the
method be dissected in our facility since any given
methodology may vary significantly from one laboratory
to another for reasons which are not always entirely
clear. In our studies, we found several components
of the serum heat-inactivation method which are affected by rather non-specific variables. For example,
such factors as the glassware, the type of water used
in buffer preparation and in which heat inactivation
is carried out, the ionic strength and pH during heat
treatment, are several of the variables which may affect the level of Hex A as defined by the O'Brien
method.

    In our laboratory, heat inactivation data at 50°
was not sufficiently accurate for widescale application. However, with inactivation of serum at a ten
fold dilution in phosphate-citrate buffer (50 mM PO_4;
40 mM citrate, Na salts) pH 4.4 at 52° for 2 and 3
hours, we can exactly reproduce the findings of
O'Brien et al.

    Additional modifications of the described assay
method were also found to be necessary. Substrate
saturation (4-methylumbelliferyl-β-D-N-acetylglu-
cosaminide, Pierce Chem. Co.) is not achieved at a
final assay concentration of 0.67 mM. Assay conditions are much more optimal at a 2.0 mM substrate
concentration. It was also found that serum hexosaminidase activity at 37° under these conditions does
not remain linear after 30 minutes. We, therefore,
have reduced the 37° serum-substrate incubation to
5-30 minutes.

    In order to apply this method to large numbers of
individuals, we felt it was critical that an automated
method be developed. Accordingly, we have devised an
automated system for serum hexosaminidase determinations in which as many as 300 individuals can be
screened per day (8). Automation critically

standardizes the assay conditions and negates day to
day technical variations or omissions which may occur
with the manual method. The assay modifications previously delineated are incorporated into the automated
system. These alterations significantly increase the
total serum hexosaminidase activity and, to a smaller
degree, affect the percentage contributed to the total
by Hex A (as determined by heat inactivation at
52°).

It is reasonable to assume that any mass screening
method will not be 100% accurate. In many ways, serum
might be considered the "clearing house or garbage
dump" for the body. It is unlikely that serum is a
primary enzyme source but rather hexosaminidase
activity measured in serum more likely represents enzyme released into the serum as the result of cellular
degradation and turnover. Moreover, one must be concerned that serum enzyme activities may be affected
by a multiplicity of factors including diet, medica-
tion, etc. Previous studies of serum hexosaminidase
and Hex A indicate that these serum activities may be
critically affected by systemic illnesses (particularly
diabetes), and importantly, pregnancy (2). For these
reasons, it was felt essential, prior to the inception
of our program, to establish a backup system for
evaluation of individuals where serum determinations
might be inaccurate. The alternative tissue sources
for enzymatic evaluation which we considered were
leukocytes and cultured skin fibroblasts. Obviously,
the latter would be an expensive and difficult method
for backup if such were needed in significant numbers
of individuals. Accordingly, we first conducted a
series of studies using leukocytes in order to evaluate
its accuracy relative to serum and its variability under those states where the serum assay is notably affected.

Again, critical dissection of the white blood cell
method with similar modifications indicated that leukocytes can be utilized as a highly accurate backup system for the serum screening method. Several factors
are critical to insure a high level of accuracy with

TABLE 1

SERUM HEXOSAMINIDASE ACTIVITY*

	TOTAL**	% HEX A (52°)		
		Mean	SD	Range
Tay-Sachs children (12)	376.4 – 926.4	0–3	–	--
Obligate heterozygotes (28)	337.7–1109.7	36.1	5.1	27.0–43.2
"Non-carriers" (100)	353.8–1146.8	56.2	4.1	50.0–70.0

*n-moles 4-methylumbelliferone produced per ml. of serum per hour at 37°C.
**range of activities

this cell type. The pH (4.4) and the protein concentration during heat inactivation, as well as those
variables previously mentioned, are critical for reproducible and accurate white cell data.

Anticipating that public education directed at
prevention of a serious genetic disorder might particularly generate responses from pregnant women, we
recognized the necessity for an accurate method for
carrier detection in pregnant females. As the data
indicates, the white blood cell method in pregnancy
as well as in non-pregnant women and men appears to
be highly accurate in reflecting the genotype of the
individual tested.

PREPARATORY STUDIES: SERUM HEXOSAMINIDASE

Table 1 depicts the results of serum hexosaminidase determinations in Tay-Sachs disease children, obligate heterozygotes, and "control individuals". It
is important to emphasize that no one can be considered
an absolute control in these studies. Definition of
an individual as a non-carrier can only be done on a
statistical basis. Only after careful evaluation of
multiple heterozygotes can statistically-based genotype assignment be given to unknown individuals.
Statistical data generated from obligate heterozygote
studies allows one to then set arbitrary ranges for
carrier/non-carrier genotype assignment. In this way,
we have defined carriers as any individuals whose
serum, on 3 consecutive duplicate determinations, show
Hex A levels between 25 and 45% of the total activity
($\pm$ 2 standard deviations of the mean for obligate
carriers). In addition, we have intentionally set an
inconclusive range (45-50% Hex A) which extends to
approximately 3 standard deviations above the mean
for obligate heterozygotes. A single inconclusive
range determination requires retesting with leukocyte
analysis. In this way, a significant number of individuals will be assigned "inconclusive" after serum
assay who will then have subsequent white cell and repeat serum analyses before definitive genotype
designation is made. This system intentionally

TABLE 2

LEUKOCYTE HEXOSAMINIDASE ACTIVITY*

	TOTAL**	% HEXOSAMINIDASE A (52°C)		
		Mean	SD	Range
Tay-Sachs children (10)	475.1–1380.2	0–7	–	--
Obligate heterozygotes (22)	449.4–1300.1	39.4	5.3	32.3–49.4
"Non-carriers" (51)	295.1–1007.2	61.6	2.9	56.0–68.5

*n-moles 4-methylumbelliferone produced per hour (37°C) per mg. soluble
  cell protein.
**range of activities

TABLE 3

SERUM AND LEUKOCYTE HEXOSAMINIDASE IN PREGNANT* AND NON-PREGNANT WOMEN

	SERUM HEX.		WBC HEX.	
	Total	% A	Total	% A
Obligate Heterozygotes				
Non-pregnant (6)	443.9- 829.9	35.6 ± 4.7	453.7-618.9	36.8 ± 3.6
Pregnant (6)**	733.4-1486.1	24.3 ± 6.5	510.9-863.8	37.4 ± 4.3
"Controls"				
Non-pregnant (59)	354.1- 926.3	57.2 ± 4.9	304.2-1007.2	61.8 ± 4.0
Pregnant (43)	561.2-1305.0	35.9 ± 11.1	469.3-1687.9	66.2 ± 6.0

*Between 6-24th menstrual week of pregnancy
**Same 6 women

overcalls inconclusives so that it becomes overly sensitive in the sense that it will not miss carriers.
An individual is deemed a non-carrier only if two consecutive determinations are greater than 3 standard
deviations above the mean for obligate heterozygotes
(>51% Hex A).

LEUKOCYTE STUDIES

Hexosaminidase levels in leukocytes from pre-
paratory studies are depicted in Table 2. A high degree of accuracy must be demanded of the white blood
cell method since this is utilized as the backup
evaluation system for serum-inconclusives, for couples
where both individuals are designated carriers by
serum assay, or in mixed couples of carrier-inconclu-
sive individuals. Moreover, because of the recognized
inaccuracy of carrier detection with serum from pregnant women, it is essential to ascertain the accuracy
of this method for genotype designation during pregnancy.

It is readily apparent in Table 2 that highly
significant differences are found in white blood cell
Hex A levels between obligate heterozygotes and individuals designated "non-carrier" by serum assay.
White cell counts and differentials were done in all
individuals. No correlation of total hexosaminidase
activity or percent Hex A was noted with either white
blood cell count or lymphocyte frequency. Total white
cells ranged from 5-13,000 per mm^3 and differentials
were all within normal limits (8-28% lymphocytes).
This, of course, does not rule out the possibility that
differential cell types may have different levels of
hexosaminidase or Hex A, but at least as applied to a
significant population with "normal white blood cell
counts and differentials", there does not appear to be
any obvious correlation.

The comparison of serum and white blood cell
testing in pregnant and non-pregnant women are shown
in Table 3. It is immediately apparent that the percentage Hex A in serum from "control" women during

TABLE 4

PRELIMINARY RESULTS OF FIRST COMMUNITY

TAY-SACHS SCREENING TEST (5/71)

DESIGNATION	INDIVIDUALS
Non-carrier	1269
Carrier	38
Inconclusive	52
TOTAL	1359

pregnancy falls into the carrier range in almost all
cases. A significant drop in percent Hex A is also
seen in the pregnant obligate carriers. In both
groups, however, the leukocyte levels appear unchanged
by pregnancy. Based on this data, we strongly suggest
that white blood cell analysis can be used in pregnancy for accurate carrier detection. We have found
two "unknown" pregnant Jewish women (out of 74 studied
to date) with white blood cell levels in the carrier
range. We believe these women are carriers of the
Tay-Sachs gene.

All of the pregnant women we have studied have
agreed to be retested after pregnancy in order to
demonstrate, as we predict, that their serum Hex A
levels will return to the non-carrier range with no
change in white blood cell levels. Several women have
already done so and, indeed, their serum determinations
are now non-carrier in type while the white cell levels
remain unchanged.

The exact explanation for the reduction in percentage Hex A (as defined by heat inactivation) during
pregnancy is not evident. It does appear, however,
that this is only a <u>relative reduction</u> of the heat-
labile Hex A due to an absolute increase in a heat
stable serum hexosaminidase during pregnancy. Total
serum hexosaminidase is known to increase with pregnancy and may be the result of hormonal effects
during this period (9). We have recently evaluated
a number of placentas from various stages of pregnancy
and do not find an increase in heat stable hexosaminidase in this tissue. Whatever the explanation, the
phenomenon does not appear to affect leukocyte levels
during pregnancy so that carrier detection can be
achieved in these cells during this period.

With this information at hand, a specific
strategy was established for couples in which the
woman was pregnant at the time of testing. No pregnant women would be screened. The husband would be
screened by serum hexosaminidase determination only
if his wife were less than 4 1/2 months into her

TABLE 5

GENOTYPE ASSIGNMENT OF RETESTED "INCONCLUSIVES"

DESIGNATION*	INDIVIDUALS
Non-carrier	41
Carrier	5
Inconclusive (persistent)	1
TOTAL	47**

*Based upon leukocyte hexosaminidase evaluations
**5 individuals initially found inconclusive were
  not retested

pregnancy. If she were pregnant more than 4 1/2 months
neither the husband or the wife would be screened.
They would be counseled appropriately that testing information could not be helpful to them in this pregnancy and that it might only serve to raise anxiety
and concern if either was tested. Analysis of sera
from the husbands of pregnant women ("pregnant husbands") is performed rapidly within the first few days
after the screening test. "Pregnant husbands" who are
found to be either carriers or inconclusives, based on
the serum assay, are contacted and they and their wives
are then asked to come to the hospital for white blood
cell and repeat serum Hex A determinations. In this
way, relatively few families require immediate follow-
up evaluation since if the "pregnant husband" were
found to be a non-carrier on serum screening, no further testing would be recommended for that couple until after the completion of pregnancy at which time it
is recommended that the wife also be screened.

THE FIRST COMMUNITY SCREENING EFFORT

After establishing the prerequisite data, and
after one year of planning and organization with the
Jewish communities of Baltimore and Washington, the
first community attempt to apply these methods was
made on May 2, 1971 in an area synagogue. A total of
1800 people came for this "genetic service" in a 7
hour screening period. Of this total, 1359 actually
had blood tests performed. The 450 people who were
not tested roughly included:

    a. 150 pregnant women ($<$4 months); only their
        husband were tested
    b. 100 pregnant women ($>$4 months)
    c. 100 husbands of women in b.
    d. 100 other individuals: unmarried, over 45
        years old, or children

All serums were coded and subsequently tested in
a double blind fashion. The results of this initial
screening are shown in Table 4. Over 98% of the
tested individuals were Jewish and of central or East

TABLE 6

CUMULATIVE RESULTS OF TAY-SACHS HETEROZYGOTE

SCREENING PROGRAM (5/2/71)

GENOTYPE ASSIGNMENT	INDIVIDUALS
Non-carrier	1315
Carrier	43*
Inconclusive	1
TOTAL	1359

*Observed heterozygote frequency: 0.0316

TABLE 7

STRATEGY FOR A COMMUNITY GENETIC SCREENING PROGRAM

PHASE   I.   INITIAL PLANNING
                 Definition of goals
                 Evaluation of methods—control studies
                 Availability and commitment of pro-
                    fessional personnel
                 Automated systems
                 Funds

PHASE   II.   PROFESSIONAL SUPPORT
                 Medical community
                 Religious community

PHASE   III.   ORGANIZATIONAL RESOURCES
                 Multi—organizational participation
                 Manpower

PHASE   IV.   VOLUNTEER TASK FORCES
                 Orientation and instruction
                 Community emissaries

PHASE   V.   PUBLIC EDUCATION
                 Medical and religious counseling
                 Brochures, newsletters, flyers
                 Telephone squads
                 Mass media
                 Personal contacts

PHASE   VI.   BEGIN MASS SCREENING

European heritage. On initial screening of the sera
obtained from 1359 people, 38 were clearly identified
as carriers and 1269 were designated as non-carriers.
Fifty-two individuals had at least one of six determinations in the inconclusive range (3.7% of total
tested). These were all assigned to the inconclusive
category in order to critically re-evaluate this
group with further testing. This is particularly important at the outset of such a screening program in
order to determine the possibility of false <u>negative</u>
carriers.

The 52 inconclusive individuals were contacted
and 47 of them have since been retested. Leukocyte
and repeat serum hexosaminidase determinations were
performed. The follow-up results of the "inconclusives" are shown in Table 5. As indicated, nearly
90% of the individuals initially inconclusive were
non-carrier on retesting. If the leukocyte levels
were clearly non-carrier and the serum still inconclusive, the individual was considered a non-carrier.
Approximately 10% were found to be carriers and one
individual of the 1359 remained inconclusive after
repeated leukocyte and serum evaluations. This was
not totally unexpected as one might anticipate a small
number of individuals to reflect genetic heterogeneity
for this locus within the population. One of the
parents of this person shows similar activity of hexosaminidase. It is likely that this individual may represent a genetic variant and further studies are
currently being conducted.

The overall results are shown in Table 6. These
findings indicate a heterozygote frequency of 0.0316
for the Tay-Sachs gene in this sample American-Jewish
population. This carrier rate is similar to the incidence previously estimated from calculations based on
Tay-Sachs disease frequency in American Jews (10, 11).

Since this initial screening effort, 8 additional
community screening programs have been conducted. To
date, approximately 7,000 individuals have been
screened. Detailed analyses of the data from these

TABLE 8

PROBLEMS IN A COMMUNITY GENETIC SCREENING PROGRAM

A. General

1. Professional personnel: commitment and
    responsibilities

    a. Delivering results

    b. Genetic counseling

2. Public education: concern vs. fear

    a. Participation of community in education

3. Pregnancy

4. Responsibility to other family members of
    identified carriers

5. Religious considerations: Orthodox Jewry,
    Roman Catholicism

6. Single vs. married-individual screening

7. Information: confidentiality

B. Specific

1. Inconclusives

2. False positives

3. Medications

4. Illnesses

screenings will be reported elsewhere. Nearly 250
carriers have been identified and perhaps, most importantly, 7 couples have now been identified as being
at risk for Tay-Sachs disease in their offspring.
None of these couples have previously had Tay-Sachs
disease in their family. These couples may now, if
they so choose, with appropriate genetic counseling
and monitoring of each pregnancy by amniocentesis, be
assisted in having only unaffected children selectively.

It is imperative to emphasize again that careful
strategy and planning for such a program must be considered before initiation in the community. Fourteen
months of preparation were carried out prior to the
initiation of the Baltimore-Washington program. The
strategic phases of this planning are outlined in
Table 7. These issues and the problems generated by
adult-oriented genetic screening have been discussed
elsewhere (12). This initial experience has raised
a number of problems, both of a general and specific
nature. Table 8 simply lists some of these issues.
These practical, logistical, and ethical problems each
require in-depth consideration and have been previously considered (12).

It is hoped that the principles, issues and con-
cepts generated by this screening program will be applicable to future programs for other genetic disorders
such as sickle cell anemia and cystic fibrosis. In
this manner, a program directed at the prevention of
the prototype sphingolipidosis may serve as a prototype for prevention of other severe, untreatable genetic disorders.

REFERENCES

1. Okada, S., and O'Brien, J.S., Science 165: 698
    (1969)
2. O'Brien, J.S., Okada, S., Chen, A., and Fillerup,
    D.L., New Eng. J. Med. 283: 15 (1970)
3. Nadler, H.L. and Gerbie, A.B., New Eng. J. Med.
    282: 596 (1970)

4. Schneck, L., Friedland, J., Valenti, C., Adachi,
    M., Amsterdam, D., and Volk, B.W., Lancet $\underline{I}$: 582,
    (1970)
5. O'Brien,J.S., Okada, S., Fillerup, D.L., Veath,
    M.L., Adornato, B., Brenner, P.H., and Leroy, J.G.
    Science $\underline{172}$: 61,(1971)
6. Kaback, M.M. (unpublished observations)
7. Kaback, M.M., and O'Brien, J.S., Soc. Ped. Res.
    Abstracts p. 283 (1971) manuscript in preparation
8. Kaback, M.M. and Lash, E., manuscript in prepara-
    tion
9. Walker, P.G., Woolen, M.D., and Pugh, D., J. Clin.
    Path. $\underline{13}$: 353, (1960)
10. Aronson, S.M., in <u>Tay-Sachs Disease</u>, B.W. Volk,
    ed. New York, Grune and Stratton (1964)
11. Myrianthopoulos, N.C., and Aronson, S.M., Amer. J.
    Hum. Gen. $\underline{18}$: 313 (1966)
12. Kaback, M.M. and Zeiger, R.S., in <u>Ethical Issues</u>
    <u>in Genetic Counseling and the Use of Genetic Know-</u>
    <u>ledge</u>, M. Harris (ed.) in press, 1971

13. The authors acknowledge the dedicated support of
    the National Capital Tay-Sachs Foundation and
    many additional organizations and individuals in
    the Baltimore-Washington communities; Donna Ger-
    man as Program Coordinator, Marguerite Sonne-
    born, Linda Reynolds, and Doctor L. Pallan for
    expert technical assistance.

METABOLIC CHANGES FOLLOWING SPLENIC TRANSPLANTATION IN A CASE OF

GAUCHER'S DISEASE

Carl G. Groth, Rolf Blomstrand, Lars Hagenfeldt,
Per-Arne Ockerman, Karin Samuelsson, Lars Svennerholm

Karolinska Institute and Royal Veterinary College,

Stockholm; University of Gothenburg and University of Lund

The fact that the highest activity of glucocerebrosidase is normally found in the spleen (2) has suggested the possibility of splenic transplantation as a means of enzyme replacement in Gaucher's disease (1). Technically successful splenic homotransplantations have been reported by Starzl and co-workers in six patients with diseases other than lipidosis (3, 9).

In Northern Sweden several related patients with juvenile Gaucher's disease have been identified; most of them die between 10 and 25 years of age (4). On January 4, 1971, we did a splenic transplantation on a patient from this group.

Case Report. The patient was a man aged 24. In infancy pancytopenia and hepatosplenomegaly were diagnosed and splenectomy was done at 2 years of age; the spleen contained typical Gaucher's cells. The growth period saw development of kyphosis, rarefaction in the long bones, and mental retardation. At 12 years psycho-motor epilepsy began and from 15 years there was progressive grand mal. Electroencephalography showed constant bilateral synchronous epileptogenic activity (4). Bone marrow aspirates contained numerous Gaucher's cells. Repeated analysis of acid phosphatase and glucocerebroside in plasma yielded high values (5, 6).

On admission to our hospital the patient was cachectic and disabled by frequent grand mal attacks, despite large doses of anti-epileptic drugs. He was, however, fully capable of meaningful communication and expressed a strong positive attitude towards the proposed treatment.

The spleen was harvested from an unrelated 26 year old male renal transplant recipient who underwent bilateral nephrectomy and

splenectomy. The ABO blood groups of the donor and recipient were
A and AB, respectively; the patients shared one lymphocyte HL-A
antigen (7), while the other three differed. The artery and vein
of the graft were anastomosed end-to-end to the right external
iliac artery and vein.

Immunosuppressive treatment with antilymphocyte globulin
(A.L.G.) (Behring-Werke, Marburg) given intravenously, azathioprine,
and prednisone were started 3-7 days before the transplantation.
Before the spleen was transferred to the recipient it was irradiated ex vivo with 300 rad for 15 minutes. Later on the transplant
was irradiated in situ.

During the first postoperative week the patient had frequent
convulsions, respiratory distress, and a striking reddening and
swelling in the abdominal wall over the graft. Wound and blood
cultures were negative. Since it seemed likely that these manifestations were due to rejection, the prednisone dose was increased.
At the same time changes in haemoglobin, bilirubin, lactate dehydrogenase, and haptoglobin indicated haemolysis. Daily blood transfusions were required to maintain an acceptable haemoglobin level.
Lymphopenia and thrombocytopenia, which first appeared during the
preoperative A.L.G. treatment, continued. After about 2 weeks the
patient's condition improved rapidly. The fever persisted but the
convulsions ceased. The reddening and tenderness of the graft disappeared, as did the haemolysis.

A technetium-99m sulphur colloid scan obtained on the first
postoperative day showed an excellent uptake of isotope in the
graft. During the following weeks the uptake diminished, and on
day 44 there was no uptake (fig. 1). Immunosuppression was augmented but when no uptake reoccurred it was rapidly reduced. The
spleen was irradiated with a betatron (500 + 1000 rad) to produce
cell death.

During the third postoperative month the patient became more
cachectic and he complained of severe skeletal pain. He became
bedridden and contracted pneumonia. Death ensued on the 90th day
after operation. Necropsy revealed organ findings typical of
Gaucher's disease. The graft was grossly well preserved, and the
vascular anastomoses were patent. Microscopic examination displayed
extensive necrosis.

Metabolic Findings. Sphingolipids in plasma were studied in
three laboratories:

Total lipid hexose with orcinol and assay of cerebroside from
thin-layer chromatograms (16, 18) (Serafimer Hospital).

Glucocerebroside by thin-layer chromatography followed by gas
chromatographic assay of total fatty acids after methanolysis,
using 19-methyl eicosanoate as an internal standard (17) (University

of Gothenburg).

Ceramide by gas chromatography and mass spectrometry (13) (Royal Veterinary College).

With the methods used the mean $\pm$ SD normal value for plasma cerebroside was 7.7 ($\pm$ 1.8) μmole per litre; the ceramide was 7.8 ($\pm$ 2.2) μmole per litre.

The plasma level N-acetyl-β-glucosaminidase (normal less than 12.5 I.U. per litre) were determined as reported by Ockerman (10-12). Total acid phosphatase activity was determined with nitro-phenyl phosphate as the substrate (14) and expressed in Bessey-Lowry units (normal range 0.13 - 0.63).

Post-mortem tissue was analysed for glucocerebroside by the methods of Svennerholm (16-18).

20-35 days before the transplantation the plasma levels of total lipid hexose and glucocerebroside were very high, while the ceramide level was normal. In one sample obtained 4 days before transplantation the total lipid hexose and cerebroside measured at Serafimer Hospital were considerably lower than earlier. During the first 3 weeks after the transplantation there was a further re-duction in the total lipid hexose. According to both methods used the postoperative cerebroside level was slightly lower than that found 3-5 weeks before operation. Ceramide levels fluctuated slightly but with no definite trend (fig. 1).

Before transplantation the acid-phosphatase activity in the serum exceeded 2 units, whereas after the operation it fell over 3 weeks, to stabilize at about 0.8 units. During the 7th week there was a rise, and shortly before death over 4 units were recorded. N-acetyl-β-glucosaminidase displayed a similar variation (fig. 1).

The percentage of Gaucher's cells in the bone marrow aspirate fell slightly for the first postoperative month from 9% before the transplantation. Death was preceded by an increase, and many of the cells were small and probably newly formed (fig. 1).

The post-mortem concentration of total lipid hexose and gluco-cerebroside in the liver was very high. A significant amount of glucocerebroside was also demonstrated in the cerebellar and cere-bral cortex, and the concentration was six times higher in the cerebellar cortex (table I). The splenic graft did not contain appreciably more total lipid hexose or glucocerebroside than the spleen from a healthy, age-matched person, according to simultane-ous analysis (table II). The fatty acid pattern of the plasma and tissue glucocerebrosides are given in table III.

Comments. To be successful, splenic transplantation in

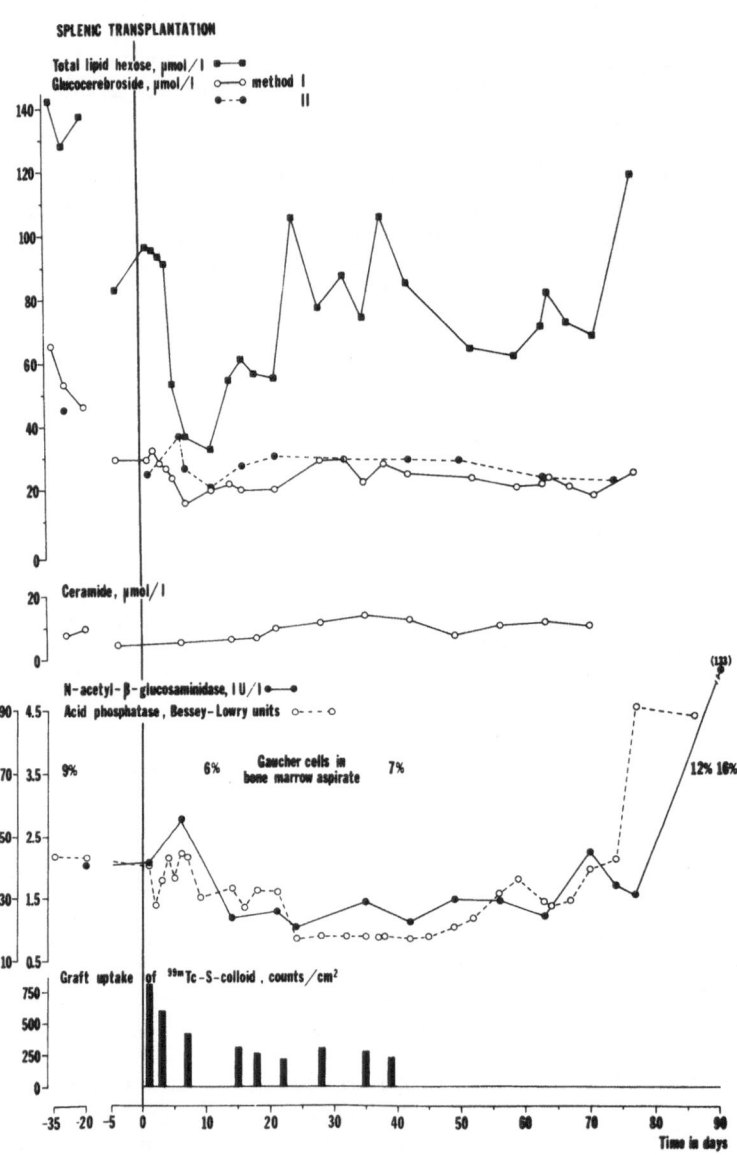

FIG. 1 -- Plasma levels of sphingolipids and lysosomal enzymes, number of Gaucher's cells found in the bone marrow, and ^{99m}Tc-S colloid uptake by the splenic graft.

TABLE I.

| | TOTAL LIPID HEXOSE | | GLUCOCEREBROSIDE | |
| | NORMAL | PATIENT | NORMAL | PATIENT |
	(μmol/g wet weight)			
Liver	0.19*	29.3	0.05*	24.2
Cerebral Cortex	---	---	NIL	0.08
Cerebellar Cortex	---	---	NIL	0.48

*Kwiterovih et al., (8)

TABLE II.

| | TOTAL LIPID HEXOSE | GLUCOCEREBROSIDE |
	(μmol/g wet weight)	
Normal Spleen	1.58	0.11
Splenic graft	2.37	0.18
Spleen in Gaucher's disease	17.3 - 39.1*	

*Suomi and Agranoff, (14)

TABLE III.   VALUES IN MOLAR %.

| | | PATIENT | | | | |
| | | PLASMA | | POST-MORTEM TISSUES | | |
FATTY ACID	NORMAL PLASMA	BEFORE TX.	32 DAYS AFTER TX.	CEREBRUM	CEREBELLUM	LIVER
16:0	12.7	16.2	11.9	17.0	7.6	8.4
16:1	0.4	1.9	0.7	4.5	1.1	0.3
18:0	2.4	5.3	3.2	41.3	20.4	3.5
18:1	2.4	3.9	1.6	6.4	1.4	0.7
20:0	2.6	2.6	2.9	4.2	5.5	5.5
22:0	18.9	12.6	11.9	4.8	12.9	27.5
22:1	7.9	6.2	8.2			
23:0	8.6	2.7	2.4	1.7	1.8	6.4
23:1	0.6	1.7	1.1			
24:0	17.9	8.7	11.8	8.4	34.7	21.4
24:1	25.5	38.3	44.4	6.7	12.4	20.2
25:0				1.0	0.6	
25:1				0.8	0.5	
26:0				1.1	0.5	
26:1				2.1	0.7	

Gaucher's disease requires that the transplant can catabolize glucocerebroside in significant amounts and that the immunological reactions can be controlled.

An analysis of the effect of the transplanted spleen on the
plasma sphingolipids is complicated by the limited time that the
graft functioned and by the fact that the lipids may well have been
affected by the other measures such as immunosuppression, blood
transfusions, and the presence of haemolysis, thrombocytopenia, and
lymphopenia. Moreover, the lower level of glucocerebroside after
operation did not accord with the time when, as judged by the isotope scan, the graft functioned. Breakdown of glucocerebroside in
the spleen might, however, not be readily reflected in the plasma
level because of the extremely large pool of the lipid in the
organs. Nonetheless, the normal level of glucocerebroside found in
the graft post-mortem indicates catabolism of any glucocerebroside
taken up.

Transplantation was followed by a significant drop in the acid-
phosphatase and glucosaminidase activities in plasma, and a slight
decrease in the number of Gaucher's cells found in the bone marrow.
Arrest of graft function was followed by a return to preoperative
levels followed by a steep rise. The temporary shift towards
normal might reflect a reduction in the influx of lipid in the
reticuloendothelial system.

The arrest of splenic graft function in our patient was probably due to rejection. Currently, more prolonged graft survival
could probably be best achieved utilizing an intrafamilial donor.

The final clinical picture, with cachexia, skeletal pain, and
convulsions, was consistent with the terminal stage in juvenile
Gaucher's disease. Moreover, the increased number of Gaucher's
cells and the striking rise in the acid phosphatase and glucosaminidase activity point to an exacerbation of the disease.

Although the patient did not benefit from the transplantation,
the spleen graft would seem to afford the most likely source of the
favorable enzyme changes recorded. Further attempts at splenic
transplantation in Gaucher's disease seem warranted.

REFERENCES

1. Brady, R.O. New Eng. J. Med. 1966, 275, 312.

2. Brady, R.O., Kanfer, J.N., Shapiro, D. J. Biol. Chem. 1965,
    240, 39.

3. Hathaway, W.E., Mull, M.M., Githens, J.H., Groth, C.G., Marchioro, T.L., Starzl, T.E. Transplantation, 1969, 7, 73.

4. Herrlin, K.-M., Hillborg, P.O. Acta Paediat. Stockh. 1962, 51, 137.

5. Hillborg, P.O., Estborn, B. Acta Paediat. Stockh. 1962, 51, 137.

6. Hillborg, P.O., Svennerholm, L. Acta Paediat. Stockh. 1960, 49, 707.

7. Kissmeyer-Nielsen, F., Thorsby, E. Transplantation Rev. 1970, 4, 115.

8. Kwiterovih, P.O., Sloan, H.R., Fredrickson, D.S. J. Lipid Res. 1970, 11, 332.

9. Marchioro, T.L., Rowlands, D.T., Jr., Rifkind, D., Waddell, W.R., Starzl, T.E., Fudenberg, H. Ann. N.Y. Acad. Sci. 1964, 120, 626.

10. Ockerman, P.A. Clinica Chim. Acta 1968, 20, 1.

11. Ockerman, P.A. Clinica Chim. Acta 1968, 21, 279.

12. Ockerman, P.A. Clinica Chim. Acta 1969, 23, 479.

13. Samuelsson, K. Scand. J. Clin. Lab. Invest. (in press).

14. Sigma Technical Bulletin No. 104, St. Louis, Missouri, 1963.

15. Suomi, W.D., Agranoff, B.W. J. Lipid Res. 1965, 6, 211.

16. Svennerholm, L. J. Neurochem. 1956, 1, 42.

17. Svennerholm, L., Stallberg-Stenhagen, S. J. Lipid Res. 1968, 9, 215.

18. Svennerholm, E., Svennerholm, L. Nature 1963, 198, 688.

STUDIES ON THE METABOLIC CONTROL OF FABRY'S DISEASE THROUGH KIDNEY

TRANSPLANTATION

Michel Philippart,[1] Stanley S. Franklin,[2] Arthur Gordon,[2] Donald Leeber,[3] and Alan R. Hull[3]

[1]Mental Retardation Center, The Neuropsychiatric Institute and Departments of Pediatrics, Neurology and Psychiatry; [2]Department of Medicine, University of California; [3]Department of Internal Medicine, University of Texas Southwestern Medical School, Dallas, Texas

INTRODUCTION

The development of the lysosome concept (7) has lately provided a theoretical background to our understanding of the pathogenesis of the so-called lipid storage disorders. A rational approach to the seemingly insurmountable problem of therapy has now become feasible on that basis. Indeed, lysosomal enzymes can be taken up by fibroblasts (22,29) and other types of cells such as those of the reticulo-endothelial system (7), kidney (25), and liver (13). As expected, the blood-brain barrier prevents extraneous enzymes from reaching the brain (1,12). This limits the value of replacement therapy to those rare lipid storage disorders with no brain involvement such as chronic Gaucher's disease (18) or minimal primary nervous lesions such as Fabry's disease (16,23).

Among the numerous functions of the lysosomes, their general role in the turnover of cell constituents has been somewhat underestimated. In this respect the metabolic disturbances secondary to the deficiency of a lysosomal enzyme strikingly illustrate the key function of these enzymes in maintaining the normal distribution of cell components. Lysosomes engulf whole cytoplasmic aliquots including organelles such as mitochondria (7). Rather than considering such phenomena as accidental, "sometimes damaging events" (7) we would like to emphasize what a straightforward mechanism this represents to renew complex and diverse molecular assemblies such as membranes. If membrane catabolism were to take place in situ, it would be exceedingly difficult to explain how the cell could adjust the amount of the numerous enzymes needed in different proportions for degradation of different types of membranes.

On the one hand the lysosomal content is part of the extracellular space, in that it is separated from the mainstream of
cytoplasmic metabolism involved in energy supply and synthesis.
On the other hand lysosomes represent a system of entry for
diverse extracellular materials such as colloids, enzymes or
endogenous proteins (7), including lysosomal enzymes (22,29).
This last property has led us to try enzyme therapy in patients
with an enzymic deficiency. Such an approach to become practical
requires purification or synthesis of proteins sufficiently similar to the deficient enzyme both in activity and structure in
order not to elicit an antibody response from the recipient. The
mode of administration should be compatible with long term
tolerance and efficiency, and adequate distribution of the
extraneous enzyme among the different tissues where it is needed.

A property of lysosomal enzymes which has not been systemat-
ically studied until recently is their occurrence in body fluids.
Although the mode of entry of these enzymes - excretion, secretion
or cellular disintegration - has not been fully explored, it has
been clearly established in tissue culture that a factor of an
undefined nature (11), possibly a lysosomal enzyme, can leave a
normal cell, diffuse into the medium surrounding it and be cap-
tured by cells deficient in this factor. Recipient cells are then
able to deal with their metabolic block. In human experiments
logically derived from such information, it was shown that serum
infusion provided the desired catabolic action in Fabry's disease
(17) and mucopolysaccharide storage (9). The amount of enzyme
which can be administrated with infusion is obviously limited.
The half-life of injected ceramide trihexosidase was only a few
days in the recipients (17). It can be expected that repeated
infusions at short intervals would rapidly elicit immune intoler-
ance in the subjects.

In order to overcome such problems we have been investigating
ways to supply patients with a permanent source of enzyme. Since
the technique of kidney transplantation has been well established,
we decided to explore whether a transplanted kidney would constitute an effective, permanent source of enzyme in patients with a
deficient lysosomal enzyme.

KEY METABOLIC PROBLEMS IN FABRY'S DISEASE

Fabry's disease is a glycolipid storage disorder (25), an
α-galactosidosis (3), resulting from an α-galactosidase deficiency
(4,5,14,24). Kidney involvement is prominent and kidney failure
is the leading cause of death in this condition (27). Glycolipid
storage in the blood vessel walls throughout the body is probably
responsible for most pathological manifestations. Vascular
involvement may be primary, but it is conceivable that a
portion of the glycolipids stored in the blood

vessels derives from the plasma. Indeed, increased levels of ceramide trihexoside (CTH) are characteristically found in the plasma of these patients (28).

Plasma CTH may arise from several sources. In the pig, old erythrocytes were shown to shed their ceramide polyhexosides into the plasma (6). In patients with Fabry's disease, part of the increased plasma CTH might originate from the possible rupture of the foam cells lining the vessel walls, thus contributing to a vicious cycle between vessel and plasma.

Urinary CTH is markedly increased (8,20), even in the new-born (19), years before the appearance of clinical symptoms and at least two decades prior to the development of kidney failure. CTH excretion may represent a useful adaptative mechanism to limit the rate of lipid accumulation inside the tissues and thus contribute to the mild, protracted course of Fabry's disease. Undoubtedly, a large proportion of urinary CTH derives from the desquamation of the foam cells observed in the glomeruli and distal tubules of the kidneys (10). Since hemodialysis results in a reduction in plasma CTH (table 1), urinary CTH may partly arise from plasma ultrafiltration. In the event of progressive kidney failure, the damaged kidney might become unable to clear the excess CTH and this might result in an overflow of kidney CTH into the plasma.

Table 1

Effect of Hemodialysis on Ceramide Trihexoside Levels
in the Plasma from Patients with Fabry's Disease
(nmoles/ml of plasma)

	Before dialysis	After dialysis
Patient A	11.3	2.6
C	1.7	1.0
D	6.1	5.1
E	3.4	2.2

KIDNEY TRANSPLANTATION IN FABRY'S DISEASE

We have studied the effect of kidney transplantation in two unrelated patients (A and B) with Fabry's disease. Detailed clinical reports will be published elsewhere (15,21). Both patients were in their mid-thirties. They had reached the stage of renal failure at the time a cadaver kidney was grafted. Patient A who still has his own non-functional kidneys was transplanted 25 months ago. Patient B was nephrectomized prior to transplantation 9 months ago.

In patient A, CTH levels in the plasma (table 2) remained close to the upper normal limits for 15 months after transplantation. The exact time of the post-operative decrease in CTH was not documented. Immunosuppressive therapy included 15 mg of prednisone (12.5 to 17.5mg)and 125mg of Azathioprine (100 to 150 mg). During the 16th month after transplantation, an episode of graft rejection prompted an increase in drug dosage (prednisone : 60mg; Azathioprine : 150mg). This was followed by a marked and persistent increase in the plasma CTH. The decrease in plasma CTH correlates well with the α-galactosidase activity in the plasma which reached 20 to 25% of the mean normal value (table 3).

Table 2

Ceramide Trihexoside Levels in the Plasma
(Fabry's Disease)
(nmoles/ml of plasma)

	Before kidney transplantation	After kidney transplantation		
		0-3 mos.	3-15 mos.	16-24 mos.
Patient A	11.3 (N.D.)	N.D.	1.5(1.0-2.4)	7.4(6.6-8.5)
Patient B	4.2 (N.D.)	4.6(0.7-9.3)	4.1(3.4-5.4)	
Untreated patients (number=25)	5.2(1.7-12.6)			
Male controls (number=13)	0.9(0.2-1.6)			

N.D. not determined

Table 3

Alpha-galactosidase Activity in Plasma(Citrate Buffer, pH5)
from Patients with Fabry's Disease
(nmoles of 4-methylumbelliferone/mg of protein/hr)

| | Before kidney transplantation | After kidney transplantation | |
		0-15 mos.	15-25 mos.
Patient A	0*	0.85-1.06	0.11-0.20
Patient B	0*	0.21-0.48**	
Untreated patients	0-0.22		
Controls (number=8)	4.26(2.43-7.91)		
Mailed controls**		(1.70-1.87)	

*Determined on frozen specimens
**Determined on refrigerated specimens (4°c)

Enzyme activity was undetectable in a frozen sample collected pre-
operatively. The difference is probably significant although the
very low activity found in some patients with Fabry's disease is
generally lost when the plasma is frozen before analysis. The
rejection episode was accompanied by a substantial and persistent
reduction in plasma α-galactosidase.

   In the urine (table 4), a progressive decrease in hydrolase
activities, including α-galactosidase, became apparent over the
months. Beta-acetylglucosaminidase, however, consistently
remained above the normal range. Daily levels of CTH excretion in
the urine fell within normal limits at all times.

   The metabolic changes might be interpreted as follows. For
more than a year following transplantation, α-galactosidase
"leaked" from the graft into the plasma. Plasma α-galactosidase
is likely to have significantly contributed to maintain plasma CTH
levels close to the normal range. Part of the CTH may have been
taken up by the graft or ultrafiltrated and catabolized by the
urinary enzyme.

Table 4

Enzyme Activity in Urine from a Patient with Fabry's Disease
Following Kidney Transplantation
(nmoles of 4-methylumbelliferone/mg of protein/hr)

| | Patient A | | | | Male Controls (number=10) |
	Jun '70	Aug. '70	Mar. '71	Aug. '71	Range
α-galactosidase *	34.1	10.3	4.6	4.7	3.1-24.1
β-galactosidase	609.1	5.8	45.3	11.7	10.2-131.6
β-glucosidase	N.D.	7.6	1.3	1.4	0.2-19.8
β-N-acetylglucosaminidase	103.4	105.8	64.3	76.9	11.6-35.8

N.D. = not determined
*The activity in 4 untreated patients with Fabry's disease
    ranged from 0 to 2.6.

The disappearance of PAS positive lipid deposits in the liver
biopsy may indicate that plasma α-galactosidase has reached organs
remote from the kidney. The disappearance of the chronic bouts of
pain also suggests a remote action on the cells involved in the
mechanism of pain. The latter has not been explained but it is not
correlated with the level of plasma CTH in our experience. The
progressive reduction in the activity of urinary hydrolases may be
regarded as the consequence of the developing rejection. The large
increase in prednisone dosage required to control graft rejection
and maintain kidney function within normal limits coincided with a
drop in plasma α-galactosidase activity and a concomitant increase
in plasma CTH levels.

The effects of kidney transplantation on patient B have been
rather disappointing. Although the patient is doing well clinically and only needs relatively low amounts of immunosuppressive drugs
(17.5mg of prednisone and 50mg of Azathioprine),the mean level of
plasma CTH (Table 2) has remained as high as before transplantation,
with the exception of a few normal values in the immediate postoperative period. Since the patient lives in another state,

α-galactosidase activity in plasma and urine could not be monitored as closely as in patient A. The refrigeration and delay before analysis entailed an appreciable loss of activity (table 3). Nevertheless, α-galactosidase activity in the plasma of patient B was 12 to 27% of the control value. This was only slightly lower than the activity found in patient A before the rejection episode. Urinary α-galactosidase was at the lower normal level, which may indicate that the graft had a limited capacity to synthesize (or excrete) the enzyme.

To understand the role of immunosuppression on hydrolase activity, we have undertaken a survey of patients transplanted for kidney disorders other than Fabry's disease. Greatly elevated activities of lysosomal hydrolases were found in the immediate post-operative period. Activities become markedly reduced several years after successful transplantation. These preliminary data point to a possible conflict between the tolerance of the graft and its ability to produce - or more specifically to excrete - lysosomal hydrolases.

The histocompatibility antigens of the cell membrane have been demonstrated in the lysosomes (2). It is thus conceivable that antibodies against the graft may disrupt the lysosome and contribute in that fashion to an increased "excretion" of hydrolases into body fluids. Prednisone, a lysosomal stabilizer (7) which has the opposite effect, limits the release of hydrolases. Therefore, it may be necessary to tolerate a low-grade rejection of the transplant to insure that an adequate amount of lysosomal enzymes will reach other tissues.

INDICATIONS FOR KIDNEY TRANSPLANTATION

A sustained clinical and biochemical reversal of the inborn error of the metabolism may be achieved through kidney transplantation in Fabry's disease. Our results, however, emphasize that major problems remain to be resolved before this procedure can be recommended as a suitable treatment for this or other similar metabolic disorders, in the absence of a definite indication such as renal failure.

Acknowledgements

We wish to thank Miss Colette Meurant and Mr. Seiji Nakatani for their helpful technical assistance.

This investigation was supported in part by funds from the State of California Department of Mental Hygiene, The Mental

Retardation Program, NPI, UCLA and research grants NB 06938, HD
04612, MCH 927, HD 00345, and HD 05615 from the National
Institutes of Health.

References

1. Austin, J.H., in <u>Inborn Disorders of Sphingolipid
    Metabolism</u>, S.M. Aronson and B.W. Volk, editors, Pergamon
    Press, New York, 359, (1967).

2. Basch, R.S. and Stetson, C.A., <u>Transplantation</u> <u>1</u>, 469, (1963).

3. Bensaude, I., Callahan, J., and Philippart, M., <u>Biochem.
    Biophys. Res. Commun.</u> <u>43</u>, 913, (1971).

4. Brady, R.O., Uhlendorf, B.W., and Jacobson, C.B., <u>Science</u> <u>172</u>,
    (1971).

5. Clarke, J.T.R., Knaack, J., Crawhall, J., and Wolfe, L.S.,
    <u>New Eng. J. Med.</u>, <u>284</u>, 233, (1971).

6. Dawson, G. and Sweeley, C.C., <u>J. Biol. Chem.</u>, <u>245</u>, No. 2,
    (1970).

7. DeDuve, C. and Wattiaux, R., <u>Ann. Rev. Physiol.</u> <u>28</u>, 435, (1966).

8. Desnick, R.J., Dawson, G., Desnick, S.J., Sweeley, C.C. and
    Krivit, W., <u>New Eng. J. Med.</u> <u>284</u>, 739, (1971).

9. DiFerrante, N., Nichols, B.L., Donnelly, P.V., Neri, G.,
    Hrgovcic, R., and Berglund, R.K., <u>Proc. Nat. Acad. Sci.</u> <u>68</u>,
    303, (1971).

10. Dubach, U.C. and Gloor, F., <u>Dtsch. Med. Wschr.</u> <u>91</u>, 241, (1966).

11. Fratantoni, J.C., Hall, C.W., and Neufeld, E.F., <u>Proc. Nat.
    Acad. Sci.</u> <u>64</u>, 360, (1969).

12. Greene, H.L., Hug, G., and Schubert, W.K., <u>Arch. Neurol.</u> <u>20</u>,
    147, (1969).

13. Hug, G. and Schubert, W.K., <u>J. Cell. Biol.</u> <u>35</u>, C1, (1967).

14. Kint, J.A., <u>Science</u> <u>167</u>, 1268, (1970).

15. Leeber, D., Philippart, M., Prati, R., Peters, P.C., and Hull,
    A.R., to be published.

16. Lou, H.O.C., and Reske-Nielsen, E., <u>Arch. Neurol</u>. <u>25</u>, 351, (1971).

17. Mapes, C.A., Anderson, R.L., Sweeley, C.C., Desnick, R.J., and Krivit, W., <u>Science</u> <u>169</u>, 987, (1970).

18. Philippart, M. and Menkes, J.H., <u>Inborn Disorders of Sphingolipid Metabolism</u>. S.M. Aronson and B.W. Volk, editors, Pergamon Press, New York, 389, (1966).

19. Philippart, M. and Franceschetti, A.T., <u>Lancet</u> <u>2</u>, 1368, 1967.

20. Philippart, M., Sarlieve, L, and Manacorda, A., <u>Pediatrics</u> <u>43</u>, 201, (1969).

21. Philippart, M., Franklin, S., and Gordon, A. to be published.

22. Porter, M.T., Fluharty, A.L., and Kihara, H., <u>Science</u> <u>172</u>, 1263, (1971).

23. Rahman, A.N. and Lindenberg, R., <u>Arch. Neurol</u>. <u>9</u>, 373, (1963).

24. Romeo, G. and Migeon, B.R., <u>Science</u> <u>170</u>, 180, (1970).

25. Straus, W., J. <u>Biophys. Biochem. Cytol</u>. <u>2</u>, 513, (1956).

26. Sweeley, C.C. and Klionsky, B., <u>J. Biol. Chem</u>. <u>238</u>, 3148, (1963).

27. Sweeley, C.C. and Klionsky, B., <u>The Metabolic Basis of Inherited Disease</u>, second edition. J.B. Stanbury, J.B. Wyngaarden, and D.S. Fredrickson, editors, McGraw-Hill Book Company, New York, 618, (1966).

28. Vance, D.E., Krivit, W., Sweeley, C.C., <u>J. Lipid Res</u>. <u>10</u>,, 188, (1969).

29. Weismann, U.N., Rossi, E.E., and Herschkowitz, N.N., <u>New Eng. J. Med</u>. <u>284</u>, 672, (1971).

THE INDUCTION OF SULFATIDE, GANGLIOSIDE AND CEREBROSIDE STORAGE IN ORGANIZED NERVOUS SYSTEM CULTURES

Jack Stern, Alex B. Novikoff and Robert D. Terry

Department of Pathology
Albert Einstein College of Medicine
Bronx, New York 10461

Although a number of animal models exist for the sphingo-lipidoses, tissue culture offers advantages in studying the development of the inclusion bodies characteristic of these diseases.

An attempt was made to induce the formation of inclusions by administering sulfatide, ganglioside and cerebroside to separate groups of long-term organotypic cultures of central and peripheral mouse and rat nervous system (7). Granules remarkably similar to those seen in metachromatic leucodystrophy (MLD) (2), Tay-Sachs disease (TSD) (11) and Krabbe's globoid leucodystrophy (KGL) (5) have been observed.

The lipids were added to the culture medium after tissues had been in vitro for 14 days. The lipid-enriched medium was replenished every 4th day. Light microscopic examination of the cultures was performed daily. Cultures were fixed for electron microscopy at timed intervals extending from 24 hours to 4 weeks after the initial administration of lipid.

Observations:

I. Cultures given 5.0 mg/ml of sulfatide demonstrated cellular alterations after 3 days, when dark granules were observed within macrophages and within the astroglia situated in the most superficial strata of the culture. With time, such granules were also observed within spinal cord neurons, oligodendroglia, dorsal root ganglion neurons and Schwann cells. These granules stained metachromatically with toluidine blue and

the cresyl-violet method of Hirsch-Peiffer (3) indicating the
presence of sulfatide. The granules also demonstrated acid
phosphatase activity, indicating their lysosomal nature (6).

Electron microscopic examination shows that in those cells
actively engaged in endocytosis, i.e., macrophages and superficial
astroglia, sulfatide is ingested by pinocytic vacuoles which fuse
with lysosomes and subsequently form "giant" lysosomes (residual
bodies) that measure up to 5 μ. The granular matrix of these
enlarged residual bodies appear transformed into numerous membranous whorls, with a 50 Å periodicity (Fig. 1). These bodies

Fig. 1   Electron micrograph of portion of a superficial
macrophage in a spinal cord culture five days after the administration of 5.0 mg/ml of sulfatide. Most of the field is occupied by
a giant lysosome (GL) with numerous membranous whorls at its
periphery (arrows). An isolated membranous figure, interpreted as
having budded from a giant lysosome, is seen at MF.

Portions of the limiting membrane of the giant lysosome and
membranous figure are seen (arrow heads). Also seen are small
parts of the nucleus (N), Golgi apparatus (G) and endoplasmic
reticulum (ER). X 37,000.

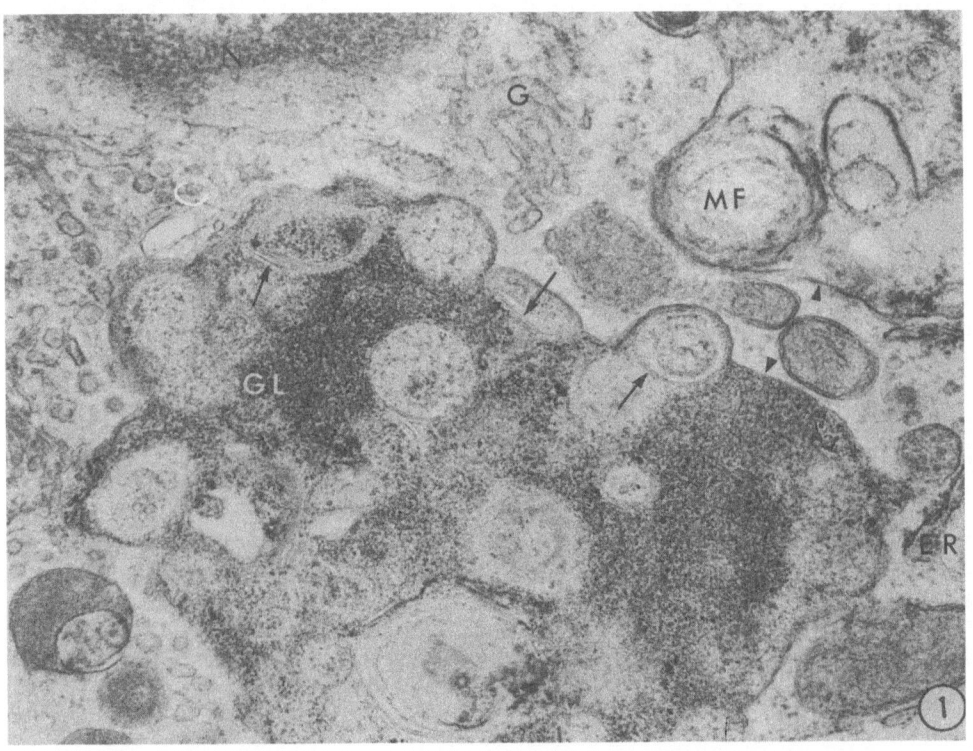

apparently bud off from the giant lysosomes as separate inclusions in the cytoplasm (Fig. 2). In those cells not actively engaged in endocytosis, i.e., spinal and dorsal root ganglion neurons, sulfatide may enter the cell, at least in part, by transport across the plasma membrane, since pinocytic vacuoles are not numerous. How such non membrane-bound lipid gains access to lysosomes is unclear. It may undergo autophagy or fuse with lysosomes. In any case, they become part of residual bodies. Membranous arrays with a 50 Å periodicity develop within the residual bodies. The inclusion bodies formed in all cell types had an average diameter of 1.0 μ and were similar, in both appearance and periodicity, to those observed in MLD (Fig. 3).

Fig. 2   A sister culture of that seen in Fig. 1, 10 days after sulfatide administration. A portion of an astroglial cell shows a giant lysosome (GL) with a membranous figure apparently budding off at the arrows. An isolated membranous figure is seen at MF. The limiting membrane (arrow heads) becomes indistinguishable from the membranous arrays in the area of the membranous figure. X 70,000.

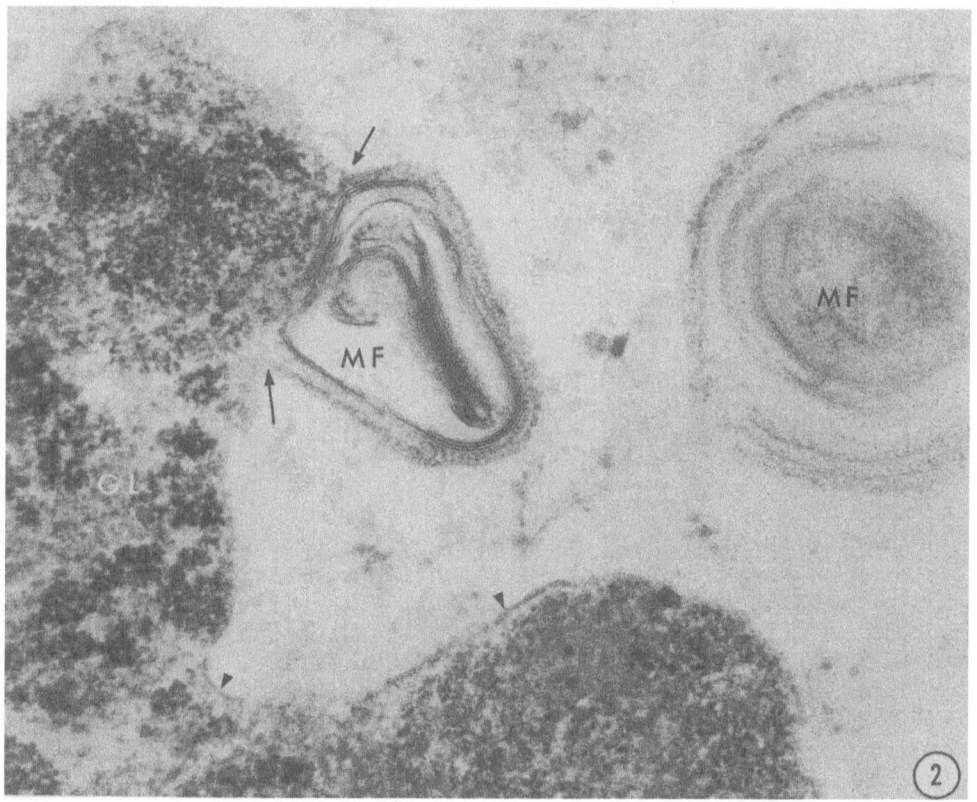

Fig. 3   Portion of the astroglial cytoplasm in a spinal cord culture which has received 5.0 mg/ml sulfatide for thirty days. Numerous membranous inclusions with a 50 Å periodicity are observed. X   50,500.

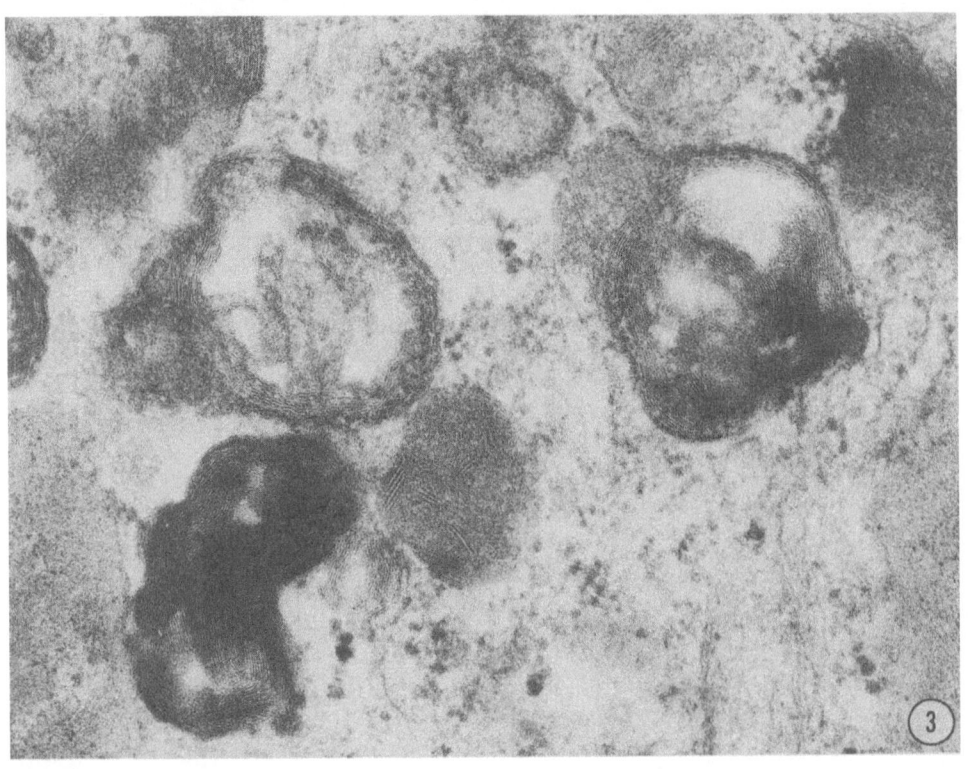

II. A mixture of whole brain ganglioside in concentrations varying from 0.1 to 5.0 mg/ml was added to a second group of cultures.

Intracellular granule formation was first observed by light microscopy 7 days after adding the ganglioside-enriched medium. As with cultures given exogenous sulfatide, the first cells to demonstrate morphological changes were the macrophages and superficial astroglia. Ten days later similar inclusions were seen within spinal cord neurons, Schwann cell and sheath cells. Such granules appeared within dorsal root ganglion neurons only after prolonged exposure to elevated concentrations of ganglioside, e.g., 5.0 mg/ml for 30 days.

Electron microscopic changes were already evident 5 days
after beginning the ganglioside feeding. The affected cells
demonstrated a slight increase in size and a marked increase in
number of lysosomes. These lysosomes displayed a variety of
round, oval or elongate forms and their matrix contained an
electron-opaque, granular stippling as well as small numbers of
lamellae aligned in parallel arrays. Within the next few days
the number of lamellae increased strikingly and assumed a circular
pattern, frequently with an inner core of matrix. Eventually
there was little or no remaining lysosomal matrix and the resulting
inclusions could be best described as "membranous bodies" (Fig. 4).
These membranous bodies measured from 1.0 to 3.0 μ in diameter with
a periodicity of about 55 Å. They bear a striking resemblance to
inclusions seen in both Tay-Sachs disease (11) (Figs. 5 and 6)
generalized gangliosidoses (1,9).

Fig. 4   Electron micrograph of two membranous bodies in an
astroglial process from a spinal cord culture which has received
2.5 mg/ml of ganglioside for 10 days. Electron-opaque granular
material is still present in parts of the lysosome (arrows). Note
a portion of the nucleus (N) of another astroglial cell and a
prominent pinocytic vesicle (PV). X   70,500.

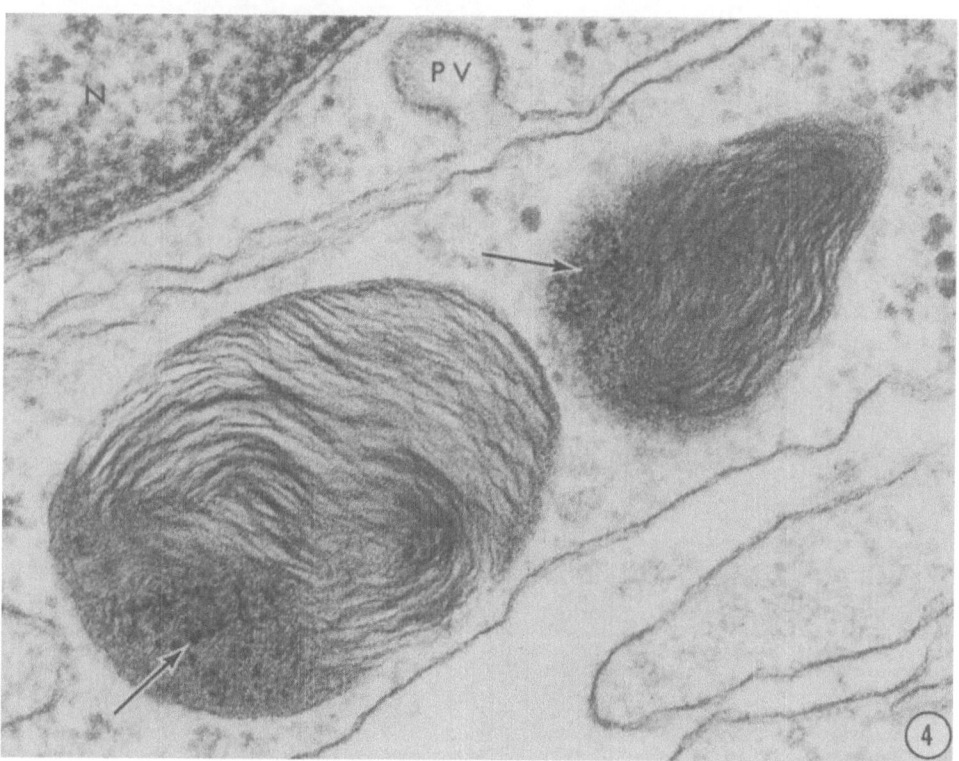

The membranous bodies demonstrated acid phosphatase activity. The sites of phosphatase activity also stained blue with the Mowry-modified Hale stain indicating the presence of sialo-mucins (4).

III. A third group of cultures was given 1.0 mg/ml of bovine galactocerebroside. Only macrophages showed changes. These were first observed, by both light and electron microscopy, 24 hours after galactocerebroside administration. The lysosomes of these cells contained straight or curved linear structures, resembling tubules, with electron-lucent centers. On cross section these tubules have a crystalline-polygonal appearance (Fig. 7). These inclusions are strikingly like those described in Krabbe's globoid leucodystrophy (5).

Fig. 5   A neuronal membranous cytoplasmic body from a patient with Tay-Sachs disease is compared with a similar membranous inclusion (Fig. 6) observed in a spinal cord neuron from a culture which received 5.0 mg/ml of ganglioside for 30 days. (Fig. 5 reprinted with permission from the Journal of Neuropathology and Experimental Neurology.) Fig. 5 X 55,000.   Fig. 6 X 60,000.

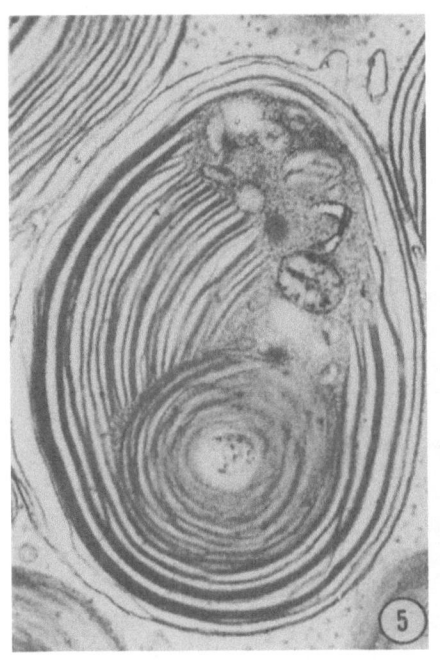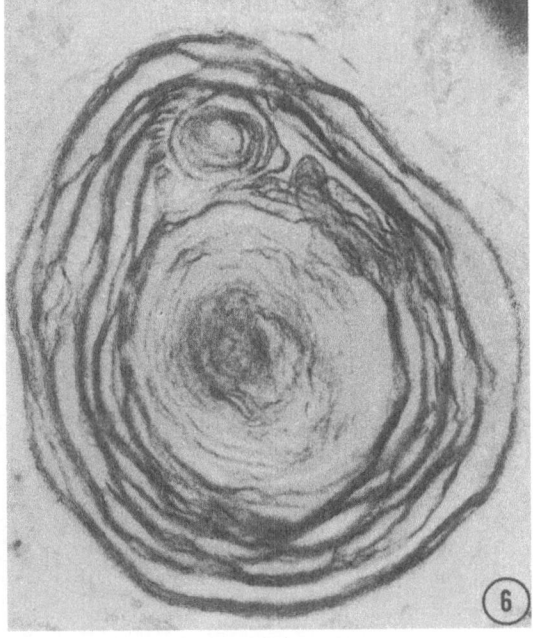

Fig. 7   Portion of a superficial macrophage in a spinal cord culture which has received 2.0 mg/ml cerebroside for 5 days. The cytoplasm demonstrates intralysosomal inclusions (arrows) and numerous pinocytic vesicles (PV). X 12,400.

Inset: Higher magnification of the "crystalline-tubular" structures in both longitudinal and transverse (arrow) section. X 25,000.

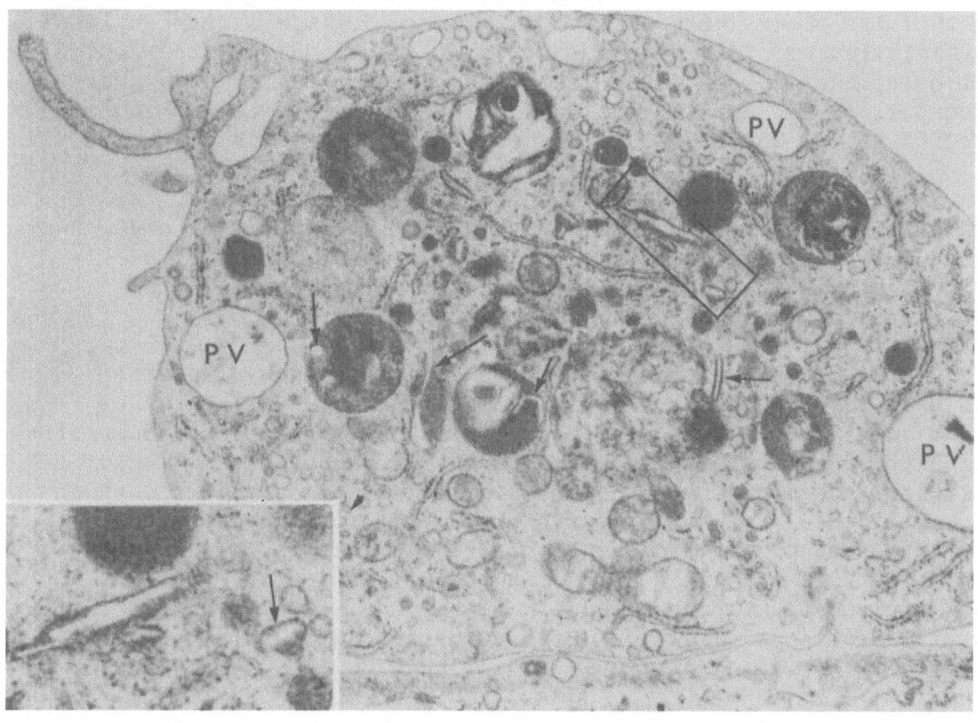

Discussion:

These experiments were designed to overload the capacity of cells in the nervous system to dispose of exogenous sulfatide, ganglioside or cerebroside. The intention was thereby to establish, in tissue culture, pathological situations analogous to those observed in three of the lipid storage disorders.

Like the granules encountered in MLD, the inclusions formed in vitro, after sulfatide administration, are seen more frequently in glial macrophages and astroglia than in spinal and dorsal root ganglion neurons. Similarly, they demonstrate acid phosphatase

activity and stain metachromatically with the cresyl-violet method
of Hirsch and Peiffer (3) indicating that these are actually
secondary lysosomes with sulfatide. These were the morphological
criteria employed to elucidate the nature of the inclusion bodies
in patients with MLD (8).

Terry and Weiss (11) described two distinct types of
membranous cytoplasmic bodies (MCB) in TSD, the compound bodies
and complex bodies. Membranous inclusions strikingly similar to
both these bodies were observed in tissue culture after ganglioside
administration. The same authors also described (11) the fusion
of pale lines to form dark lines, and whenever there was a group of
dense lines the outer lines were pale. The in vitro membranous
bodies showed both these features. They also resembled the in vivo
inclusions in other respects. Both types of inclusions were found
in the same cell. The membranes of the Golgi apparatus, the
endoplasmic reticulum and other structures were neither continuous
with nor in close apposition to the membranous bodies. These
findings are also applicable to the inclusions formed after
sulfatide or cerebroside administration.

Cellular alterations after the administration of bovine
cerebroside were observed only in macrophages. Unlike the
membranous bodies formed after sulfatide or ganglioside administration these inclusions assumed a tubular configuration which appear
as a polygonal-crystal in cross section and are similar to those
seen in human KGL. These structures were usually embedded in
membrane-bound, electron-dense homogenous material. Acid phosphatase staining has identified these structures as lysosomes.
The twisted tubules described in both human KGL (12) and in rat
brain injected with human KGL cerebroside (10) were not observed.
The characteristic multinucleated-globoid cells were also not
observed.

A number of generalized phenomena was observed in all three
cases. The first cells to demonstrate intracellular granule
formation were macrophages and astroglia. This phenomenon is
probably related to the fact that both these cell types are actively
engaged in pinocytosis and both are situated in the uppermost strata
of the culture and therefore have the most immediate access to the
culture medium. Secondly there appears to be critical lipid concentration necessary for the formation of inclusion bodies. Below
this level none is formed; presumably the cells can catabolize the
lipid at concentrations below this threshold.

However, it was observed that in the cases of sulfatide and
ganglioside, even at these low concentrations, the lysosomes
contained electron-opaque granular stippling (Fig. 4) similar to
that seen at earlier time intervals with higher ganglioside levels.
This opaque material probably represents the exogenous lipid and

possibly other materials at a stage prior to its alignment in membranous arrays. At this stage, the exogenous lipids may have combined with other molecules, lipid or proteins, available from either the nutrient medium or from within the cell.

In all cases, there was a gradual decrease in both size and number of cytoplasmic inclusions when cultures were returned to normal medium. This suggests that hydrolytic enzymes were still active within the inclusion bodies and whatever conformational or bonding changes may have occurred did not inhibit enzymatic activity.

In conclusion, we have shown that when exogenous sulfatide, ganglioside or cerebroside is administered to cultured nervous tissue, it is taken up by a variety of cells. Granular cytoplasmic inclusions are formed if appropriately high concentrations of lipid are used. These inclusions have been shown to demonstrate acid phosphatase activity and, in two cases, stain positively in histochemical procedures for the particular lipid added to the medium. Electron microscopy reveals a striking similarity between the in vitro inclusion bodies and those observed in the human disease.

We are grateful to Dr. Murray B. Bornstein, in whose laboratory the tissue culture work was done.

This study was supported by NIH Predoctoral grant 5 F01 GM 47252-02, a grant from the Philadelphia Chapter of the National Tay-Sachs and Allied Disease Association, Inc., NIH grants NS 08952, NS 06735 and CA 06576.

The data in this paper are from a thesis to be submitted in partial fulfillment for the degree of Doctor of Philosophy in the Sue Golding Graduate Division of Medical Sciences, Albert Einstein College of Medicine, Yeshiva University.

1. Gonatas, N. K. and Gonatas, J. Ultrastructural and biochemical observations on a case of systemic late infantile lipidosis and its relationship to Tay-Sachs disease and gargoylism. J. Neuropath. Exp. Neurol. 24:318, 1965.

2. Grégoire, A., Périer, O. and Dustin, P. Metachromatic leukodystrophy, an electron microscopic study. J. Neuropath. Exp. Neurol. 25:617, 1966.

3. Hirsch, T. von and Peiffer, J. Über histologische Methoden in der Differential diagnose von Leucodystrophien und Lipidosen. Arch. Psychiat. Nerven Kr. 194:88, 1955.

4. Mowry, R.W. Improved procedure for the staining of acidic
    polysaccharides by Müllers colloidal (Hydrous) ferric oxide
    and its combination with the Feulgen and the Periodic Acid-
    Schiff reactions. Lab. Invest. 7:566, 1958.

5. Nelson, E., Aurebeck, G., Osterberg, K., Berry, J., Jabbour,
    J. T., and Bornhofen, J. Ultrastructural and chemical studies
    on Krabbe's disease. J. Neuropath. Exp. Neurol. 22:414, 1963.

6. Novikoff, A.B. Lysosomes and related particles. In: The Cell.
    Edited by Brachet, J. and Mirsky, A.E. New York, Acad. Press,
    1961.

7. Peterson, E.R., Crain, S.M. and Murray, M.R. Differentiation
    and prolonged maintenance of bioelectrically active spinal cord
    cultures (rat, chick and human). Z. Zellforsch. 66:130, 1965.

8. Résibois, A. Electron microscopic study of metachromatic
    leucodystrophy. III. Lysosomal nature of the inclusions.
    Acta Neuropath. (Berlin) 13:149, 1969.

9. Suzuki, K., Suzuki, K. and Chen, G.C. Morphological, histo-
    chemical and biochemical studies on a case of systemic late
    infantile lipidosis (Generalized Gangliosidosis). J. Neuropath.
    Exp. Neurol. 27:15, 1968.

10. Suzuki, K. Ultrastructural study of experimental globoid cells.
    Lab. Invest. 23:612, 1970.

11. Terry, R.D. and Weiss, M. Studies in Tay-Sachs disease.
    II. Ultrastructure of the cerebrum. J. Neuropath. Exp. Neurol.
    22:18, 1963.

12. Yunis, E.J. and Lee, R.E. The ultrastructure of Globoid (Krabbe)
    Leukodystrophy. Lab. Invest. 21:415, 1969.

NUTRITIONAL SUPPORT, INCLUDING INTRAVENOUS ALIMENTATION, FOR THE

INFANT WITH WOLMAN'S DISEASE

Allen C. Crocker, Joseph N. Fisher, and
Robert M. Filler

Departments of Medicine and Surgery, Children's
Hospital Medical Center; Departments of Pediatrics
and Surgery, Harvard Medical School, Boston,
Massachusetts

Wolman's disease was identified 15 years ago as a hereditary syndrome involving an inborn error of lipid metabolism. The visible expression of this handicap is an accumulation of ester cholesterol and triglyceride in foam cells in the viscera, and a resultant severe compromise in general body nutrition and development, for the homozygously affected infant. An early terminology for the condition, "Primary familial xanthomatosis with involvement and calcification of the adrenals" (Wolman et al, 1961), pointed out the remarkable adrenal changes; the significance of the functional effects from this pathology has remained uncertain. Although Wolman's disease appears to be uncommon, a world-wide distribution is now documented, without an apparent increase in gene frequency in any particular population group. Families have been reported from Israel (both Jewish and Arab), Japan, New Zealand, England, Belgium, Canada (Toronto, Montreal), and the United States (Boston, Philadelphia, Cleveland, Los Angeles, Albany, and Charleston, W. Va.)

There are certain features about this lipidosis which suggest that careful planning of a basic therapeutic program may hold higher prospects of success than in the usual "sphingolipidosis" circumstance. First, the lipids involved in the tissue deposition are of a less structural, more dynamic sort, usually associated with energy stores and transport. Second, the central nervous system handicap seems relatively mild and inconstant, perhaps again because the basic sphingolipids are not altered. And, third, the fatal evolution of the clinical course in the typical patient (the very young infant) seems dominated by secondary aspects— particularly a severe nutritional failure deriving from the packing of intestinal villi with foam cells, a chronic diarrhea,

661

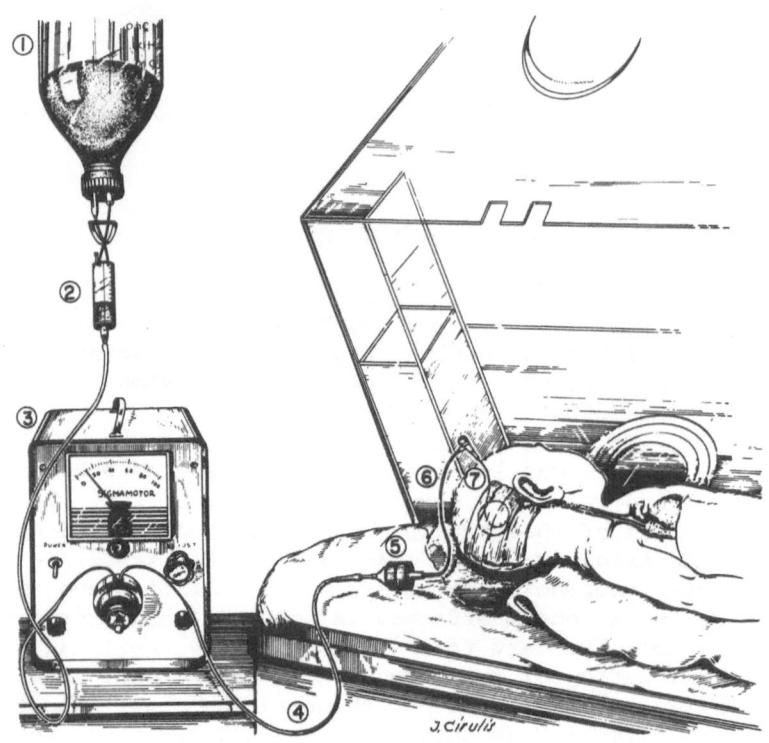

Fig. 1. System for long-term intravenous alimentation
("Lifeline"). 1. Amino acid-glucose infusate. 2. Calibrated
burette. 3. Constant infusion pump. 4. Disposable tubing with
a compressible section which adapts to pump head. 5. Millipore
filter. 6. "T" connector. 7. Silicone rubber intravenous catheter.
(Reprinted with permission of PEDIATRICS, Vol.46, Pg. 456, 1970)

fibrosis of the liver, and, possibly, alterations in adrenocor-
tical function. Support programs attempted to date, employing
cholestyramine, d-thyroxine, clofibrate, feeding with medium-chain
triglycerides, corticosteroid supplements, and agents to depress
intestinal hyperactivity, have not had critically useful effects.
On conceptual grounds, it would seem potentially valuable to offer
these infants oral feeding of the most simplified type, or, even
more strategically, complete parenteral alimentation which would
by-pass the handicapped intestinal and hepatic functions.

    Experience in the last several years has developed a scheme
for the intravenous feeding of small infants which can meet their

total nutritional requirements for continuing periods (Filler and Eraklis, 1970). This is based on the use of a fat-free solution containing protein hydrolysate (3.0% protein) and 20% glucose, with adjustment of electrolytes as appropriate, and addition of a multivitamin mixture, vitamin B_{12}, phytonadione, folic acid, and, occasionally blood plasma (and iron injections). With a typical maximal daily fluid infusion of 135 ml/kg, the infant receives 110 calories per kilogram. This hypertonic solution is delivered by a constant infusion pump through a silicone rubber catheter which reaches to the superior vena cava, installed surgically via a jugular vein from a distant skin entry site (Fig. 1). At the Children's Hospital in Boston, 109 infants have been fed to date by this route, for periods of up to 3 months, with provision of conditions which allowed weight gain and tissue repair. As could be anticipated, the critical problem involves infection, and in 16 children abrupt discontinuance of the infusion program was necessary because of septicemia (commonly with infection by yeast organisms).

An infant with Wolman's disease (Patient D.D., now to be identified as Da.D.) was reported in detail from this hospital (Crocker et al, 1965). The birth of an affected sibling (Di.D.) of this child stimulated the formation of a new therapeutic plan which might hopefully improve on the desultory course experienced by the first patient. "Di.D." was born in December 1969, from the fourth pregnancy of a mother who was healthy except for inactive tuberculosis (she had received p-amino salicylic acid and isonia-zid during the pregnancy). The birth weight was 9 lbs, 5 1/2 oz., and there were no clinical difficulties in the newborn period. On the second day of life it was confirmed that she had a soft liver edge palpable 6 cms below the costal margin, calcification of the adrenals easily visible by x-ray, and conspicuous vacuolization of the lymphocytes on smear of the peripheral blood. At the parents' request, a trial of normal infant care was begun, with the post-ponement of special feeding programs until clinical indications required such. On a prepared infant formula, during the first 4 weeks, she was relatively content, but the stools gradually increased in number and vomiting began. Her indigestion was then approached by the use of a soy formula, and initially she did quite well on this--regaining her birth weight for the first time (maximum weight: 9 lbs, 6 oz., at 6 weeks of age) and showing some developmental gains. After that time she rapidly became more troubled, however, with increasing weakness, loose stools, vomit-ing, and cough. Nutramigen (R) feeding, including by means of gavage, did not assist, and she was admitted to the hospital at 7 weeks of age for what was to be the remainder of her life. Her weight was then 9 lbs 2 oz., her liver was 6 and the spleen 2 cms below the costal margin, and her performance was like that of a one-month-old child (Figure 2).

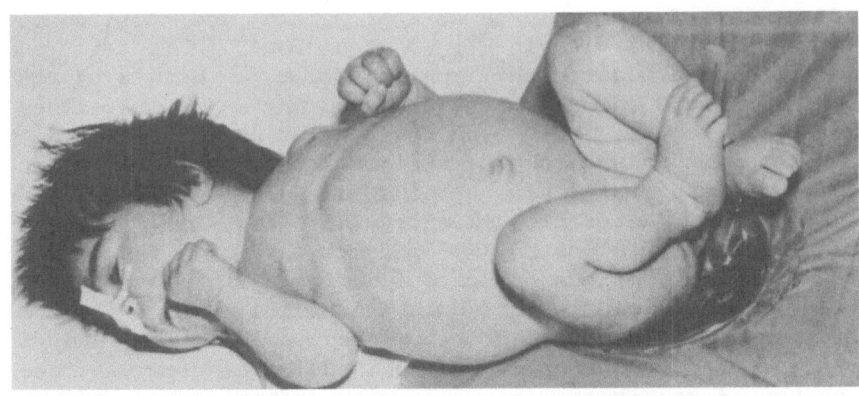

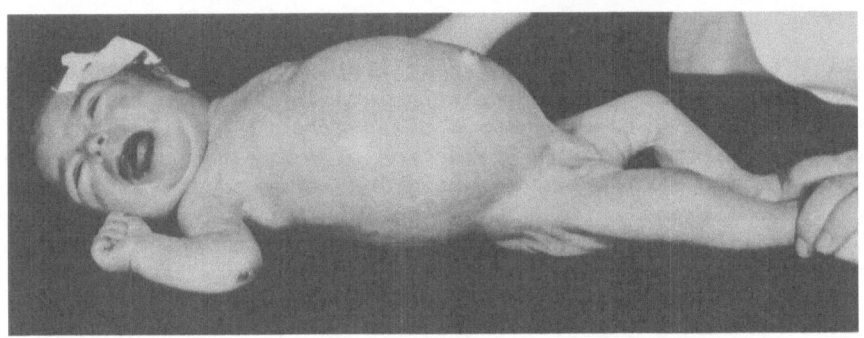

Fig. 2. Patient Di.D., at 7 1/2 weeks (upper) and 13 weeks
(lower) of age, with progressive enlargement of the abdominal
viscera and loss of subcutaneous tissue.

        For the first 19 days that Di.D. was in the hospital an
attempt was made to accommodate to her intestinal handicap by the
use of a low-residue feeding (Vivonex 100 (R)) in varying concentrations, first by the oral route and then by slow gavage (pump)
infusion, with codeine for intestinal sedation. It was soon found
that whenever her intake exceeded 60 calories/kg/day a serious
diarrhea developed, plus irregular vomiting, with the volume of
stool and vomitus together averaging about a third of the fluid
intake. On this program, she showed a net loss of 65 grams of
body weight for the 2 1/2 week period. The serum protein level
rose from 3.8 to 5.2 gms%, serum lipids remained low (cholesterol
level 96 to 108 mgms%), serum pH averaged 7.37, and SGOT levels
were 75-300 units. Urinary measures of 17-ketosteroids and
hydroxycorticoids were at the usual low level for this age period;

serum electrolytes were entirely normal, and hypoglycemia was not identified. Several small transfusions were given. At this time, the liver was 8 and the spleen 4 cms below the costal margin. A duodenal biopsy demonstrated the expected accumulation of foam cells in the lamina propria, and a liver biopsy had abundant foam cell formation. It was then agreed that oral feeding held almost no prospect of allowing adequate nutrition for growth, and it was decided to begin parenteral alimentation by the "lifeline" as described above.

The venous catheter was installed on the 20th day of the hospital admission, and she was then begun on a series of 3-day balance periods to evaluate her utilization of calories, nitrogen, and electrolytes. Clinical progress was satisfactory for the first two weeks, but penicillin-resistant Staphylococci were recovered from the blood on the 10th day of the catheter usage. This persisted for 3 days, in spite of oxacillin administration, followed then by heavy growth of Candida tropicalis. The child became toxic-appearing, and a striking increase in the size of the liver and spleen occurred (each 10 cms below the costal margin). On the 16th day of total intravenous alimentation, the catheter was removed.

Di.D. lived for 12 more days, although with almost constant difficulty from complications of the disease and its management. Despite the removal of the catheter her blood culture remained positive for Candida. Her feeding was entirely by conventional intravenous drips, plus the use of small blood transfusions. She developed generalized edema, associated with a serum protein level of 3.7 gms%, showing some improvement after albumin administration. The extent of her hepatosplenomegaly first decreased (liver 7 and spleen 6 cms below the costal margin), and then gradually increased (to an eventual maximum of 11 and 12 cms, respectively) (Fig. 2). In the last two days she became jaundiced, and gram-negative rods were cultured from her blood. She died with seizures and decreasing responsiveness.

Four 3-day balance periods on the lifeline were recorded before complications interfered with the observations. As is shown in Table 1, a positive nitrogen balance was indeed achieved under these circumstances, to the extent of nearly one gram per day, which compares favorably with the gains found possible for other depleted infants not limited by the metabolic handicap of Wolman's disease (Filler et al, 1969). Coordinate studies showed that a generally positive balance was also present for sodium, potassium, chloride, calcium, phosphorus, and magnesium, and there was no evidence of selective failure of retention of any electrolyte. Three hundred grams of body weight gain occurred. Serum lipid levels rose somewhat (cholesterol 160 mgms%). In the interval before the septicemia became critical, the degree of

Table 1

Metabolic Balance Studies
(patient on complete intravenous alimentation)

period	I	II	III	IV
(3-day periods--all data given as total for the 3 days)				
intake volume (ml)	1426	1694	1638	1876
urinary volume (ml)	1015	1050	1110	1110
urinary creatinine (mg)	125	139	114	175
N I T R O G E N (grams)				
intake	6.42	7.62	7.37	8.44
urine	3.28	4.09	3.79	5.73
stool	0.38	0.10	0.22	0.05
balance	2.76	3.43	3.36	2.46

visceromegaly had not significantly changed. Personal developmental progress was obscured although special efforts had been
made by the nursing personnel to provide varied contact and stimulation.

Di.D. died at 13 1/2 weeks of age, compared to 16 1/2 weeks
for her sibling, Da.D. The autopsy findings showed similar ana-
tomic changes. There was a mixed gram-negative bacillus infection
of the blood stream (Klebsiella, E.coli, Psuedomonas), chronic
pneumonitis, focal endocarditis, and a generalized lymphoid depletion. There was severe portal fibrosis in the liver, and vacuolization of hepatocytes. Atrophy of the intestinal mucosa was present, and depletion of the pituitary acidophilic cells. The
adrenals weighed 10 grams each, with areas present of necrosis
and patchy calcification. The central nervous system had no specific abnormalities, including no distension of the neurones of
the cortex or the sympathetic ganglia. The characteristic foam
cells of Wolman's disease occurred in abundance in the bone marrow, liver, spleen, lungs, lymph nodes, gastro-intestinal tract
(Fig. 3), and thymus. Tissue lipid studies (Table 2, Fig. 4)
showed elevations of cholesterol level in liver, spleen, and cortical gray matter generically comparable to, but quantitatively

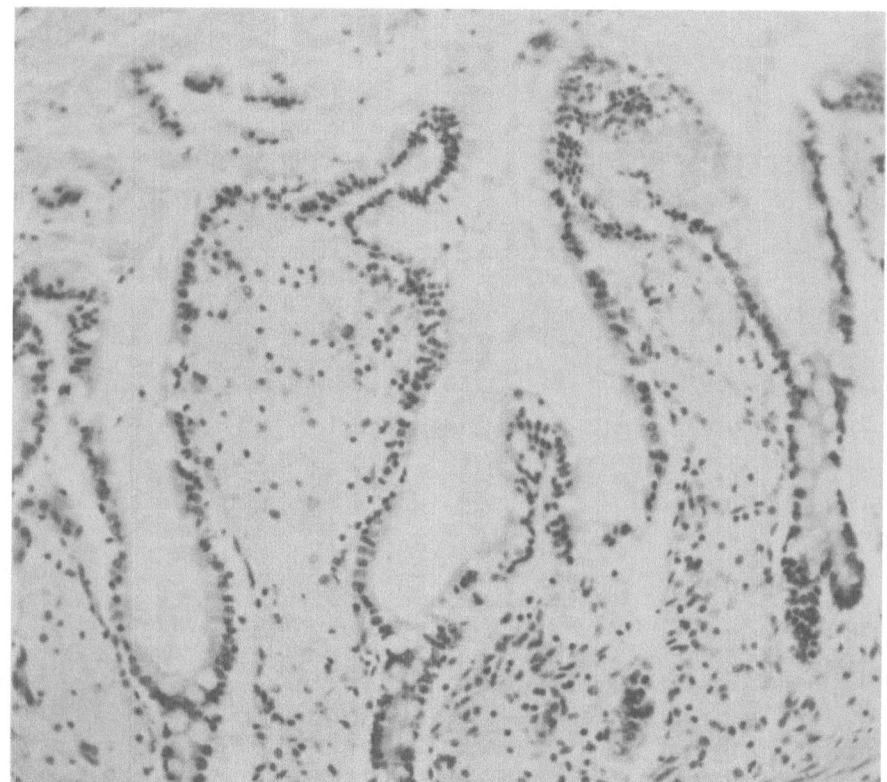

Fig. 3. A section of small intestine from Pt. Di.D., showing
aggregations of foam cells in the individual villi.

somewhat milder than, those found in Da.D. There was an intense
increase in neutral fat in the liver.

     It is difficult to establish final conclusions about the
relevance of therapeutic efforts of this sort to the over-all
clinical needs of the Wolman's disease infant. It had been hoped
that an equilibrium period of secured nutritional gains could be
utilized for observation of the uncomplicated course of the illness, including effects on the central nervous system. One could
also have anticipated that this model system of special support
could have been employed for trials of enzyme-inducing agents or
replacement programs. The provision of supplements of normal
human serum, so frequently mentioned currently as a potential
source of normal enzymes or other corrective factors, was actually
carried out indirectly, with transfusions given to this child
about once weekly. The total experiment was obviously subverted
by complications of the technique, involving an unusually rapid

Table 2

Tissue Lipid Analyses on Patients Da.D. and Di.D.
(in grams per 100 grams of fresh weight of tissue)

	Pt. Da.D.	Pt. Di.D.	normals
L I V E R			
total lipids	16.4*	17.9	3-4.5
phospholipids	1.54	1.31	1.5-2.5
sphingomyelin	0.25	0.33	0.2-0.3
cholesterol	4.60	3.08	0.3-0.4
neutral fat (approx.)	9½	13	1
S P L E E N			
total lipids	6.34	4.62	2-3.5
phospholipids	1.62	1.17	1-2
sphingomyelin	0.30	0.35	0.2-0.4
cholesterol	1.80	0.94	0.3-0.5
neutral fat (approx.)	2½	2	½
C E R E B R U M			
GRAY MATTER			
total lipids	3.88	5.34	4.3-5.8
phospholipids	2.42	2.10	2.2-3.6
sphingomyelin	0.35	0.46	0.4-0.8
cholesterol	0.97	0.88	0.4-0.6
WHITE MATTER			
total lipids	4.70	5.35	4.4-12.1
phospholipids	2.38	2.05	2.2-5.5
sphingomyelin	0.38	0.36	0.5-1.3
cholesterol	1.21	1.04	0.6-1.5

* - underlined figures indicate significant
    elevation in lipid level

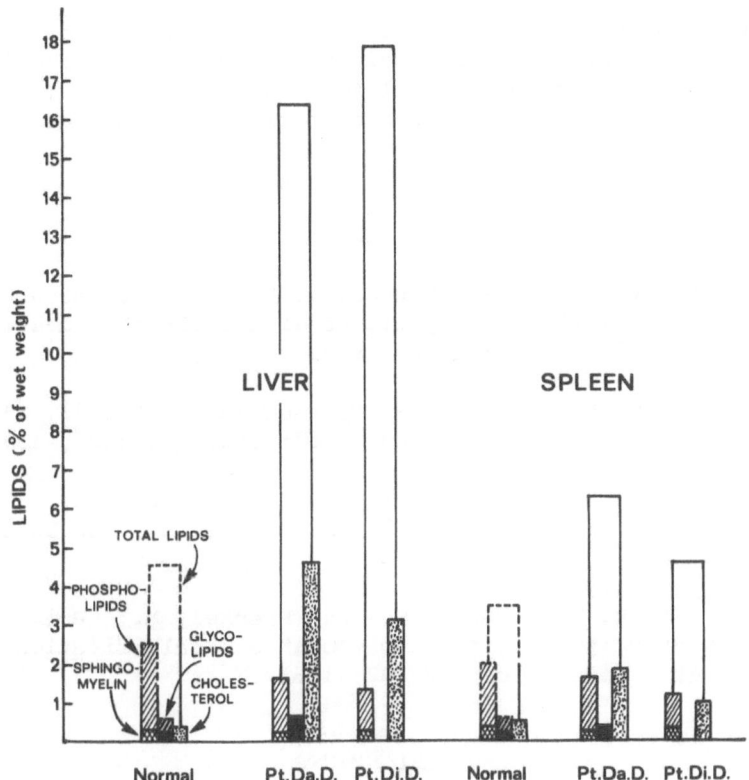

Fig. 4. Graphic representation of the tissue lipid abnormalities in the liver and spleen of the "D" patients.

and definitive interference by blood stream infection. It is possible that better fortune might prevail for other similar infants in the future, with the opportunity then to assess additional therapeutic trials.

SUMMARY

A patient with Wolman's disease, the second child to be involved from this family, was admitted to the hospital at 7 weeks of age for a program of special nutritional supports. During the first 2 1/2 weeks an unsuccessful attempt was made to quiet intestinal hyperactivity and achieve weight gains by the use of a low residue feeding. Following this, she was carried on complete parenteral alimentation, using a central venous catheter. On the latter program she was able to establish a positive nitrogen balance, and a small weight gain, but blood stream infection

(Candida) limited the possibility of continuing this technique. She died two weeks later, with tissue findings as expected for the basic syndrome. Further consideration seems justified regarding the application of parenteral feeding of this sort for metabolically handicapped infants where special treatment goals can be formulated.

REFERENCES

Crocker, A.C., Vawter, G.F., Neuhauser, E.B.D., and Rosowsky, A.: Wolman's disease; three new patients with a recently described lipidosis. Pediatrics, 35:627, 1965.

Filler, R.N., and Eraklis, A.J.: Care of the critically ill child: intravenous alimentation. Pediatrics, 46:456, 1970.

Filler, R.N., Eraklis, A.J., Rubin, V.G., and Das, J.B.: Long-term total parenteral nutrition in infants. New Eng.J.Med., 281:589, 1969.

Wolman, M., Sterk, V.V., Gatt, S., and Frenkel, M.: Primary familial xanthomatosis with involvement and calcification of the adrenals. Pediatrics, 28:742, 1961.

ACKNOWLEDGEMENTS

These studies were supported by the Children's Hospital Medical Center Mental Retardation and Human Development Research Program (HD 03-0773), a grant (RR-128) from the General Clinical Research Centers Program of the Division of Research Resources, National Institute of Health, and a grant from the McGaw Laboratory, Glendale, California. Appreciation is also expressed to Dr. Byron D. Roseman, of Chelmsford, Massachusetts, for his referral of this patient and his assistance in her care.

PRECOCIOUS PUBERTY IN TAY-SACHS DISEASE[1]

Richard Relkin, M.D.

Dept. of Medicine & Isaac Albert Research Inst., Kings-

brook Jewish Medical Center, Brooklyn, N.Y., 11203, USA

Various neurologic causes of sexual precocity have been reported. Among these have been destructive pineal tumors (6,19,25),
hamartomas or hyperplasia of the tuber cinereum (8,14,31), hypothalamic tumors (34,36,40,48,53), tumors of the optic chiasm (12), en-
cephalitis (16), miliary tuberculosis and tuberous sclerosis (55),
the Sturge-Weber syndrome, porencephalic cysts, brain damage, cranio-
stenosis, microcephaly, arrested hydrocephalus, and so-called idiopathic cases in which non-specific, but grossly abnormal electroen-
cephalograms have been found (27). In addition, at this institution
it has been noted that children with Tay-Sachs disease not uncommon-
ly manifest premature thelarche and/or pubarche (unpublished observations). In an effort to elucidate the pathogenesis of these complete and incomplete forms of precocious puberty, as well as to detect any other hitherto unsuspected hormonal abnormalities, detailed
endocrine evaluations of 2 female children with Tay-Sachs disease
were carried out.

Case Reports

Case 1. P.K., during the period of this study, was a 3 8/12-3
11/12 yr old girl who was born of Jewish parents of East-European
descent. At 7 months of age the child was noted to have slow psychomotor development and was diagnosed as having Tay-Sachs disease. At
admission the patient was 22 months of age and showed the classic
clinical findings of Tay-Sachs disease, including bilateral cherry-
red maculae. An electroencephalogram (EEG) performed at the time of

[1]This work was supported in part by a grant from the National Tay-
Sachs and Allied Disease Association, Inc.

admission revealed bilateral cerebral dysfunction, i.e., 1-3 cycles
per sec with very high voltage (50-100 mV). The patient had developed coarse, stiff pubic hair at the age of approximately 2 yr. At
the age of 3 8/12 yr the labia minora were developed, and there was
no evidence of axillary hair, breast development, or abnormality of
the clitoris; menses had not been observed. Excessive fine hair was
observed on the limbs. Hepatomegaly, splenomegaly and lymphadenopathy were not present. Rectal examination was negative. Liver
chemistries were normal. A lateral roentgenogram of the skull revealed a normal sella turcica and the bone age was 4 2/12 yr. A
vaginal smear revealed a slight estrogen effect. The patient died
from bronchopneumonia at the age of 4 yr; an autopsy was performed.

Case 2. M.H., during the period of this study, was a 4 3/12-4
1/2 yr old girl who was also a descendant of East-European parents.
She was noted to have psychomotor deterioration at the age of 5
months, after which time typical symptoms of Tay-Sachs disease developed and the patient was admitted to this institution. At the age of
2 yr an EEG revealed a pattern identical to that described for patient P.K. By the age of 3 yr the patient had developed coarse axillary and pubic hair. At the age of 4 3/12 yr the labia minora were
developed, breast tissue was palpable and the clitoris was normal;
menses had not been observed. Excessive fine hair was present on the
limbs. Hepatosplenomegaly and lymphadenopathy were not observed.
Rectal examination was negative. Neither in this patient nor the
preceding case was it possible to accurately measure height because
of spasticity and/or contractures. Liver chemistries were normal.
A lateral roentgenogram of the skull revealed a normal sella turcica
and the bone age was 5 9/12 yr. A vaginal smear revealed a moderate
estrogen effect. The patient died at the age of 5 1/12 yr; an autopsy was not performed.

Three other female patients with Tay-Sachs disease, who died before this study was begun, also manifested premature pubarche with or
without premature thelarche. One of these girls (H.P.) represented a
more florid example of these changes than the other 2, or than the 2
girls reported above, and a photograph is therefore included (see
fig. 1).

Materials and Methods

The patients were catheterized (with consent), and refrigerated
24 hr urine samples were collected from 8 A.M. to 8 A.M. Adequacy
of urine collections was checked by creatinine determinations and
was adequate in all instances. Urinary 17-hydroxycorticoids (17-OH-
CS) were determined by the method of Silber and Porter (46), and urinary 17-ketosteroids (17-KS) were measured by the method of Drekter
et al.(13). The urinary estrogens, estrone (E_1), 17β-estradiol (E_2),
and estriol (E_3) were determined by the method of Brown et al.(9) and
urinary testosterone by the method of Ibayaski et al.(21); both are

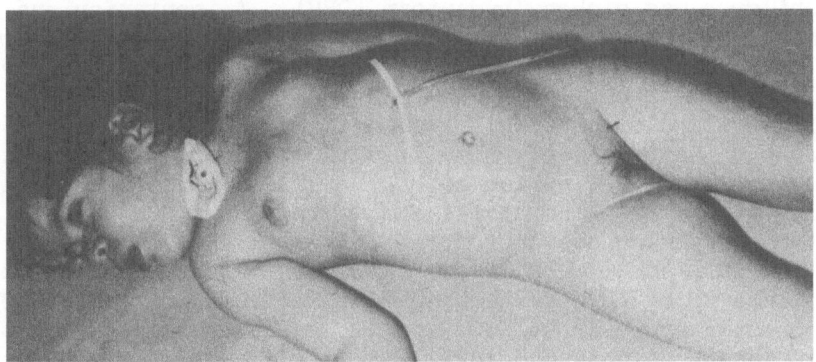

Figure 1

recovery analyses which yielded 85-90% recovery. Control urines for
estrogen and testosterone determinations were collected (by catheter,
with consent, or catchbag when necessary) in the manner described
above from 3 female children (aged 2 2/12 to 3 8/12 yr) with Tay-
Sachs disease who did not manifest any evidence of puberty, as well
as from 6 normal female children aged 3 9/12 to 4 8/12 yr. Urinary
pregnanediol and pregnanetriol were determined by the method of Tietz
(50). Plasma cortisol was measured by the method of Mattingly (30).
Duplicate samples were measured for all steroids except urinary 17-KS
and plasma cortisol. All testosterone values were checked by having
duplicate samples measured by New England Nuclear Company, Cambridge,
Massachusetts. Aside from the latter substantiative analyses all
steroid analyses were performed by Universal Diagnostic Laboratories,
Brooklyn, New York.

    Protein-bound iodine (PBI) was determined by the method of Bark-
er et al.(4). Radioactive iodine (RAI^{131}) uptake was determined at
24 hr using a standard collimated counter; doses used were 5-10 uCi.

    Plasma human growth hormone (HGH) assays were performed in the
laboratory of Dr. Seymour M. Glick. Plasma samples were deep frozen
and analyzed at a later date according to the radioimmunoassay method
of Glick et al.(17), using Wilhelmi preparation 705A as a standard
(from National Pituitary Agency).

    Plasma follicle stimulating hormone (FSH) and luteinizing hor-
mone (LH) levels were determined in the laboratory of Dr. Brij B.
Saxena. Plasma samples were drawn at 8 A.M. and then deep frozen and
analyzed at a later date according to the radioimmunoassay method as
described by Saxena et al.(42,43).

    Bone age was estimated from radiographs of wrists and hands, by
comparison with standards in the atlas of Greulich and Pyle (18).

    Throughout the period of the study the only medication received

by the children was diphenylhydantoin (DPH). Alimentation and oral
drug administration was achieved in both children by gastrostomy
feeding. There were no incidents of aspiration pneumonitis during
the period of the study.

Adrenal stimulation. This was performed at first using 15 U AC-
TH per sq M of surface area, dissolved in physiologic saline and giv-
en intravenously over a period of 6 hr. Plasma cortisol was measured
just prior to the test and at the end of the test. On the day before
the test and again on the day of the test urine was collected for determination of 17-KS, 17-OHCS, and estrogens. The second stimulation
test utilized 20 mg ACTH gel per sq M of surface area administered
intramuscularly every 12 hr for 3 days. Following collection of a
control urine to be measured for 17-KS, 17-OHCS, testosterone and estrogens, test urines were collected on the 1st, 2nd and 3rd day of
ACTH administration.

Adrenal suppression. Dexamethasone 1.25 mg per 100 lb of body
weight per day, to be administered as an oral suspension in divided
doses over a period of 7 days, was the basic regime formulation.
However, because of the known propensity of DPH to stimulate microsomal enzyme activity and hence to enhance the hepatic conjugation
and biliary excretion of the drug (22,54), resulting in falsely negative suppression responses, the dosage administered to the 2 girls
was doubled. Urine for 17-OHCS was collected on the 3rd day of dexamethasone administration and urine for 17-OHCS, 17-KS, testosterone
and estrogens on the 7th day.

Gonadal stimulation. This test consisted of the continued administration of dexamethasone as described above with the addition of
3,000 IU per day of human chorionic gonadotropin (HCG) given intramuscularly for 3 days. Urine for 17-OHCS, 17-KS, testosterone and
estrogens was collected on the 3rd day. Human menopausal gonadotropin (HMG; Pergonal) could not be obtained.

Metyrapone test. The dosage regimen was based on a basic formulation of 300 mg per sq M of surface area given as an oral suspension
every 4 hr for 6 doses. However, because of the effect of DPH in
producing subnormal steroid responses in the oral test as a result of
accelerated hepatic conjugation of metyrapone (32) the dose of the
latter was doubled. Urine for 17-OHCS, 17-KS, testosterone and estrogens was collected the day after metyrapone administration.

Medroxyprogesterone suppression. Twenty-five mg of medroxyprogesterone acetate (MPA) was administered as an oral suspension every
6 hr for 14 days. Urine for testosterone and estrogens was collected
on the last day of the test.

Glucagon stimulation of HGH (33). After obtaining a fasting
blood sample for HGH level 1 mg of glucagon was injected intramuscularly. Subsequent samples were drawn at 60, 120, 150 and 180 minutes
and analyzed for HGH content.

Serum and urine osmolality. These were determined both under
control conditions as well as during a modified dehydration procedure described by the author (38). These determinations were accompanied by measurement of serum electrolytes and urinary sodium excre-

tion.

Results

PBI and RAI uptake. For case 1 (P.K.) the values were 5.9 ug%
and 24.1% respectively, and for case 2 (M.H.) 4.2 ug% and 15.1%. The
normal range for PBI in this laboratory is 3.5-8 ug%, and for RAI uptake 15-45%. Thus, values for PBI and RAI were normal in both patients.

FSH and LH levels. In case 1 FSH was 28 mIU[2] per ml plasma and
LH 11 mIU per ml plasma; for case 2 the values were, FSH 14 mIU per
ml plasma and LH 15 mIU per ml plasma. The normal mean for children
for FSH in the laboratory where the assays were performed is 10.1,
with a range of 5.6-18.5; for LH the mean is 10.2 with a range of
2.5-15 (42).

Steroid Values. Tables 1 and 2 give the results of all the
steroid tests. As can be seen, 2 of the first 3 control values for
17-OHCS in case 1 and all of the first 3 control values for 17-OHCS
in case 2 were low (normal 1.5-4.0 mg per 24 hr). The same first 3
control specimens contained elevated levels of 17-KS (normal 0.4-1.5
mg per 24 hr).

Both cases manifested elevated testosterone levels. The normal
range is 0-0.9 ug per 24 hr.

Elevated control levels of both E_2 and E_3 were also found in
both cases (respective normals 0-1.3 and 0-0.9 ug per 24 hr), while
the values for E_1 were normal (normal 0-0.5 ug per 24 hr). The reason for the absence of a corresponding elevation of E_1 levels was not
ascertained.

The respective control values for pregnanediol and pregnanetriol
for case 1 were 0.2 and 0.1, and for case 2 0.02 and 0.4 mg per 24 hr
(respective pregnanediol and pregnanetriol normals 0.02-0.4 and 0.01-
0.5 mg per 24 hr).

Control values for plasma cortisol were within the normal range
of 6-26 ug%.

Adrenal stimulation. Following the administration of ACTH iv
plasma cortisol rose from 2½ to 4 times the control values, while
urinary 17-OHCS values barely doubled, and 17-KS levels rose approximately 50%. ACTH iv also brought about an approximate doubling of
the values for E_2 and a rise of approximately 50% in E_3 values; E_1
levels in this and the studies to follow underwent minimal changes,
if any at all. When the test was repeated with ACTH im essentially
the same observations were made on the 2nd day of ACTH, except that

[2]Milli-International Units of Second International Reference Preparation of Human Menopausal Gonadotropin.

Table 1. Urinary steroid values and plasma cortisol in case 1 (P.K.)

Dates of Collection	Conditions	Plasma Cortisol (ug %)	17-OHCS (mg/24 hr)	17-KS (mg/24 hr)	Testosterone (ug/24 hr)	Estrogens (ug/24 hr)+		
						E₁	E₂	E₃
12/22-23/69	control		1.1	1.8		0.1	14.5	10.2
1/13/70	pre-ACTH iv	20						
1/13/70	post-ACTH iv	51						
1/12-13/70	pre-ACTH iv		1.6	1.8		0.2	14.0	11.3
1/13-14/70	day ACTH iv		3.5	2.9		0.1	31.5	18.6
2/4-5/70	control				7.2	0.1	15.0	10.8
2/18-19/70	14th day MPA*				1.9	0.0	4.6	3.1
3/1-2/70	control		1.3	2.3	8.1	0.2	12.9	9.6
3/3-4/70	2nd day ACTH im		3.1	4.2	23.8	0.3	30.8	18.1
3/4-5/70	3rd day ACTH im		3.3	4.0	11.8	0.0	10.5	11.3
3/7-8/70	3rd day dexamethasone		1.1					
3/11-12/70	7th day dexamethasone		0.8	3.0	3.6	0.0	6.7	5.0
3/14-15/70	3rd day dexamethasone + HCG**		0.7	1.9	2.0	0.2	7.7	5.8
3/15-16/70	control		1.6	3.1	20.7	0.3	34.0	27.1
3/16-17/70	control		1.4	2.5	13.3	0.1	20.5	15.3
3/18-19/70	day after metyrapone		3.3	3.7	7.7	0.1	13.2	11.0

*MPA=medroxyprogesterone acetate
**HCG=human chorionic gonadotropin
+E₁=estrone, E₂=17β-estradiol, E₃=estriol

Table 2. Urinary steroid values and plasma cortisol in case 2 (M.H.)

Dates of Collection	Conditions	Plasma Cortisol (ug %)	17-OHCS (mg/24 hr)	17-KS (mg/24 hr)	Testosterone (ug/24 hr)	Estrogens (ug/24 hr)+		
						E₁	E₂	E₃
12/22-23/70	control		1.3	2.8		0.1	19.4	16.0
1/13/70	pre-ACTH iv	15						
1/13/70	post-ACTH iv	61						
1/12-13/70	pre-ACTH iv		1.1	1.9		0.1	22.0	18.1
1/13-14/70	day ACTH iv		2.4	2.7		0.2	42.3	29.4
2/4-5/70	control				6.3	0.1	20.2	16.8
2/18-19/70	14th day MPA*				2.0	0.0	6.5	4.9
3/1-2/70	control		1.2	2.6	5.9	0.1	18.9	17.6
3/3-4/70	2nd day ACTH im		2.7	3.6	14.8	0.1	41.0	33.5
3/4-5/70	3rd day ACTH im		1.6	2.2	5.3	0.0	21.6	15.3
3/7-8/70	3rd day dexamethasone		0.9					
3/11-12/70	7th day dexamethasone		0.7	2.3	2.9	0.0	10.7	10.0
3/14-15/70	3rd day dexamethasone + HCG**		0.8	1.4	2.6	0.2	11.9	11.1
3/15-16/70	control		0.9	2.9	4.0	0.1	17.1	15.0
3/16-17/70	control		1.1	3.2	15.9	0.2	39.6	35.8
3/18-19/70	day after metyrapone		0.9	1.6	7.0	0.1	22.3	17.5

*MPA=medroxyprogesterone acetate
**HCG=human chorionic gonadotropin
+E₁=estrone, E₂=17β-estradiol, E₃=estriol

the E$_3$ levels approached or reached 100% increments. These changes were accompanied by a rise of approximately 250-300% in the levels of testosterone, based on an average of the 2 initial control values. No steroid values were obtained the first day of im ACTH due to loss of the specimens.

Adrenal suppression and gonadal stimulation. With the use of dexamethasone, values on the 7th day for 17-OHCS fell to levels approaching 50% of the highest of the first 3 control values; levels on the 3rd day of the test revealed less evidence of suppression. The value for 17-KS on the 7th day of dexamethasone revealed essentially no change compared to the initial control levels, and in case 1 was actually higher. At the same time, compared with the initial control values, the testosterone levels fell by an average of approximately 45%, E$_2$ levels 50-55%, and E$_3$ levels 50-60%. When HCG was added, while continuing adrenal suppression, testosterone levels either fell further or remained almost constant. With HCG the values for E_2 and E_3 rose by approximately 15% in case 1, and 10% in case 2.

Metyrapone test. In patient 1 the 17-OHCS values on the day following administration of this drug more than doubled; however, this normal response was not observed in patient 2.

HGH levels after glucagon. A normal response is defined as a HGH level of at least 7.0 ng per ml at some time during the test; by this criterion both subjects responded normally.

Serum and urine osmolality. Control values of serum osmolality fell between 286 and 293 mOsm per kg in both subjects, while those of urinary osmolality fell between 205 and 370 mOsm per kg. When the modified dehydration procedure was used both patients manifested a progressive rise in urine osmolality without a tendency to plateau, the test being terminated when osmolality exceeded 600 mOsm per kg; vasopressin was not used as it was felt that the response of endogenous vasopressin (ADH) secretion to dehydration, as well as renal ADH-responsiveness were adequate. The finding of normal serum electrolytes and urinary sodium, taken together with normal serum osmolality ruled out a state of inappropriate secretion of ADH.

Light and electron microscopy. Fig. 2 is a representative area of the hypothalamus of case 1 seen under light microscopy. In this figure ballooned neuronal cells with peripherally displaced, or absent nuclei are seen. The Nissl bodies are decreased in number and have a perinuclear location. In fig. 3, an electron photomicrograph reveals a diffuse accumulation in the cytoplasm of a hypothalamic neuron of the typical membranous cytoplasmic bodies (MCB) of Tay-Sachs disease. Fig. 4 is an electron photomicrograph of the pineal gland of case 1. The diffuse ganglioside accumulation found in the pinealocytes has taken the form of oval cytoplasmic inclusion bodies which are surrounded by a single membrane and contain either parallel membranes or small compound bodies; typical MCB were not found.

As for the pituitary in case 1, electron microscopic examination (fig. 5) revealed MCB (not shown in figure), as well as parallel membranous structures similar to those observed in the pineal. Both of these morphologic types of ganglioside accumulation were sparsely distributed in the 3 main cell types of the anterior pituitary, as well as in the posterior part of the gland.

The ovaries measured 1.6 and 1.8 cm in greatest diameter. Histologically they contained several cystic follicles, the largest of which measured 1.1 cm in greatest size (fig. 6). These cystic follicles were lined by granulosa and theca cells, some of the latter appearing minimally luteinized (fig. 7)

Discussion

FSH and LH levels. It can be seen that the FSH level in case 1

was abnormally high, comparable to values for adult females in the
luteal phase (mean 21.1, range 16.8-31.7). The levels of FSH and LH
in case 2 are well above the normal mean for children; taken together

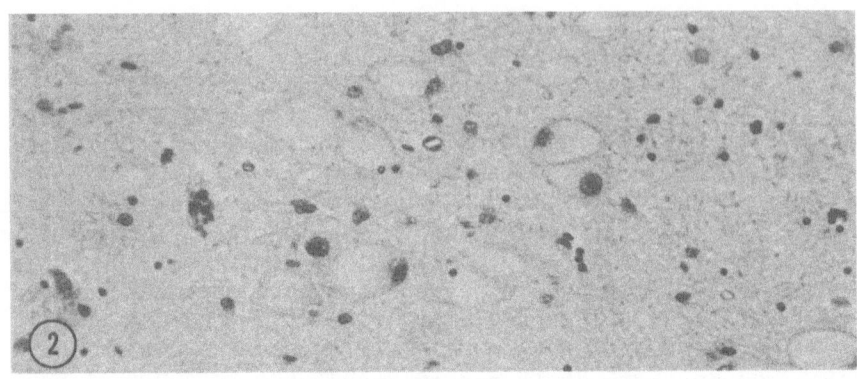

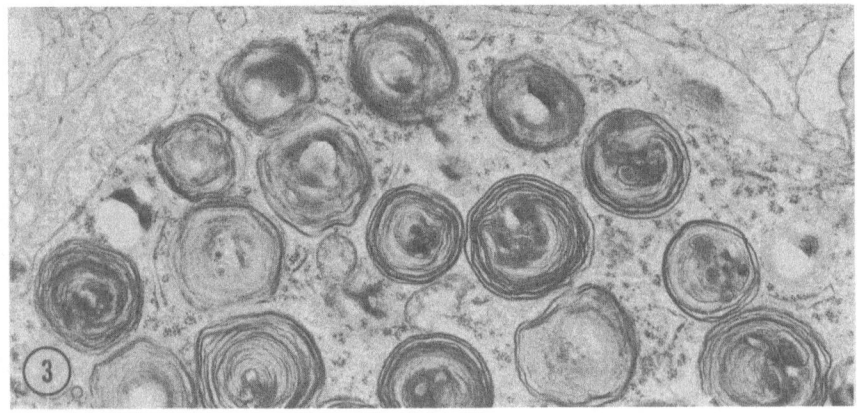

Fig. 2. Hypothalamus. Nissl stain, x125.
Fig. 3. Hypothalamus. x17,500.
Fig. 4. Electron photomicrograph of a portion of a pinealocyte show-
         ing cytoplasmic inclusion bodies which are oval and are sur-
         rounded by a single membrane. These structures contain ei-
         ther parallel membranes (straight arrows) or small compound
         bodies (curved arrows). x19,800.
Fig. 5. Pituitary. Electron photomicrograph of a portion of an aci-
         dophilic cell showing membrane-bound cytoplasmic bodies
         (straight arrows) which contain irregularly arranged or par-
         allel membranes. Various sizes of secretory granules
         (curved arrows) are also seen in the cytoplasm. M (mitochon-
         dria). N (nucleus). x21,000.
Fig. 6. Ovaries. Hematoxylin-eosin stain, x3.
Fig. 7. Wall of largest cyst revealing layer of granulosa cells (G)
         (detachment from theca interna is an artifact). Point of ar-
         row falls between two theca interna cells which reveal early
         luteinization. Hematoxylin-eosin stain, x 375.

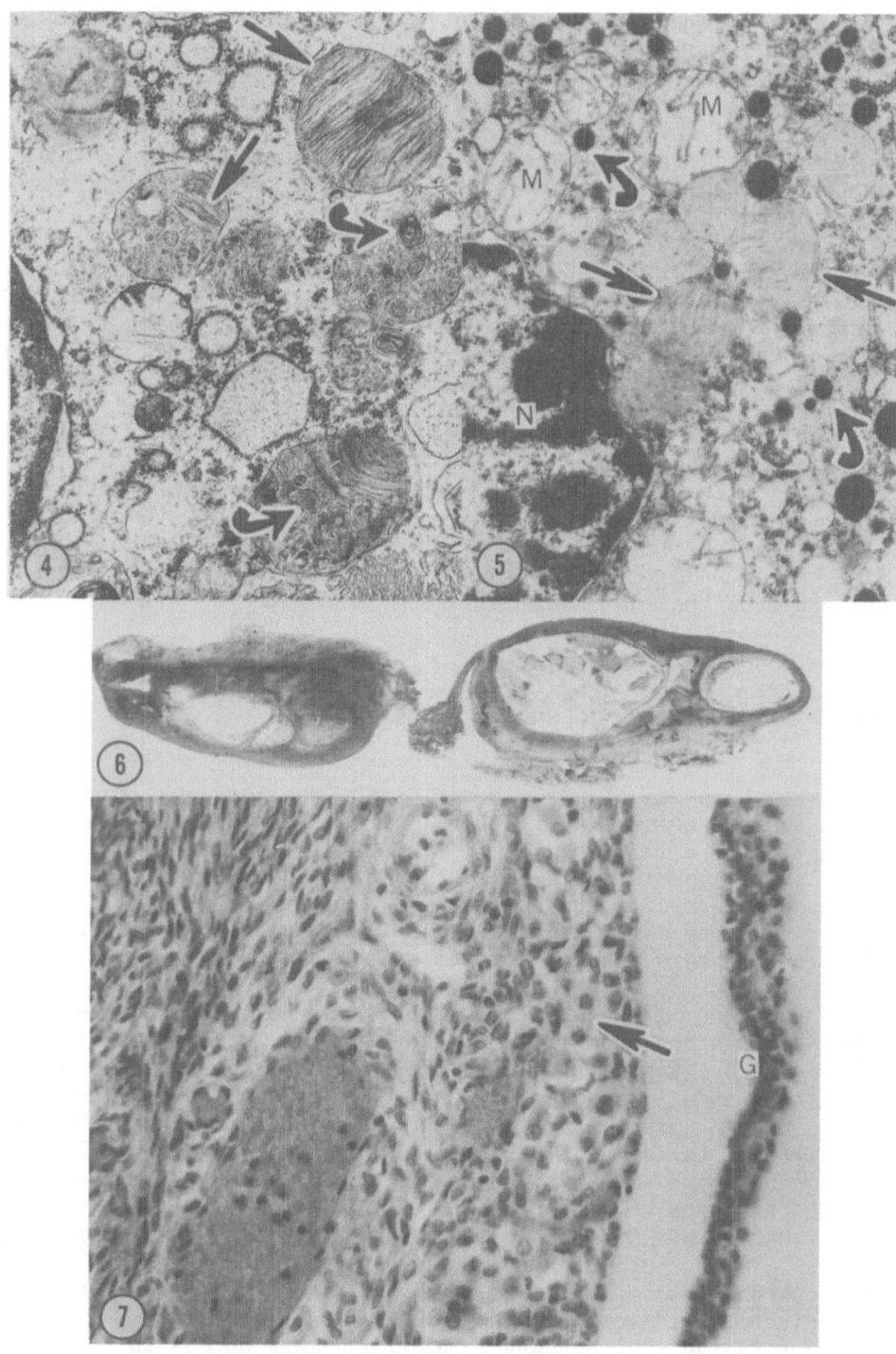

these values fall well within the normal range for adult females in the follicular phase (for FSH the mean for follicular phase values is 14.9 with a range of 7-27.2, and for LH the mean is 14.6 with a range of 6-27.2). Though the LH level in case 1 is in this same follicular range, it falls much closer to the mean for children.

Steroid values. The baseline values of testosterone in both cases fell in the normal range of 2.8-10 ug per 24 hr for adult females reported by Wegienka et al.(52).

In view of the adequate control levels of plasma cortisol a reason was sought for the low, or low normal control values obtained for urinary 17-OHCS. As urine collection, judged by volume and creatinine content was adequate, a possible explanation may be that the children did not retain or absorb the protein in their feedings. This would result in a decreased renal clearance of cortisol metabolites (45) in the face of adequate blood levels, and implies a diminished cortisol secretion rate.

Adrenal stimulation. Aside from the absence of confirmatory clinical stigmata, the normal baseline levels and response to ACTH of plasma cortisol, as well as the modest rise in 17-KS in response to ACTH, would tend to rule out any type of hydroxylase deficiency as the cause of the low baseline levels of urinary 17-OHCS and their modest response to ACTH.

The greater rise in E_3 levels following ACTH im versus ACTH iv is possibly related to the greater length of time of adrenal stimulation.

On the third day of ACTH im administration there was an unexpected uniform decrease in all steroid levels in both patients, with the exception of a further minimal increase in the level of 17-OHCS in case 1. It appears as if the adrenals had become exhausted under the 3 day stimulus of ACTH.

Adrenal suppression and gonadal stimulation. In both girls all testosterone appears to have originated in the adrenals.

The response of E_2 and E_3 levels to HCG, taken together with the estrogen response to ACTH and dexamethasone, would indicate that the estrogens originated mainly in the adrenals, and to a lesser degree in the gonads. In observing the relatively small estrogenic response to HCG in cases 1 and 2, it should be remembered that HCG is relatively weak in terms of FSH equivalent, being predominantly luteinizing in nature (2). It has been ascertained that for every 1000 IU of HCG there are 2 IU of FSH (2nd IRP) (3). Thus, in the total dose of 9,000 IU of HCG there were 18 IU of FSH. This is approximately 25% of the 75 IU of FSH in a usual dose of Pergonal (HMG).

Metyrapone test. The normal response to metyrapone in case 1 would indicate an intact pituitary-adrenal feedback system. The lack of response to the drug by case 2 might possibly be due to the fact that the rise of steroids occurred on the 1st day and was missed, and possibly due to a dose of metyrapone which, though doubled, was insufficient to evoke a response. In both cases, with the exception of the values for 17-OHCS, it was noted that the two control collections preceding this test was characterized by a rebound phenomenon with an overshooting of original control values, either on the first day (case 1) or the second (case 2); this was most evident in the levels of testosterone and estrogens. The subsidence of these exaggerated levels seems to have left the adrenals incapable of responding to metyrapone with an increased output of sex steroids, the values in both subjects for these latter falling near or within the original control ranges at the same time that there was a satisfactory response in 17-OHCS and 17-KS levels in case 1.

MPA suppression. While it might be hoped that the information obtained with MPA suppression would help define the origin of the sex steroids, MPA has been shown to suppress not only FSH and LH (41) but, more recently, ACTH as well (29). MPA has also been shown to blunt the response to metyrapone (29); although a month elapsed between its discontinuation and the metyrapone test, its prior administration might offer a third possible reason for the poor response to metyrapone in patient 2, as the effect of MPA on the pituitary-adrenal axis does not abate immediately.

Light and electron microscopy. As regards the absence of typical MCB in the pineal, it has been shown that lipid cytosomes have characteristic molar ratios of cholesterol, ganglioside, phospholipid and proteolipid (49). Therefore, it has been proposed that their ultrastructual appearance is the visual expression of the chemical environment of the cell (44). Since the appearance of these lipid cytosomes vary according to the tissue in which they are found (1,51), it is thus not surprising that their ultrastructual appearance in the pinealocyte differs from that found in a CNS neuron.

Though cystic ovarian follicles have been observed throughout prepuberty, those measuring 1 cm or larger are found only occasionally (37). Unfortunately, cyst fluid was not analyzed for estrogen content. It is of some interest to note that the last time a large cystic follicle was observed in a Tay-Sachs child, the child also manifested precocious puberty (unpublished observation). It is perhaps of even greater interest to note that polycystic ovaries have been induced in rats by exposing them to continuous light (the physiologic equivalent of ablating the pineal gland) (47).

Clinical. Several clinical points remain to be commented upon. Case 1 and 2, as well as patient H.P. (shown in fig. 1) manifested excessive limb hirsuitism secondary to chronic DPH administration, and the question might arise as to whether this drug could produce significant axillary and/or pubic hair growth; actually, this has been shown not to occur with DPH (7,28).

In case 1, the presence of only a slight estrogen effect on vaginal smear and the absence of breast tissue in the face of elevated estrogen levels is puzzling. It might be postulated that this was

the result of lesser target tissue responsiveness to estrogens as
contrasted with case 2. It should be noted that case 1 did manifest
development of the labia minora, an estrogen effect. This would
point to a difference in responsiveness to estrogens by the breast
tissue and vaginal mucosa in the two cases.

Conclusions

The foregoing study presents evidence for a disturbance in both
gonadotropin and adrenal sex-steroid secretion. That the adrenal abnormality is not secondary to a local phenomenon would seem to be resolved by the failure to observe abnormal lipid bodies in the adrenals of case 1 when they were examined by electron microscopy; the
same was true of the ovaries. There is evidence that in idiopathic
precocious puberty there is increased production of FSH and LH (23),
and a selective increase in adrenal androgen secretion (10). The
factor(s) that modifies adrenal steroidogenesis in precocious puberty
is unknown, but may involve a blockade of adrenal 3β-ol dehydrogenase
by gonadal estrogen.

As the pinealocytes of one of the pubescent cases was shown to
contain abnormal lipid whereas non-pubescent cases were almost devoid
of such infiltration, and as the pineal has been shown to act on the
hypothalamus to inhibit release of gonadotropin-releasing factors
(11,35), accumulations of abnormal lipid in this gland might explain
in part the early appearance of puberty on the basis of an interference with the production and secretion of melatonin and other pineal
indoleamines. Furthermore, as it has been demonstrated in rats that
removal of the pineal is associated with an increased secretion of
aldosterone and corticosterone (24), it was proposed that infiltration of the pineal with abnormal lipid might remove a tonic inhibition over adrenal testosterone and estrogen (or precursor(s)) synthesis. However, work on rats recently completed in this laboratory
appears to have disproved this theory. If the pineal has any part
in the onset of precocious puberty in Tay-Sachs disease its role
would seem to be primarily concerned with gonadotropin secretion.

In the early phases of this study it was hypothesized that infiltration of the hypothalamus with Tay-Sachs lipid resulted either
in irritation of cells containing gonadotropin-releasing factors or
destruction of cells containing gonadotropin-releasing-inhibitor factors (39). A gonadotropin-inhibiting center located in the posterior
hypothalamus has been postulated in man (5) and in rats an FSH-inhi-
biting center has been found in the anterior hypothalamus (20). Releasing factors presumably are secreted throughout prepuberty, the
advance towards sexual maturity being a reduction in the sensitivity
of the hypothalamus to the inhibitory effects of circulating estrogen
or testosterone (26). However, as the hypothalamus is not only diffusely, but apparently equally infiltrated with abnormal lipid in

both pubescent and non-pubescent Tay-Sachs cases, it is difficult to assign a decisive role to either of the two alternatives suggested, or to explain, on either basis, why some children with Tay-Sachs disease undergo pubertal changes and others do not. Possibly a factor such as infiltrative destruction of the amygdaloid complex (15) might in itself, or in conjunction with hypothalamic infiltration, explain the precocious puberty on the basis of interference with the stria terminalis or its connections in the hypothalamus.

In view of the significantly greater degree of Tay-Sachs lipid accumulation in all cells of the anterior pituitary of the pubescent versus non-pubescent cases, it might be postulated that the pituitary pathology itself set in motion the events leading to the endocrinopathy observed here. However, this would not explain the absence of alteration in secretion of HGH and TSH. Furthermore, aside from the secretion of prolactin, when isolated from hypothalamic inhibition, the pituitary has not been generally known to secrete trophic hormones autonomously.

Thus, it is impossible at this point to state with certainty the exact determinants which cause puberty in some Tay-Sachs children and not in others.

Acknowledgments

The author wishes to express his gratitude to Brij B. Saxena, Ph.D., Associate Professor of Biochemistry, Cornell University College of Medicine, for performing the gonadotropin determinations; to Seymour M. Glick, M.D., Chief of Medical Services, Coney Island Hospital division of Maimonides Medical Center, for the growth hormone assays; to Linden Badal, R.N., nurse in charge of the Tay-Sachs ward, for his fastidious supervision of the investigational protocol; to Klaus Wellman, M.D. for interpretation of the ovarian pathology; to Larry Schneck, M.D. for his encouragement and advice in studying these patients; to Bruno W. Volk, M.D. for his unflagging interest and advice in this study; to Mr. Herbert A. Fishler for preparing the photomicrographs; and especially to Masazumi Adachi, M.D. without whose invaluable assistance this study could not have been completed.

References

1. Adachi, M., Volk, B.W., Schneck, L., Torii, J. Arch Path 87:228, 1969
2. Albert, A., Derner, I. J Clin Endocr 20:1225, 1960
3. Albert, A. J Clin Endocr 29:1504, 1969
4. Barker, S.B., Humphrey, M.J., Soley, M.H. J Clin Invest 30:55, 1951
5. Bauer, H.G. J Clin Endocr 14:13, 1954

6. Bing, J.F., Globus, J.H., Simon, H. J Mt Sinai Hosp 4:935, 1938
7. Bray, P.F. Pediatrics 23:151, 1959
8. Bronstein, I.P., Luchan, J.A., Mavrelis, W.B. J Dis Child 64: 211, 1942
9. Brown, J.B., Bulbrook, R.D., Greenwood, F. J Endocr 16:49, 1957
10. Castells, S., Neurwirth, J.S., Orti, E. (in press)
11. Clementi, F., de Virgilis, G., Fraschini, F., Mess, B. In Uyeda, R. (ed.) Electron Microscopy Vol. 2, Biology, Tokyo, Maruzen Co., Ltd., 1966, p. 539
12. Clemont, R., Puech, P., Delon, J. Bull Soc Med Hosp Paris 58: 333, 1942
13. Drekter, I.J., Pearson, S., Bartczak, E., McGavack, T.H. J Clin Endocr 7:795, 1947
14. Driggs, M., Spatz, H. Virchow Arch Path Anat 305:567, 1939
15. Elwers, M., Critchlow, V. Am J Physiol 198:381, 1960
16. Ford, F.R., Guild, H. Bull Johns Hopkins Hosp 60:192, 1937
17. Glick, S.M., Roth, J., Yalow, R.S., Berson, S.A. Nature 199:784, 1963
18. Greulich, W.W., Pyle, S.I. Radiographic Atlas of Skeletal Development of the Hand and Wrist, 2nd ed., Stanford University Press, Stanford, California, 1959
19. Heubner, O. Deutsche med Wchnschr 24:214, 1898
20. Horowitz, S., van den Werff ten Bosch, J.J. Acta Endocr (Kobenhavn) 41:301, 1962
21. Ibayaski, H., Nakamura, N., Tanioca, T., Nabaco, K. Steroids 3: 559, 1964
22. Jubiz, W., Meikle, A.W., Levinson, R.A., Mizutani, S., West, C. D., Tyler, F.H. New Eng J Med 283:11, 1970
23. Kenny, F.M., Midgley, A.R., Jr., Jaffe, R.B., Garces, L.Y., Vazquez, A., Taylor, F.H. J Clin Endocr 29:1272, 1969
24. Kinson, G., Wahid, A.K., Singer, B. Gen Comp Endocr 8:445, 1967
25. Kitay, J.I. J Clin Endocr 14:622, 1954
26. Kulin, H.E., Grumbach, M.M., Kaplan, S.L. Science 166:1012, 1969
27. Liu, N., Grumbach, M.M., de Napoli, R.A., Morishima, A. J Clin Endocr 25:1296, 1965
28. Livingston, S., Petersen, D., Boks, L.L. J Pediat 47:351, 1955
29. Mathews, J.H., Abrams, C.A.L., Morishima, A. J Clin Endocr 30: 653, 1970
30. Mattingly, D. J Clin Path 15:374, 1962
31. McCullagh, E.P., Rosenberg, H.S., Norman, N. J Clin Endocr 20: 1286:1960
32. Meikle, A.W., Jubiz, W., Matsukura, S., West, C.D., Tyler, F.H. J Clin Endocr 29:1553, 1969
33. Mitchell, M.L., Byrne, M.J., Sanchez, Y., Sawin, C.T. New Eng J Med 282:539, 1970
34. Morley, T.P. J Clin Endocr 14:1, 1954
35. Motta, M., Fraschini, F., Martini, L. Proc Soc Exp Biol Med 126: 431, 1967
36. Piotti, A. Acta Endocr (Kobenhavn) 10:66, 1952
37. Potter, E.L. Pathology of the Fetus and Infant, 2nd ed., Year

Book Med. Publ., Inc., Chicago, Ill., 1961, p. 469

38. Relkin, R. Ann N Y Acad Sci 151:880, 1968
39. Relkin, R., Schneck, L. Clin Res 18:370, 1970
40. Richter, R.B. J Neuropath Exp Neurol 10:368, 1951
41. Rifkind, A.B., Kulin, H.E., Cargille, C.M., Rayford, P.C., Ross, G.T. J Clin Endocr 29:506, 1969
42. Saxena, B.B., Demura, H., Gandy, H.M., Peterson, R.E. J Clin Endocr 28:519, 1968
43. Saxena, B.B., Leyendecker, G., Chen, W., Gandy, H.M., Peterson, R.E. Acta Endocr (Kobenhavn) 63:185, 1969. Supplimentum 142
44. Schneck, L., Adachi, M., Friedland, J., Amsterdam, D., Valenti, C., Volk, B.W. VIth Internation Congress of Neuropathology, Masson et Cie, Ed. 1970, p. 1130
45. Schteingart, D.E., Conn, J.W. Ann N Y Acad Sci 131:388, 1965
46. Silber, R.H., Porter, C.C. J Biol Chem 210:932, 1954
47. Singh, K.B. Am J Obstet Gynec 105:274, 1969
48. Stotÿn, C.P.J., Nauta, W.J.H. J Nerv Ment Dis 111:207, 1950
49. Suzuki, K., Suzuki, K., Kamoshita, S. J Neuropath Exp Neurol 28:25, 1969
50. Tietz, N.W. In Workshop Manual Gas Chromatographing in Clinical Chemistry, Chicago Med. Sch. & Mt. Sinai Hosp. Chicago, Ill., 1967, p. 13
51. Volk, B.W., Wallace, B.J. Am J Path 49:203, 1966
52. Wegienka, L.C., Bower, B.F., Shinsako, J., Elattar, T.M., Hane, S., Mimica, N., Demertze, E., Stutheit, J.E., Forsham, P.H. Analyt Biochem 18:203, 1967
53. Weinberger, L.M., Grant, F.C. Arch Int Med 67:762, 1941
54. Werk, E.E., Jr., Choi, Y., Sholiton, L., Olinger, C., Haque, N. New Eng J Med 281:32, 1969
55. Wilkins, L. The Diagnosis and Treatment of Endocrine Disorders in Childhood and Adolescence, 3rd ed. Springfield, Charles C. Thomas, 1965, p. 227

SUMMARY REMARKS

George A. Jervis

Institute for Basic Research in Mental Retardation

Staten Island, New York

As in previous symposia, the major part of the presentations was devoted to that group of sphingolipidoses that was considered in the past under the heading of "Amaurotic Idiocies." New clinical, pathological and biochemical data justify a different nosological interpretation. Infantile amaurotic idiocy (Tay-Sachs disease) considered in the recent past as a characteristic disease entity, includes at present three different conditions: 1) Classical Tay-Sachs disease or GM_2-gangliosidosis I; 2) Landing's disease or GM_1-gangliosidosis, which was the object of the presentations by Wolfe et al and by Landing himself; and 3) Sandhoff's disease or GM_2-gangliosidosis II. This last condition, a newcomer, was discussed extensively by several investigators, Jatzkewitz and Sandhoff from the Max-Planck Institute where the disease was identified, Kolodny from Harvard University and Desnick and colleagues from the University of Minnesota. From these reports, originating in various parts of the world, the disease can apparently be differentiated from Tay-Sachs disease by its pathology (because of the involvement of lung, spleen and hematopoietic system) and by enzymatic characteristics (lack of total hexosaminidase), but neither by the clinical features nor by chemical differences of the deposited gangliosides.

The juvenile, adult and late infantile groups of "amaurotic idiocies" once known under various eponyms, Batten, Bielschowsky, Spielmeyer, Vogt, Kufs, are also rapidly undergoing a more scientific classification. At present one can distinguish biochemically the juvenile GM_1-gangliosidosis first described by Berry and later by O'Brien from the juvenile GM_2-gangliosidosis described by Seitelberger. Thus far, these two diseases appear

to be rare. A third and larger group is apparently identifiable
from a pathologic, clinical and biochemical point of view under
the term ceroidosis. An interesting presentation at the symposium was given by Siakotos and his co-workers from Indiana University on the separation of ceroid from lipofuscin on the basis
of density, ultrastructural and fluorescent characteristics,
cation composition and enzymatic pattern. Although ceroidosis
seems to develop mostly during the juvenile age, infantile and
adult forms of the disease probably do occur.

The congenital form of Tay-Sachs disease first recorded by
Norman a few years ago deserves further investigation. Adachi,
Volk and Schneck presented pathological data of a case of early
Tay-Sachs disease which may well be similar to Norman's patient.
In this respect, the paper of Schneck, Volk and Adachi was of
great interest. They showed morphological and chemical data
documenting the onset of Tay-Sachs disease in fetal life. Their
material originated from abortions following intrauterine diagnosis of Tay-Sachs disease.

The hallmark of the symposium was the discussion of the
findings by Okada and O'Brien and by Brady that the enzymatic
defect in Tay-Sachs disease consists of inactivity of hexosaminidase A. From the data presented by various investigators, including the teams of workers at the Isaac Albert Research Institute,
New York, Johns Hopkins Hospital and Toronto University, it is
now apparent that the test is sufficiently standardized to permit
a reasonably reliable identification of the homozygote in utero
and of subjects homozygous and heterozygous for the Tay-Sachs
gene. The practical bearing of these findings to genetic counseling cannot be overstressed. It is hopefully expected that the
number of children affected by Tay-Sachs disease will soon show
a significant decrease.

This superb accomplishment is the direct result of basic
studies on the metabolism of sphingolipids. Reports on these
studies were perhaps more numerous in previous symposia. However,
in the present symposium basic biochemistry was well represented
by the papers of Gatt, Lowden and Sloan on the enzymes of lipid
metabolism and the presentations of Roseman, Kanfer, Burton and
his group on various aspects of sphingolipid turnover.

Aside from "amaurotic idiocies" other forms of neurolipidoses
were considered in this as in previous symposia.

Krabbe's disease, better known as globoid cell leukodystrophy,
appears to be the most common form of sphingolipidoses in Sweden
and on the basis of numerous Swedish cases Svennerholm was able to
confirm the findings of a low content in cerebrosides and sulfa-

tides of the brain white matter. He reported, in addition, on an
increase of all gangliosides and on some peculiarities of their
fatty acid pattern. Suzuki and collaborators re-emphasized their
recent discovery that the enzymatic defect is not due to inactivity of cerebroside-sulfatide sulfotransferase but rather is due
to a deficiency in galactocerebroside-beta-galactosidase. He also
presented data indicating that prenatal diagnosis in utero of the
enzymatic defect is possible. According to his findings it is
possible to identify the heterozygous condition although the margin in enzymatic activity between normal and heterozygote is
rather small. Finally, he described Krabbe's disease in dogs.
This well known condition is pathologically quite similar to the
human form. The same enzymatic defect is present in both human
and dog tissues, but curiously enough the activity of the specific
galactosidase is not decreased in the canine type. Preceeding
these presentations on Krabbe's disease there was a useful general
paper by Radin on the metabolism of galacto-and gluco-cerebrosides.

New data on metachromatic leukodystrophy were presented by
Austin and collaborators. Neuwelt, the speaker for the group,
noted that the defect of arylsulfatase, which is characteristic
of the disease, varies in the various forms of the condition. He
gave practical indications on the purification of the enzymatic
system and of its determination in the urine of patients. Difficulties of identification of the heterozygous state were stressed
and a new immunological approach to the determination of arysul-
fatase was suggested. The difficulties in the approach to the
determination of arylsulfatase was suggested. The difficulties in
the prenatal diagnosis of metachromatic leukodystrophy was indicated also by Kaback. He observed that amniotic fluid is normally
quite low in arylsulfatase. In addition, the difference in enzyme
activity between heterozygous and homozygous conditions is so
narrow that a wrong diagnosis cannot be avoided. A new exceptional variant of metachromatic leukodystrophy was documented by
Moser. It is characterized by deficiency of arylsulfatase A, B
and C, by increase of cholesterol sulfate and almost complete absence of steroid sulfate. This case is thus far unique.

The mucopolysaccharidoses are justifiably included in the
family of sphingolipidoses because of their association with
sphingolipids in several conditions. A pithy general discussion
on the group of mucopolysaccharidoses was presented by Dorfman,
a pioneer in the study of these diseases. Neufeld described and
amplified on her well known experiments of the "curative" effect
on cell cultures from mucopolysaccharidosis patients which is
brought about by infusion of normal human serum. At the closing
of the session on mucopolysaccharidoses, Hers gave a lucid expo-
sition of his hypothesis of lysosomal disease in which mucopolysaccharidoses and sphingolipidoses may be grouped together.

Some aspects of Niemann-Pick disease were discussed by Lowden with emphasis on its prenatal diagnosis. This is possible because of the absence of sphingomyelinase. However, the test does not discriminate between the classical severe infantile form (type A) which is extremely rare and the non-neurological type B or the mild juvenile form. He, therefore, doubts that the prenatal diagnosis would have practical significance.

The characterics of phytanic acid disease (Refsum's syndrome) a form of ataxic polyneuritis due to lack of an oxidase of this fatty acid, were described by Steinberg. The disease is amenable to dietary therapy since phytanic acid is not formed in the body but derives entirely from alimentary phytal.

A number of interesting individual instances of sphingolipidoses were presented. A new variant of Farber's granulomatosis somewhat similar to that described by Crocker in the last symposium was discussed by Samuelsson and Zetterstrom. There was no mental retardation, no involvement of liver and spleen and the course was protracted. Lipid composition of the granulomatous tissue was, however, identical with that of the classical form.

Groth, Samuelsson and Svennerholm discussed a patient with Gaucher's disease in whom splenic transplantation was performed. The possible therapeutic results of normal plasma infusion in a case of Fabry's disease were reported by Sweeley. Philipart discussed the data of another patient with Fabry's disease who underwent kidney transplant and received plasma infusion.

The possibilities of tissue culture techniques in the study of sphingolipidoses was beautifully illustrated by the papers of Stern and Terry, Menkes, and Hug and collaborators. Of considerable practical interest were the discussions of Landing and Rouser on the diagnosis of various lipidoses by means of biochemical analysis of tissue obtained by biopsy or at autopsy. Precious diagnostic hints were liberally interspersed in their presentations.

In comparison to previous symposia, the genetics of Tay-Sachs disease received scanty attention. The only contribution was that of Myrianthopoulos and Aronson who advanced the intriguing hypothesis that heterozygous individuals for the Tay-Sachs gene may show a peculiar resistance to tuberculosis and thus would confer on them some selective advantage. Bits of significant genetic information were obtained in other papers. For instance Kaback, in his large survey of the Baltimore Jewish population for enzymatic deficiency of hexosaminidase A, found partial deficiency in a higher percentage than previously surmised.

Only those few of us who have been interested in lipidoses
for many years and have attended the four symposia organized by
the Isaac Albert Research Institute are in a position to appreciate the remarkable development in our knowledge of sphingolipidoses from the time of the first symposium to the present
meeting. Dr. Sachs' work at the end of the last century firmly
established the clinical and pathological foundations of Tay-
Sachs disease, but it was only some 50 years later that biochemists became interested in sphingolipidoses. At the first symposium in 1958, Klenk presented his masterly work on gangliosides
and since then the biochemists have unquestionably dominated the
field of sphingolipidoses. At the present symposium a new trend
toward a clinical orientation was apparent. The wide application
of enzymological methods to the diagnosis, the increased emphasis
on clinical description of phenotypes and on pathological features of individual cases were indicative of this trend. Moreover, for the first time one heard a number of papers concerned
with treatment or possibilities of treatment.

In this respect, the few here present who have known Bernard
Sachs cannot help but pay homage to his memory. He was a dedicated physician but always well aware that only basic research
in biochemistry, genetics and pathology was indispensable to
solve the clinical problems of the disease that bears his name.
The contribution of basic sciences is certainly far from exhausted but is sufficiently developed today to justify some
cautious clinical applications. It is indeed the beginning of
Dr. Sachs' hopeful prediction.